CARDIAC SURGERY ESSENTIALS

for Critical Care Nursing

THIRD EDITION

Sonya R. Hardin, PhD, CCRN, NP-C, FAAN
Professor and Dean, School of Nursing, University of Louisville
Louisville, Kentucky

Roberta Kaplow, PhD, APRN-CCNS, AOCNS, CCRN
Clinical Nurse Specialist, Emory University Hospital
Atlanta, Georgia

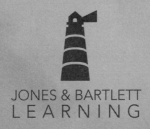

JONES & BARTLETT
LEARNING

D1364343

World Headquarters
Jones & Bartlett Learning
5 Wall Street
Burlington, MA 01803
978-443-5000
info@jblearning.com
www.jblearning.com

Jones & Bartlett Learning books and products are available through most bookstores and online booksellers. To contact Jones & Bartlett Learning directly, call 800-832-0034, fax 978-443-8000, or visit our website, www.jblearning.com.

17531-8

Production Credits
VP, Product Management: Amanda Martin
Director of Product Management: Matthew Kane
Product Manager: Teresa Reilly
Product Assistant: Christina Freitas
Project Specialist: Alex Schab
Digital Project Specialist: Rachel Reyes
Director of Marketing: Andrea DeFronzo
Product Fulfillment Manager: Wendy Kilborn
Composition: S4Carlisle Publishing Services
Project Management: S4Carlisle Publishing Services

Cover Design: Kristin E. Parker
Text Design: Kristin E. Parker
Rights & Media Specialist: John Rusk
Media Development Editor: Troy Liston
Cover Image (Title Page, Part Opener, Chapter Opener):
 © LeslieLauren/iStock/Getty Images; © 13UG13th/iStock/
 Getty Images
Printing and Binding: McNaughton & Gunn
Cover Printing: McNaughton & Gunn

Library of Congress Cataloging-in-Publication Data
Names: Hardin, Sonya R., editor. | Kaplow, Roberta, editor.
Title: Cardiac surgery essentials for critical care nursing / [edited by]
 Sonya Hardin & Roberta Kaplow.
Description: 3rd editon. | Burlington, MA : Jones & Bartlett Learning, [2020]
 | Includes bibliographical references and index.
Identifiers: LCCN 2018049396| ISBN 9781284175318 | ISBN 9781284154214 (eISBN)
Subjects: | MESH: Heart Diseases--nursing | Cardiac Surgical
 Procedures--nursing | Critical Care Nursing--methods
Classification: LCC RC674 | NLM WY 152.5 | DDC 616.1/20231--dc23 LC record available at
 https://lccn.loc.gov/2018049396

6048

Printed in the United States of America
23 22 21 20 19   10 9 8 7 6 5 4 3 2 1

This book is dedicated to Jack, Eleanor, Susan, Dave, Jessie, Pauline, James, Bria, and Adam. We are indeed grateful for your love, support, patience, and encouragement as we worked on the production of this book.

A special thanks to James Perron, our medical illustrator, who was responsive to all of our late-hour requests and for his patience with our attention to detail. He was a true asset to the development of this book.

Brief Contents

Contents

Preface

Postoperative care of the cardiac surgery patient is both challenging and dynamic. Changes in technology, new research findings, the advent of minimally invasive procedures, and the development of off-pump procedures now afford patients of advanced age and with higher levels of acuity the opportunity to undergo procedures for which they were deemed unsuitable candidates not so long ago. Hence, patients with more—and more significant—comorbidities are receiving care in the immediate postoperative period in the intensive care unit (ICU).

Patients who undergo cardiac surgery are at risk for several adverse events not only related to their preoperative condition, but also as a result of effects of the surgical procedure and anesthesia. This requires ICU nurses to demonstrate high levels of clinical judgment, clinical inquiry, and caring practices to effectively manage patients and help optimize outcomes. High-level competency as a facilitator of learning is also required as nurses prepare their patients to undergo cardiac surgery. Clearly, ICU nurses, as members of a multidisciplinary team, play a pivotal role in promoting 10-year survival and high quality of life for patients who undergo cardiac surgery.

This updated *Third Edition* is updated to address the needs of both new and experienced nurses who care for patients in the ICU immediately following cardiac surgery. The purpose of this book is twofold. First, it is designed to prepare the nurse who is first learning to care for patients undergoing cardiac surgery. It addresses significant changes in cardiac surgery and the nursing responsibilities required to meet the needs of these acutely ill patients. Second, the book provides advanced knowledge and a scientific basis for care for nurses who have mastered the essential knowledge and skills necessary to care for this patient population, but who now seek to develop a more in-depth knowledge base about advances in this dynamic field and strategies to optimize patient outcomes. The emphasis throughout the book is on providing an evidence-based foundation for care of patients during the vulnerable period immediately following cardiac surgery. A number of chapters in the book will also prove useful to nurses who work in other areas in which there are acute and critically ill patients, as many of the concepts discussed here can be translated into care of patients other than those who have undergone cardiac surgery.

Because this book uses a comprehensive approach to address the needs of patients in the immediate postoperative period following cardiac surgery, it can also be used to help prepare nurses who plan to take the Cardiac Surgery Certification (CSC®) subspecialty exam offered by the American Association of Critical-Care Nurses.

In addition to updating the text based on the changes in cardiac surgery that have occurred in the past few years, four new chapters have been added based on needs of patients, families, and readers. These chapters address nutritional issues, post-ICU care, psychological and spiritual support, and rehabilitation care following cardiac surgery. We sincerely hope the readers find this information helpful and that it augments patient outcomes.

Throughout the book, Clinical Inquiry Boxes highlight research findings that have implications for nursing practice. Other features that promote critical thinking and provide application of content are the Case Studies and Critical Thinking Questions that follow the respective chapter content. To further enhance critical thinking and for nurses preparing for the CSC exam, the Self-Assessment Questions found at the end of each chapter can be used as practice questions. New in this edition are rationales for the correct answers to the multiple choice questions.

Contributors

Antonia Ash, MSN, RN, CCRN
Charge Nurse, CVICU
Emory University Hospital
Atlanta, Georgia

Kathy Lee Bishop, PT, DPT
Program Manager
Emory St. Joseph's Cardiac Rehabilitation
    Program
Program Director
Emory University Acute Care Residency Program
Assistant Professor
Emory University School of Medicine
Atlanta, Georgia

Mary Jane Bowles, DNP, RN, CCRN, CNS-BC
Clinical Nurse Specialist
Mary Washington Healthcare
Fredericksburg, Virginia

**Courtenay W. Brown, MSN, APRN-CCNS,
    CCRN, PCCN**
Clinical Nurse Specialist, Cardiovascular
    Intermediate Care
Emory University Hospital
Atlanta, Georgia

Susan K. Chase, EdD, RN, FNP-BC, FNAP
Associate Dean for Graduate Affairs
    and Professor
College of Nursing
University of Central Florida
Orlando, Florida

Becky Dean, MSN, APRN, ACNS-BS, CCRN
Unit Director in Cardiology
Emory University Hospital
Atlanta, Georgia

**Judy Dillworth, PhD, RN, FCCM, CCRN-K,
    NEA-BC**
Magnet Program Coordinator
St. Francis Hospital
Roslyn, New York

Carrie L. Griffiths, PharmD, BCCCP
Assistant Professor of Pharmacy
Clinical Pharmacist-Critical Care
Wingate University School of Pharmacy
Wingate, North Carolina

Muna Hassan Hammash, PhD, RN
Assistant Professor
School of Nursing
University of Louisville
Louisville, Kentucky

Sonya R. Hardin PhD, CCRN, NP-C, FAAN
Dean and Professor
School of Nursing
University of Louisville
Louisville, Kentucky

**Kari Hatfield, MSN, RN, AGACNP-BC,
    PCCN, CCRN**
ICU Nurse
Grady Memorial Hospital
Atlanta, Georgia

**Roberta Kaplow, PhD, APRN-CCNS,
    AOCNS, CCRN**
Clinical Nurse Specialist
Emory University Hospital
Atlanta, Georgia

Joyce King, PhD, RN, FNP, CNM, FACNM
Professor Emeritus
Emory University
Atlanta, Georgia

Barbara "Bobbi" Leeper, MN, RN-BC, CNS M-S, CCRN, FAHA
Clinical Nurse Specialist, Cardiovascular Services
Baylor University Medical Center
Dallas, Texas

Julie Miller, BSN, RN, CCRN-K
Clinical Practice Specialist
American Association of Critical-Care Nurses
Aliso Viejo, California

Elizabeth C. Mitchell, MSN, MSPH, RN, AGACNP-BC
Nurse Practitioner, Critical Care
Wellstar Pulmonary and Critical Care Medicine
Marietta, Georgia

Vicki Morelock, MN, APRN-CNS, ACCNS-AG, CCRN
Clinical Nurse Specialist, Cardiothoracic Surgery ICU
Emory University Hospital Midtown
Atlanta, Georgia

Malissa Mulkey, MSN, APRN, CCNS, CCRN, CNRN
Neuroscience Clinical Nurse Specialist
Duke University Hospital
Durham, North Carolina

Noreen O. Peyatt, MSN Ed, RN-BC
Clinical Nurse Specialist
Emory University Hospital
Atlanta, Georgia

Tobias P. Rebmann, ACNP
Christus Trinity
Cardiovascular Associates of East Texas
Tyler, Texas

Dalton Skipper, MSN, ACNPC-AG, CCRN, SCRN
Education Coordinator, Enterprise Staffing Pool
Emory University Hospital
Tucker, Georgia

Shelley K. Welch, MSN, RN, CCRN-CSC
Staff Development Educator, Cardiology
Trinity Mother Frances Hospitals and Clinics
Tyler, Texas

Amy M. Wimsatt, MSN, RN
Associate Professor
University of Louisville
School of Nursing-Owensboro Extension
Owensboro, Kentucky

Alison Yam, MS, AGPCNP-BC, AGCNS-BC, APRN
Clinical Nurse Specialist, Cardiology
Emory University Hospital
Atlanta, Georgia

Mary Zellinger, MN, APRN-CCNS, ANP-BC, CCRN-CSC
Clinical Nurse Specialist, Cardiovascular ICU
Emory University Hospital
Atlanta, Georgia

All medications discussed in the text have been recommended in the medical literature. Nevertheless, the package insert for each drug should be consulted for manufacturer recommendations regarding use, dosage, and administration. Because new information continues to be brought forth by the FDA and through results of clinical trials, it is advisable to stay informed of new information emerging.

Hospital regulations should be followed regarding abbreviations, hospital policy on medication dosing, and new changes emerging in practice.

CHAPTER 1

Clinical Judgment in Critical Care

Susan K. Chase

▶ Introduction

The critical care unit provides a location for continuous monitoring of unstable patients as well as a context for the use of invasive technology that supports basic life processes for acute and critically ill patients. Learning about technology and mastering its safe use are often the foci of basic critical care education and orientation. Aside from its technology, the more basic value of a critical care unit is the level of clinical judgment that occurs there. The thinking processes of clinicians from a variety of disciplines are essential to safe and effective care. The potential for optimal outcomes is enhanced when clinical judgments occur with the nurse synthesizing and interpreting multiple, often conflicting sources of data (Curcio, 2017).

Working in a critical care area is both exciting and rewarding, but it is also demanding and challenging. Nurses in critical care are central for rapid response to potentially life-threatening conditions and key in humanizing technological care. Since critical care units were first developed, both the monitoring of and the early response to changes in patients' conditions by nurses have revolutionized care. Nurses in critical care areas must

make rapid and accurate decisions about diagnostic and treatment approaches in an independent way, which may include the use of protocols or standard orders. The nurse must constantly judge whether the standard protocols or orders are appropriate for a specific patient. This chapter describes the processes used by critical care nurses as they make these decisions. It will be useful to new critical care nurses as they learn to provide safe care. It will also be useful to experienced critical care nurses who wish to improve their processes of thinking and communicating.

The thinking processes used by critical care nurses (CCNs) differ quite dramatically from the schoolbook description of the "nursing process." The linear process of collecting information, forming a decision, choosing an action, and evaluating that action is rarely used in real-world practice. In critical care, multiple conditions are assessed simultaneously, a variety of actions and interventions are carried out concurrently, and the condition of the patient changes constantly. There is never just one single diagnosis or condition that is "resolved." Patients' conditions are constantly changing, and continual monitoring is required. Because the thinking work of CCNs is not a linear process, this chapter is likewise not linear. It deals in general terms with phases of the "thinking work" of nursing, but acknowledges that thinking and acting often overlap in real life.

Clinical judgment is one of the eight nurse competencies of the American Association of Critical-Care Nurses (AACN) Synergy Model for Patient Care (Curcio, 2017). Clinical judgment is defined as the use of clinical reasoning, which includes decision making, critical thinking, and achieving a global grasp of a situation, coupled with nursing skills acquired through a process of integrating education, experimental knowledge, and evidence-based guidelines (AACN, 2002).

▶ Clinical Judgment Processes

Research has provided a window into how humans think and make decisions. Several models can help clinicians to understand their decision-making processes, to thus become more efficient and reduce errors in judgment. The three models that are useful in critical care are information processing, intuition, and decision analysis (Chase, 2004). Each model contributes a unique perspective to decision making, and clinicians can choose which model to apply based on matters of individual style. The nature of specific problems may also determine which model is useful in a particular situation.

Information Processing

The information processing model uses the analogy of the human brain working like a computer as it processes new information that becomes available. It also relies on the assumption that an "optimal" diagnosis can be made by taking into account the data that are available in the problem situation. The possible diagnoses or problems that might be present for a patient are called "hypotheses" before they are confirmed. There are usually multiple competing hypotheses to explain a particular pattern of data. For example, a nurse

may notice that a patient with diabetes has a serum glucose level above baseline. This finding might be a result of several causes—a faster than expected glucose infusion, a new infection, or a missed insulin dose, among other possibilities. Each of these possibilities is a hypothesis. Further data collection can help to narrow the options by ruling out certain problems or increasing the likelihood of another explanation. In the example just given, if the nurse notes cloudiness in urine and an elevation of body temperature, then the probability increases that the hypothesis of infection is correct. This, in turn, directs further action by the nurse. More data can be collected, such as a urinalysis and urine culture, to rule in (confirm) a urinary tract infection.

The information processing model focuses on the reevaluation of competing hypotheses based on new data (David, 2015). In critical care areas, nurses frequently work independently in choosing further data to be collected to support a hypothesis. Units may have protocols that authorize the nurse to proceed with further data collection without obtaining orders from a provider. This relative autonomy increases the necessity for CCNs to exercise appropriate judgment. It would not be appropriate judgment for the nurse to run expensive tests if the data do not warrant it. Judgment includes the decision to do things or not to do them. An economy of practice occurs when all appropriate actions—but only appropriate actions—are taken. To make the choice of further diagnostic testing, all information present must be considered.

In real life, nurses frequently need to act before all information necessary to confirm a diagnosis is available. If a condition that is suspected is particularly critical, such as impending respiratory failure, actions to support the patient must be taken even before a full understanding of the reason for such failure is obtained. To wait to offer support until the patient is in full respiratory failure is to miss the opportunity to offer timely interventions that support the patient's function. At times, by taking the most appropriate actions for the most likely problem and then noting the patient's response to those measures, the diagnosis is either confirmed or refuted. If the treatment approach does not work, additional reasons for the patient's problems must be investigated. New data must be considered to help develop a picture that answers the question, "What's going on with this patient?"

In any clinical situation, certain diagnoses or problems are possible, and some are more likely than others. Critical care units are places where monitoring equipment allows for the collection of a wider range of data than in less acute settings. Critical care nurses are the constant collectors and evaluators of clinical data. Early in their careers, nurses new to critical care may focus on the compilation of data through the use of new or unfamiliar equipment such as electrocardiography, monitoring systems that reflect and record hemodynamic parameters through the use of a pulmonary artery catheter, or continuous blood pressure through intra-arterial lines. It is appropriate that new nurses focus on perfecting their skills in managing and interpreting data from these systems. The assembly of information is just one small aspect of critical care nursing, however. The data obtained from monitoring systems represent key components to be utilized in understanding the full clinical picture presented by the patient.

Nurses collect and evaluate data to arrive at a diagnosis. Even after an initial medical diagnosis of acute myocardial infarction (AMI) is made, for example, the CCN has many diagnostic options to consider. Patients with AMI may develop dysrhythmias, cardiogenic shock, pulmonary edema, or anxiety. Early detection of these conditions can lead to early and more effective treatment and better outcomes. As more data are collected, they change the likelihood of recognizing each of the possible complications that might occur. A normal respiratory rate and arterial blood gas values within normal limits for the patient's age, for instance, indicate that respiratory failure is not imminent. Even simple data, such as vital signs, offer a view of the wholeness of the patient and change the diagnostic possibilities. A normal respiratory rate might indicate that the patient is not in impending respiratory failure or experiencing anxiety. Standard support and monitoring will

likely be sufficient to detect any changes in patient status. A rapid respiratory rate or restlessness in the patient should cause the nurse to set up different levels of support and to collect additional data.

Managing Data

In real life, multiple conditions may occur concurrently, and one finding (e.g., vital sign, hemodynamic parameter, lab value, assessment finding) may provide evidence for a variety of conditions. Because so much information is collected and used to form judgments in acute and critical care settings, flowsheets—either written on paper or assembled electronically—are used to organize and present the many pieces of information. Recognition of any condition depends on seeing patterns in the wide range of data available. Additionally, flowsheets enable health care providers to see how data points change over time. Individual values in isolation are not reflective of the whole person, nor are they reflective of the direction that a particular patient's condition is taking. Is the patient becoming more stable or less stable? Is mechanical ventilation providing adequate support of physiologic function, or is the patient so agitated or distressed by being unable to speak that expenditure of unnecessary energy is occurring? Is the patient failing to respond to any treatment approach such that multiple organ dysfunction syndrome is occurring? Experienced CCNs develop routine approaches to data collection that support recognition of patterns in the data. Seeing the whole of a situation comes with experience. It can lead to intuition, the topic of the next subsection.

Intuition

Once the nurse is oriented to critical care, the patterns of human response to challenges faced in critical situations become more evident and easily recognizable. Eventually, the nurse is able to see the wholeness of a situation. The pieces of data are not seen discretely, but rather as patterns indicative of the whole. The nurse may simply look at the patient and recognize impending loss of stability or the loss of the will to live. At times, experienced nurses will see a pattern or feel a "gut" response to a clinical situation that allows them to "know" the situation of the patient without spending time processing individual pieces of data. Of course, to provide the data that an interdisciplinary team needs to set up a treatment plan, nurses must generate data and check on those "gut" feelings they have about the patient. What is interesting is that the intuition precedes the action. Nurses can develop their intuitive skills by discussing their "hunches" about patients, by analyzing which indicators led them to their intuitive sense, and by checking their own accuracy. Experienced nurses can do this in unit nursing rounds or in clinical case discussions.

The AACN Synergy Model for Patient Care recognizes that as nurses gain expertise, they move from Level 1, which focuses on data collection, following decision trees, and using standard protocols, to Level 3, where nurses are able to see the wholeness of situations quickly. A sense of understanding of the direction of processes is part of the competency of these nurses. At Level 5, nurses synthesize large amounts of data and help the entire team to recognize the "big picture" of what is happening with the patient (Pate, 2017).

Decision Analysis

Decision analysis is an approach to decision making based on mathematical models that take into consideration the likelihood of specific responses given action options. What is the likelihood that a patient who is intubated will develop pneumonia? What is the likelihood that the same intubation will allow for physiologic support during response from trauma or surgery? On a larger scale, if a new closed system suction device is used, what will be the reduced cost of care if the rate of a ventilator-associated condition is reduced? Decision analysis uses frequency and cost data to weigh options in care. It can be used for either individuals or groups of patients. Many current guidelines for practice are based on this kind of mathematical analysis. Electronic records and large dataset analytic techniques will support improved decision analysis in

the near future. Nurses can participate in the use of decision analysis and remind the team of the "whole person" view.

▶ Relationship-Centered Caring in Critical Care

All nursing is carried out in the setting of relationships. Despite the fact that many critically ill patients are intubated and unable to speak, nurses form relationships with their patients and their families. Such relationships are not just "being nice"; rather, they are central to coming to know patients and how they respond to the challenges of illness. Critical care nurses learn to recognize the patterns of patient responses. How one patient responds to the physical challenge of weaning from mechanical ventilation differs from how another patient responds. For example, one patient may become tachypneic in response to the increased work of breathing during weaning, whereas another patient may experience an increased heart rate. Recognizing and communicating patient response patterns are important to excellence in critical care nursing. Recognizing the patterns of how patients respond to challenges can help the nurse decide when in the day is best to provide physical care or to attempt a weaning trial. If a patient did not sleep the previous night, for example, then rest before weaning may result in a better response.

The relationships formed by nurses also extend to patients' families. Family members can provide needed comfort and a quiet presence, or they can spread their own anxiety to the patient. Supporting the family and managing their responses and connection to the patient are important interventions for optimal outcomes. Additionally, family members can assist CCNs in coming to know their patients, thereby helping ensure that the nurses can understand what matters most to the patients.

Now that we have explored the various ways of thinking that can be used in clinical judgment situations, we will see how CCNs can use these models in day-to-day practice.

▶ Day-to-Day Practice

The use of specialized equipment to allow for the continuous collection of data related to a patient's status was discussed in the previous section. The quality of the data being collected and recorded is a central issue in its use. If an intra-arterial line is improperly calibrated, the readings will be consistent—but they will be consistently inaccurate, which can lead to improper treatment plans being established. Critical care nurses learn during orientation how to set up monitoring systems in anticipation of patient admission to the unit, and they learn routines of validating systems as they assume responsibility. In many units, technicians are available to set up lines and equipment, but verifying the accuracy of readings is the responsibility of the nurse. In addition, over time, readings can drift for various reasons such as lines moving, patient position changes, or mechanical equipment problems. Experienced nurses learn to constantly assess the reliability of the data they collect. If the data pattern does not match the apparent condition of the patient, the nurse rechecks the source of the data for accuracy. The adage, "Treat the patient, not the numbers," is good to remember regardless of whether the numbers are accurate. Other data that might not be reliable include arterial blood gas values if the sample is not read immediately if the patient has leukocytosis. Serum chemistry values may also be inaccurate depending on the quality of the sample, any delay in analysis, or the precision of the analysis.

Establishing and verifying the data collection and monitoring systems are important first steps in critical care judgment. The next step is establishing regular monitoring routines. Most critical care units have unit-specific routines for data collection, and some establish routines for monitoring particular types of clinical problems. These routines are important because a patient's status may change frequently in critical care, and regular monitoring allows the nurse to detect changes early, when intervention can prevent clinical deterioration. The nurse should consider, however, that each decision about data collection also has its own cost. For example, frequent blood draws over time can result in noticeable blood loss, particularly in pediatric settings. Awakening a patient hourly for days and nights in a row can result in sleep deprivation, which prevents healing and can lead to delirium. Sending samples for lab analysis costs the patient and the entire system financially as well.

The timing of data collection is one judgment that nurses should make by considering the entire situation of the patient. Additionally, unit protocols for assessment should be periodically reviewed after considering published reports and patient data. At which phase of recovery from major surgery is the patient most likely to have specific complications? When would data collection be appropriately timed to detect a specific complication? At what time should a sample be collected so that results are available for team rounds? Unit-level practice committees can address questions such as these.

Too often, data collection becomes a mindless routine. The numbers are generated and the flowsheet is completed (either written or electronically), but no one really considers what the data mean. This situation represents a failure of the nurse to exert clinical judgment. It results in wasted energy and resources, and it does not protect the patient. Several ways that the CCN can be thoughtful about the data that are routinely collected are discussed next.

Trending and Knowing the Patient

Electronic or paper flowsheets are developed for specific critical care units to help organize data for processing purposes. By seeing how individual data bits change over time, "trends" can be detected. These trends are more important in determining the status of the patient than any individual piece of data would be. Has the blood pressure been making a slow decline over the past 2 hours? Is this patient's heart rate generally slower than baseline? Identifying such patterns helps to determine the clinical significance of a change in any data readings. For a patient with a normally slow heart rate, a new rate of 80 might be worrisome; for another patient, a rate of 80 would not be a reason for clinical concern. Flowsheets on paper or on a screen also allow the nurse to see how readings of one parameter change along with other parameters. Blood pressure readings that are gradually decreasing but remain in the acceptable range might not be of concern. However, if the urine output is dropping during the same period, a condition of low cardiac output must be considered as a possible hypothesis. Additional data about recent fluid loss, rates of fluid replacement, and an assessment for crackles in lungs would be needed. Critical care nurses spend much of their time collecting data. This is not the end task, however; it is only the beginning. Taking time to reflect on the "movement" or trend of the data is essential for critical care clinical judgment. In an interview study of intensive care nurses who were asked about pain management in intensive care, respondents reported that their personal knowledge of the patient and his or her unique characteristics weighed more on their judgment about pain management than the use of a scoring system did, largely due to a reduced ability for the patient to communicate directly (Wøien & Bjørk, 2013).

Even in critical care, contextual patient-related factors are important in coming to know the patient. The AACN Synergy Model for Patient Care points out patient characteristics that are part of each encounter. Central to critical care are consideration of patient stability and the predictability of the course of recovery. Other key characteristics include patient resiliency, vulnerability, complexity, and resource availability. The Synergy Model also incorporates a consideration of the patient's ability to participate in decision making and care (Kaplow, 2017). Clearly, coming to know the patient involves more than simply gathering physiologic data.

Common Trajectories

Making sense of data requires knowing not only the individual patient, but also pathophysiology and having an understanding of the workings of the body's compensatory mechanisms for a variety of critical care conditions. Nurses know, for their own particular specialty unit—be it cardiovascular surgical, trauma, coronary

care, neurosurgical, medical, transplant, or some other unit—the particular problems patients typically face in that unit. Critical care judgments are formed through a blend of knowing individual patients and knowing the trajectories that patients are likely to experience in a particular setting. In individual orientation programs or staff meetings, the particularities of units can be discussed and a common understanding developed by nurses or, even more powerfully, an interdisciplinary team.

A trajectory is a predictable path or sequence of events that is commonly seen in a particular setting. For example, following open heart surgery for coronary revascularization with cardiopulmonary bypass, patients commonly require vasopressor administration to maintain blood pressure to support patency of newly implanted vessels. In addition, patients may experience tachycardia that can decrease cardiac output. Patients may be mechanically ventilated and have multiple chest tubes and pacing wires implanted directly in the myocardium. They will have central vascular access to facilitate fluid and medication administration. A common trajectory includes improvement in hemodynamic stability so that weaning the patient from vasopressors can occur on the first night following surgery. A decrease in the effects of anesthesia can lead to weaning from mechanical ventilation by the morning after surgery (if not extubated before then), and a gradual reduction in chest tube drainage can be noted as blood vessels heal. Deviation from this expected trajectory, such as decreased oxygenation when weaning from mechanical ventilation is attempted or continued blood loss from chest tubes, indicates that this particular patient will require an individualized approach to support. Experienced CCNs recognize patients' progress along specific trajectories. A sense of how the patient is progressing down the predictable path of recovery is one way the CCN sees patterns and senses the wholeness of the situation.

Surveillance

In critical care areas, nurses use a type of thinking that assesses for problems that do not yet exist. This is a different style of thinking than problem identification. It is a continual scanning for signs that a problem is developing. This method of thinking requires several kinds of knowledge, data collection, and processing. Critical care nurses who wait until a problem becomes obvious before they intervene have missed a chance to prevent a cascade of events.

Knowledge that supports effective surveillance includes a deep understanding of the physiologic responses to the critical care setting and to the particular patient problems being addressed. Knowing that tracheal intubation exposes a patient to risk of ventilator-associated conditions, the CCN with a high level of clinical judgment monitors arterial blood gas results, breath sounds, airway pressures, and vital signs. Waiting until pneumonia is fully evident would result in risk of hemodynamic instability and sepsis, both of which can lead to longer intensive care unit (ICU) stays or death. Regular data collection for evidence of stability or signs of problems is essential to the process of surveillance. Most important, though, is the nurse's ability to recognize patterns that indicate deviation from the normal trajectory.

Investigating Problems

Experienced CCNs read their "gut" reactions. When patient responses indicate that things are going as predicted, nurses can alter their vigilance. Conversely, if the patient is not following the predicted trajectory, then the nurse appropriately considers other data sources and discusses possible meanings of this divergent pattern with the treatment team. The nurse does not "rest" until the picture becomes clearer. Even "hunches" about what is going on can be explored and discussed until the patient's picture becomes clearer and data indicate an appropriate direction for decision.

One practice that CCNs use is that of "running possibilities." This process is a form of hypothesis generation, referred to earlier in this chapter. What could be a possible explanation for this finding? Could this person have an unusual presentation of a treatable problem? What if we try a treatment option for a while and see how the patient responds? This sort of thinking frequently happens in conversation with other nurses or health care providers (Chase, 1995).

Research has shown that CCNs focus on individual and contextual variables when assessing and planning care. A study of factors affecting pain assessment using both the Behavioral Pain Score (BPS) and physiologic variables was conducted with cardiovascular surgery patients. Patients were assessed before and after turning and suctioning. Findings reflected that BPS scores were significantly associated with higher disease status levels (Ito, Teruya, Kubota, Yorozu, & Nakajima, 2017). The study concluded that in assessing pain, disease severity is an important covariant, reflecting the Synergy Model as earlier described.

Communicating Findings

Nurses in critical care have more autonomy than nurses in many other practice settings regarding data collection and treatment decisions, such as weaning from various types of support. Critical care nurses do not work in isolation, however, and they contribute to excellence in patient care by working collaboratively with a team of other health care providers. One skill that CCNs develop is effective communication of their impressions of a patient's status to other members of the team. Many nurses have had the frustrating experience of believing that the patient needs to be managed in a certain way, but other members of the team do not agree. When the direction of the care and support differs, nurses are obligated to clarify, verify, and question the appropriateness of the treatment plan if they believe that harm will come to the patient. Learning to communicate data and impressions in ways that allow others to understand the basis for the CCN's judgment can minimize this source of frustration.

Assembly of data into patterns that have meaning will assist CCNs in communicating their overall impressions. Calling a health care provider and offering random bits of data will often not result in a positive response. The nurse can better organize this process by coming to know the types of data that individual clinicians value. For example, even if the findings are not abnormal, the amount of chest tube drainage will be important to a cardiothoracic surgeon. When working with new interdisciplinary teams of providers, an anticipatory question can help to establish communication, such as, "Is there any particular parameter that you want us to pay special attention to this evening?" or "I've noticed a downward trend in blood pressure. Is there a level at which you want us to notify you?" Then, should a call be necessary, it has a context. This kind of communication requires "forward thinking."

One method that has been established in health care settings to assist with the assembly of data into meaningful patterns is the Situation–Background–Assessment–Recommendation (SBAR) technique. This framework facilitates communication among health care providers by providing a focused approach for communicating essential patient information in a usable context so that accurate care decisions can be made (Institute for Healthcare Improvement, 2018).

By understanding the competing hypotheses for the patient's condition, the CCN will be better able to present data in a way that assists the entire team in making good decisions. One kind of data that must be considered is "pertinent negative" data—that is, showing that certain data are normal to reduce the likelihood of one of the diagnostic options. For example, if the blood pressure is trending down, but breath sounds and arterial blood gas results are normal, that combination of findings would decrease the likelihood of left ventricular failure and increase the likelihood that the patient is volume depleted. The breath sounds and arterial blood gas results should be reported even though they are normal, because they assist the other clinicians to understand the whole picture: They are "pertinent" even though they are normal.

Mobilizing the Team

Sometimes CCNs may detect that the patient's condition is changing rapidly and they must assemble the necessary team members to respond appropriately. To do so, the nurse may need to page respiratory therapy, anesthesia, or other airway management teams, as well as the primary provider. Making the decision to mobilize the team can be a daunting one for new CCNs. Experienced nurses and leaders can assist the new CCN in making this decision in a timely fashion. On the one hand, waiting until the situation becomes obvious would be dangerous for the patient. On the other hand, if the nurse calls in the team unnecessarily, that decision has costs, both financial and personal. It is possible that the CCN's clinical judgment was at a lower level in the AACN Synergy Model and that the call came prematurely or in error.

To deal with such issues, CCNs can discuss the process of mobilizing the team on individual units and reflect on how the process went: Did the nurse assemble sufficient data to generate the calls? Was the potential patient problem severe enough to warrant the call? Was the presentation of findings sufficiently clear? Did other members of the team respond appropriately? In hindsight, would any aspect of the patient's care be managed differently?

Team Decision Making

Ultimately, the critical care process is a team process. Data support the idea that good communication on a unit results in better patient outcomes (AACN, 2016; Flicek, 2012; Tulsky, 2016). Units vary widely in how effectively communication occurs. Several possible problems can occur that the CCN should be aware of and try to correct.

The first consideration is nurse-to-nurse communication. Are experienced nurses helpful to new orientees, or do they require new nurses to "pay their dues"? This kind of bullying should be recognized as such and should be dealt with by other observing staff and unit leadership. Other nurse-to-nurse difficulties can come at change-of-shift report, where one shift does not help establish the new shift nurses' understanding of patient baseline due to emotionally charged communication.

Other issues that arise may relate to whether the patient unit is orderly, with supplies on hand and with essential data already assembled. Small things like this can lead to difficult communication and ultimately can result in poor nursing care.

Additional nurse-to-nurse difficulties can happen at the time of patient transfer. It is essential to the clinical judgment process that open and clear communication be established between patient care areas. By sharing with health care providers in the new unit what the patient's clinical course or trajectory has been, how this patient is unique, and which approaches have worked best, better clinical judgment is promoted on the new unit.

The health care team involves many disciplines and individual technicians. These teams can come to decisions for action using different processes and standards. It sometimes seems as if different disciplines use different languages to describe patient data and situations. Critical care nurses need to learn to be flexible in communication so that essential meaning of data can be communicated to support patient care (Chase, 1995).

Choosing Interventional Approaches

Much of our consideration thus far has focused on clinical judgment as it relates to the status of the patient, patient stability, patient movement along a recovery trajectory, patient comfort, or the identification of problems. Judgment is also required regarding how best to respond to the issues that are identified in the assessment process. All management choices should be goal oriented and contextually appropriate. The AACN Synergy Model provides for a way of matching the CCN's competencies to the patient's needs: The model is built around a connection between nurse competencies and patient characteristics, driven by patient factors, nurse judgment, and system support and integration (Hardin & Kaplow, 2017). Even given the same medical condition, the CCN's response to the patient should reflect numerous factors, including those described in the Synergy Model. For example, a patient who has high levels of resiliency, as evidenced by return to baseline data after treatments, can be expected to recover more quickly and need less aggressive support than a

patient who, because of long-standing concurrent conditions, might not be capable of rallying. A patient with few external resources might require aggressive advocacy on the part of the CCN.

Goal-Oriented Decisions

In line with the concept of trajectory, CCNs should always have a goal in mind when planning specific nursing actions. If the goal is stability, then support of basic physiologic functioning will support that goal. If the goal is to increase participation in care so as to support the patient–family unit, then adjusting visiting times to allow for prolonged contact might be chosen, provided that patient stability is not compromised. The CCN can then reflect on the effectiveness of those interventions in accomplishing the goal.

Critical care nurses can actively support the unit in developing documentation systems that include goals and nursing actions. If a patient is anxious about how the family is responding to critical illness, for example, being able to see and be with a family member can reduce stress and the related catecholamine release that can have negative effects on the cardiovascular system. Nursing actions can have real effects on overall patient status. Promoting comfort and dignity for patients is a requirement for humanistic care and healing.

Supporting the Dying

As discussed earlier, the experienced CCN develops a sense of the big picture of the patient's condition and the direction of the trajectory. Often, critically ill patients have life-threatening conditions that can result in death. Death sometimes happens during aggressive resuscitative efforts. Frequently, however, an impending death is recognized by at least one member of the team. The goals of care may then shift to allow for patient comfort and family communication. The transition to caring for the dying patient can be one that provides the ultimate meaningful contribution on the part of the staff. Too often, however, an impending death is a time of competing goals, shifting direction of care, and difficult communication among team members.

The CCN can assist in the dying process by maintaining a consideration of "Where are we going?" Asking that question during team meetings can assist the entire team in addressing the futility of care. The patient's and family members' goals will also need to be determined as part of this process, and it is often the nurse who assists in clarifying these values (Hiltunen, Medich, Chase, Peterson, & Forrow, 1999).

A review of studies using the shared decision-making (SDM) intervention for end-of-life situations in critical care units showed that few studies included all elements of SDM, which include understanding the problem, hearing options, and considering values, among other elements. Two studies showed that ICU length of stay was reduced after offering SDM. The study points out that even when the health care team and the family understand the gravity of the situation, time may be required to clarify options and come to acceptance (Kryworuchko, Hill, Murray, Stacey, & Fergusson, 2013). More research needs to be done on how to support patients, families, and health care teams through this difficult process. Critical care nurses are key players in this conversation.

▶ Summary

A CCN is not a technician. As a professional nurse, the CCN's focus of care is on the whole person and family at a particularly vulnerable time. The focus of care on the physical problems patients face in critical care is obvious. More is known by clinicians about the functioning of the human body of patients in a critical care unit than by providers in almost any other environment of the health care system. Critical care nurses learn over time, however, that more is going on in a critical care unit than simply the care of physical bodies. Critically ill patients are whole human beings. Their fear or trust, will to live, ability to participate in care, and family support can make a real difference in patient outcomes. Ultimately, the clinical judgments made by CCNs are pivotal to providing

care to acutely and critically ill patients. Nurses are essential to the process of providing care by virtue of their perspective on meeting the needs of the whole patient. These needs can be based on the eight patient characteristics outlined in the Synergy Model. Nurses' constant presence provides for a way of seeing and knowing the person who is experiencing critical illness. Growing in ability to form exquisitely appropriate clinical judgments is a lifetime challenge—but it is one that is rewarding to both patient and nurse.

References

American Association of Critical-Care Nurses. (2002). *Competency level description for nurse characteristics.* Aliso Viejo, CA: AACN Certification Corporation.

American Association of Critical-Care Nurses. (2016). *AACN standards for establishing and sustaining healthy work environments: A journey to excellence* (2nd ed.). Retrieved from http://www.aacn.org/wd/hwe/docs/hwestandards.pdf.

Chase, S. K. (1995). The social context of critical care clinical judgment. *Heart & Lung, 24*(2), 154–162.

Chase, S. K. (2004). *Clinical judgment and communication in nurse practitioner practice* (pp. 22–50). Philadelphia: F.A. Davis.

Curcio, K. (2017). Clinical judgment. In S. R. Hardin & R. Kaplow (Eds.), *Synergy for clinical excellence: The AACN synergy model for patient care* (2nd ed., pp. 67–73). Burlington, MA: Jones and Bartlett Learning.

David, I. (2015). *Information processing therapy.* Retrieved from https://www.learning-theories.com/information-processing-theory.html.

Flicek, C. L. (2012). Communication: A dynamic between nurses and physicians. *MEDSURG Nursing, 21*(6), 385–387.

Hardin, S. R., & Kaplow, R. (Eds.). (2017). *Synergy for clinical excellence: The AACN synergy model for patient care* (2nd ed.). Burlington, MA: Jones and Bartlett Learning.

Hiltunen, E., Medich, D., Chase, S., Peterson, L., & Forrow, L. (1999). Family decision making for end of life treatment: The SUPPORT nurse narratives. *The Journal of Clinical Ethics, 10*(2), 126–134.

Institute for Healthcare Improvement. (2018). *SBAR toolkit.* Retrieved from http://www.ihi.org/resources/Pages/Tools/sbartoolkit.aspx.

Ito, Y., Teruya, K., Kubota, H., Yorozu, T., & Nakajima, E. (2017). Factors affecting pain assessment scores in patients on mechanical ventilation. *Intensive and Critical Care Nursing, 42*, 75–79.

Kaplow, R. (2017). Participation in decision making. In S. R. Hardin & R. Kaplow (Eds.), *Synergy for clinical excellence: The AACN synergy model for patient care* (2nd ed., pp. 53–58). Burlington, MA: Jones & Bartlett Learning.

Kryworuchko, J., Hill, E., Murray, M. A., Stacey, D., & Fergusson, D. A. (2013). Interventions for shared decision-making about life support in the intensive care unit: A systematic review. *World Views on Evidence-Based Nursing, 10,* 3–16.

Pate, M. F. (2017). Introduction. In S. R. Hardin & R. Kaplow (Eds.), *Synergy for clinical excellence. The AACN synergy model for patient care* (2nd ed., pp. 3–10). Burlington, MA: Jones & Bartlett Learning.

Tulsky, J. A. (2016). *How effective communication can improve patient care—and reduce physician burnout.* Retrieved from http://www.accupost.com/issues/january-25-2016/how-effective-communication-can-improve-patient-care-and-reduce-physician-burnout.

Wøien, H., & Bjørk, I. T. (2013). Intensive care pain treatment and sedation: Nurses' experiences of the conflict between clinical judgment and standardised care: An explorative study. *Intensive and Critical Care Nursing, 29,* 128–136.

Web Resource

Synergy Concept Map: https://www.youtube.com/watch?v=Z-M3VsFnD64

CHAPTER 2

Cardiovascular Anatomy and Physiology

Susan K. Chase

▶ Introduction

The heart is a muscular organ located beneath the sternum, between and slightly anterior to the lungs, in a section of the thorax known as the mediastinum. The mediastinum also contains the great blood vessels—the vena cavae, the pulmonary artery, and the aorta—as well as the esophagus, the trachea, the thoracic duct, and (in children) the thymus gland. **FIGURE 2.1** illustrates the location of the heart.

The heart is surrounded by the pericardium, a dual-layer sac that is minimally elastic. This sac allows for smooth movement of the cardiac muscle within the pericardium. If fluid or blood fills the pericardium, it puts pressure on the heart from the outside and prevents normal filling of heart chambers. The main function of the heart is to pump blood throughout the lungs and the systemic circulation, thereby allowing for the delivery of oxygen and nutrients to the body cells and for the transport of waste products to processing or removal organs. Other functions of the cardiovascular system relate to the vascular endothelium and the blood itself. The blood consists of cells that support the body's ability to fight off

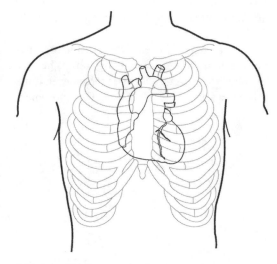

FIGURE 2.1 The heart and its location in the thoracic cavity.

infection as well as chemicals such as hormones that control processes of bodily systems. The vascular endothelium is active in controlling the diameter and tone of the blood vessels. In addition, the heart releases hormones that assist in controlling blood flow and pressures.

▶ Chambers and Valves of the Heart

The structure of the heart supports its functions. The heart consists of four chambers, each with muscular walls (**FIGURE 2.2**). It also has four valves that control the direction of blood flow through these chambers. The two upper chambers of the heart are the atria; the two lower chambers are the ventricles. The terminology of "upper" and "lower" refers to a conceptual picture of the heart, with the most anterior chambers of the heart being the right and left ventricles. The muscle walls of the four chambers vary widely in thickness. Because the left ventricle must pump blood into the systemic circulation, which has relatively higher pressure than the pulmonary system, the wall of the left ventricle is the thickest (13–15 mm). The muscle wall of the right ventricle is only 3 to 5 mm thick. The atria have the thinnest walls (2–5 mm).

The tip of the left ventricle is positioned anterior and to the left in the mediastinum. When the left ventricle contracts, its tip is forced even more anteriorly toward the chest wall. This movement can be palpated as the point of maximal impulse (PMI). The PMI is normally located in the midclavicular line at the fifth intercostal space, but can sometimes vary. Abnormalities in the shape and size of the heart, for example, can alter the position and location of the heart itself. A distended abdomen can flatten and elevate the level of the heart. Hyperextended lungs can depress the level of the heart. Enlargement of the heart can cause the PMI to shift to the left in the chest. Noting the position of the PMI can therefore give some indication of the size or position of the heart (Goldberg, 2015).

Although most of the heart tissue is muscle, this organ also has a fibrous band that separates the atria from the ventricles and contains the four cardiac valves, which are made up of connective tissue. The cardiac valves consist of fibrous rings to which valve leaflets are attached. The tricuspid valve contains three flat valve leaflets. The mitral valve has two flat leaflets that resemble the pointed shape of a bishop's miter. The pulmonic and aortic valves each have three leaflets that are termed *semilunar* because of their crescent-like shape. The tricuspid and mitral valves (collectively termed the *atrioventricular [AV] valves* because of

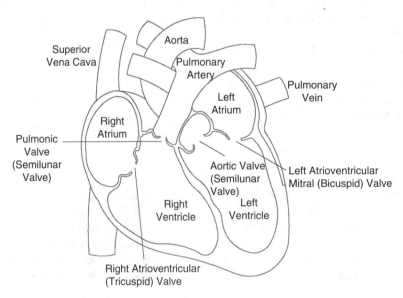

FIGURE 2.2 Chambers of the heart and valves.

their location) are attached to chordae tendinae, which are connected on their opposite ends to papillary muscles in the ventricles. The muscles prevent the valve leaflets from being pushed backward into the atria when pressure rises in the ventricular chambers during ventricular contraction. Proper functioning of the valves depends on all these features being intact. The valves themselves are covered with epithelial tissue.

The right and left sides of the heart are divided by the septa. The interatrial septum consists of the fossa ovalis (the sealed foramen ovale that normally closes in the postpartum period) and the muscular walls of the right and left atria. The interventricular septum is formed by the ventricular muscle in the lower portions and by the upper membranous section (Marieb & Hoehn, 2016).

▶ Blood Flow Through the Heart and Major Blood Vessels

Blood flow is determined by a pressure gradient. It flows from areas of higher pressure to those of relatively lower pressure. The four heart valves support "one-way" flow of blood through the heart. The right atrium receives blood from the body through the superior and inferior vena cavae as well as from the coronary sinus, which returns the blood that has circulated through the heart muscle itself. Blood enters the right atrium during atrial relaxation (and ventricular systole). When the pressure in the right ventricle decreases during its resting phase (ventricular diastole), the tricuspid valve opens, allowing the blood flow from the right atrium to the right ventricle. Contraction of the right atrium near the end of ventricular diastole forces additional blood into the right ventricle. After the right ventricle fills with blood, the muscle wall contracts, increasing the pressure in its chamber, which in turn forces the tricuspid valve to close. As pressures continue to increase, blood is forced out of the right ventricle across the pulmonic valve and into the pulmonary artery. The pulmonary artery transports the still unoxygenated blood into the pulmonary vascular system. At the end of right ventricular systole, the pressures in the right ventricle decrease and the pulmonic valve closes, preventing blood in the pulmonary artery from returning to the right ventricle. Blood from the right atrium then refills the ventricle for the next systole.

In the pulmonary system, the blood circulates through a series of arteries, capillaries, and veins. In the thin-walled capillaries of the pulmonary circuit, red blood cells exchange carbon dioxide for oxygen. The oxygenated blood then returns to the left atrium, driven by the pressure differential: Pressures in the left ventricle are lower than in the pulmonary vascular system. Oxygenated blood returning from the pulmonary vein enters the resting left atrium. When the left atrium pressure rises higher than the pressure in the resting left ventricle, the mitral valve opens. Blood then passes to the left ventricle across the mitral valve. The contraction of the left atrium forces additional blood into the left ventricle. Finally, as the left ventricle contracts, the pressure there increases and forces the mitral valve closed and the aortic valve open. Blood passes from the left ventricle to the systemic circulation across the aortic valve. It flows to the cardiac muscle itself through the right and left coronary arteries, which arise from the lower aorta, just above the aortic valves. At the end of left ventricular systole, with decreased pressure in the left ventricle, the aortic valve closes.

Each of the cardiac chambers has its own range of normal fluid pressures, which depend on the force of contraction of the muscle walls and the position of the cardiac valves in that chamber. Each chamber has a phase when its walls are contracting (systole) and a phase when the muscle is resting (diastole). Most of the time, the words *systole* and *diastole* are used to refer to the phases of the ventricles. Under normal circumstances, due to the electrical control system of the heart, the atria contract together and the ventricles contract together.

It is useful to be able to picture the heart during systole and diastole when interpreting heart sounds. During ventricular systole, the AV valves are closed and the semilunar valves are open; blood flows through the latter valves into the pulmonary and systemic circulation. During ventricular diastole, the semilunar valves close and the AV valves open, with blood flowing through the latter valves from the atria to the ventricles. Unexpected sounds heard during ventricular systole could result from tight or "stenotic" semilunar valves (aortic or pulmonic) or from incompetent or "regurgitant" AV valves (mitral or tricuspid). Obstruction to forward flow can be called *stenotic,* and backward flow of blood is due to an incompetent valve and can be called *regurgitant*. This also causes an unexpected sound. These sounds are best heard after heart sound S_1 and before heart sound S_2. Unexpected sounds heard during ventricular diastole are heard after S_2 and before the following S_1 heart sound. These sounds can be related to mitral/tricuspid stenosis or aortic/pulmonic insufficiency (regurgitation). Heart sounds can further be differentiated by noting the area on the chest wall where they are heard most prominently. For example, a sound can be referred to as a *systolic aortic murmur* when it is heard between S_1 and S_2 in the upper right border of the sternum. That murmur is often caused by aortic stenosis. **TABLE 2.1** summarizes the murmur differentiations.

Cardiac surgery often involves the replacement or repair of cardiac valves. The heart and lungs of patients with long-term valve disorders have often adapted to changes in pressure and blood flow and may result in dysfunction even after the valve has been repaired. Patients may need support until physiology returns to more normal responses.

Being able to think spatially will assist the nurse in making sense of cardiovascular assessment data. The cardiac cycle in **FIGURE 2.3** shows the simultaneous events of cardiac function, including pressure changes in individual vessels and chambers and electrical activity, which will be discussed in this chapter.

TABLE 2.1 Murmur Differentiation

Valve	Stenosis	Insufficiency
Tricuspid and Mitral	Diastolic	Systolic
Pulmonic and Aortic	Systolic	Diastolic

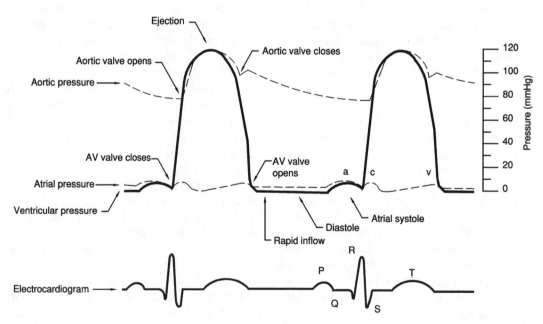

FIGURE 2.3 The cardiac cycle.

▶ Coronary Arteries

Normally we think of tissue perfusion in the body as occurring during systole, but because the pressure in the muscle tissue during ventricular systole is so high, the coronary arteries are perfused during ventricular diastole. The left main coronary artery divides fairly quickly into the left anterior descending (LAD) artery and the circumflex artery (**FIGURE 2.4**). The right coronary artery (RCA) supplies most of the right atrium and ventricle and the sinoatrial (SA) node (in 60% of people), the AV node (in 80%–90% of people), and part of the bundle branches. The LAD artery supplies the left atrium and ventricle, including the ventricular septum. The circumflex artery supplies the posterior portion of the left ventricle and the left atrium. The blood supply to the SA node in 40% of the population is received through the left circumflex artery. The venous return of the heart leads to the great coronary vein, which parallels the circumflex artery and eventually returns to the right atrium. People can vary somewhat in terms of the arrangement and area that the coronary arteries supply. Coronary angiography can reveal the individual's unique configuration. With age and stress, vessels may become narrowed due to plaque and thickening of the arterial walls. Collateral circulation may then develop, as blood is drawn from nearby arterioles to supply areas that might otherwise not be perfused adequately because of blockages to primary blood sources. If collateral circulation is well developed, blockage of a major artery may not cause as much damage as it would for a person with no collateral circulation (Marieb & Hoehn, 2016).

▶ Cardiac Lymphatic System

The heart produces a certain amount of lymphatic drainage that flows through the pretracheal lymph node and eventually empties into the superior vena cava. Blockage of lymph flow can affect pressures in the heart itself related to congestion. The return of lymph to the systemic circulation is critical to prevent interstitial edema. Also of importance is that cardiac lymph fluid contains hormones (atrial

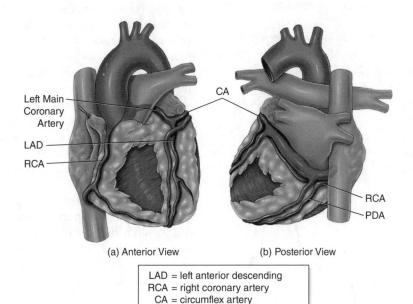

Left Main Coronary Artery
LAD
RCA
CA
RCA
PDA

(a) Anterior View   (b) Posterior View

LAD = left anterior descending
RCA = right coronary artery
CA = circumflex artery
PDA = posterior descending artery

FIGURE 2.4 Diagram of coronary circulation.

natriuretic peptide) and adrenergic neurons (norepinephrine) that can be used as markers for myocardial edema, reperfusion injury, and myocardial damage (Marieb & Hoehn, 2016).

▶ Pressure of Blood in Major Blood Vessels

The pressure of the blood in major blood vessels varies related to cardiac events. Monitoring the pattern of pressure variation is an important part of postoperative care for cardiac surgery patients. Pressure waves in the great veins and the right atrium are given codes (letters) to assist in the interpretation of waveforms (**FIGURE 2.5**). For example, the "v" wave represents filling of the atrium from systemic veins. The "x" descent follows the "v" wave and represents change in shape of the atrium as a result of ventricular emptying. The "a" wave represents increased right atrial pressure caused by atrial contraction and is followed by the "y" descent, which represents a decrease in pressure as the tricuspid valve opens. The slight rise in right atrial (RA) pressure, called the "c" wave, represents the increase in pressure coming from the ventricle that causes the tricuspid valve to close.

Arterial pressure increases rapidly with ventricular systole and attains the pressure represented by the systolic blood pressure. The dicrotic notch of the arterial waveform represents closure of the aortic valve. This closure maintains the

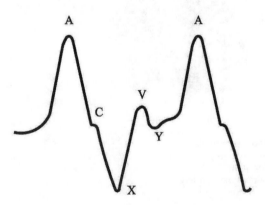

FIGURE 2.5 Pressure waveforms.

pressure of the system circuit at the level represented by the diastolic blood pressure.

▶ Electrical Control of Cardiac Muscle

Cardiac muscle cells are unique in the body for a number of reasons. First, unlike skeletal muscle cells, they are capable of automaticity. That is, cardiac muscle cells do not require stimulation from an outside force, such as a nerve, to initiate an action potential to cause contraction. Second, cardiac muscle cells are interconnected in weblike fashion with separation only by intercalated discs, which allows for impulses to pass through the entire section of the heart like a wave.

Action potentials occur when the polarity (i.e., electrical charges) across the cell membrane changes rapidly. In the resting state, outside the cell membrane there are more positive ions (sodium ions, which are present in the largest number, but also calcium and magnesium ions) as compared with the positive charges inside the cell. Potassium is the chief intracellular cation (positive ion), and there exist relatively more anions (negative ions) inside the cell from proteins and other sources. The cell membrane is therefore "polar"—similar to the scheme used to power a flashlight battery, which has more positive ions on one side than on the other. An action potential spreads to neighboring cardiac cells like a wave. Depolarization causes a change in electrical charge across the cell membrane. It occurs as ions are allowed to cross the cell membrane by ion channels. Normally, action potentials precede muscle contraction.

The atria and ventricles are separated by thick fibrous tissue that supports the four heart valves. This fibrous tissue prevents action potentials from being transmitted between the atria and ventricles. The exception to this barrier occurs in the AV junction, or the AV node. Electrical impulses pass from atria to ventricles across this specialized set of tissues (**FIGURE 2.6**). To support simultaneous contraction of the thick ventricular muscle walls, specialized conduction tissue transmits electrical

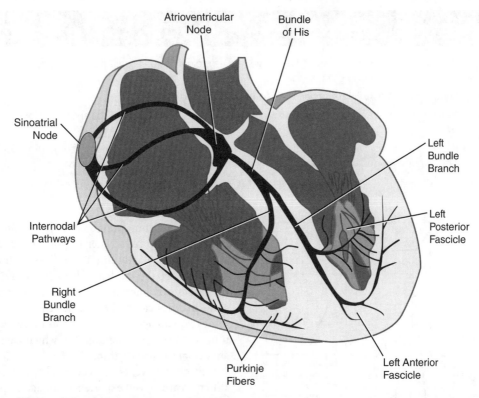

Sinoatrial Node

Atrioventricular Node

Bundle of His

Left Bundle Branch

Left Posterior Fascicle

Internodal Pathways

Right Bundle Branch

Purkinje Fibers

Left Anterior Fascicle

FIGURE 2.6 Electrical conduction system of heart.

impulses through the bundle branches and the Purkinje fibers; the atria have similar transmission fibers. The electrical impulse from the atria is slowed at the AV node, a delay that allows for the atria to contract and empty blood into the ventricles before the action potential moves through the ventricles.

Each cell of the heart is capable of initiating an action potential, but different areas of the heart have different basic rates of discharging. Under normal conditions, the SA node, which is located in the right atrium, has the fastest rate; depolarization occurs there approximately 60 to 100 times per minute. Cells of the AV node can depolarize 40 to 60 times per minute unless a more frequent impulse, such as from the SA node, is transmitted through them. Ventricular cells can initiate an action potential 20 to 40 times per minute. This activity is protective to the heart: If something happens to prevent normal action potentials from

reaching the ventricle, the heart will still beat. The SA node is normally in control of the heart rate because it has the fastest intrinsic rate.

BOX 2.1 provides a closer look at the various phases of action potentials to help explain these events and explain how certain medications can affect them. Action potentials for the SA and AV nodes have a more gradual increase than those for the atria or ventricles, as depicted in **FIGURE 2.7**. The SA and AV node impulses are more tightly controlled by the slow calcium channels than by the sodium channels. Calcium channel blockers can slow heart rate by slowing the transport of calcium across the cell membrane (McCance & Huether, 2014).

A refractory period occurs after the action potential, before the resting concentrations of ions have fully returned to normal. New impulses that reach the tissue during this period will not be transmitted, or potentially can establish abnormal

BOX 2.1 Action Potential Phases

Phase 0: Depolarization. Sodium ions cross the cell membrane rapidly through sodium channels, causing the polarity of the cell membrane to change rapidly.

Phase 1: Rapid Repolarization. Potassium ions "leak" outside the cell.

Phase 2: Plateau. Opening of slower calcium channels allows cations to enter the cell, balancing the loss of potassium ions.

Phase 3: Rapid Repolarization. At the end of the action potential, the channels close and the cell returns to its resting state by pumping sodium ions out of the cell and bringing potassium ions back inside.

Phase 4: Resting State. This phase is diastole where cells remain resting until an electrical impulse occurs.

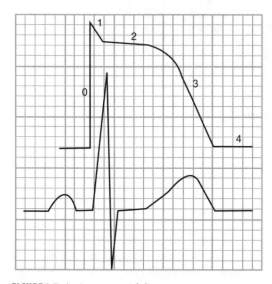

FIGURE 2.7 Action potential diagram.

sodium-potassium pump activity, sodium ions build up in the cell. Water (a polar molecule) is attracted to the sodium ion. As a result, internal structures of the cardiac cell swell, resulting in the release of internal cell enzymes. Electrolyte abnormalities can make cardiac cells more prone to develop an action potential and more likely to initiate a transmittable impulse, which causes an abnormal cardiac rhythm.

Electrical events precede mechanical events. When a cardiac cell experiences an action potential, it contracts. As the wave of electrical activity passes through the cardiac muscle wall, the muscle contracts in a wavelike fashion. For this reason, cardiac function is often monitored by electrocardiography. The nurse must be aware that damaged cardiac muscle may not respond with full-force contraction even if the electrocardiogram tracings appear normal.

rhythm patterns. Reestablishing the normal concentration gradient of electrolytes across the cell membrane is referred to as the *sodium-potassium pump*. It requires working against the concentration gradient and the expenditure of energy. As much as two-thirds of the cardiac cell's energy as stored in adenosine triphosphate (ATP) molecules is spent in supporting the sodium-potassium pump. Any loss in energy for the cardiac cell, which may be due to decreased perfusion of oxygen-rich blood to the myocardium, results in interruption of this essential pump fairly quickly. Such a disruption affects the cell's ability to return to normal polarity. Without

▶ Cardiac Output, Preload, and Afterload

As mentioned, the heart functions to pump oxygenated blood to cells, organs, muscles, and tissues and deoxygenated blood back from the systemic circulation. Some concepts have been developed that assist clinicians in understanding overall cardiac function. Cardiac output (CO) is a measure of the amount of blood that is ejected by the heart each minute. Stroke volume (SV) represents the amount of blood that is ejected from the left ventricle with one contraction. Cardiac output, then, is the product of the stroke volume and the heart rate (HR), which is beats per minute:

$$CO = SV \times HR.$$

Stroke volume is influenced by the amount of blood in the ventricle and by the force of contraction of the ventricle. It can also be affected if the aortic valve restricts flow out of the left ventricle. The ejection fraction (EF) is the percentage of the volume of the left ventricle that is ejected with each contraction. A normal EF is in the range of approximately 65% to 70%, where this value reflects the efficiency of the left ventricle in pumping blood forward into the systemic circulation.

Preload (sometimes referred to as left ventricular end-diastolic pressure) is the pressure found in the left ventricle at the end of diastole. The Frank-Starling law states that stretched muscle fibers produce a more powerful contraction; thus when the left ventricle is fully filled, a more powerful contraction becomes possible. Conditions that prevent filling of the ventricle with blood—such as hypovolemia, dehydration, or external pressure on the heart from fluid in the pericardium—will reduce both the volume of blood in the ventricle and the ventricle's ability to pump blood forward. Nevertheless, the Frank-Starling law reaches its limit when cardiac chambers are overstretched. The resulting contraction is not as effective as it would have been with slightly less stretch. The overstretching can eventually result in a lower CO. Preload can also be affected by blood that was not ejected during the previous systole. A low EF can increase preload and overstretch the ventricle.

Afterload is the resistance against which the left ventricle must pump to move blood forward. The pressure of the arterial systemic circulation produces afterload. Smooth muscle tone in arterioles can increase the resistance to blood flow and increase afterload. Medications can also alter the amount of resistance that arteriolar smooth muscle generates. For example, arterial vasodilators decrease afterload, whereas vasoconstrictor agents, which may have been given to increase systemic blood pressure, can increase preload, afterload, or both. Chronic, uncontrolled hypertension can lead to left ventricular hypertrophy, a thickening of the ventricle wall due to increased workload.

▶ External Control of the Heart

Nervous system control of the heart comes through the autonomic nervous system and can cause rapid changes in heart activity. The autonomic nervous system consists of sympathetic and parasympathetic nerve fibers. The sympathetic nervous system controls the body's "fight or flight" mechanisms, quickly preparing the total organism to resist an attack.

The parasympathetic system governs the "rest and refresh" responses to stress and has nerves that function more individually. The vagus nerve has the chief parasympathetic influence on the heart by affecting primarily the SA and AV nodes slowing the heart rate and increasing the conduction block at the AV node. Parasympathetic nerve fibers release acetylcholine, which slows the heart—a function sometimes termed *cholinergic*.

Sympathetic stimulation increases heart rate and contractility, affecting all parts of the heart. Sympathetic nerve fibers release norepinephrine, which has a profound effect by increasing cardiac contractility and vascular resistance. Additionally, the medulla of the adrenal glands is part of the sympathetic nervous system and can stimulate the release of epinephrine into the systemic circulation—a function sometimes termed *adrenergic*. Receptors for adrenergic neurotransmitters can be classified as either alpha (α) or beta (β) receptors. Receptors can be further subclassified as α_1 and α_2, or as β_1 and β_2. Dopamine is another neurotransmitter that affects the cardiovascular system. **TABLE 2.2** summarizes the locations and actions of the various receptors.

The activity of the sympathetic neurotransmitters is determined by the location and type of receptors in various tissues. In this way, the same chemical can have different effects in different locations. The heart is rich in β_1 receptors, so that effect is most prevalent for the heart. The systemic circulation has relatively more α receptors, so that effect is more predominant there. Epinephrine stimulates all types of adrenergic receptors, but norepinephrine has little effect on β_2 receptors. Dilation of α_2 coronary blood vessels

TABLE 2.2 Autonomic Receptors and Cardiovascular Function

Location	Adrenergic Receptor Type	Adrenergic Effect	Vagus Nerve Cholinergic Effect
Sinoatrial (SA) node	β_1, β_2	Increased rate	Decreased rate, arrest
Atrial tissue	β_1, β_2	Increased contractility and conduction velocity	Decreased contractility, shorter action potential
Atrioventricular (AV) node	β_1, β_2	Increased automaticity and conduction velocity	Decreased conduction velocity and automaticity
Purkinje fibers	β_1, β_2	Increased automaticity and conduction velocity	No receptors
Ventricles	β_1, β_2	Increased contractility	No receptors
Coronary	$\alpha_1, \alpha_2, \beta_2$	Constriction, dilation	Dilation
Skin	α_1, β	Constriction	Dilation
Skeletal muscle	α, β_2	Constriction, dilation	No receptors
Cerebral	α_1	Constriction (slight)	No receptors
Pulmonary	α_2	Constriction, dilation	
Renal	α_1, β_1	Constriction, dilation	

is promoted by epinephrine, but not norepinephrine (McCance & Huether, 2014).

▶ Systemic Circulation

Blood is pumped from the left ventricle into the aorta, the largest artery in the body. The aorta rises from the aortic valve and heads superiorly and to the right, which explains why one listens for aortic valve heart sounds at the first intercostal space on the right sternal border. Arteries branch from the aorta beginning at the aortic arch and continue until the aorta itself branches into the two iliac arteries at the level of the abdomen.

Multiple systemic arteries branch off from the aorta as it passes through the body. Arteries then branch into a series of increasingly smaller units until they become the smallest of all blood vessels, the capillaries. The capillaries eventually collect into venules, which combine to form veins, which return blood to the heart through the inferior and superior vena cavae.

The entire circulatory system is lined with endothelial cells that are active in controlling local conditions through the release of chemicals. The types of blood vessels have unique characteristics that affect their function. Arteries have thicker walls containing three layers, including a smooth muscle layer. The constriction of the smooth muscle surrounding the arteries is controlled by the action of chemicals such as epinephrine or norepinephrine. The outer layer of the artery consists of connective tissue. Veins have more narrow walls with a thinner muscle layer. The venous system can expand to create a reservoir of blood that can be mobilized if needed to support circulation. Venous blood is squeezed up from the legs through skeletal muscle contraction; the large veins of the leg have internal valves that prevent blood from flowing down by gravity.

The endothelial layer of cells constitutes the capillary wall. Capillaries have incredibly thin walls; the varying spaces between the cells that line them allow for fluid and blood cells to pass through the capillary cell membranes or through the spaces between the cells. In the brain, however, the extremely tight junctions between the endothelial cells force all fluid to go through these cells. In contrast, capillaries found in other parts of the body have relatively more open spaces between endothelial cells that allow for easier exchange of fluid and dissolved chemicals; this kind of openness is found in the liver, for example. Certain conditions, such as inflammation or sepsis, can result in widened spaces, leading to a condition euphemistically called *leaky capillaries*. Precapillary sphincters—smooth muscle cells that control the smallest arterioles—control blood flow to capillary networks. Under normal circumstances, local acidosis causes opening of a precapillary sphincter to an area, thereby increasing its blood supply. Blood flow is not uniform in all body tissues. The body can shift blood flow to areas of demonstrated need as reflected by local acidosis.

Pressures in the arterial system can be measured by use of a sphygmomanometer or by direct arterial cannulation. Pressures in the capillary network are lower than arteriolar pressures; venous pressures are even lower, supporting venous return. As with blood flow through the heart, blood flow in the periphery is determined by control of pressures and resistance to flow. Resistance to blood flow comes in the form of pressure in vessels, which is partly determined by smooth muscle tone and blood vessel length. In general, the key principle governing blood flow can be summarized as "the greater the resistance, the lower the flow." Resistance to flow can also be increased if the blood is more viscous, such as occurs with polycythemia. Blood flow can also be affected by the shape and internal smoothness of the blood vessels.

Blockage of arteries can cause decreased blood flow to areas of the body normally supplied by these arteries. Blockage can be caused by gradual increase in formation of smooth muscles from hyperinsulinism or by the accumulation of plaque from hypercholesterolemia. When plaques rupture, they cause a break in the endothelial lining of the vessel and a blood clot forms, further blocking the artery. Cardiac surgery often involves revascularization of arteries that have been blocked over time. One can expect that the basic process that affected coronary artery flow likely will affect flow in other areas of the body.

▶ Systemic Control of Blood Pressure

In addition to acting through the sympathetic nervous system, which can increase the blood pressure by increasing vascular resistance, the body can control blood pressure through other chemical pathways. The kidneys autoregulate their blood flow so that pressures at the glomerulus are sufficiently high to maintain filtration. If the kidneys detect decreased blood flow, they also release renin. Renin leads to a production of angiotensin I, which is later converted to angiotensin II. Angiotensin II increases systemic vascular resistance by causing vasoconstriction. It also stimulates the release of aldosterone from the adrenal glands. Aldosterone, a mineralocorticoid, causes sodium—and therefore water—retention. If the cause of renal blood flow decrease is blood loss, these compensatory mechanisms are helpful. Conversely, if low CO is caused by pump failure, then these mechanisms actually work against cardiac function by increasing afterload and water retention. Angiotensin-converting enzyme (ACE) inhibitors block this pathway, and guidelines now recommend their use both for heart failure and following myocardial infarction.

The body's water levels are regulated by antidiuretic hormone (ADH), a chemical released from the posterior pituitary gland. When diuresis slows, the amount of free body water increases. This effect then reduces the concentration (osmolality) of dissolved substances in the body. Baroreceptors in the left atrium, the aortic arch, and the carotid artery are sensitive to fluid volume and will send messages to increase ADH production when pressures are low.

Natriuretic peptides are released by parts of the body in response to plasma volume changes. They stimulate diuresis, systemic vasodilation and increased glomerular filtration rate. These proteins include atrial natriuretic peptide (ANP), brain natriuretic peptide (BNP), and C-type natriuretic peptide (CNP). BNP levels can reflect overall ventricular function (McCance & Huether, 2014).

▸ Disorders of Major Blood Vessels

Sometimes, as a result of long-standing high pressure inside arteries or because of turbulent flow caused by irregularities in the internal shape of the artery, weaknesses may develop in the arterial wall. An aneurysm is a widening in an artery that can completely surround the artery or that can consist of an outpouching at one part of the circumference of the artery. When aneurysms rupture, they cause rapid blood loss from the artery into surrounding tissues and a reduction in blood flow to areas normally supplied by the artery.

The aorta is prone to aneurysm development because it sustains the highest pressures in the vascular system. When an aneurysm involves all three levels of the arterial wall, it is termed a *true aneurysm*. This type of aneurysm typically involves the entire circumference of the vessel. Other aneurysms form between the layers of the artery, particularly following vascular surgery. In this case, blood leaks through the endothelial and tunica media layers and collects under the adventitia.

Aneurysms are usually undetectable until they threaten to rupture or actually do rupture. Symptoms depend on the location of the aneurysm. A widening aneurysm can result in decreased blood flow to small arteries in the area. A ruptured aneurysm causes pain, which can often be *referred*, meaning the pain is perceived in an area of the body different from where the actual injury is located. Thoracic aneurysms can cause dyspnea or dysphagia due to pressure on the esophagus and lung tissue. An abdominal aortic aneurysm can result in ischemia to tissues normally supplied by blood from the area below the aneurysm.

Diagnosis of aneurysms may be made through ultrasonography and by using imaging technologies such as computed tomography (CT) or magnetic resonance imaging (MRI). The goals of treatment are to reduce blood loss by reducing blood pressure until surgical repair can be accomplished. Asymptomatic aneurysms are sometimes detected on chest radiograph or by abdominal palpation of a pulsatile mass.

The decision to make a surgical repair, either through intravascular approach or as an open surgery, depends on the relative risk of the repair itself compared with the risk of the aneurysm's rupture. If, for example, the renal arteries are compromised by the location of the aneurysm, then the intravascular repair may not be possible. The age of the patient and the size of the aneurysm are factored into this decision. Intravascular approaches to supporting the integrity of the artery have been developed that allow for much quicker recovery by patients. The location of the aneurysm is key to understanding the symptoms produced by the arterial defect.

▸ Summary

By understanding the anatomy and physiology of the cardiovascular system, the nurse is able to make reasoned responses to patient problems. Concepts such as cardiac output and electrophysiology will be daily concerns of the CCN. Accurate assessment of cardiovascular function and early detection of problems are essential to providing high-quality care. Cardiovascular conditions remain the leading cause of death in the United States. Nurses caring for acute and critically ill patients will be needed who are experts in the care of patients with these conditions.

Self-Assessment Questions

1. You have a patient who is scheduled to have a coronary artery bypass graft. On physical exam, you note that the PMI is located at the left axilla. This assessment finding more than likely indicates
   A. cardiac tamponade.
   B. left axis deviation.
   C. tension pneumothorax.
   D. ventricular hypertrophy.
2. Blood flowing through the pulmonic valve is leaving the
   A. right ventricle.
   B. left ventricle.
   C. right atrium.
   D. left atrium.
3. The Frank-Starling law illustrates the relationship between
   A. vasoactive agent administration and hemodynamic response.
   B. sympathetic response and parasympathetic response.
   C. fluid status and cardiac function.
   D. acetylcholine and degree of bradycardia.
4. In the presence of increased afterload, which agents are useful in lowering resistance to cardiac ejection?
   A. Vasodilator agents
   B. Anticholinergic agents
   C. Vasoconstrictor agents
   D. Beta blockers
5. Decreased left ventricular preload can occur in the setting of
   A. cardiac tamponade.
   B. hypovolemia.
   C. cardiogenic shock.
   D. hypoxemia.
6. Angiotensin II increases systemic vascular resistance by causing
   A. vasoconstriction.
   B. parasympathetic stimulation.
   C. aldosterone release.
   D. production of renin.

7. Common signs of thoracic aneurysms include
   A. hypertension and cough.
   B. dyspnea and dysphagia.
   C. pleuritic chest pain and shortness of breath.
   D. bradycardia and jugular venous distention.
8. Atrial natriuretic protein is released when pressure is detected in the
   A. left atrium.
   B. left ventricle.
   C. right atrium.
   D. right ventricle.
9. Which neurotransmitter is released by the sympathetic nerve fibers, resulting in a profound effect on cardiac contractility and on vascular resistance?
   A. Angiotensin
   B. Acetylcholine
   C. Norepinephrine
   D. Dobutamine
10. Administration of a beta blocker will result in which of the following outcomes?
    A. Increased cardiac output
    B. Vasoconstriction
    C. Decreased contractility
    D. Compensation by dopaminergic receptors

Answers to Self-Assessment Questions

1. D. **ventricular hypertrophy**
   Rationale: If there is a change in shape or size of the left ventricle, there can be a change in the position and location of PMI. With ventricular hypertrophy, there is enlargement of the left ventricle. As a result, the PMI location may be altered.
2. A. **right ventricle**
   Rationale: Blood flows from the right ventricle, through the pulmonic valve, and into the pulmonary artery.
3. C. **fluid status and cardiac function**
   Rationale: The Frank-Starling law states that stretched muscle fibers produce a more powerful contraction. If there is more

filling of the left ventricle, there will be a greater force of contraction, up to a point.

4. A. **vasodilator agents**
   Rationale: When vessels are dilated, there is a decrease in the amount of work the heart must do to eject blood.

5. B. **hypovolemia**
   Rationale: When hypovolemia exists, less blood will return to the left ventricle; thus there is a decrease in left ventricular preload.

6. A. **vasoconstriction**
   Rationale: Angiotensin II is a potent vasoconstrictor. Vasoconstriction increases the amount of work the heart must do to eject blood (i.e., increased afterload).

7. B. **dyspnea and dysphagia**
   Rationale: Dyspnea and dysphagia from thoracic aneurysms occur due to pressure on the lung tissue and esophagus, respectively.

8. C. **right atrium**
   Rationale: Atrial natriuretic peptide is synthesized, stored, and released from atrial distention.

9. C. **norepinephrine**
   Rationale: Norepinephrine release causes β_1 receptor stimulation as well as α_1 receptor stimulation. Stimulating β_1 receptors results in increased heart rate, blood pressure, contractility, and cardiac output; α_1 receptor stimulation results in vasoconstriction.

10. C. **decreased contractility**
    Rationale: Stimulating β_1 receptors results in increased heart rate, blood pressure, contractility, and cardiac output. Logically, if β_1 receptor stimulation is blocked with the administration of beta blockers, a decrease in all four of these parameters should be anticipated.

References

Goldberg, C. (2015). *A practical guide to clinical medicine.* Retrieved from https://meded.ucsd.edu/clincalmed/heart.htm.

Marieb, E. N., & Hoehn K. N. (2016). The cardiovascular system. In E. N. Marieb & K. N. Hoehn (Eds.), *Human anatomy and physiology* (10th ed., pp. 579–607). Boston, MA: Pearson Publishers.

McCance, K. L., & Huether, S. E. (2014). *Pathophysiology: The biologic basis for disease in adults and children* (7th ed.). St. Louis, MO: Elsevier Mosby.

Web Resources

The Auscultation Assistant provides heart sounds, heart murmurs, and breath sounds to help medical students and others improve their physical diagnosis skills: http://www.med.ucla.edu/wilkes/intro.html

Basic cardiac assessment is a video demonstration: http://www.youtube.com/watch?v=dp5m2tXHDmA

MediavisonFilms. Cardiac Anatomy HD part 1 uses a pig's heart to display structures of a heart: https://www.youtube.com/watch?v=960_mAShiXQ

MediavisonFilms. Cardiac Anatomy HD part 2 uses a pig's heart to display structures of a heart: https://www.youtube.com/watch?v=Vr-DAhgq75w

Thought CO. The Anatomy of the Heart provides multiple views of cardiac anatomy with video of blood circulation: https://www.thoughtco.com/heart-anatomy-373485

The University of Minnesota Atlas of Human Cardiac Anatomy has diagrams, some using 3-D projections and MRI images: http://www.vhlab.umn.edu/atlas/

CHAPTER 3

Indications for Cardiac Surgery

Judy Dillworth

▶ Introduction

The heart has captivated the interest of human beings for centuries as the foundation of life and emotions. Technically, the first surgery on a human beating heart was performed in the early 1900s, but major advancements in cardiac surgery were achieved with the development of surface hypothermia and extracorporeal circulation in the mid-20th century. With advances in pharmacotherapy and innovations in technology such as minimally invasive and robotic surgical techniques, cardiac surgery has emerged as a dynamic and flourishing medical and nursing specialty. Thousands of individuals benefit from cardiac surgery each year. The evolution of surgical techniques presents exciting and varied challenges for critical care nurses and interdisciplinary team members. The purpose of this chapter is to review the types of cardiac surgery and their indications.

▶ Surgery for Ischemic Heart Disease

There are an estimated 92.1 million adult Americans, half of whom are 60 years of age and older,

diagnosed with one or more types of cardiovascular disease (CVD) (Benjamin et al., 2017). By 2030, 44% of the U.S. population is projected to have CVD (Benjamin et al., 2017). According to the National Health and Nutrition Examination Survey (NHANES), from 2011 to 2014, approximately 16.5 million American adults 20 years and older have coronary heart disease (CHD), also known as coronary artery disease (CAD). There are three major strategies used to treat significant coronary artery stenosis and prevent further ischemic damage: goal-directed medical therapy (GDMT), percutaneous revascularization, and surgical revascularization. Medical therapies include oral agents, aspirin, beta (β) blockers, lipid-lowering therapy, angiotensin-converting enzyme (ACE) inhibitors, and aldosterone antagonists, which control hypertension and treat symptoms of cardiac dysfunction (Yancy et al., 2013). The goals of percutaneous and surgical revascularization are to alleviate symptoms of angina and restore blood flow and oxygen delivery to the myocardium. Percutaneous coronary intervention (PCI), also known as percutaneous transluminal coronary angioplasty (PTCA), is a nonsurgical procedure in which an arterial catheter and various mechanical techniques (e.g., balloon angioplasty, drug eluting stents [DES]) are used to increase the diameter of narrowed

---

Original contributions from Kristine J. Peterson

coronary arteries and improve blood flow. Surgical revascularization, more frequently referred to as coronary artery bypass grafting (CABG), involves the attachment of sections of arterial or venous vessels from the aorta to the coronary artery. The goal of CABG surgery is to create new pathways that "bypass" the stenosis, improve blood flow to the coronary arteries, and relieve chest pain. Inpatient CABG procedures in the United States have steadily declined since 1998, due in part to the clinical relevance and rapid growth of PCI procedures (Benjamin et al., 2017). A customized approach is used to make decisions regarding the type of revascularization modality that is most appropriate for each individual patient.

Medical Therapy Versus Surgical Revascularization

Management of chronic stable ischemic heart disease includes either GDMT alone or GDMT supplemented with revascularization, such as PCI or CABG (Fihn et al., 2015). GDMT is recommended as an initial treatment for all patients with stable CAD. Revascularization with PCI or CABG is recommended for patients with symptoms or significant CAD (Iqbal et al., 2015). Because atherosclerosis continues to progress, GDMT is maintained postrevascularization to reduce adverse outcomes (Iqbal et al., 2015). Early trials demonstrated a survival benefit of CABG over medical therapy in patients with stable angina and high risk (Hillis et al., 2011). High-risk patients were identified by the severity of angina or ischemia, the number of diseased vessels, and the presence of left ventricular (LV) dysfunction. Hueb and colleagues' (2010) Medicine, Angioplasty or Surgery Study (MASS II) compared the 10-year survival of patients with multivessel CAD, stable angina, and preserved ventricular function with the treatment received. That is, patients who received medical treatment were more likely to have a subsequent myocardial infarction, need for revascularization, or cardiac death when compared to patients who had CABG surgery. Additionally, patients reported that CABG surgery was more effective in relieving angina than medical therapy. The 2011 American College of Cardiology Foundation/American Heart Association (ACCF/AHA) Guideline for Coronary Artery Bypass Graft Surgery supports the recommendations of CABG surgery for multivessel disease but does not recommended treatment of single-vessel disease with CABG surgery unless there is proximal left anterior descending (LAD) involvement (Hillis et al., 2011).

Percutaneous Versus Surgical Revascularization

Different strategies of myocardial revascularization include CABG, balloon angioplasty, PCI with bare metal stents (BMS), and first and second generation drug eluting stents (DES) (Costa et al., 2015). The first percutaneous coronary intervention procedure was performed in 1977. Many clinical trials have compared short- and long-term outcomes of PCI and surgical revascularization (Buszman et al., 2016; Fanari, Weiss, Zhang, Sonnad, & Weintraub, 2015; Palmierini et al., 2017). The Synergy Between Percutaneous Coronary Intervention with TAXUS drug-eluting stent and Cardiac Surgery (SYNTAX) score is an anatomically based tool, developed from other tools, that uses angiographic findings to define the complexity of CAD, predict mortality, and guide decision making in the selection of the revascularization modality (CABG versus PCI) (Costa et al., 2015). The SYNTAX score is determined by the location, severity, and extent of coronary stenosis. A lower SYNTAX score indicates a less complicated anatomic CAD (Levine et al., 2011). The SYNTAX score, evaluated in the landmark SYNTAX trial (Farooq, Brugaletta, & Serruys, 2011) has been established as an independent predictor of major adverse cardiac and cerebrovascular events (MACCE) following PCI (Farooq et al., 2013). The SYNTAX trial was a prospective, multicenter, randomized trial comparing PCI and CABG for patients with complex left mainstem or triple vessel CAD. In the SYNTAX trial (Serruys et al., 2009), 1,800 patients were randomized for PCI or CABG. Those patients suitable for only one treatment were entered into a nested PCI or CABG registry. The investigators validated CABG as the standard of care for these patients, resulting in significantly less MACCE at 12 months. This was due in large part to significantly higher revascularization rates in the patients treated with PCI (p=0.002). The incidence of stroke was higher in the CABG patients.

In a systematic review of 13 randomized control trials (RCTs) and 5 meta-analyses of patient status following the SYNTAX trial, Deb and colleagues (2013) concluded that PCI and CABG are both reasonable in patients with extensive coronary disease. The researchers recommended CABG for patients with complex disease and unprotected left main disease (ULMD), multivessel disease, diabetes and multivessel disease, or LV dysfunction and considered PCI for patients with less complex disease or surgical risk. The researchers corroborated conclusions that revascularization was higher after PCI, while incidence of stroke was higher after CABG. Head and colleagues (2014) also concluded CABG to have better outcomes for patients with triple vessel disease in their 5-year follow-up of the SYNTAX trial since patients who received PCI were at increased risk for repeated revascularization. Because patients treated with PCI were less likely to have a stroke than patients treated with CABG, PCI was recommended for patients with low SYNTAX scores. The recommendation for CABG in patients with significant stenosis in multivessel disease (e.g., three major coronary arteries or in both the proximal LAD and another major coronary artery) was therefore endorsed in the 2011 ACCF/AHA/Society for Cardiovascular Angiography (SCAI) Guideline for Percutaneous Coronary Intervention (Levine et al., 2011).

Buszman and colleagues (2016) studied 105 patients who received either PCI with stenting (n=52) or CABG (Nn=53) using the SYNTAX score for unprotected left main coronary artery stenosis. At a 10-year follow-up, patients treated with PCI tended to have a higher ejection fraction than patients post-CABG, but there was no statistical difference in mortality, myocardial infarction (MI), stroke, or repeated revascularization rates. Similarly, Cavalcante and colleagues (2016) compared PCI and CABG for treatment of ULMD in 1,305 patients. The incidence of MACCE was 28.3% in the PCI group compared to 23% in the CABG group. While death, MI, and stroke rates were similar in both studies, Cavalcante's team found patients who received a CABG to have less need for revascularization.

In a meta-analysis of 4,686 patients, Palmerini and colleagues (2017) concluded that PCI with DES may be an acceptable alternative to CABG for ULMD. When comparing patients post-PCI and -CABG at 39 months, there was no significant difference in the risk for cardiac and all-cause mortality, MI, or stroke. However, an interaction effect suggested a relatively lower mortality with PCI in patients with a low SYNTAX score and a relatively lower mortality with CABG in patients with a high SYNTAX score. Upadhaya and colleagues (2017) used a meta-analysis to compare clinical outcomes of PCI with DES to CABG. From five RCTs and 4,595 patients, the researchers reported significant differences in MACCE (p<0.0001) and repeat revascularization (p<0.00001) favoring CABG. As in other studies, there were no significant differences in MI, stroke, or cardiac and all-cause mortality. Since clinical outcomes in selected patients are similar, PCI is suggested to be a reasonable alternative therapy for CABG in selected patients with stenosis and low or medium complexity of coexisting coronary artery disease, even though revascularization rates are higher after PCI than CABG. Similar to Palmerini's team review, Upadhaya and colleagues (2017) recommended CABG for patients with ULMD and higher SYNTAX scores (≥33). The 2011 ACCF/AHA/SCAI Guideline for Percutaneous Coronary Intervention also recommended CABG for treatment of left main CAD, although PCI is suggested for patients with increased surgical risk and anatomy amenable to PCI (Levine et al., 2011).

The 2013 ACCF/AHA ST-segment elevation myocardial infarction (STEMI) guidelines recommended a limited role for CABG in the acute phase of STEMI (O'Gara et al., 2013). CABG is recommended for failed PCI and for anatomy not amenable to PCI in the setting of STEMI with high-risk factors such as ongoing or recurrent ischemia, severe heart failure, or cardiogenic shock. The guidelines also recommended CABG for STEMI at the time of surgical repair of mechanical defects (e.g., a ventricular septal defect or mitral valve repair). The same guidelines also recommended consideration of emergency CABG for STEMI in patients who are not in cardiogenic shock and are not candidates for PCI or fibrinolytic therapy (O'Gara et al., 2013).

▶ Indications for Coronary Artery Bypass Grafting

The ACCF/AHA Task Force on Practice Guidelines has established recommendations for CABG surgery to improve survival and to relieve symptoms (Hillis et al., 2011). For decisions regarding revascularization, procedures that promote survival are generally given greater consideration. CABG is recommended as the treatment of choice for patients with significant stenosis and unacceptable angina despite GDMT.

The ACCF/AHA recommendations are categorized into three classes: I, II, and III. Class I indicates that evidence or general agreement exists that the intervention is effective, or both. Class II indicates that conflicting evidence or a divergence of opinion exists about the efficacy of the intervention, or both. Class II is further divided into Class IIa and Class IIb: Class IIa indicates that evidence/opinion is in favor of the intervention's efficacy, whereas Class IIb interventions have less efficacy as established by evidence/opinion. For Class III interventions, evidence and/or general opinion suggest that the intervention is not beneficial and may be harmful.

The strength of the level of evidence for specific interventions is also identified according to the type or presence of research. For example, Level of Evidence A indicates that findings from multiple RCTs or meta-analyses supported use of an intervention. Level of Evidence B indicates that a single randomized trial or a series of nonrandomized trials supported an intervention. Level of Evidence C is assigned to those interventions supported by consensus opinion of experts, case studies, or standards of care (Fihn et al., 2014; Hillis et al., 2011). Levels of recommendations for each patient population are provided in **TABLES 3.1, 3.2**, and **3.3**.

CABG in Diabetics

Over the past 30 years, the incidence of diabetes mellitus (DM) in patients requiring CABG

surgery has markedly increased (Hillis et al., 2011). Patients with diabetes, especially those who are insulin dependent, have higher rates of perioperative morbidity and mortality and a reduced long-term survival rate compared to those patients without diabetes. As such, GDMT is recommended for patients with stable ischemic heart disease (SIHD) and DM, according to the 2014 American College of Cardiology/AHA/American Association for Thoracic Surgery/Preventive Cardiovascular Nurses Association/SCAI/Society of Thoracic Surgeons (ACC/AHA/AATS/PCNA/SCAI/STS) Focused Update of the Guideline for the Diagnosis and Management of Patients with Stable Ischemic Heart Disease (Fihn et al., 2015). When symptoms compromise the patients' quality of life, revascularization should be considered (Fihn et al., 2015). CABG surgery is recommended over PCI as the treatment of choice for patients with DM and multivessel disease (Fihn et al., 2015; Farkouh et al., 2012; Verma et al., 2013). This recommendation is based on the results of the Future Revascularization Evaluation in Patients with Diabetes Mellitus: Optimal Management of Multivessel Disease (FREEDOM) trial, which enrolled 1,900 patients at 140 international centers and randomly assigned CABG or PCI with DES to patients with DM and multivessel disease (Farkouh et al., 2012). Patients with DM and multivessel CAD had significantly lower rates of MI ($p<0.001$) and death of any cause ($p=0.049$) when treated with CABG surgery as compared to patients who received PCI (Farkouh et al., 2012). However, the incidence of stroke was more frequent in patients post-CABG (Farkouh et al., 2012). Verma and colleagues (2013) conducted a meta-analysis of eight RCTs comparing CABG and PCI outcomes for patients with DM. The meta-analysis included 7,468 participants, of whom 3,612 patients had diabetes. Four studies used PCI with BMS and four studies used PCI with DES. At 5 years, diabetic patients treated with CABG had a lower all-cause mortality than patients treated with PCI ($p=0.002$). The researchers found no differences in outcome for patients who received BMS or DES (Verma et al., 2013). The 2011 ACCF/AHA guideline for CABG surgery recommends CABG over PCI for patients with DM and multivessel disease.

TABLE 3.1 2011 Guideline for Coronary Artery Bypass Graft Surgery: Revascularization to Improve Survival

Clinical or Anatomic Setting	Recommendation	Class of Recommendation	Level of Evidence
UPLM or complex CAD	Heart team approach to treatment	I	C
	Calculation of STS and SYNTAX scores	IIa	B
UPLM	CABG	I	B
	PCI—for SIHD when both of the following are present: ■ Anatomic conditions associated with a low risk of PCI procedural complications and a high likelihood of good long-term outcome (e.g., a low SYNTAX score of ≤22, ostial or trunk left main CAD) ■ Clinical characteristics that predict a significantly increased risk of adverse surgical outcomes (e.g., STS-predicted risk of operative mortality ≥5%)	IIa	B
	PCI—for STEMI when distal coronary flow is TIMI flow grade <3 and PCI can be performed more rapidly and safely than CABG	IIa	C
	PCI—for SIHD when both of the following are present: ■ Anatomic conditions associated with a low to intermediate risk of PCI procedural complications and intermediate to high likelihood of good long-term outcome (e.g., low–intermediate SYNTAX score of <33, bifurcation left main CAD) ■ Clinical characteristics that predict an increased risk of adverse surgical outcomes (e.g., moderate–severe COPD, disability from prior stroke, or prior cardiac surgery; STS-predicted risk of operative mortality >2%)	IIb	B

(continues)

TABLE 3.1 2011 Guideline for Coronary Artery Bypass Graft Surgery: Revascularization to Improve Survival *(continued)*

Clinical or Anatomic Setting	Recommendation	Class of Recommendation	Level of Evidence
	PCI—harm for SIHD in patients (versus performing CABG) with unfavorable anatomy for PCI and who are good candidates for CABG	III	B
Three-vessel disease with or without proximal LAD artery disease	CABG	I	B
	CABG—multivessel with diabetes	IIa	B
	CABG—patients with complex three-vessel CAD (e.g., SYNTAX >22) who are good candidates for CABG	IIa	B
	PCI	IIb	B
Two-vessel disease with proximal LAD artery disease	CABG	I	B
	CABG—multivessel with diabetes	IIa	B
	PCI	IIb	B
Two-vessel disease without proximal LAD artery disease	CABG—with extensive ischemia	IIa	B
	CABG—multivessel with diabetes	IIa	B
	CABG—without extensive ischemia; of uncertain benefit	IIb	C
	PCI	IIb	B
One-vessel disease with proximal LAD artery disease	CABG with LITA (formerly LIMA)	IIa	B
	PCI	IIb	B

Clinical or Anatomic Setting	Recommendation	Class of Recommendation	Level of Evidence
One-vessel disease without proximal LAD artery disease	CABG—harm	III	B
	PCI—harm	III	B
LV dysfunction	CABG—EF 35% to 50%	IIa	B
	CABG—EF <35% without significant left main CAD	IIb	B
	PCI	Insufficient data	
Survivors of sudden cardiac death with presumed ischemia-mediated VT	CABG	I	B
	PCI	I	C

*CABG, coronary artery bypass graft; CAD, coronary artery disease; COPD, chronic obstructive pulmonary disease; COR, class of recommendation; EF, ejection fraction; LAD, left anterior descending; LIMA, left internal mammary artery; LITA, left internal thoracic artery; LOE, level of evidence; LV, left ventricular; N/A, not applicable; PCI, percutaneous coronary intervention; SIHD, stable ischemic heart disease; STEMI, ST-segment elevation myocardial infarction; STS, Society of Thoracic Surgeons; SYNTAX, Synergy between Percutaneous Coronary Intervention with TAXUS and Cardiac Surgery; TIMI, thrombolysis in myocardial infarction; UA/NSTEMI, unstable angina/non–ST elevation myocardial infarction; UPLM, unprotected left main disease; VT, ventricular tachycardia.
Reproduced from Hillis, L. D., Smith, P. K., Anderson, J. L., Bittl, J. A., Bridges, C. R., Byrne, J. G., . . . Winneford, M. D. (2011). 2011 ACCF/AHA guideline for coronary artery bypass graft surgery. *Journal of the American College of Cardiology, 58*(24), e140.

TABLE 3.2 2011 Guideline for Coronary Artery Bypass Graft Surgery: Revascularization to Improve Symptoms with Significant Anatomic (>50% Left Main or >70% Non–Left Main CAD) or Physiological (FFR <0.80) Coronary Artery Stenoses

Clinical Setting	Recommendation	Class of Recommendation	Level of Evidence
>1 significant stenoses amenable to revascularization and unacceptable angina despite GDMT	CABG	I	A
	PCI	I	A

(continues)

TABLE 3.2 2011 Guideline for Coronary Artery Bypass Graft Surgery: Revascularization to Improve Symptoms with Significant Anatomic (>50% Left Main or >70% Non–Left Main CAD) or Physiological (FFR <0.80) Coronary Artery Stenoses _(continued)_

Clinical Setting	Recommendation	Class of Recommendation	Level of Evidence
>1 significant stenoses and unacceptable angina in whom GDMT cannot be implemented because of medication contraindications, adverse effects, or patient preferences	CABG	IIa	C
	PCI	IIa	C
Previous CABG with >1 significant stenoses associated with ischemia and unacceptable angina despite GDMT	PCI	IIa	C
	CABG	IIb	C
Complex three-vessel CAD (e.g., SYNTAX score >22) with or without involvement of the proximal LAD artery and a good candidate for CABG	CABG—preferred over PCI	IIa	B
Viable ischemic myocardium that is perfused by coronary arteries that are not amenable to grafting	TMR as an adjunct to CABG	IIb	B

*CABG, coronary artery bypass graft; CAD, coronary artery disease; COPD, chronic obstructive pulmonary disease; FFR, fractional flow reserve; GDMT, guideline-determined medial therapy; LAD, left anterior descending; PCI, percutaneous coronary intervention; SYNTAX, Synergy between Percutaneous Coronary Intervention with TAXUS and Cardiac Surgery; TMR, transmyocardial laser revascularization.
Reproduced from Hillis, L. D., Smith, P. K., Anderson, J. L., Bittl, J. A., Bridges, C. R., Byrne, J. G., . . . Winneford, M. D. (2011). 2011 ACCF/AHA guideline for coronary artery bypass graft surgery. _Journal of the American College of Cardiology, 58_(24), e141.

TABLE 3.3 2011 Guideline for Coronary Artery Bypass Graft Surgery: Indications for Coronary Artery Bypass Graft Surgery in Other Settings

Class of Recommendation and Level of Evidence	Recommendation	Clinical Setting
IB	Emergency CABG	Patients with acute MI in whom: ■ Primary PCI has failed or cannot be performed, and ■ Coronary anatomy is suitable for CABG, and ■ Persistent ischemia of a significant area of myocardium at rest and/or hemodynamic instability refractory to nonsurgical therapy is present

Class of Recommendation and Level of Evidence	Recommendation	Clinical Setting
IB	Emergency CABG	Patients with acute MI and surgical repair of a postinfarction mechanical complication of MI, such as ventricular septal rupture, mitral valve insufficiency because of papillary muscle infarction and/or rupture, or free wall rupture
IB	Emergency CABG	Patients with acute MI with cardiogenic shock and who are suitable for CABG irrespective of the time interval from MI to onset of shock and time from MI to CABG
IC	Emergency CABG	Patients with acute MI and life-threatening ventricular arrhythmias (believed to be ischemic in origin) in the presence of left main stenosis ≥50% and/or 3-vessel disease
IIaB	CABG	Patients with acute MI and multi-vessel CAD with recurrent angina or MI within the first 48 hours of STEMI presentation as an alternative to a more delayed strategy
IIaB	CABG PCI	Patients >75 years of age with ST-segment elevation or left bundle branch block who are suitable for revascularization irrespective of the time interval from MI to onset of shock
IIIC—harm	CABG	Patients with persistent angina and a small area of viable myocardium who are stable hemodynamically
IIIC—harm	CABG	Patients with no reflow (successful epicardial reperfusion with unsuccessful microvascular reperfusion)
IB	CABG	Patients with life-threatening ventricular arrhythmias in resuscitated sudden cardiac death or sustained ventricular tachycardia thought to be caused by significant CAD (≥50% stenosis of left main coronary artery and/or ≥70% stenosis of 1, 2, or all 3 epicardial coronary arteries) and resultant myocardial ischemia
III	CABG	Patients with ventricular tachycardia with scar and no evidence of ischemia

*CABG, coronary artery bypass graft; CAD, coronary artery disease; MI, myocardial infarction; PCI, percutaneous coronary intervention; STEMI, ST-segment elevation myocardial infarction.

Reproduced from Hillis, L. D., Smith, P. K., Anderson, J. L., Bittl, J. A., Bridges, C. R., Byrne, J. G., . . . Winneford, M. D. (2011). 2011 ACCF/AHA guideline for coronary artery bypass graft surgery. *Journal of the American College of Cardiology, 58*(24), e123–e210.

Additionally, the use of an interdisciplinary heart team approach is suggested in decision making to ensure the appropriate treatment modality is used (Hillis et al., 2011).

CABG in Patients with Concomitant Carotid Disease

Patients with concomitant cerebrovascular and coronary heart disease have a higher incidence of left main coronary disease and a reduced left ventricular ejection fraction and subsequently a higher risk for perioperative stroke when compared with patients who have isolated coronary heart disease (Lazar, Wilson, & Messe, 2016). Cerebrovascular complications are among the most feared consequences of CABG surgery. The ACCF/AHA guideline for CABG surgery recommends the evaluation of patients with significant carotid artery disease by a multidisciplinary team consisting of a cardiologist, cardiac surgeon, vascular surgeon, and neurologist and the use of coronary artery duplex scanning in select high-risk patients (e.g., ≥65 years, PAD, history of cerebrovascular disease, hypertension, DM) (Hillis et al., 2011).

The perioperative stroke rate is reported to be twice as high for patients with bilateral versus unilateral carotid atherosclerotic disease (Fairman, 2016). In a review of 350 patients, Shishehbor and colleagues (2013) compared three treatment strategies: (1) staged carotid endarterectomy (CEA)–open heart surgery (OHS), (2) combined CEA-OHS, and (3) staged carotid artery stenting (CAS)–OHS. They concluded that short-term mortality, stroke, and MI were similar for staged CAS-OHS and combined CEA-OHS, and both were better than staged CEA-OHS. However, at 12 months, the same outcomes favored staged CAS-OHS. Aydin, Ozen, Sarikaya, and Yukseltan (2014) reported a case series of 110 patients who underwent simultaneous CEA and CABG. They concluded that this strategy results in low morbidity and mortality. Chiariello and colleagues (2015) studied 132 consecutive patients for whom concomitant CAD with stenting and CABG were performed and similarly reported low mortality and freedom from neurologic events up to 10 years postsurgery. Sharma, Deo, Park, and Joyce (2014)

conducted a meta-analysis of staged and combined CEA-CABG surgery. There were 25,021 patients (n=7,552 staged; n=17,469 combined) in 12 observational studies. The researchers reported insignificant differences in early mortality and postoperative stroke. While there appears to be consensus that staged and combined CEA-CABG surgery could be used interchangeably, the ideal surgical strategy depends on the patient's clinical condition and preference.

Minimally Invasive Myocardial Revascularization

Minimally invasive surgery has become increasingly common with several advantages, including less postoperative pain, lower complication rates, and early recovery (Hillis et al., 2011). Approaches to CABG other than the traditional median sternotomy and use of cardiac arrest with cardiopulmonary bypass (CPB), also known as on-pump CABG, include the minimally invasive direct coronary artery bypass (MIDCAB), which uses an entry other than a median sternotomy; the off-pump CABG (OPCAB), performed on the beating heart with stabilizing devices; and newer hybrid approaches to CABG (Hillis et al., 2011). Based on earlier studies indicating that both on- and off-pump CABG reduced morbidity and mortality rates, the 2011 ACCF/AHA guideline for CABG (Hillis et al., 2011) suggests either approach. The technique used is dependent on the skill of the surgeon and the avoidance of aortic manipulation, which are important factors in reducing the risk of neurologic complications (Hillis et al., 2011).

Since the publication of the ACCF/AHA Guideline for Coronary Artery Bypass Graft Surgery Guidelines (Hillis et al., 2011), Nardi and colleagues (2014) compared clinical outcomes for OPCAB patients (n=166) and on-pump CABG patients (n=203) 4 years postoperatively. They concluded that MACCE and repeat revascularization were similar in both groups but freedom from cardiac death was better after on-pump CABG. Fudulu and colleagues (2016) reported comparable early and late survival for both off-pump and conventional CABG upon review of several RCTs and meta-analysis. Patients undergoing OPCAB grafting appeared to have less postoperative renal dysfunction, bleeding, transfusion requirements, and respiratory complications, with similar perioperative myocardial infarction rates and higher repeat revascularization rates compared to patients undergoing on-pump CABG. Fudulu and colleagues (2016) recommended OPCAB for high-risk patients. Filardo and colleagues (2017) performed a meta-analysis of 73 studies (42 RCTs, 31 observational studies) and 1.2 million patients to determine the efficacy and effectiveness of on- versus off-pump CABG techniques in the general elective CABG patient population at various timeframes. The results indicated that OPCAB offered an initial advantage of operative safety and lower short-term mortality at 1 year but poorer survival at 5 years (Filardo et al., 2017). Off-pump coronary artery bypass is discussed in more detail in Chapter 6.

Minimally invasive direct coronary artery bypass provides revascularization on a beating heart in a less invasive manner and suggests reduction in complication risks such as infection and stroke (Kikuchi & Mori, 2017). Studies have compared patient outcomes of minimally invasive (e.g., MIDCAB) and conventional approaches to CABG and have reported no significant differences in graft patency or long-term survival. Advantages of MIDCAB include less tissue trauma, improved body image, and shorter recovery periods and hospital stays (Reser, Holubee, Caliskan, Guidotti, & Maisano, 2015; Rogers et al., 2013, 2017). Dieberg, Smart, and King (2016) conducted a systematic review and meta-analysis of eight studies (n=596 patients), with the conclusion that MIDCAB contributed to shorter operation times (p=0.008) and fewer intensive care unit (ICU) days (p=0.009). There was no significant difference in ventilator and hospital days, or the incidence of complications such as MI or stroke.

▶ Transmyocardial Laser Revascularization

Myocardial revascularization, or laser revascularization, is an alternative procedure for patients with ischemic CHD who have small coronary arteries or diffuse coronary artery disease/stenosis

or were determined to be ineligible for PCI or CABG procedures because previous approaches were unsuccessful (Soran, 2016). Patients with CHD and refractory angina despite maximal medical and interventional therapy may be eligible for revascularization. However, severe, diffuse CHD may not be amenable to complete revascularization, leaving the myocardium at risk even after such a procedure is attempted. Incomplete revascularization is a predictor of adverse events (Soran, 2016).

Options to treat refractory CHD include angiogenesis, genetic therapies, and transmyocardial laser revascularization (TMLR). These strategies involve various means of creating new pathways for blood to reach the myocardium. TMLR is a procedure in which a high-energy laser beam is applied to the left ventricle to create transmyocardial channels that direct blood flow from the ventricle to the myocardium. Open and percutaneous TMLR have been performed for patients with end-stage coronary artery disease (CAD), refractory to GDMT and who are not suitable candidates for alternative surgical interventions. Because a variety of nuclear imaging modalities can be used, the published literature related to TMLR procedures is limited and inconsistent. However, there is evidence of improved refractory angina and no difference in survival rate when compared to other treatments (Hillis et al., 2011; Iwanski et al., 2017).

▶ Surgery for Valve Disease

Patients with valvular heart disease (VHD) may present with a heart murmur, physical symptoms, or incidental findings of valvular abnormalities on chest imaging or noninvasive testing. Severity of VHD is determined by multiple criteria, including a history and physical examination, chest x-ray, electrocardiogram, and transthoracic echocardiogram (TTE). The treatment goal of valve surgery is to improve symptoms and/or prolong survival (Nishimura et al., 2014).

The 2017 Focused Update of the 2014 AHA/ACC Guideline for the Management of Patients

With Valvular Heart Disease recommends either surgical aortic valve replacement (AVR) or transcatheter aortic valve replacement (TAVR) for treatment of symptomatic patients with severe aortic stenosis (AS) or Stage D heart disease, based on an integrated assessment of the patients' procedural risk, comorbidities, frailty, values, and preferences. TAVR is recommended for patients with severe symptomatic AS who are ineligible for surgical AVR because of a prohibitive surgical risk, but are expected to survive at least 1 year postintervention (Nishimura et al., 2017). The Society of Thoracic Surgeons/American College of Cardiology Transcatheter Valve Therapy (STS/ACC TVT) registry provides annual data regarding patient outcomes and trends for this rapidly evolving technology. From the initial approval of TAVR by the U.S. Food and Drug Administration in 2011 through 2016, almost 55,000 TAVRs were performed for high-risk patients with a median age of 83 years (Grover et al., 2017). Clinical outcomes of patients postoperative-TAVR from 2013 to 2015 included a decrease in postoperative atrial fibrillation (AF) and bleeding, a decrease in hospital mortality from 5.7% to 2.9%, and a decrease in 1-year mortality from 25.8% to 21.6% (Grover et al., 2017). However, there was an increase in post-TAVR pacemaker insertion from 8.8% to 12.0% (Grover et al., 2017).

Valvular disease can occur due to congenital or acquired factors. Most valvular diseases are chronic and with symptoms appearing over time, after many structural changes have occurred. Congenital valvular disease originates with abnormal embryonic development and leads to structural defects, which may affect one or all four valves. Acquired valvular disease occurs most frequently in mitral and aortic valves and are due to high pressures on the left side of the heart. Acquired valvular disease results from inflammatory (or rheumatic) or degenerative disease processes. Rheumatic heart disease is uncommon in the United States but remains an important cause of morbidity and mortality in low- and middle-income countries (Benjamin et al., 2017). The incidence of infective endocarditis (IE) has not increased in the past decade (Benjamin et al., 2017). Mitral valve replacement is indicated before

a full course of antibiotics is completed for patients who have IE, valve dysfunction, and symptoms of heart failure (Nishimura et al., 2017). Decisions regarding medical or surgical management (repair or replacement) are made by weighing the risks and benefits of each treatment modality. Since VHD-related complications include asymptomatic irreversible ventricular dysfunction, pulmonary hypertension, stroke, and AF, a review of the indications and appropriate timing for surgical intervention should be made collaboratively by a heart team consisting of cardiologists, cardiothoracic surgeons, and infectious disease specialists (Nishimura et al., 2014, 2017). Valve surgery is discussed in detail in Chapter 5.

▶ Surgical Management of Arrhythmias

Sinus node dysfunction (SND), first described in 1968, refers to abnormalities in the sinus node and atrial pulse formation. Sinus node dysfunction is primarily a disease of the elderly and includes persistent sinus bradycardia, paroxysmal or persistent sinus arrest, with escape rhythms in the atrium, AV junction, or ventricular myocardium (Epstein et al., 2013). Permanent pacemaker implantation is the only effective treatment for patients with second- and third-degree AV block associated with arrhythmias or other medical conditions that result in syncope and documented symptomatic bradycardia (Epstein et al., 2013).

Tachy-brady syndrome describes the condition in which paroxysmal AF and sinus bradyarrhythmias suddenly oscillate from one to the other. Patients experience lightheadedness, syncope, palpitations, and other symptoms associated with a very slow or fast heart rate. This syndrome is treated with a cardiac pacemaker to reestablish effective circulation and normalize hemodynamic parameters (Homoud, 2016).

Durrer, Schoo, Schuilenburg, and Wellens (1967) first reported the successful initiation and termination of a tachycardia when they induced and successfully terminated atrioventricular reentrant tachycardia (AVRT). Advancements in understanding of arrhythmia initiation and propagation as well as surgical techniques created a role for surgical ablation for tachyarrhythmias. Many arrhythmias, including AVRT, atrial tachycardia, atrial flutter, AF, and ventricular tachycardia (VT) have been mapped and ablated using catheter techniques with varying degrees of success (Chinitz, Eckart, & Epstein, 2018).

Options for management of patients with ventricular arrhythmias are individualized to the presentation of each patient (e.g., syncope, stage of HF, LV function, spontaneous or induced ventricular arrhythmia) and include antiarrhythmic agents, catheter ablation, and surgery. When catheter ablation and/or medications fail to control the arrhythmia or produce intolerable side effects, an implanted pacemaker may be useful to treat or prevent recurrent ventricular tachycardia and supraventricular tachycardias (SVTs) (Epstein et al., 2013). A variety of pacing techniques, including programmed stimulation and short bursts of rapid pacing, may be used to terminate reentrant rhythms, including atrial flutter, paroxysmal reentrant SVT, and VT (Epstein et al., 2013). Implantable cardioverter-defibrillator (ICD) therapy is not indicated when VF or VT is responsive to surgical or catheter ablation. Indications for ICDs, cardiac resynchronization therapy (CRT) devices, and combined ICDs and CRT devices are expected to continuously evolve as new trials are conducted (Epstein et al., 2013).

Atrial Fibrillation

Atrial fibrillation is a supraventricular tachyarrhythmia with an uncoordinated and ineffective atrial contraction. This common cardiac rhythm disturbance is often associated with structural heart disease and other comorbidities (January et al., 2014). Symptoms of AF range from nonexistent to severe (e.g., fatigue, palpitations, hypotension, syncope, heart failure); fatigue is the most prevalent. According to the Centers for Disease Control and Prevention (CDC; 2017), approximately 2.7 to 6.1 million people in the United States have AF, which is responsible for 15% to 20% of ischemic strokes and contributes to a significant societal health care burden (CDC, 2017).

The incidence of AF increases with age and more than 12 million people in the United States are anticipated to have AF by 2050 (Oral & Latchamsetty, 2014).

Atrial fibrillation is a complex, multifactorial arrhythmia involving both arrhythmogenic triggers and an altered atrial substrate that maintains the arrhythmia. In addition, AF remodels the atria and perpetuates the AF (Oral & Latchamsetty, 2014). Since pulmonary veins frequently trigger AF, catheter-based and surgical techniques have been developed to isolate them. Treatment approaches are selected based on patient symptoms and classification. There are four classifications of atrial fibrillation based on the duration and persistence of episodes: (1) paroxysmal (AF that terminates spontaneously within 7 days of onset), (2) persistent (continuous sustained AF >7 days), (3) long-standing persistent (continuous sustained AF >12 months), and (4) permanent (January et al., 2014). Goals of therapy for AF consist of symptom alleviation, rate and rhythm control, and anticoagulation to prevent thromboembolism and stroke (Calkins et al., 2017; January et al., 2014).

The goal of antiarrhythmic medications is to maintain sinus rhythm. Antiarrhythmic medications provide first line therapy for paroxysmal and persistent AF, but are limited by their inconsistent efficacy and side effects (January et al., 2014). Treatment of AF is discussed in detail in Chapter 15.

Thromboembolic risk in AF is multifactorial. It involves left atrial mechanical dysfunction, blood stasis in the left atrial appendage, a hypercoagulable state, and elevated C-reactive protein levels (Oral & Latchamsetty, 2014). Surgery for AF is indicated when GDMT is ineffective and clinical symptoms interfere with the patients' lifestyle or ability to work. Because catheter and surgical ablation of AF are complex procedures, the benefits and risks of each need to be carefully assessed for each patient (Calkins et al., 2017). The purposes of the surgical approach are to isolate the pulmonary veins, modify the left atrial substrate, and decide the fate of the left atrial appendage (Zembala & Suwalski, 2013). The Maze procedure, originally a cut-and-sew procedure using a median sternotomy and CPB, was introduced by James Cox in 1987 (Zembala & Suwalski, 2013). The Maze procedure surgically induces scar formation and interrupts the transmission of the electrical impulses that cause AF. The Maze procedure has since evolved to include radiofrequency ablation (RFA), freezing, and ultrasonic energy. For example, the Cox Maze IV procedure uses radiofrequency, cryoablation to create the Maze III lines of ablation, or both; and can be done with a thoracoscopic approach. Procedures that involve both atria have been most effective in controlling AF (Kouchoukos, Blackstone, Hanley, & Kirklin, 2013).

The FAST trial was the first randomized trial comparing catheter ablation and minimally invasive surgical ablation of AF (Boersma et al., 2012). The investigators randomized 124 patients to catheter ablation or surgical ablation. Surgical ablation included RFA of pulmonary veins, ablation of the ganglionic plexi, and left atrial appendage exclusion. Freedom from atrial arrhythmias without pharmacotherapy at 12 months was significantly better with surgical ablation than catheter ablation, although adverse events associated with the procedure were greater with surgical ablation. Surgery for documented AF may be performed in conjunction with mitral valve surgery (Kouchoukos et al., 2013). Ad, Suri, and Gammie (2012) analyzed data on surgical AF ablations using the Society of Thoracic Surgeons Adult Cardiac Surgery Database. There were 91,801 surgical ablations documented over the 5 years reviewed, of which 4,893 (5.3%) were stand-alone procedures. Over the 5 years reviewed, a significant increase in stand-alone surgical ablations was noted. Operative mortality and stroke rates were similar in both the on- and off-pump bypass groups. The off-pump bypass group had significantly less bleeding reoperations, shorter ventilation, and shorter hospital stays. Ad and colleagues concluded that both on- and off-pump bypass approaches were safe and surgical ablation should be considered as a viable alternative to catheter-based ablation.

In a systematic review of surgical ablation versus catheter ablation, Kearney and colleagues (2014) reviewed seven studies and found significantly higher rates of freedom from AF after surgical ablation, with comparable rates of complications and higher rates for pacemaker implantation. This systematic review examined RCTs of surgical ablation at the time of mitral valve surgery. They found the combination of surgical ablation with mitral valve surgery did not change MACCE but significantly increased long-term freedom from AF when compared to patients without surgical ablation. The 2014 AHA/ACC/Heart Rhythm Society (HRS) Guideline for the Management of Patients With Atrial Fibrillation (January et al., 2014) recommends initial treatment of the underlying heart disease and comorbidities. Atrial fibrillation catheter ablation is recommended for symptomatic paroxysmal AF for failed rhythm control despite treatment with a minimum of one class I or III antiarrhythmic medication. The AHA/ACC/HRS guideline suggests surgical ablation to be reasonable for patients undergoing cardiac surgery and provides conditional recommendations for stand-alone surgical ablation as the primary therapy for patients who are not well managed by other treatments.

Surgical Management of Ventricular Tachycardia

Ventricular arrhythmias, particularly sustained VT, commonly occur in patients who survive acute myocardial infarction (AMI); the incidence in this patient population is approximately 3.5% (Podrid & Ganz, 2016). After evaluation to identify the cause of the MI and exclusion of completely reversible causes, ICD therapy is recommended in patients with nonischemic dilated cardiomyopathy, who are survivors of cardiac arrest due to hemodynamically unstable sustained VT or VF (Epstein et al., 2013).

Indications for surgery for VT are ill defined and largely dependent on the surgeon's judgment. There is consensus that VT caused by ischemic heart disease is most amenable to surgical therapy. Yet, surgical interventions for VT have failed to demonstrate a positive effect on long-term mortality to date (Kouchoukos et al., 2013). In the ACCF/AHA Guideline for Coronary Artery Bypass Graft Surgery, CABG surgery is not recommended for patients with VT, scarring, and without evidence of ischemia. Coronary artery bypass graft is a class IB recommendation for patients with resuscitated cardiac arrest thought to be due to significant or multivessel coronary artery disease and ischemia (Hillis et al., 2011).

▸ Surgical Therapies for Heart Failure

Following an MI, both the infarcted and noninfarcted areas undergo pathologic changes such as thinning and fibrous replacement, which alter the size and shape of the ventricle and ultimately lead to heart failure (HF). The ACCF/AHA stages of HF are fourfold (A, B, C, D) and reflect risk factors and cardiac structure abnormalities associated with HF (Yancy et al., 2013). Structural heart disease is only present in patients with stages B, C, or D. Interventions are identified for each respective stage and include GDMT to improve symptoms, treat structural heart disease, and reduce morbidity and mortality. Temporary or permanent mechanical circulatory support (MCS) devices are surgically implanted assist devices considered for patients with stage D HF refractory to GDMT, who may or may not be eligible for heart transplantation and cannot be weaned from intravenous inotropes (Lietz et al., 2013). Heart transplantation continues to be the gold standard for patients with advanced or refractory HF, but there is a limited supply of donor hearts and not all patients are eligible for transplantation (Ammirati et al., 2014). Accordingly, other surgical options have been developed. The left ventricular assist device (LVAD) has been used as a bridge to transplant, destination therapy, as a bridge to decision for patients with potentially reversible/treatable conditions, and occasionally as a bridge to recovery for whom ventricular recovery is expected after a period of time (Miller & Guglin, 2013). Cardiac transplantation is discussed in detail in Chapter 19.

▸ Cardiac Transplantation

The 5-year survival of end-stage HF patients posttransplant is 71.7% (Yancy et al., 2013). The primary limitation to heart transplantation is the growing gap between the number of potential recipients and the number of available donors. Given this mismatch in supply and demand, LVADs are increasingly being considered as a temporary or permanent alternative for treatment (Fanaroff, DeVore, Mentz, Daneshmand, & Patel, 2014). For more detail on cardiac transplantation, see Chapter 19.

Heart-Lung Transplantation

Heart-lung transplantation is the preferred procedure for selected patients with concomitant end-stage HF and end-stage pulmonary disease. Combined heart-lung transplantation is reserved for patients with end-stage cardiopulmonary and septic lung disease and for whom surgery is the only option (Mallidi, Anand, & Robbins, 2018). The procedure reached its peak in the 1990s. Since then, however, due to improvements in single- and double-lung transplant techniques as well as donor allocation to critically ill heart recipients, the number of procedures has declined substantially. According to the International Heart and Lung Transplantation Registry, there have been 4,745 total heart-lung transplants performed in the United States from 1981 through June 2016 (Yusen et al., 2016). The three most common indications for heart-lung transplantation are complex congenital heart disease with Eisenmenger syndrome, idiopathic pulmonary arterial hypertension, and cardiomyopathy (Singer, 2017).

▸ Surgery for Adult Congenital Heart Disease

Congenital heart defects can vary in size and severity, ranging from tiny pinholes that may resolve spontaneously to major malformations that require multiple surgical procedures to correct (Benjamin et al., 2017). Over the past 30 years, advancements in surgical techniques have improved the life expectancy and quality of life of infants born with congenital heart defects, with an estimated 85% of patients surviving into adulthood (Benjamin et al., 2017; Warnes et al., 2008). From 1999 to 2014, the number of age-adjusted deaths attributed to congenital heart defects in black, white, and Hispanic males and females decreased (Benjamin et al., 2017). According to the National Center for Health Statistics since 1979, trends in age-adjusted death rates for all congenital heart defects declined 39% and tended to occur progressively at older ages (Benjamin et al., 2017). This means that there is a growing generation of adults with CHD who are at risk for the development of ischemic strokes and chronic multisystem disease, thus presenting lifelong care requirements and management challenges. Coordination of care by adult congenital cardiovascular specialists is therefore recommended. ACC/AHA 2008 Guidelines for the Management of Adults with Congenital Heart Disease are the most recent and provide recommendations for the care of adult patients with congenital heart defects with particular attention to atrial septal defects, ventricular septal defects, atrioventricular septal defects, and patent ductus arteriosus (Warnes et al., 2008).

There are two categories of adult congenital heart disease. The first is secondary congenital heart disease, which refers to a previously treated disease and is more common than primary congenital heart disease. Primary congenital heart disease in the adult consists either of previously unknown and untreated disease or newly diagnosed anomalies. The most common of these are the atrial septal defect (ASD) and bicuspid aortic valve congenital heart disease (Kouchoukos et al., 2013). For the purposes of this chapter, this section focuses on management of ASDs.

Most ASDs with a diameter of 8 mm or less close spontaneously in childhood; those with a diameter of 5 mm or less should be followed closely due to the risk of paradoxical embolism (Connolly, 2015). A paradoxical embolism occurs when a venous clot, typically of the lower extremity, passes through the ASD to the arterial system. Patients with small ASDs and a normal-sized right ventricle (RV) are generally asymptomatic and do not require treatment until the individual reaches

adulthood. The ASD often becomes evident in patients with symptoms of AF and reduced exercise tolerance. Chronic left-to-right shunting may cause RV failure, tricuspid regurgitation, atrial arrhythmias, paradoxical embolization, and cerebral abscesses, which result in irreversible pulmonary hypertension and ultimately lead to right-to-left shunting (Burke, 2018; Connolly, 2015).

Surgical closure of an ASD is recommended for patients who experience paradoxical embolism or atrial arrhythmias, regardless of the size of the ASD, and right ventricular enlargement (Kouchoukos et al., 2013). ASDs may be closed by patch under cardiopulmonary bypass or via percutaneous closure using a closure device.

Studies have demonstrated good outcomes from surgical closure of ASDs. Mortality appears to be related to the degree of pulmonary artery hypertension (Humenberger et al., 2011; Kouchoukos et al., 2013). Humenberger and colleagues (2011) reviewed outcomes of 236 consecutive patients having transcatheter closure of their ASD. Better survival rates were reported in patients with less functional impairment and lower pulmonary artery pressures (PAP). The researchers also found that ASD closure at any age resulted in a significant decrease in symptoms, RV size, and PAP. Given that PAP increases with age, an ASD should be closed when the diagnosis is made (Humenberger et al., 2011; Kouchoukos et al., 2013).

▶ Hypertrophic Cardiomyopathy

According to the AHA 2017 Heart and Stroke Update, cardiomyopathy is a common cause of sudden cardiac death, second to CAD in the United States. Cardiomyopathy can be genetic or acquired from another disease, primarily CAD. There are four main types of cardiomyopathy: (1) dilated cardiomyopathy, (2) hypertrophic cardiomyopathy (HCM), (3) restrictive cardiomyopathy, and (4) stress-induced cardiomyopathy. Cardiomyopathy can progress to arrhythmias, blood clots, heart valve disease, and heart failure. Patients diagnosed with cardiomyopathy may not require treatment until symptoms develop. The goal of treatment is to control symptoms, reduce complications, and prevent progression of the disease. HCM is one of the most common causes of sudden death in competitive young athletes (Benjamin et al., 2017).

From 1990 to 2010, cardiomyopathy and myocarditis contributed to an 11.4% increase in years patients lived with a disability (from 5 to 6 years) and a 40.8% increase in global number of deaths from 286,800 to 403,900 (Benjamin et al., 2017). Cardiomyopathies and their resultant systolic and diastolic HF remain the main cause of cardiovascular morbidity and mortality in both children and adults and are a frequent indication for cardiac transplantation (Benjamin et al., 2017). Patients with HCM who receive a heart transplant have a survival rate of 75% to 100% at 5 years and 61% to 94% at 10 years (Mehra et al., 2016).

HCM is a common genetic cardiovascular disease characterized by abnormal myocytes leading to hypertrophy without dilatation and preserved systolic function (Schoen & Padera, 2018). While HCM has a variable course, patients are most commonly treated for impaired diastolic filling and/or obstruction of the LV outflow tract (Schoen & Padera, 2018). Treatment includes pharmacologic therapy, dual-chamber pacing, surgery, and chemical ablation (Maron, 2017). Patients with HF and no outflow obstruction are initially treated with pharmacologic therapy. Beta blockade is the standard first line therapy and verapamil (Calan®) and disopyramide (Norpace®) are added to treat patients with symptoms of HF, but without outflow obstruction (Gersh et al., 2011). Dual-chamber pacing was introduced in the 1990s. Pacing was thought to change the geometry of ventricular contraction and lead to reduced LV outflow tract obstruction and symptomatic improvement. Data failed to show significant reductions in the outflow tract obstruction or exercise tolerance. The 2011 ACCF/AHA Task Force on Practice Guideline for the Diagnosis and Treatment of Hypertrophic Cardiomyopathy recommends septal reduction surgery in most cases, with IIbB recommendations for pacing patients who are symptomatic despite medical therapy and who are not considered candidates for septal reduction surgery (Gersh et al., 2011). Pacemakers and ICDs are recommended in these instances to help control arrhythmias and reduce symptoms (Gersh et al., 2011).

For patients with HCM who develop significant drug-refractory LV outflow tract obstruction, the recommended treatment is surgical LV myectomy and/or mitral valve replacement (Gersh et al., 2011; Kouchoukos et al., 2013; Maron, 2017). Septal myectomy involves excision of the thickened section of subaortic septal muscle with or without mitral valve repair/replacement. A perioperative transesophageal echocardiography (TEE) is used to determine the amount of tissue to be excised. The myectomy procedure has been known to be safe and effective in providing excellent hemodynamic results with improved quality of life (Gersh et al., 2011; Kouchoukos et al., 2013; Maron, 2017).

Systolic anterior motion (SAM) of the mitral valve has been shown to be a major determinant of the amount of outflow obstruction. Depending on the degree of SAM and obstruction, MVR is recommended. The 2011 guideline lists an IC recommendation for septal reduction in patients whose symptoms are refractory to pharmacologic therapy and who have demonstrated outflow tract obstruction (Gersh et al., 2011). The AHA guidelines do not recommend septal reduction surgery for patients who are asymptomatic and have normal exercise tolerance or in those who are controlled with medical therapy (Gersh et al., 2011).

Chemical ethanol septal ablation is a nonsurgical procedure that relieves outflow obstruction by infusing ethanol into the first septal branch of the left anterior descending coronary artery by way of an angioplasty catheter (Maron, 2017). Studies of this approach indicate that ethanol ablation creates a myocardial scar and reduces outflow tract obstruction, increases exercise capacity, and improves symptoms (Maron, 2017). In an observational series of 177 patients who had ethanol septal ablation, long-term survival was no different from surgical septal myectomy (Sorajja et al., 2012). Ethanol ablation is not recommended for asymptomatic or medically controlled patients or for adults under 40, if myectomy is a viable option (Gersh et al., 2011).

Heart transplantation is recommended as a last resort for patients with severe heart failure and nonobstructive HCM. Patients with LV dilation and systolic dysfunction should receive particular attention (Gersh et al., 2011).

▶ Other Cardiac Surgeries: Pericardial Surgery

Bleeding and cardiac tamponade are known complications after cardiac surgery and require immediate intervention. It is possible for blood and clots to accumulate in the mediastinal space and impair ventricular filling (cardiac tamponade). When patients exhibit signs of tamponade, including a sudden decrease or cessation of chest tube output, tachycardia, narrowing pulse pressure, and decreased cardiac index, the fluid around the heart must be drained as quickly as possible. Emergency interventions include pericardiocentesis (needle aspiration) and/or creation of a pericardial window (partial resection of the pericardium) to allow fluid to drain into the pleural or peritoneal space and prevent reaccumulation of pericardial fluid.

▶ Cardiac Tumors

Primary cardiac tumors are extremely rare, resemble many other cardiovascular diseases, and are often discovered incidentally during evaluation for another problem (Gaasch & Vander Salm, 2017; Spartalis et al., 2017). Myxomas are the most common of the primary cardiac tumors. Myxomas can occur in all four chambers of the heart with 75% benign and 75% occurring in the left atrium (Spartalis et al., 2017). These tumors cause obstruction of blood flow, mimicking mitral stenosis or mitral regurgitation. Myxomas can be detected by echocardiography, MRI, and/or CT scan (Gaasch & Vander Salm, 2017). Depending on the size, location, and characteristics of the tumor and its position in the heart, patients may present with signs of HF and/or central nervous system (CNS) embolization (Spartalis et al., 2017). Patients have reported dyspnea, fever, weight loss, fatigue, weakness, arthralgia, and myalgia. Malignant cardiac tumors are often accompanied by hemorrhagic pericardial effusion. Simple or complex surgical resection is the recommended treatment for benign myxomas and malignant cardiac tumors, respectively. Surgical resections have a high success rate and should be electively performed when the diagnosis is made (Spartalis et al., 2017). Mortality and complications from surgery are low. Recurrences are rare and occur in less than 3% of patients (Kouchoukos et al., 2013).

▶ Summary

This chapter described the various cardiac surgical procedures and their associated indications based on the most recent evidence.

🔍 CASE STUDY

C. P. is a 57-year-old male with a 4-year history of coronary artery disease. He underwent angioplasty and stenting to the left posterior descending artery and an obtuse marginal 2 years ago. He reports increased symptoms over the past 2 weeks, including more frequent episodes of chest pain on exertion that is relieved with rest. He underwent coronary angiography, which revealed proximal left anterior descending artery and right coronary artery occlusion of 95%. He also had diffuse atherosclerosis. Transesophageal echocardiogram revealed an ejection fraction of 40% with septal dyskinesis and left ventricular hypokinesis. He has normal RV systolic function.

C. P.'s medical history is significant for end-stage renal disease secondary to polycystic kidney disease; he undergoes hemodialysis three times weekly. His medical history is also significant for hypertension and hypercholesterolemia. C. P.'s medications include daily aspirin, an angiotensin-converting enzyme inhibitor, and a statin.

C. P. underwent a CABG procedure with a left internal thoracic artery graft to the left anterior descending artery and a radial artery graft to the right coronary artery. The operation was uneventful, and the patient was transferred to the intensive care unit in stable condition. He had a smooth recovery. His only postoperative complication was self-limiting hyperglycemia. He was extubated within 4 hours and transferred to the progressive care unit the next morning. C. P. was discharged to home on postoperative day 6. His discharge instructions included consumption of a low-fat, low-cholesterol diet and outpatient cardiac rehabilitation. He was given an appointment for the hospital's "Living with Heart Disease" class and was discharged on his preadmission medications. He was to follow up with his surgeon in 2 weeks and his primary care physician in 4 weeks.

Critical Thinking Questions

1. Why did the physician recommend CABG procedure instead of stenting?
2. What were the indications for CABG on this patient?
3. What was the likely etiology of self-limiting hyperglycemia?

Answers to Critical Thinking Questions

1. C. P. had contraindications for PTCA. Specifically, he had multivessel disease with diffuse atherosclerosis and impaired LV function.
2. Two-vessel disease with proximal left anterior descending artery disease.
3. The hyperglycemia was likely related to increased catecholamines.

Self-Assessment Questions

1. For which of the following rhythms is the use of catheter ablation techniques indicated?
   A. Accelerated junctional rhythm
   B. Atrial tachycardia
   C. Mobitz II
   D. Ventricular fibrillation
2. For which of the following is transmyocardial laser revascularization indicated as a sole therapy?
   A. Ejection fraction 40% refractory to medical therapy or surgical revascularization
   B. Stage IV angina responsive to medical therapy
   C. Irreversible ischemia of the LV free wall
   D. Transmyocardial laser revascularization is no longer indicated.
3. For which of the following patients with atrial fibrillation is a surgical intervention indicated? A patient who:
   A. doesn't want the risk of life-threatening side effects of pharmacotherapy.
   B. has cardiomyopathy secondary to tachyarrhythmias.
   C. has supraventricular tachycardia unresponsive to medical therapy.
   D. is not compliant with pharmacotherapy.
4. Which of the following patients is most likely to be successfully treated with surgical therapy for ventricular tachycardia? A patient with:
   A. diffuse myocardial damage.
   B. cardiomyopathy.
   C. irreversibly damaged myocardium.
   D. frequent episodes of hyperkalemia.

5. For which of the following patients with heart failure is revascularization indicated? A patient with:
   A. pulmonary hypertension.
   B. RV dysfunction.
   C. right-sided heart failure.
   D. ejection fraction of 10%.

6. For which of the following patients is percutaneous coronary intervention recommended? A patient with:
   A. diabetes and multivessel disease.
   B. unprotected left main disease.
   C. left ventricular dysfunction.
   D. surgical risk.

7. Which of the following patients has an indication for cardiac transplantation? A patient with:
   A. pulmonary vascular resistance over 5 U/m^2.
   B. diabetic neuropathy.
   C. active sarcoidosis.
   D. ischemic heart disease with intractable angina.

8. For which of the following patients is a heart-lung transplant indicated? A patient with:
   A. bilirubin 2.6 mg/dL with glomerular filtration rate 40 mL/min.
   B. cystic fibrosis.
   C. body mass index 42 kg/m^2.
   D. COPD with heart failure.

9. Which of the following is a sequela of chronic right-to-left shunting?
   A. Mitral regurgitation
   B. LV failure
   C. Ventricular dysrhythmias
   D. Pulmonary hypertension

10. The nurse should anticipate that the initial treatment for hypertrophic cardiomyopathy with sinus node dysfunction is:
    A. beta blocker.
    B. dual-chamber pacing.
    C. calcium channel blocker.
    D. mitral valve replacement.

Answers to Self-Assessment Questions

1. **D. ventricular fibrillation**
   Rationale: Catheter ablation is mostly used to treat a condition called supraventricular tachycardia (SVT), ventricular tachycardia, and ventricular fibrillation, which occurs because of abnormal conduction fibers in the heart.

2. **D. transmyocardial laser revascularization is no longer indicated**
   Rationale: Transmyocardial laser revascularization is not indicated as a sole therapy. A recent meta-analysis found no significant difference with use to extend survival rates. However, both CO_2 and Ho:Yag laser systems demonstrated a decrease in angina at 3, 6, and 12 months.

3. **B. has cardiomyopathy secondary to tachyarrhythmias**
   Rationale: Management of AF and/or atrial flutter is geared toward avoidance of thromboembolic events, reduction of symptoms, and avoidance of arrhythmia-induced cardiomyopathy. Control of heart rate can be met through either a rate control strategy with atrioventricular (AV) nodal blocking agents (or ablation and pacer implant in cases of multiple drug failures) or maintenance of sinus rhythm (rhythm control strategy).

4. **C. irreversibly damaged myocardium**
   Rationale: There are three treatment options for VT, although many patients require a combination: implantable cardiac defibrillator (ICD), antiarrhythmic medications, or catheter ablation.

5. **D. an ejection fraction of 10%**
   Rationale: Patients with preserved effort tolerance but with multivessel CAD, lower EF, and higher end-systolic volume index were most likely to benefit from CABG with respect to long-term survival.

6. D. **surgical risk**

Rationale: The AWESOME trial tested the hypothesis that PCI is a safe and effective alternative to CABG surgery for patients with refractory ischemia and high risk of adverse outcomes.

7. D. **ischemic heart disease with intractable angina**

Rationale: Cardiac transplantation is the treatment of choice for many patients with end-stage heart failure who remain symptomatic despite optimal medical therapy.

8. B. **cystic fibrosis**

Rationale: Patients with cystic fibrosis and end-stage bronchiectasis require replacement of both lungs to avoid the complications of allograft contamination. The best treatment for these patients is double-lung transplantation; however, in patients with compromised cardiac function, a heart-lung transplant is indicated.

9. D. **pulmonary hypertension**

Rationale: Over a long period, the increased blood flow through the lungs provokes a hypertensive reaction in the pulmonary vasculature that effectively increases the pressure in the right ventricle and atrium.

10. A. **beta blocker**

Rationale: A symptomatic patient with resting or provocable LV outflow tract obstruction is initially treated with negative inotropic or chronotropic therapy to help alleviate obstruction. Beta blockers can mitigate symptoms and reduce outflow tract obstruction. Verapamil has been shown in a few cases to cause death when a patient with HCM has elevated arterial pressure and LV outflow tract obstruction. A dual-chamber pacemaker may be an option in select patients. These would be individuals with medically refractory symptomatic obstruction.

CLINICAL INQUIRY BOX

Question: What is the effect of diabetes on graft patency 1 year following CABG?

Reference: Singh, S. K., Desai, N. D., Petroff, S. D., Deb, S., Cohen, E. A., Radhakrishnan, S., . . . Fremes, S. E. (2008). The impact of diabetic status on coronary artery bypass graft patency: Insights from the Radial Artery Patency Study. *Circulation, 118,* 5222–5225.

Objective: To determine the impact of diabetes on graft patency 1 year following CABG.

Method: Multicenter randomized trial. Follow-up with angiography was made 1 year following CABG.

Results: A total of 561 patients were enrolled. A comparison of the saphenous vein and radial artery was made. Thirty-three of 230 (14.4%) of the grafts were occluded in patients with diabetes. This compared to 63 of 650 (9.7%) of patients who did not have diabetes. Saphenous vein grafts were statistically more often occluded in patients with diabetes (19% versus 12%). Fewer radial artery grafts were occluded in patients with diabetes.

Conclusions: Occlusion occurred more often in patients with diabetes as compared to those without diabetes. This was attributed to more frequent saphenous vein graft failures in patients with diabetes.

Data from Singh, S. K., Desai, N. D., Petroff, S. D., Deb, S., Cohen, E. A., Radhakrishnan, S., . . . Fremes, S. E. (2008). The impact of diabetic status on coronary artery bypass graft patency: Insights from the Radial Artery Patency Study. Circulation, 118, 5222–5225.

References

Ad, N., Suri, R. M., & Gammie, J. S. (2012). Surgical ablation of atrial fibrillation trends and outcomes in North America. *The Journal of Thoracic and Cardiovascular Surgery, 144,* 1051–1060.

Ammirati, E., Oliva, F., Cannata, A., Contri, R., Colombo, T., Martinelli, L., & Frigerio, M. (2014). Current indications for heart transplantation and left ventricular assist device: A practical point of view. *European Journal of Internal Medicine, 25*(5), 422–429.

Aydin, E., Ozen, Y., Sarikaya, S., & Yukseltan, I. (2014). Simultaneous coronary artery bypass grafting and carotid endarterectomy can be performed with low mortality rates. *Cardiovascular Journal of Africa, 25,* 130–133.

Benjamin, E. J., Blaha, M. J., Chiuve, S. E., Cushman, M., Das, S. R., . . . On behalf of the American Heart Association Statistics Committee and Stroke Statistics Subcommittee. (2017). Heart disease and stroke statistics 2017 update: A report from the American Heart Association. *Circulation, 135*(10), e146–603.

Boersma, L. V., Castella, M., van Boven, W., Berruezo, A., Yilmaz, A., Nadal, M., . . . Mont, L. (2012). Atrial fibrillation catheter ablation versus surgical ablation treatment (FAST): A 2-center randomized clinical trial. *Circulation, 125*(1), 25–30.

Burke, R. P. (2018). Surgery for adult congenital heart disease. In L. H. Cohn (Ed.), *Cardiac surgery in the adult* (5th ed., pp. 1215–1224). New York, NY: McGraw-Hill Medical.

Buszman, P. E., Buszman, P. P., Banasiewicz-Szkrobka, I., Milewski, K. P., Zurakowski, A., Orlik, B., . . . Bochenek, A. (2016). Left main stenting in comparison with surgical revascularization: 10-year outcomes of the (left main coronary artery stenting) LE MANS trial. *JACC Cardiovascular Interventions, 9*(4), 318–327.

Calkins, H., Hindricks, G., Cappato, R., Kim, Y. H., Saad, E. B., Aguinaga, L., . . . Yamane, T. (2017). 2017 HRS/EHRA /ECAS/APHRS/SOLAECE expert consensus statement on catheter and surgical ablation of atrial fibrillation. *Heart Rhythm, 14*(10), e275–e444.

Cavalcante, R., Sotomi, Y., Lee, C. W., Ahn, J. M., Farooq, V., Tateishi, H., . . . Serruys, P. W. (2016). Outcomes after percutaneous coronary intervention or bypass surgery in patients with unprotected left main disease. *Journal of the American College of Cardiology, 68*(10), 999–1009.

Centers for Disease Control and Prevention. (2017). *Atrial fibrillation fact sheet*. Retrieved from https://www .cdc.gov/dhdsp/data_statistics/fact_sheets/fs_atrial_ fibrillation.htm.

Chiariello, L., Nardi, P., Pellegrino, A., Saitto, G., Chiariello, G. A., Russo, M., . . . Versaci, F. (2015). Simultaneous carotid artery stenting and heart surgery: Expanded experience of hybrid surgical procedures. *The Annals of Thoracic Surgery, 99*(4), 1291–1297.

Chinitz, J. S., Eckart, R. E., & Epstein, L. M. (2018). Interventional therapy for atrial and ventricular arrhythmias. In L. H. Cohn (Ed.), *Cardiac surgery in the adult* (5th ed., pp. 1147–1166). New York, NY: McGraw-Hill Medical.

Connolly, H. W. (2015). *Indications for closure and medical management of atrial septal defects in adults*. Retrieved from https://www.uptodate.com/contents /indications-for-closure-and-medical-management-of -atrial-septal-defects-in-adults/abstract/1.

Costa, F., Ariotti, S., Valgimigli, M., Kolh, P., Windecker, S., & Task Force on Myocardial Revascularization of the European Society of Cardiology (ESC) and the European Association for Cardio-Thoracic Surgery (EACTS). (2015). Perspectives on the 2014 ESC/EACTS guidelines on myocardial revascularization: Fifty years of revas-cularization: Where are we and where are we heading? *Journal of Cardiovascular Translational Research, 8*(4), 211–220.

Deb, S., Wijeysundera, H. C., Ko, D. T., Tsubota, H., Hill, S., & Fremes, S. E. (2013). Coronary artery bypass graft surgery vs percutaneous interventions in coronary revascularization. A systematic review. *Journal of the American Medical Association, 310*(19), 2086–2095.

Dieberg, G., Smart, N. A., & King, N. (2016). Minimally invasive cardiac surgery: A systematic review and meta-analysis. *International Journal of Cardiology, 223*, 554–560.

Durrer, D., Schoo, L., Schuilenburg, R. M., & Wellens, H. J. (1967). The role of premature beats in the initiation of and the termination of supraventricular tachycardia in the Wolff–Parkinson–White syndrome. *Circulation, 36*, 644–662.

Epstein, A. E., DiMarco, J. P., Ellenbogen, K. A., Estes III, N. A., Freedman, R. A., Gettes, L. S., . . . Heart Rhythm Society. (2013). 2012 ACCF/AHA/HRS focused update incorporated into the ACCF/AHA/HRS 2008 guidelines for device-based therapy of cardiac rhythm abnormalities: A report of the American College of Cardiology Foundation/American Heart Association Task Force on Practice Guidelines and the Heart Rhythm Society. *Journal of the American College of Cardiology, 61*(3), e6–e75.

Fairman, R. M. (2016). *Carotid endarterectomy*. Retrieved from http://www.uptodate.com/contents/carotid-endarterectomy.

Fanari, Z., Weiss, S. A., Zhang, W., Sonnad, S. S., & Weintraub, W. S. (2015). Comparison of percutaneous coronary intervention with drug eluting stents versus coronary artery bypass grafting in patients with multivessel coronary artery disease: Meta-analysis of six randomized controlled trials. *Cardiovascular Revascularization Medicine: Including Molecular Interventions, 16*(2), 70–77.

Fanaroff, A. C., DeVore, A. D., Mentz, R. J., Daneshmand, M. A., & Patel, C. B. (2014). Patient selection for advanced heart failure therapy referral. *Critical Pathways in Cardiology, 13*(1), 1–5.

Fang, J. C., Ewald, G. A., Allen, L. A., Butler, J., Westlake Canary, C. A., Colvin-Adams, M., . . . Givertz, M. M. (2015). Advanced (stage D) heart failure: A statement from the Heart Failure Society of America Guidelines Committee. *Journal of Cardiac Failure, 21*(6), 519–534.

Farkouh, M. E., Domanski, M., Sleeper, L. A., Siami, F. S., Dangas, G., Mack, M., . . . FREEDOM Trial Investigators. (2012). Strategies for multivessel revascularization in patients with diabetes. *The New England Journal of Medicine, 367*(25), 2375–2384.

Farooq, V., Brugaletta, S., & Serruys, P. (2011). The SYNTAX score and SYNTAX-based clinical risk scores. *Seminars in Thoracic and Cardiovascular Surgery, 23*(2), 99–105.

Farooq, V., Serruys, P. W., Zhang, Y., Mack, M., Ståhle, M., Holmes, D. R., . . . Mohr, F. W. (2013). Short-term and long-term clinical impact of stent thrombosis and graft occlusion in the SYNTAX trial at 5 years. *Journal of the American College of Cardiology, 62*, 2360–2369.

Fihn, S. D., Blankenship, J. C., Alexander, K. P., Bittl, J. A., Byrne, J. G., Fletcher, B. J., . . . Society of Thoracic Surgeons. (2015). 2014 ACC/AHA/AATS/PCNA/SCAI/ STS focused update of the guideline for the diagnosis and management of patients with stable ischemic heart disease: A report of the American College of Cardiology/American Heart Association Task Force on Practice Guidelines, and the American Association for Thoracic Surgery, Preventive Cardiovascular Nurses Association, Society for Cardiovascular Angiography and Interventions, and

Society of Thoracic Surgeons. *The Journal of Thoracic and Cardiovascular Surgery, 149*(3), e5–e23.

Filardo, G., Hamman, B. L., da Graca, B., Sass, D. M., Machala, N. J., Ismail, S., . . . Grayburn, P. A. (2017). Efficacy and effectiveness of on- versus off-pump coronary artery bypass grafting: A meta-analysis of mortality and survival. *The Journal of Thoracic and Cardiovascular Surgery.* doi:S0022-5223(17)31786-5

Fudulu, D., Benedetto, U., Pecchinenda, G. G., Chivasso, P., Bruno, V. D., Rapetto, F., . . . Angelini, G. D. (2016). Current outcomes of off-pump versus on-pump coronary artery bypass grafting: Evidence from randomized controlled trials. *Journal of Thoracic Disease, 8*(Suppl 10), S758–S771.

Gaasch, W. H., & Vander Salm, T. J. (2017). *Cardiac tumors.* Retrieved from https://www.uptodate.com/contents/cardiac-tumors.

Gersh, B. J., Maron, B. J., Bonow, R. O., Dearani, J. A., Fifer, M. A., Link, M. S., . . . Yancy, C. W. (2011). 2011 ACCF/AHA guideline for the diagnosis and treatment of hypertrophic cardiomyopathy: A report of the American College of Cardiology Foundation/American Heart Association Task Force on Practice Guidelines. *Circulation, 124*(24), e783–e831.

Grover, F. L., Vemulapalli, S., Carroll, J. D., Edwards, F. H., Mack, M. J., Thourani, V. H., . . . STS/ACC TVT Registry. (2017). 2016 annual report of the Society of Thoracic Surgeons/American College of Cardiology Transcatheter Valve Therapy Registry. *Journal of the American College of Cardiology, 69*(10), 1215–1230.

Head, S. J., Davierwala, P. M., Serruys, P. W., Redwood, S. R., Colombo, A., Mack, M. J., . . . Mohr, F. W. (2014). Coronary artery bypass grafting vs. percutaneous coronary intervention for patients with three-vessel disease: Final five-year follow-up of the SYNTAX trial. *European Heart Journal, 35*(40), 2821–2830.

Hillis, L. D., Smith, P. K., Anderson, J. L., Bittl, J. A., Bridges, C.R., Byrne, J. G., . . . Winneford, M. D. (2011). 2011 ACCF/AHA guideline for coronary artery bypass graft surgery. *Journal of the American College of Cardiology, 58*(24), e123–e210.

Homoud, M. (2016). *Sick sinus syndrome: Clinical manifestations, diagnosis and evaluation.* Retrieved from https://www.uptodate.com/contents/sick-sinus-syndrome-clinical-manifestations-diagnosis-and-evaluation?source=search_result&search=brady+tachy&selectedTitle=3%7E142.

Hueb, W., Lopes, N., Gersh, B. J., Soares, P. R., Ribeiro, E. E., Pereira, A. C., . . . Ramires, J. A. (2010). Ten-year follow-up survival of the medicine, angioplasty, or surgery study (MASS II): A randomized controlled clinical trial of 3 therapeutic strategies for multivessel coronary artery disease. *Circulation, 122*(10), 949–957.

Humenberger, M., Rosenhek, R., Gabriel, H., Rader, F., Heger, M., Klaar, U., . . . Baumgartner, H. (2011). Benefit of atrial septal defect closure in adults: Impact of age. *European Heart Journal, 32*(5), 553–560.

Iqbal, J., Zhang, Y. J., Holmes, D. R., Morice, M. C., Mack, M. J., Kappetein, A. P., . . . Serruys, P. W. (2015). Optimal medical therapy improves clinical outcomes in patients undergoing revascularization with percutaneous coronary intervention or coronary artery bypass grafting: Insights from the synergy between percutaneous coronary intervention with TAXUS and cardiac surgery (SYNTAX) trial at the 5-year follow-up. *Circulation, 131*(14), 1269–1277.

Iwanski, J., Knapp, S. M., Avery, R., Oliva, I., Wong, R. K., Runyan, R. B., . . . Khalpey, Z. (2017). Clinical outcomes meta-analysis: Measuring subendocardial perfusion and efficacy of transmyocardial laser revascularization with nuclear imaging. *Journal of Cardiothoracic Surgery, 12,* 37. doi:10.1186/s13019-017-0602-8

January, C. T., Wann, L. S., Alpert, J. S., Calkins, H., Cigarroa, J. E., Cleveland Jr., J. C., . . . ACC/AHA Task Force Members. (2014). 2014 AHA/ACC/HRS guideline for the management of patients with atrial fibrillation: Executive summary: A report of the American College of Cardiology/American Heart Association Task Force on Practice Guidelines and the Heart Rhythm Society. *Circulation, 130*(23), 2071–2104.

Kappetein, A. P., Mohr, F. W., Feldman, T. E., Morice, M. C., Holmes, D. R., Ståhle, E., . . . Colombo, A. (2011). Comparison of coronary bypass surgery with drug-eluting stenting for the treatment of left main and/or three-vessel disease: 3-year follow-up of the SYNTAX trial. *European Heart Journal, 17,* 2125–2134.

Kearney, K., Stephenson, R., Phan, K., Chan, W. Y., Huang, M. Y., & Yan, T. D. (2014). A systematic review of surgical ablation versus catheter ablation for atrial fibrillation. *Annals of Cardiothoracic Surgery, 3*(1), 15–29.

Kikuchi, K., & Mori, M. (2017). Minimally invasive coronary artery bypass grafting: A systematic review. *Asian Cardiovascular & Thoracic Annals, 25*(5), 364–370.

Kouchoukos, N. T., Blackstone, E. H., Hanley, F. L., & Kirklin, J. K, (2013). *Kirklin/Barratt-Boyes cardiac surgery* (4th ed.). Philadelphia, PA: Elsevier.

Lazar, H., Wilson, C., & Messe, S. (2016). *Coronary artery bypass grafting in patients with cerebrovascular disease.* Retrieved from https://www.uptodate.com/contents/coronary-artery-bypass-grafting-in-patients-with-cerebrovascular-disease.

Levine, G. N., Bates, E. R., Blankenship, J. C., Bailey, S. R., Bittl, J. A., Cercek, B., . . . Society for Cardiovascular Angiography and Interventions. (2011). 2011 ACCF/AHA/SCAI guideline for percutaneous coronary intervention. A report of the American College of Cardiology Foundation/American Heart Association Task Force on Practice Guidelines and the Society for Cardiovascular Angiography and Interventions. *Journal of the American College of Cardiology, 58*(24), e44–e122.

Lietz, K., Deng, M., Feldman, D., Kaan, A., Pamboukian, S. V., Rame, J. E., Teuteberg, J. J. (2013). The 2013 International Society for Heart and Lung Transplantation Guidelines for Mechanical Circulatory Support: Executive summary task force 1: Selection of candidates for mechanical circulatory support and risk management prior to implantation for fixed comorbidities. *The Journal of Heart and Lung Transplantation, 32*(2), 157–187.

Mallidi, H., Anand, J., & Robbins, R. C. (2018). Lung transplantation and heart–lung transplantation. In L. H. Cohn (Ed.), *Cardiac surgery in the adult* (5th ed., pp. 1331–1360). New York, NY: McGraw-Hill Medical.

Maron, M. S. (2017). *Hypertrophic cardiomyopathy: Clinical manifestations, diagnosis and evaluation.* Retrieved from https://www.uptodate.com/contents/hypertrophic -cardiomyopathy-clinical-manifestations-diagnosis-and -evaluation.

Mehra, M. R., Canter, C. E., Hannan, M. M., Semigran, M. J., Uber, P. A., Baran, D. A., . . . Zuckermann, A. (2016). The 2016 International Society for Heart Lung Transplantation listing criteria for heart transplantation: A 10-year update. *The Journal of Heart and Lung Transplantation, 35*(1), 1–23.

Miller, L., & Guglin, M. (2013). Patient selection for ventricular assist devices: A moving target. *Journal of the American College of Cardiology, 61*(12), 1209–1221.

Nardi, P., Pellegrino, A., Bassano, C., Mani, R., Chiariello, G. A., Zeitani, J., . . . Chiariello, L. (2014). The fate at mid-term follow-up of the on-pump vs. off-pump coronary artery bypass grafting surgery. *Journal of Cardiovascular Medicine, 16*(2), 125–133.

Nishimura, R. A., Otto, C. M., Bonow, R. O., Carabello, B. A., Erwin III, J. P., Fleisher, L. A., . . . Thompson, A. (2017). 2017 AHA/ACC focused update of the 2014 AHA/ACC guideline for the management of patients with valvular heart disease: A report of the American College of Cardiology/American Heart Association Task Force on Clinical Practice Guidelines. *Journal of the American College of Cardiology, 70*(2), 252–289.

Nishimura, R. A., Otto, C. M., Bonow, R. O., Carabello, B. A., Erwin III, J. P., Guyton, R. A., . . . American Heart Association. (2014). 2014 AHA/ACC guideline for the management of patients with valvular heart disease: A report of the American College of Cardiology/American Heart Association Task Force on Practice Guidelines. *The Journal of Thoracic and Cardiovascular Surgery, 148*(1), e1–e132.

O'Gara, P. T., Kushner, F. G., Ascheim, D. D., Casey Jr., D. E., Chung, M. K., de Lemos, J. A., . . . Yancy, C. W. (2013). 2013 ACCF/AHA guideline for the management of ST-elevation myocardial infarction: A report of the American College of Cardiology Foundation/American Heart Association Task Force on Practice Guidelines. *Journal of the American College of Cardiology, 61*(4), e78–e140.

Oral, H., & Latchamsetty, R. (2014). Atrial fibrillation: Paroxysmal, persistent, and permanent. In D. P. Zipes & J. Jalife (Eds.), *Cardiac electrophysiology: From cell to bedside* (6th ed., pp. 739–754). Philadelphia, PA: Elsevier.

Palmerini, T., Serruys, P., Kappetein, A. P., Genereux, P., Riva, D. D., Reggiani, L. B., . . . Stone, G. W. (2017). Clinical outcomes with percutaneous coronary revascularization vs coronary artery bypass grafting surgery in patients with unprotected left main coronary artery disease: A meta-analysis of 6 randomized trials and 4,686 patients. *American Heart Journal, 190*, 54–63.

Podrid, P. J., & Ganz, L. I. (2016). *Pathogenesis of ventricular tachycardia and ventricular fibrillation during acute myocardial infarction.* Retrieved from http://www.uptodate .com/contents/pathogenesis-of-ventricular-tachycardia -and-ventricular-fibrillation-during-acute-myocardial -infarction.

Reser, D., Holubec, T, Caliskan, E, Guidotti, A., & Maisano, F., (2015) Left anterior small thoracotomy for minimally invasive coronary artery bypass grafting. *Multimedia Manual of Cardio-Thoracic Surgery,* doi: 10.1093/mmcts/mmv022

Reser, D., Walser, R., van Hemelrijk, M., Holubec, T., Weber, A., Plass, A., . . . Maisano, F. (2017). Long-term outcomes after minimally invasive aortic valve surgery through right anterior minithoracotomy. *The Thoracic and Cardiovascular Surgeon, 65*(3), 191–197.

Rogers, C. A., Pike, K., Angelini, G. D., Reeves, B. C., Glauber, M., Ferrarini, M., . . . Murphy, G. J. (2013). An open randomized controlled trial of median sternotomy versus anterolateral left thoracotomy on morbidity and health care resource use in patients having off-pump coronary artery bypass surgery: The sternotomy versus thoracotomy (STET) trial. *The Journal of Thoracic and Cardiovascular Surgery, 146*(2), 306–316, e1–e9.

Schoen, F. J., & Padera, R. F. (2018). Cardiovascular pathology. In L. H. Cohn (Ed.), *Cardiac surgery in the adult* (5th ed., pp. 99–156). New York, NY: McGraw-Hill Medical.

Serruys, P. W., Morice, M. C., Kappetein, A. P., Colombo, A., Holmes, D. R., Mack, M. J., . . . SYNTAX Investigators. (2009). Percutaneous coronary intervention versus coronary-artery bypass grafting for severe coronary artery disease. *The New England Journal of Medicine, 360*(10), 961–972.

Sharma, V., Deo, S. V., Park, S. J., & Joyce, L. D. (2014). Meta-analysis of staged versus combined carotid endarterectomy and coronary artery bypass grafting. *The Annals of Thoracic Surgery, 97*(1), 102–109.

Shishehbor, M. H., Venkatachalam, S., Sun, Z., Rajeswaran, J., Kapadia, S. R., Bajzer, C., . . . Blackstone, E. H. (2013). A direct comparison of early and late outcomes with three approaches to carotid revascularization and open heart surgery. *Journal of the American College of Cardiology, 62,* 1948–1956.

Shroyer, A. L., Grover, F. L., Hattler, B., Collins, J. F., McDonald, G. O., Kozora, E., . . . The ROOBY Study Group. (2009). On-pump versus off-pump coronary-artery bypass surgery. *The New England Journal of Medicine, 361,* 1827–1837.

Singer, L.G. (2017). *Heart-lung transplantation.* Retrieved from http://www.uptodate.com/contents/heart-lung -transplantation.

Sorajja, P., Ommen, S. R., Holmes Jr., D. R., Dearani, J. A., Rihal, C. S., Gersh, B. J., . . . Nishimura, R. A. (2012). Survival after alcohol septal ablation for obstructive hypertrophic cardiomyopathy. *Circulation, 126*(20), 2374–2380.

Soran, O. (2016). Alternative therapy for medically refractory angina: Enhanced external counterpulsation and trans-myocardial laser revascularization. *Heart Failure Clinics, 12*(1), 107–116.

Spartalis, M., Tzatzaki, E., Spartalis, E., et al. (2017). Atrial myxoma mimicking mitral stenosis. *Cardiology Research, 8*(3), 128–130.

Upadhaya, S., Baniya, R., Madala, S., Subedi, S. K., Khan, J., Velagapudi, R. K., . . . Bachuwa, G. (2017). Drug-eluting stent placement versus coronary artery bypass surgery for unprotected left main coronary artery disease: A meta-analysis of randomized controlled trials. *Journal of Cardiac Surgery, 32*(2), 70–79.

Verma, S., Farkouh, M. E., Yanagawa, B., Fitchett, D. H., Ahsan, M. R., Ruel, M., . . . Friedrich, J. O. (2013). Comparison of coronary artery bypass surgery and percutaneous coronary intervention in patients with diabetes: A meta-analysis of randomised controlled trials. *The Lancet: Diabetes & Endocrinology, 1*(4), 317–328.

Warnes, C. A., Williams, R. G., Bashore, T. M., Child, J. S., Connolly, H. M., Dearani, J. A., . . . Webb G. D. (2008). ACC/AHA 2008 guidelines for the management of adults with congenital heart disease: A report of the American College of Cardiology/American Heart Association Task Force on Practice Guidelines (writing committee to develop guidelines on the management of adults with congenital heart disease). *Circulation, 118*(23), e714.

Yancy, C. W., Jessup, M., Bozkurt, B., Butler, J., Casey Jr., D. E., Drazner, M. H., . . . Wilkoff, B. L. (2013). 2013 ACCF/AHA Guideline for the management of heart failure: A report of the American College of Cardiology Foundation/American Heart Association Task Force on Practice Guidelines. *Journal of the American College of Cardiology, 62*(16), e147–e239.

Yusen, R. D., Edwards, L. B., Dipchand, A. I., Goldfarb, S. B., Kucheryavaya, A. Y., Levvey, B. J., . . . International Society for Heart and Lung Transplantation. (2016). The registry of the International Society for Heart and Lung Transplantation: Thirty-third adult lung and heart-lung transplant report-2016; focus theme: Primary diagnostic indications for transplant. *The Journal of Heart and Lung Transplantation, 35*(10), 1170–1184.

Zembala, M. O., & Suwalski, P. (2013). Minimally invasive surgery for atrial fibrillation. *Journal of Thoracic Disease, 5*, S704–S712.

CHAPTER 4

Preoperative Cardiac Surgery Nursing Evaluation

Roberta Kaplow, Sonya R. Hardin

▶ Introduction

The primary goal of a preoperative assessment is evaluation of perioperative risk. An in-depth assessment assists in minimizing surgical risk and potential morbidity and mortality. The literature supports the preoperative optimization of a patient's cardiovascular status as part of the effort to improve patient outcomes (Zhan, Purcell, & Bush, 2015). An evaluative screening identifies special needs that may require modification of the patient's course of treatment before, during, and after surgery.

▶ Risk Factors of Morbidity and Mortality Following Cardiac Surgery

The major risk factors for adverse outcomes of cardiac surgery include factors in all three phases of hospitalization (preoperative, intraoperative, and postoperative). A number of risk assessment tools (Parsonnet, Dean, & Bernstein, 1989) score risk factors for morbidity and mortality, such as advanced age, emergency surgery, previous cardiac surgery, dialysis dependency, creatinine level of 2 mg/dL or higher, and preoperative renal insufficiency (Bhukal et al., 2012). EuroSCORE II factors include age, gender, renal impairment, poor mobility, chronic obstructive pulmonary disease (COPD), extracardiac arteriopathy, diabetes on insulin, neurologic dysfunction, previous cardiac surgery, serum creatinine, active endocarditis, critical preoperative state, cardiac factors (e.g., unstable angina, left ventricular [LV] dysfunction, recent myocardial infarction [MI], and pulmonary hypertension), previous cardiac surgery (e.g., emergency, other than isolated coronary artery bypass graft [CABG], thoracic aorta, and postinfarct septal rupture), urgency of procedure, weight of the intervention, and New York Heart Association (NYHA) score (EuroSCORE. org, n.d.). The EuroSCORE II is an interactive calculator whereby a nurse can input information for a final score. This tool can be found online.

Numerous risk assessment tools have been developed to predict mortality in patients undergoing heart surgery. Some of these scoring tools include the Parsonnet, Cleveland Clinic, French, Euro, Pons, and Ontario Province Risk scores (Eamer et al., 2018). The Parsonnet score has been found to be predictive in the oldest of old individuals who require cardiac surgery (Tomaras, 2017). Prolonged hospital stays and increased mortality are associated with higher scores.

Research has demonstrated a decreased incidence of physical and psychological problems that adversely affect recovery when preoperative education of patients is completed. Evidence further indicates that preoperative patient education results in increased patient compliance, resulting in decreased length of hospital stay (LOS) (Edwards, Mears, & Barnes, 2018).

▶ Nursing Assessment

Nursing assessment prior to cardiac surgery typically begins during an outpatient visit, but may occur during an acute inpatient admission. The latter situation may occur in patients with conditions that increase their operative risk. Components of the preoperative assessment include information from the patient, family, and medical records, and the physical exam. Baseline information is obtained about the patient's clinical history, including the type of heart disease, associated symptoms, resource availability, stability, and ability to participate in care and decision making. The level of resilience is determined when the nurse ascertains the degree of compensation the patient has developed.

Preoperative Patient Interview

The purpose of a patient interview is to review past medical and surgical histories and to conduct a systems evaluation to identify processes that may affect the outcome of a patient's cardiac surgery. The interview helps the nurse evaluate patient and family knowledge as well as determine educational needs related to the planned procedure. Understanding of the underlying illness, planned surgical course, and willingness and ability to adhere to the surgical regimen are also evaluated. Put simply, the nurse is responsible for the overall assessment of the patient's physical and psychological readiness for surgery. Data suggest that cardiac surgery patients who receive preoperative education with or without coping strategies as opposed to routine preoperative preparation experience less emotional distress, have better physical and psychological recovery, and experience fewer hypertensive episodes postoperatively (Powell et al., 2016).

During the patient interview, the nurse should seek to discover any information that can affect perioperative risk and postoperative management. Several risk factors have been identified in the literature as influencing the mortality of cardiac surgery patients. **TABLE 4.1** lists many of these comorbid conditions.

The nurse should also inquire if the patient has any history of gastrointestinal bleeding, peptic ulcer disease, or bleeding diathesis. Any of these conditions may affect the antiplatelet regimen following revascularization or the choice of a valvular prosthesis. Likewise, the nursing evaluation should gather information on the presence of cardiac risk factors as well as presence of associated medical diseases such as COPD, cerebrovascular or other peripheral arterial occlusive disease, and hypertension.

The patient's baseline sleep patterns should be determined. Patients who undergo CABG procedures are at risk of developing sleep disturbances postoperatively. The presence of anxiety and depression should be assessed as well, because these psychosocial conditions may develop in the postoperative cardiac surgery patient (Gonçalves et al., 2016).

Obstructive Sleep Apnea

Presence of obstructive sleep apnea (OSA) is typically assessed for by surgical and anesthesia providers prior to surgery. The diagnosis of OSA can impact postoperative outcomes after cardiac surgery. In some instances providers may decide to offer elective surgery to treat OSA with continuous positive airway pressure (CPAP) several weeks prior to surgery. The literature supports OSA patients sleeping in the lateral, prone, or sitting position to improve apnea–hypopnea index

TABLE 4.1 Factors That May Affect Cardiac Surgery Patient Mortality

Alcohol use	Tobacco use
Diabetes	Elevated serum creatinine (≥2 mg/dL)
Chronic airway disease	Previous cardiac surgery
Recent MI (<90 days)	Low left ventricular ejection fraction (<30%)
Chronic heart failure	Pulmonary hypertension
Unstable angina	Depression
Obesity	Hypoalbuminemia
Active endocarditis	Procedure urgency
Ventricular septal rupture	Critical preoperative condition
Dialysis	Advanced age (>70 years)
Preoperative GFR	African American race
Preoperative functional status	Ascending aortic aneurysm
Aortic regurgitation	Atrial fibrillation
Coronary artery disease	Aortic valve endocarditis
Female gender	Aortic valve surgery
Tricuspid valve surgery	Reoperation
CABG with valve repair	

CABG, coronary artery bypass grafting; GFR, glomerular filtration rate; MI, myocardial infarction
Data from Carr et al., 2015; Fortes et al., 2016; LaPar et al., 2014

scores. Nurses should be aware that concurrent administration of sedative agents increases the risk of respiratory depression and airway obstruction. Supplemental oxygen should be used postoperatively until peripheral capillary oxygen saturation (SpO$_2$) monitoring shows that individuals can maintain an airway with their CPAP mask as was used in the home environment (American Society of Anesthesiologists, 2014).

Nutrition Evaluation

The preoperative evaluation should also look for indicators of nutritional deficiency. In particular, malnutrition is a risk factor associated with significant morbidity and mortality in surgical patients. During the nursing evaluation, it is essential that all cardiac surgery patients undergo nutritional screening to identify malnourished or at-risk patients to ensure that an adequate nutritional plan is included as part of the patient's care.

The Malnutrition Universal Screening Tool (MUST) has been found to predict postoperative complications in cardiac surgery patients (Lomivorotov et al., 2013). The MUST tool includes the variables of body mass index (BMI), weight loss in the last 3 to 6 months, and the effect of lack of nutritional intake for greater than 5 days due to acute disease process. A score of 3 or greater indicates malnutrition. Malnutrition is observed in 1.2% to 46.4% of patients having cardiac surgery (Ringaitiené et al., 2016).

In addition to the nutritional assessment screens available, unintentional weight loss, protein-calorie malnutrition, laboratory findings (e.g., anemia, hypoalbuminemia, prealbumin, vitamin B$_{12}$ deficiency, other vitamin and mineral deficiency), and low BMI are among the variables suggesting nutritional deficiency (Stoppe et al., 2017). Patients with hypoalbuminemia (<2.5 g/dL) should have their nutritional status optimized 1 to 4 weeks prior to cardiac surgery, because they are at great risk for sepsis and respiratory failure. Enhanced nutrition is also essential to promote wound healing and meet postoperative metabolic demands (Stoppe et al., 2017). This can be accomplished with dietary enhancement or enteral feeding if no contraindications are present. Patients who are undergoing cardiac surgery and who have a low BMI (<20 kg/m^2) and hypoalbuminemia (<2.5 g/dL) are at increased risk of postoperative morbidity and mortality (Montazerghaem, Safaie, & Samiei, 2014). Further, patients with hypoalbuminemia are at increased risk for developing sternal wound infections, postoperative anemia, infection from the saphenous vein graft harvest site, renal failure, increased risk of postoperative atrial fibrillation (AF), increased hospital LOS, and prolonged ventilatory support (Lazar, Salm, Engelman, Orgill, & Gordon, 2016). Conversely, patients with a high percentage of body fat have a greater risk for sternal wound infection (Thelwall, Harrington, Sheridan, & Lamagni, 2015).

Discharge Planning

To begin proactive discharge planning, the patient's living arrangements are assessed. Many patients need assistance at discharge owing to limited social and financial resources. Early discharge planning alleviates stressors and anxiety for both the patient and family (Sharif, Moshkelgosha, Molazem, Najafi Kalyani, & Vossughi, 2014). Discharge to rehabilitative units either in long-term care or subacute care units can be easily predicted. Strong predictors include use of an intra-aortic balloon pump, emergency surgery, older age, long postoperative stays, poor nutritional state, comorbidities, and descending thoracic aorta procedures (Almashrafi, Alsabti, Mukaddirov, Balan, & Aylin, 2016).

Physical Assessment

Cardiac Assessment

For patients undergoing cardiac surgery, assessment of the cardiovascular system will likely be more extensive than assessment of other body systems. Blood pressure, temperature, peripheral pulses, and weight are recorded. Blood pressure readings should be obtained from both arms. Blood pressure difference between arms is associated with increased morbidity and mortality (Clark, 2015) and subclavian artery stenosis (Epperla et al., 2017). This condition may eliminate the possibility of using the internal mammary artery for grafting (Epperla et al., 2017). It has been suggested that

stenting the subclavian artery will make the vessel suitable for CABG (Che et al., 2016).

Auscultation of the heart and carotid arteries will provide essential baseline information. Heart sounds should be evaluated in terms of rate, rhythm, and presence of extra sounds, murmurs, gallops, or rubs. Identification of aortic regurgitation (AR) is a significant finding, because this condition may be exacerbated during cardiopulmonary bypass (CPB) and lead to acute LV distention (Gaasch, Otto, & Yeon, 2018). Aortic regurgitation is identified with the presence of an early diastolic murmur that can be heard at the second and third intercostal spaces (ICSs) at the right sternal border and at the second and fourth ICSs at the left sternal border. The murmur of AR usually decreases in intensity (decrescendo) and disappears before the S$_1$ heart sound (McGee, 2018).

A carotid bruit is a sound associated with turbulent flow and may indicate arterial stenosis. Auscultation of the carotid arteries is performed from the base of the neck to the angle of the jaw while breath holding. A bruit is usually most audible in the upper third of the carotid near the bifurcation (McGee, 2018).

As noted in Chapter 3, perioperative stroke rate is reported to be twice as high for patients with bilateral versus unilateral carotid atherosclerotic disease (Mohler & Fairman, 2014). Accordingly, carotid endarterectomy is recommended before CABG in patients with high-grade carotid stenosis and for whom coronary revascularization is not urgent or concurrently with CABG in patients who have an urgent need for revascularization (i.e., those with severe left main coronary heart disease, diffuse coronary heart disease without satisfactory collateral circulation, or unstable angina) (Lazar, Wilson, & Messé, 2014).

Peripheral vascular assessment is performed to help determine the extent of peripheral perfusion. Components of this evaluation include determining the presence and strength of pulses in all extremities, capillary refill time, extremity and nailbed color, and temperature. Calculating the ankle-brachial index helps evaluate the arterial blood flow to the lower extremities; steps to determine this index appear in Chapter 10.

The results of this calculation are then used to rate degree of peripheral artery disease and will help determine if the saphenous vein is suitable for use during cardiac surgery (Tomoaki, 2018).

A cardiac assessment further entails determining presence of varicose veins. Presence of significant numbers of lower extremity varicosities may indicate the need to use upper-extremity vessels (e.g., radial artery) as conduits during CABG.

Pulmonary Assessment

Postoperative pulmonary complications contribute significantly to morbidity and mortality. A thorough pulmonary assessment, including identification of associated risk factors, is pivotal so that implementation of strategies to mitigate complications can begin in a timely fashion or risk of complications can be anticipated (Miskovic & Lumb, 2017).

Lung auscultation provides information about respiratory rate and breath sounds, and the presence of crackles or wheezing. Presence of crackles indicates fluid in the alveoli, which may require diuresis prior to surgery. Presence of decreased breath sounds or adventitious sounds may be related to an undiagnosed condition that may increase the risk of postoperative pulmonary complications or to underlying heart or lung disease. In either case, optimizing the patient's clinical condition preoperatively is indicated (Ruff & O'Gara, 2018).

A patient's smoking history should be determined. Some data suggest that patients who smoke are more likely to experience pulmonary adverse events following cardiac surgery (Miskovic & Lumb, 2017). Long-term effects of smoking following cardiac surgery are also emphasized in the literature. Patients should be counseled on smoking cessation 4 to 8 weeks prior to cardiac surgery to avoid these long-term effects. Quitting smoking a few days prior to cardiac surgery likely has no benefit and may result in increased secretions (Ruff & O'Gara, 2018). Preoperative cardiac surgery patients should be assessed for preexisting pulmonary disease to help anticipate potential postoperative conditions. Specifically,

a history of pulmonary hypertension and COPD are two predictors of pulmonary complications following cardiac surgery (Ruff & O'Gara, 2018). Patients with COPD, bronchitis, poor control of asthma symptoms, productive cough, or lower respiratory tract colonization are also more likely to develop postoperative complications (Ruff & O'Gara, 2018). It is recommended that patients with COPD who are undergoing cardiac surgery have preoperative pulmonary function testing (Miskovic & Lumb, 2017).

Abdominal Assessment

A preoperative abdominal assessment is important to determine the presence of an abdominal aortic aneurysm (AAA), which is a potential contraindication of the use of an intra-aortic balloon pump (Ali & Abu-Omar, 2018). (Intra-aortic balloon pump therapy is discussed in detail in Chapter 10.)

Ultrasound is the preferred method to screen for presence of an AAA. It has high sensitivity and specificity levels. Abdominal palpation is not recommended for determining presence of an AAA as it is not an accurate assessment (Agency for Healthcare Research and Quality, 2014).

Neurologic Assessment

A patient who is undergoing cardiac surgery may develop neurologic impairment during the intraoperative or postoperative period. A baseline assessment will help facilitate identification of changes in neurologic status. Baseline data can help prevent unnecessary testing that might otherwise be performed to evaluate postoperative neurologic symptoms, which in fact might have been present preoperatively. The risk for postoperative delirium has been reported to be 11.5% in cardiac surgery patients. Risk factors include longer cross-clamping time, diabetes, gastritis or ulcer problems, volume received in the operating room, amount of time on mechanical ventilation in the intensive care unit (ICU), highest postoperative temperature in the ICU, amount of sodium received in the ICU, AF, and advanced age (Francis, Aminoff, & Wilterdink, 2018).

▶ Preoperative Assessment of Heart Disease

Typically, patients undergoing cardiac surgery have coronary artery disease (CAD). In fact, increasing numbers of patients who are undergoing cardiac surgery have several comorbid conditions and have a higher operative risk. Resource utilization after cardiac surgery is higher in patients with risk, especially in the elderly. In one study, elderly patients used more medications (e.g., inotropic agents, antimicrobials, antiarrhythmic therapy), blood products, interventions (e.g., renal replacement therapies, resternotomy, or sternal rewiring), and implantation of devices (e.g., intra-aortic balloon pump, pulmonary artery catheter, permanent pacemaker, ventricular assist device), and their ICU and hospital LOS were also higher (Tam & Petsikas, 2014).

A baseline assessment of underlying heart function is essential to identify those patients at risk during the intraoperative period. Data specific to heart function as well as the presence and extent of comorbidities such as COPD, diabetes, and hypertension should be collected. The patient history should include determination of when cardiac comorbidities (e.g., MI) occurred and whether associated complications are present (e.g., heart failure, ischemia, dysrhythmias) (Sannakki, Sannakki, Echebarria, & Patteril, 2018).

The relationship between CAD and valvular disease is discussed in Chapter 5. Patients with valvular heart disease are vulnerable to additional intraoperative and postoperative risk. A preoperative cardiac assessment for these patients should evaluate the impact of valvular disease on ventricular function.

Cardiac History

Nursing evaluation includes assessment of the current level of symptoms. During the patient interview, any increase in intensity or frequency of symptoms should be relatively easy to uncover. The interview is used to identify the degree of the patient's associated functional impairment and to observe for indications that heart function is inadequate during exertion. Several classification systems can be used to assess the functional status of patients with heart disease; these systems evaluate angina, heart failure, and other aspects of heart disease. For example, the Canadian Cardiovascular Society's (CCS) functional classification system is used for the evaluation of angina; the New York Heart Association's (NYHA) classification is used to evaluate heart failure (Christensen, 2014; Dumitru, 2018).

Preoperative evaluation of a patient's current medical status should include a cardiac history. Specifically, the presence and severity of symptoms of CAD should be determined. In addition to assessing presence of risk factors for CAD (e.g., tobacco, hypertension, diabetes, hyperlipidemia), obtaining a list of the patient's current medications and patient adherence will provide essential information. Severity of pain should be rated on a 0 to 10 scale. Characteristics of angina patterns should be described in terms of onset; location; duration; character; precipitating, aggravating, and alleviating factors; and frequency. From this information, health care providers can decide whether the patient has stable or unstable angina. Existence of a previous or recent MI and presence of dysrhythmias or palpitations are also essential pieces of information. Signs of pulmonary edema or pulmonary hypertension or other associated cardiovascular, peripheral vascular, or valvular heart disease should be identified as well. The surgeon should be notified of significant findings and, if possible, preoperative hospital admission is anticipated.

Dyspnea is another symptom of heart disease to be evaluated in the preoperative cardiac surgery patient; it usually results from inadequate tissue oxygen delivery. Patients may report difficult, labored, or uncomfortable breathing. Some of the more common causes of dyspnea include heart failure, cardiac ischemia, asthma, COPD, and pneumonia. If dyspnea is noted, determination of whether it has a cardiac or pulmonary etiology is vital. Indices of a cardiac etiology include a history of dyspnea on exertion, paroxysmal nocturnal dyspnea, orthopnea, and chest pain. Physical findings may include jugular venous distention, S_3 gallop, ascites, and peripheral edema. Radiologic studies may reveal cardiomegaly (D'Ambra & Diprose, 2018). Dyspnea is commonly observed in patients with valvular disease; it may also be experienced by patients with ventricular dysfunction.

Orthopnea is the sensation of breathlessness when the patient is lying in a position of rest. It is relieved by sitting or standing. With worsening cardiac disease, orthopnea often develops such that the patient needs to elevate the head of the bed with more than one pillow to breathe comfortably while recumbent.

Serological Testing

In addition to patient history, preoperative testing with serological and other diagnostic methods should be performed. Data from these tests will help determine surgical and postoperative risk and define the presence or extent of any new or known comorbid conditions.

Laboratory data that may be collected preoperatively include complete blood count (CBC); coagulation profile; liver, renal, and thyroid function; electrolytes; and albumin level. Identifying the presence of anemia or infection is an important consideration when evaluating cardiac patients, because there are always risks of intraoperative bleeding and dilutional effects with bypass procedures. Attaining and maintaining a hematocrit greater than 35% is recommended. In addition, CBC data will help suggest presence of an infection from an elevated white blood cell count. Preoperative treatment of infection should be implemented. It is recommended that surgery not be delayed because of the infection unless implantation of prosthetic material is planned. Preoperative anemia is associated with increased risk of noncardiac complications and increased morbidity and mortality during cardiac surgery (Ruff & O'Gara, 2018). If CBC results reveal thrombocytopenia, a decision as to whether the patient should receive heparin should be made, because thrombocytopenia may be an indication of heparin-induced thrombocytopenia (HIT). Further testing must be done to confirm HIT. If a patient tests positive for HIT, an alternative anticoagulation method should

be considered for CPB. For example, bivalirudin (Angiomax®), a direct thrombin inhibitor, has been used in cardiac surgery patients requiring bypass (Shore-Lesserson et al., 2018).

Patients will be heparinized during bypass procedures. Any coagulopathies should be corrected (e.g., with fresh frozen plasma or platelet transfusion, administration of vitamin K) prior to surgery to minimize risk of postoperative bleeding (Shore-Lesserson et al., 2018).

Assessment of liver function should be conducted to help predict how medications, including anesthetic agents, will be metabolized. The value in optimizing a patient's nutritional status preoperatively was discussed earlier; albumin level is one component of that assessment.

Renal dysfunction is common in patients awaiting cardiac surgery and is a predictor of postoperative morbidity and mortality. Perioperative management includes minimizing use of nephrotoxic agents and maintaining perfusion to the kidneys (Leung & Ragbir-Toolsie, 2017). Sometimes a patient develops acute kidney injury (AKI) following cardiac surgery. The 30-day mortality rate increases dramatically with this complication. Risk factors for the development of AKI following cardiac surgery have been identified. These include female gender, COPD, diabetes, peripheral vascular disease, renal insufficiency, heart failure, LV ejection fraction less than 35%, need for emergent surgery, presence of cardiogenic shock that requires use of an intra-aortic balloon pump, left main CAD, and total circulatory arrest (Nadim et al., 2018). These data speak to the essential nature of a comprehensive patient assessment prior to cardiac surgery.

The overall mortality rate from AKI following cardiac surgery is reported to be as high as 80%, depending on development of multiple organ dysfunction, increase in serum creatinine, and need for renal replacement therapies. The high mortality rate is attributed primarily to infection; other factors such as immune dysregulation, platelet dysfunction, and issues related to being on hemodialysis (e.g., hemodynamic instability, infections of the vascular access devices, and ventricular ectopy) have been implicated as well (Nadim et al., 2018).

Although thyroid function tests are not part of the usual preoperative assessment, data suggest that hypothyroidism is overlooked in cardiac surgery patients. Postoperative cardiac surgery patients with hypothyroidism are reported to have a longer LOS in the ICU and hospital, higher incidence of postoperative AF, and higher long-term mortality rates (Worku, Tortolani, Gulkarov, Isom, & Klein, 2015). These data provide justification for preoperative thyroid function testing.

Maintaining serum glucose levels within a normal range decreases the rate of cardiac surgery complications. Effective treatment and monitoring of these data for the cardiac surgery patient should begin in the preoperative setting. Data suggest that presence of hyperglycemia in cardiac surgery patients increases mortality, postoperative AF, LOS, and infection rates (Hulst et al., 2018).

Diagnostic Studies

In addition to laboratory tests, other diagnostic procedures may potentially be performed for the preoperative cardiac surgery patient. Results of these tests will provide information about cardiac anatomic and physiologic issues and pulmonary status, help identify those patients who may be at higher risk (and the degree of risk) with surgery, alert the surgeon that preoperative "fine-tuning" may be necessary, or suggest that modifications of fluids or medications (or both) intraoperatively may be anticipated. Some of the diagnostic procedures that may be performed for these purposes include echocardiography, computed tomography (CT), magnetic resonance imaging (MRI), radionuclide scanning, cardiopulmonary exercise testing, cardiac catheterization, and pulmonary function tests (Ruff & O'Gara, 2018).

Echocardiography may be performed to discover any cardiac anatomic irregularities that might affect surgery. Results of an echocardiogram (ECG) may reveal conditions such as decreased ejection fraction (EF) or right ventricular (RV) function, presence of aortic stenosis or insufficiency, or mitral insufficiency. These data may be used to reevaluate the surgical plan, identify intraoperative risk, or devise a plan to optimize the patient's clinical status as much as possible prior to surgery. Data from echocardiography are important because decreased EF is associated with poor survival following revascularization (Silvestry, 2018).

Computed tomography may be performed to identify any cardiac anatomic irregularities that might affect the surgical outcome. A literature review suggested that use of preoperative CT has resulted in surgery being canceled up to 13% of the time and use of preventive intraoperative strategies (e.g., not using a midline approach, initiating bypass procedures before resternotomy, and peripheral vascular exposure) results in surgery cancellation. A lower incidence of intraoperative injury is also reported with preoperative CT scanning (Padma & Sundaram, 2014). As part of the preoperative evaluation, MRI may be performed to identify any cardiac anatomic irregularities, assess cardiac function and perfusion, and evaluate valves and blood vessels. Cardiac MRI (CMR) creates cardiac images while the heart is beating, thereby providing both still and moving images of the heart and major blood vessels. Heart structure and function can be evaluated. Chamber size and damage from MI may be determined through use of this technology as well (Bucciarelli-Ducci, Baritussio, & Auricchio, 2016).

Cardiopulmonary exercise testing (CPET) may be performed to determine a patient's fitness for surgery. It assesses the heart's functional reserve—that is, the amount of work the heart is able to do in extraordinary conditions (Birkey et al., 2018). During this noninvasive evaluation, concomitant cardiac and ventilatory effects of exercise are assessed. Gas exchange, heart rate, and blood pressure measurements, along with ECG evaluation, provide information on actual energy expenditure and stroke volume during exercise. The oxygen extraction from each beat is also measured at varying work intensities. Cardiopulmonary exercise testing is increasing in acceptance in Europe because of its precise evaluation of postoperative morbidity (Birkey et al., 2018).

Cardiac catheterization is considered the gold standard for the diagnosis of CAD. In the case of the cardiac surgery patient, it is performed to evaluate coronary anatomy and efficacy of cardiac contractility (Olade, Safl, & Badero, 2016). Data such as baseline right atrial, pulmonary artery systolic, diastolic, and occlusive pressures, as well as pulmonary vascular resistance, ejection fraction, and cardiac output, will help determine LV and RV function, augment valve function data, and assist with intraoperative and postoperative hemodynamic management. Administration of fluids and vasoactive agents and the choice of the operative procedure itself are guided by these data. A cardiac catheterization may sometimes reveal the presence of an LV mural thrombus, which places the patient at risk for a stroke in the intraoperative or postoperative period. In patients with valvular heart disease, cardiac catheterization may be used to estimate the degree of regurgitation. Unlike echocardiography, which provides an indirect measurement of the pressure gradient, cardiac catheterization provides for a direct measurement of this parameter (Ruff & O'Gara, 2018).

Pulmonary function tests (PFTs) may be performed on patients who have preexisting lung disease (e.g., COPD). As noted earlier in this chapter, patients with a history of COPD are at greater risk for developing postoperative complications and requiring prolonged intubation. Data from a preoperative arterial blood gas sample can help guide postoperative weaning (Ponomarev et al., 2017).

Even patients with healthy lungs may have pulmonary complications after cardiac surgery. Issues include decreased functional residual capacity following general anesthesia and neuromuscular blocking agent administration; decreased vital capacity from sternotomy and intrathoracic manipulation, atelectasis, intravascular lung water, and increased capillary permeability leading to leakage; and increased extravascular lung water secondary to the inflammatory response associated with CPB. Lung function may also be compromised due to fluid overload from blood and fluid administration (Ponomarev et al., 2017).

Pulmonary function tests have been helpful to reclassify COPD before cardiac surgery. In one study, data provided from PFTs were used to determine prognosis after cardiac surgery (Ponomarev et al., 2017).

Given that carotid artery stenosis is a risk factor for stroke following CABG, a preoperative carotid ultrasound should be considered. Patients with a carotid bruit or a history of cerebrovascular accident are at greater risk for developing this complication. Assessment of the carotid arteries preoperatively may decrease the postoperative risk of stroke (Ko, 2018).

Patients who are undergoing cardiac surgery should receive a preoperative dental examination. This is especially true of patients who will be receiving a prosthetic heart valve. These patients are at increased risk for infective endocarditis or prosthetic valvular endocarditis (Jay et al., 2018).

Other recent data suggest that delaying cardiac surgery to have dental work may be associated with adverse events or death. The authors of one study noted that patients who required dental work tended to be sicker (Jay et al., 2018). In that study, six patients (2.9%) died between dental surgery and the planned cardiac procedure; 10 (4.8%) had major adverse outcomes before cardiac surgery, including acute coronary syndrome or stroke. Postoperatively, there was an increased time on mechanical ventilation and renal failure.

Medications

A comprehensive review of the patient's current medication profile and concomitant medical and surgical histories is essential to assist with preoperative planning and prevent intraoperative and postoperative complications. Although some medications may be withheld before cardiac surgery, many others are continued or adjusted during the preoperative period, particularly those used to manage hypertension or heart disease (Ruff & O'Gara, 2018).

Nitrates

Nitrates should be continued up to the time of surgery to avoid an ischemic event. Further, preoperative administration of a nitrate or other vasodilator (e.g., prostacyclin, nitric oxide) may be indicated to decrease pulmonary vascular resistance (PVR) (Ruff & O'Gara, 2018).

Inotropes

If patients have a history of PVR that results in RV dysfunction, preoperative administration of an inotropic agent may be indicated. Agents such as dobutamine (Dobutrex®) or milrinone (Primacor®) may be used. Patients who are awaiting heart transplant may have low cardiac output preoperatively as well. Patients with low cardiac output before transplant have higher mortality rates as compared to patients with acceptable hemodynamics. Preoperative administration of an inotrope improves hemodynamics before heart transplantation, bringing mortality statistics equal to other transplant recipients (Kouchoukos, Blackstone, Hanley, & Kirklin, 2013).

Beta Blockers

Discontinuing beta adrenergic blocking agents can result in a hypersympathetic state that could precipitate myocardial ischemia, infarction, rebound hypertension, tachycardia, or dysrhythmias. As such, they should be continued in patients who are already taking these agents (Lomivorotov, Efremov, Abubakirov, Belletti, & Karaskov, 2018). As noted in Chapter 15, the incidence of AF following cardiac surgery varies with the procedure performed. In one study, of the patients who underwent aortic valve replacement, CABG, or off-pump coronary artery bypass (OPCAB), 74%, 44%, and 35%, respectively, developed postoperative AF (Lomivorotov et al., 2018). The patients who developed AF in this study were older, more often female, had a lower EF, and were less likely to be smokers. Other identified risk factors include greater age, history of hypertension or AF, and heart failure. Preoperative prophylactic administration of beta blockers has reportedly decreased the incidence of AF by 70% to 80% in patients who undergo CABG. Some researchers suggest that sympathetic tone, which is augmented during cardiac surgery, is diminished when beta blockers are taken.

It is further suggested that beta blockers not be initiated before surgery in patients who are not currently taking them as this practice has been found to be harmful. Worse cardiac outcomes occurred when beta blocker–naïve patients were started on therapy preoperatively (Lomivorotov et al., 2018). If a beta blocker must be started, it is recommended that it be started several weeks before surgery to allow time for dose adjustments and to

check for adverse events (Ruff & O'Gara, 2018). It has been further suggested that beta blockers be tapered or changed to short-acting agents to help patients avoid potential intraoperative myocardial depression (Lomivorotov et al., 2018).

Angiotensin-Converting Enzyme (ACE) Inhibitors and Angiotensin Receptor Blockers (ARBs)

While most cardiac medications are not held in the preoperative cardiac surgery patient, ACE inhibitors are typically held on the morning of surgery. Use of ACE inhibitors preoperatively in CABG surgery has uncertain findings as intraoperative hypotension and vasoplegia have been reported (Sannkki et al., 2018). The American College of Physicians' guidelines on perioperative management of hypertensive patients recommend continuing ACE inhibitors "with caution," and to avoid hypovolemia in patients maintained on ACE inhibitors during surgery (Nishimura et al., 2017). Based upon the most recent ACC/AHA guidelines, it is reasonable to continue these agents (ACEI and ARBs) perioperatively. If they are withheld before surgery, it is reasonable to restart the medication when clinically feasible.

Calcium Channel Blockers (CCBs)

Patients should continue to take their calcium channel blocker up to and including the day of surgery. One exception may be in cases of poor hemodynamics (e.g., hypotension, arrhythmias). A short-acting CCB may be substituted (e.g., diltiazem [Cardizem®]) (Lomivorotov et al., 2018).

Anticoagulants

Medications affecting hemostasis or bleeding are discontinued in preparation for cardiac surgery. Specifically, warfarin (Coumadin®) is held 5 days prior to surgery so that the international normalized ratio (INR) reaches a level less than 2.0 (Ruff & O'Gara, 2018). Patients who are at risk for developing thrombosis should receive intravenous heparin when the INR reaches subtherapeutic levels (Lomivorotov et al., 2018).

Clopidogrel (Plavix®) is held 5 to 10 days before surgery to decrease the risk of excessive intraoperative bleeding, transfusion requirements, and reoperations. Patients can be transfused with platelets if bleeding is a postoperative issue (Ruff & O'Gara, 2018).

Aspirin irreversibly inhibits platelet function. Recent data suggest, however, that there is no difference in 30-day and 1-year mortality, MI, or stroke at 30 days in patients who continued aspirin therapy before CPB surgery (Guay & Ochroch, 2014). In another study, up to a 20% increase in bleeding was reported. There was no difference in severity of bleeding or mortality between patients taking aspirin and those who were not. It is recommended that low-dose aspirin be continued unless the risk of bleeding outweighs the benefit (Ruff & O'Gara, 2018).

Glycoprotein IIb/IIIa inhibitors (e.g., eptifibatide [Integrilin®], tirofiban [Aggrastat®]) are antiplatelet drugs. They should be discontinued 4 to 6 hours before surgery (Ruff & O'Gara, 2018).

The use of heparin before CPB surgery has two rationales. First, heparin provides prophylaxis against development of a venous thrombotic event (VTE). Second, heparin can serve as a substitute for aspirin. Potential safe alternatives for heparin during cardiac surgery include low-molecular-weight heparin (LMWH), recombinant hirudin (Lepirudin®), and the organic chemical argatroban (Ruff & O'Gara, 2018). Some data suggest that LMWH does not increase postoperative blood loss when it is withheld shortly before cardiac surgery (Ruff & O'Gara, 2018).

Bivalirudin, a short-acting direct thrombin inhibitor (DTI), should be discontinued 3 hours before cardiac surgery. Long-acting DTIs (e.g., hirudin [Refludan®, Revasc®] and argatroban [Acova®]) should be discontinued earlier and unfractionated heparin given in its place (Ruff & O'Gara, 2018).

Clinically silent deep vein thrombosis (DVT) develops during hospitalization in nearly 50% of patients after myocardial revascularization. Low-dose subcutaneous heparin and LMWH given once a day reduce the incidence of DVT to approximately 35% and 18% of controls, respectively (Ruff & O'Gara, 2018).

Hypoglycemics

Patients with diabetes are at increased risk of complications following surgery. This is due to hormonal and inflammatory stressors that can occur with surgery and anesthesia (Duggan, Carlson, & Umpierrez, 2017). Preoperatively, the patient's blood sugar should be made as stable as possible. This is typically done with subcutaneous insulin. Patients who have not taken insulin in the past should be placed on a sliding scale to correct the blood sugar. Low-dose basal insulin may be added to patients with hyperglycemia. Basal insulin analogs are preferred because of their consistent action and decreased risk of hypoglycemia. For patients already receiving insulin, it is recommended that the basal insulin be continued with a possible decrease of 20% to 30% of the dose and sliding scale insulin, as needed. Patients who take combination insulin or premixed insulin types should receive an estimate of the basal dose. Delivery of 40% to 50% of that dose can be administered as basal insulin. Sliding-scale insulin may be added as needed (Leung & Ragbir-Toolsie, 2017).

Patients who are taking oral hypoglycemic agents for type 2 diabetes should have these agents withheld preoperatively for several days because of the risks associated with them. This is especially true of metformin (Glucophage®), which is known to contribute to the development of postoperative lactic acidosis if there is a decrease in renal function (DeFronzo, Fleming, Chen, & Bicsak, 2016). Metformin should be held 1 to 2 days before surgery if administration of intravenous contrast is anticipated or if hemodynamic instability is anticipated (as this latter condition leads to decreased renal perfusion).

Thiazolidinediones (e.g., pioglitazone [Actos®], rosiglitazone [Avandia®]) induce fluid retention and should be discontinued a few days before surgery. Glucagon-like peptide 1 (GLP-1) agonists (e.g., exenatide [Byetta®]) have the potential to decrease gastric motility and delay gastrointestinal recovery following surgery. As such, it is recommended that GLP-1 agonists be held on the day of surgery. Gliptins or dipeptidyl peptidase 4 (DPP-4) inhibitors (e.g., alogliptin [NESINA®], linagliptin [Tradjenta®], saxagliptin [Onglyza®], sitagliptin [Januvia®]) may be continued so long as there are no associated significant side effects. However, because of their mechanism of action, these agents should not be needed if the patient is nil per os (NPO) (Ruff & O'Gara, 2018).

Patients with type 1 diabetes must continue to receive their basal insulin replacement in the preoperative period. Sliding scale insulin may be used to correct elevated blood sugar levels (Ruff & O'Gara, 2018).

Long-acting insulin is usually discontinued preoperatively as well. In contrast, insulin glargine (Lantus®), a long-acting basal insulin, may be continued during the surgical period (Sudhakaran & Surani, 2015). Other patients who receive insulin therapy may have their dose withheld on the day of surgery, with medication levels being regulated based on blood glucose monitoring.

Statins

In addition to lowering lipids, statins decrease vascular inflammation, augment endothelial function, and stabilize atherosclerotic plaque (Hearps & Du Toit, 2017). Data suggest that continuing statin therapy in patients undergoing cardiac or vascular surgery decreases cardiac risk. Stopping statins abruptly results in a rebound effect. During this time, there is an increased cardiac risk. Data suggest that statin therapy should be continued through the day of surgery (Ruff & O'Gara, 2018). Administration of a statin prior to cardiac surgery is associated with a 38% decrease in mortality, and decreased incidence of AF and stroke (Ruff & O'Gara, 2018).

Herbal Remedies

Use of herbal remedies can cause increased risk of bleeding and drug interactions. While the medication profile obtained during the preoperative evaluation should include information about the use of herbal remedies, more is being learned about potential interactions between these supplements and other medications every day. As this growing knowledge base has significant clinical implications for the cardiac surgery patient, no herbal remedies should be taken for at least 2 weeks prior to surgery. Garlic, ginseng, echinacea, ginkgo biloba, St. John's wort, valerian, kava, flavonoids, and grapefruit juice are all known to decrease platelet activity. Ginseng may also cause hypoglycemia. Kava and valerian may cause an enhanced sedative effect of anesthetic agents. St. John's wort may cause increased metabolism of many of the drugs used in the perioperative period (Sultan, Viqar, Ali, Tajik, & Jahangir, 2015). Herbal remedies should be stopped at least 1 to 2 weeks before surgery (Rabins & Phipps, 2016).

▶ Management of High-Risk Patients

Ventricular Dysfunction

Preoperative cardiac surgery patients with heart failure and a history of hypertension, ischemia, hypertrophic cardiomyopathy, or acute valvular dysfunction are at risk for, and should be assessed for, ventricular dysfunction. High morbidity and mortality rates are associated with cardiac surgery in patients who have severe LV dysfunction and clinically significant heart failure secondary to ischemic or valvular heart disease (Carr et al., 2015; Fortes et al., 2016). Patients with LV dysfunction and valvular disease (e.g., mitral regurgitation, aortic stenosis) require preoperative management of their hemodynamic status.

The presence of heart failure may cause surgery to be delayed while health care providers attempt to improve the patient's cardiac function and decrease surgical risk. Data suggest that patients who are undergoing a CABG procedure who had an LV ejection fraction (LVEF) less than 20% have almost four times the in-hospital mortality rates, were less likely to be discharged home, and had a higher incidence of postoperative respiratory failure, acute kidney injury, and sepsis than patients with an LVEF greater than 40%. A preoperative cardiac evaluation of these patients may include positive emission tomography, dobutamine echocardiogram, dobutamine MRI, or delayed enhancement MRI (Ruff & O'Gara, 2018). Therapy focuses on maintaining adequate preload and afterload. Medication or the intra-aortic balloon pump (IABP) may be used to augment afterload reduction. In such a case, the nursing evaluation focuses on identifying and optimizing the patient's unstable hemodynamic status.

Coronary artery bypass grafting-associated mortality is higher in patients who had a recent MI (i.e., within the past 3–7 days). It is recommended that surgery be delayed for at least that amount of time. Patients who sustained an anterior wall MI should be evaluated for presence of an LV thrombus with transesophageal echocardiogram. An inferior wall MI decreases right ventricular function. These patients undergoing CPB may develop hemodynamic consequences exacerbated during CPB procedures. A recovery of 4 weeks is recommended (Ruff & O'Gara, 2018).

Patients with peripheral vascular disease or a carotid bruit should be further evaluated with carotid Doppler to determine if and when carotid revascularization should be performed (Ruff & O'Gara, 2018).

▶ Summary

Patients who present for cardiac surgery have higher levels of complexity than in the past. Often, because of comorbid or concomitant conditions, surgical procedures are combined, creating potentially higher levels of vulnerability and instability. An in-depth preoperative evaluation of the patient's history and cardiac status, along with collection of laboratory data and possibly invasive and noninvasive procedures, is critical to prevent poor outcomes postoperatively. Early detection of potential complications can improve outcomes and help ensure a successful recovery. Critical care nurses are in a unique position to utilize clinical inquiry techniques and critical thinking skills to uncover those risk factors and data that can redirect interventions to become more individual specific.

🔍 CASE STUDY

K. P. is a 72-year-old frail female with a history of hypertension, heart failure (with an LVEF of 20%), and 3-vessel disease. She is scheduled for CABG. She is admitted preoperatively for evaluation and to control her blood pressure. Her medication profile includes losartan 50 mg daily, enalapril 2.5 mg twice daily, and furosemide 40 mg daily. K. P. reports that she also takes St. John's wort for depression and ginkgo biloba to help prevent memory loss. Both of these supplements were encouraged by her daughter. Her preoperative albumin level is 2.2 g/dL.

Critical Thinking Questions

1. Given the history of this patient, which potential postoperative problem might the nurse expect?
2. What medications should the nurse anticipate being administered and held in preparation for this patient's surgery?
3. What should the patient be told about her taking herbal supplements?

Answers to Critical Thinking Questions

1. Given that K. P. is frail and her albumin level is low, she is showing indications of nutritional deficiencies that could affect her recovery.
2. K. P.'s ACE inhibitor will be held on the morning of surgery as its continuation may result in intraoperative hypotension by augmenting the effects of anesthesia. The ARB that K. P. is receiving will likely be discontinued 24 hours before surgery as these agents have a longer half-life. The furosemide will likely be held the day of surgery to prevent electrolyte depletion during and after surgery.
3. St. John's wort and gingko biloba will need to be stopped immediately. Ideally, a week should pass prior to surgery. St. John's wort is of concern because of the numerous drug–drug interactions associated with this supplement; it is a known CYP3A4 inducer. As such, it will decrease levels of other drugs that are metabolized by this enzyme system. Gingko biloba is of concern because it inhibits platelet-activating factor; this puts K. P. at increased risk for bleeding.

Self-Assessment Questions

1. Which is the primary goal of an assessment before cardiac surgery?
    A. Select the anesthetic agent to be used
    B. Predict postoperative complications
    C. Determine perioperative risk
    D. Improve patient outcomes

2. Which patient is at greatest risk for adverse outcomes of cardiac surgery?
    A. 55-year-old male with elevated low-density lipoproteins
    B. 48-year-old male with HbA_{1c} 5.5%
    C. 70-year-old female with creatinine 2.1 mg/dL
    D. 61-year-old female with LVEF 45%

3. An 80-year-old patient is being evaluated for cardiac surgery. Presence of which puts the patient at greatest mortality risk?
    A. Cardiogenic shock
    B. Acute kidney injury
    C. Left ventricular aneurysm
    D. Second reoperation required

4. Which is evaluated during a nursing interview before cardiac surgery?
    A. Understanding of education materials provided
    B. Willingness to adhere to the surgical regimen
    C. Ability to pay the hospital bill after discharge
    D. Preference for type of procedure to be performed

5. A patient is to undergo emergent cardiac surgery. Preoperative evaluation revealed an albumin level of 2.1 g/dL and body mass index of 19 kg/m². For which should the nurse anticipate having to monitor postoperatively?
    A. Excessive clotting
    B. Respiratory failure
    C. Ventricular dysrhythmias
    D. Sternal wound infection

6. Upon preoperative assessment for cardiac surgery, the nurse notes presence of an early diastolic murmur at the second and third intercostal spaces at the right sternal border. Which should be anticipated in the postoperative period following cardiopulmonary bypass?
    A. Papillary muscle rupture
    B. Left ventricular distention
    C. Cardiogenic shock
    D. Right bundle branch block

7. Which condition puts the patient at greatest risk for cognitive impairment following cardiac surgery?
    A. Anxiety disorder
    B. COPD
    C. Abdominal aortic aneurysm
    D. Atrial fibrillation

8. Dyspnea is noted on cardiac assessment. Which is most likely present?
    A. Valvular disease
    B. Pericardial effusion
    C. 2-vessel occlusion of 80%
    D. Aortic aneurysm

9. Which set of electrolytes places the patient at greatest risk for development of dysrhythmias following cardiac surgery?

	Potassium (mEq/L)	Magnesium (mg/dL)
A.	5.2	1.6
B.	3.1	4.0
C.	3.2	1.5
D.	5.1	4.1

10. Which medication should the nurse anticipate being discontinued at least a day before cardiac surgery?
    A. Nitroglycerin (Tridil®)
    B. Metoprolol (Lopressor®)
    C. Enalapril (Vasotec®)
    D. Milrinone (Primacor®)

Answers to Self-Assessment Questions

1. C. **determine perioperative risk**
    Rationale: Perioperative assessment is conducted to gather information on the perioperative risk. During a perioperative assessment, the nurse can confirm presence, progression, and severity of cardiac symptoms.

2. C. **70-year-old female with creatinine 2.1 mg/dL**
   Rationale: A 70-year-old female with creatinine 2.1 mg/dL is at greatest risk. This is because in using the EuroSCORE, being over 60 years of age, female, and having an elevated serum creatinine will increase the overall score and risk of major complications, duration of critical care, and resource utilization.

3. A. **cardiogenic shock**
   Rationale: While all four of the answers increase risk, cardiogenic shock is the most common cause of in-hospital death in patients with acute coronary syndrome.

4. B. **willingness to adhere to the surgical regimen**
   Rationale: The evaluation of the patient's willingness to adhere to surgical regimen is the best option. Preoperatively and postoperatively, patients will be asked to stop smoking, and change lifestyle. Such changes in diet, medication, and physical activity can be overwhelming to a patient. Establishing support systems to help patients be successful in the management of their health condition is important for success.

5. B. **respiratory failure**
   Rationale: Serum albumin is used to quantify nutritional status and underlying disease. Extremely low body mass index increases morbidity and mortality with cardiac surgery. An increased risk of pneumonia is seen with this population.

6. B. **left ventricular distention**
   Rationale: Diastolic murmurs generated by regurgitant flow back through the semilunar valves are loudest in intensity at the left (pulmonic valve) and right (aortic valve) sternal border in the second intercostal space. A diastolic murmur in the left second or third ICS in the right sternal border is from an aortic valvular regurgitation. This often results in left ventricular distention.

7. D. **atrial fibrillation**
   Rationale: Atrial fibrillation increases the risk of cognitive impairment postoperatively. Atrial fibrillation is associated with an increase in stroke, silent infarcts, microbleeds associated with oral anticoagulants, and cerebral hypoperfusion, all of which play a role in cognitive impairment.

8. A. **valvular disease**
   Rationale: Dyspnea on cardiac assessments is most likely due to valvular disease. Many patients do not recognize symptoms that may develop gradually and attribute them to fatigue and dyspnea from aging or deconditioning.

9. C. **3.2 / 1.5**
   Rationale: Low potassium and magnesium levels are associated with abnormal heart rhythms. Magnesium deficiency is frequently associated with hypokalemia. Coadministration of magnesium is essential for correcting the hypokalemia.

10. C. **enalapril (Vasotec)**
    Rationale: Enalapril (Vasotec), an ACE inhibitor, is stopped due to the risk of hypotension during surgery requiring more vasopressors and acute kidney injury seen postoperatively.

CLINICAL INQUIRY BOX

Question: How can malnutrition prior to cardiac surgery be assessed more accurately?

Reference: Ringaitienė, D., Gineitytė, D., Vicka, V., Žvirblis, T., Šipylaitė, J., Irnius, A., & Ivaškevičius, J. (2016). Preoperative risk factors of malnutrition for cardiac surgery patients. *Acta Medica Lituanica, 23*(2), 99–109.

Objective: To determine whether phase angle (PA) is a marker of malnutrition in low-risk cardiac surgery patients.

(continues)

CLINICAL INQUIRY BOX   *(continued)*

Methods: A prospective study was performed with 342 patients. These patients were classified into two groups: Low PA and normal PA. Associations between low PA and low fat-free mass index and outcomes were made. The nutritional state was evaluated using bioelectrical impedance analysis.

Results: Low PA was detected in 61 patients and was associated with higher rates and risk of postoperative mortality in univariate regression analysis.

Conclusions: A low preoperative PA is an indicator of malnutrition and determines adverse outcomes after cardiac surgery. Further research is needed to evaluate clinical applications of the PA, such as a more accurate identification of malnourished cardiac surgery patients.

References

Agency for Healthcare Research and Quality. (2014). *Screening for abdominal aortic aneurysm*. Retrieved from https://www.ahrq.gov/professionals/clinicians-providers/guidelines-recommendations/guide/section2.html.

Ali, J. M., & Abu-Omar, Y. (2018). The intra-aortic balloon pump and other methods of mechanical circulatory support. *Surgery (Oxford), 36*(2), 68–74.

Almashrafi, A., Alsabti, H., Mukaddirov, M., Balan, B., & Aylin, P. (2016). Factors associated with prolonged length of stay following cardiac surgery in a major referral hospital in Oman: A retrospective observational study. *British Medical Journal Open, 6*, e010764. doi:10.1136/bmjopen-2015-010764

American Society of Anesthesiologists Committee on Standards and Practice Parameters and the Task Force on Perioperative Management of Obstructive Sleep Apnea. (2014). Practice guidelines for the perioperative management of patients with obstructive sleep apnea. *Anesthesiology, 120*(2), 1–19.

Bhukal, I., Solanki, S. L., Ramaswamy, S., Yaddanapudi, L. N., Jain, A., & Kumar, P. (2012). Perioperative predictors of morbidity and mortality following cardiac surgery under cardiopulmonary bypass. *Saudi Journal of Anaesthesia, 6*, 242–247.

Birkey, T., Dixon, J., Jacobsen, R., Ginde, S., Nugent, M., Yan, K., . . . Kovach, J. (2018). Cardiopulmonary exercise testing for surgical risk stratification in adults with congenital heart disease. *Pediatric Cardiology*. doi:10.1007/s00246-018-1918-4

Bucciarelli-Ducci, C., Baritussio, A., & Auricchio, A. (2016). Cardiac MRI anatomy and function as a substrate for arrhythmias. *EP Europace, 18*(4), iv130–iv135.

Carr, B. M., Romeiser, J., Ruan, J., Gupta, S., Seifert, F. C., Zhu, W., . . . Shroyer, A. L. (2016). Long-term post-CABG survival: Performance of clinical risk models versus actuarial predictions. *Journal of Cardiac Surgery, 31*(1), 23–30.

Che, W., Dong, H., Jiang, X., Peng, M., Zou, Y., Qian, H., . . . Gao, R. (2016). Stenting for left subclavian artery stenosis in patients scheduled for left internal mammary artery-coronary artery bypass grafting. *Catheterization and Cardiovascular Interventions, 87*(Suppl 1), S1579–S1588.

Christensen, B. (2014). *Canadian Cardiovascular Society grading system for stable angina*. Retrieved from https://emedicine.medscape.com/article/2172431-overview.

Clark, C. E. (2015). Difference in blood pressure measurements between arms: Methodological and clinical implications. *Current Pharmaceutical Design, 21*(6), 737–743.

D'Ambra, M. N., & Diprose, P. (2018). *Anesthesia for cardiac valve surgery*. Retrieved from https://www.uptodate.com/contents/anesthesia-for-cardiac-valve-surgery.

DeFronzo, R., Fleming, A., Chen, K., & Bicsak, T. A. (2016). Metformin-associated lactic acidosis: Current perspectives on causes and risk. *Metabolism, 65*(2), 20–29.

Duggan, E. W., Carlson, K., & Umpierrez, G. E. (2017). Perioperative hyperglycemia management: An update. *Anesthesiology, 126*(3), 547–560.

Dumitru, I. (2018). *Heart failure*. Retrieved from https://emedicine.medscape.com/article/163062-overview.

Eamer, G., Al-Amoodi, M., Holroyd-Leduc, J., Rolfson, D. B., Warkentin, L., & Khadaroo, R. G. (2018). Review of risk assessment tools to predict morbidity and mortality in elderly surgical patients. *American Journal of Surgery*. doi: 10.1016/j.amjsurg.2018.04.006

Edwards, P. K., Mears, S. C., & Barnes, C. L. (2018). Preoperative care of the TKA patient. *Journal of Knee Surgery, 31*(7), 618–624.

Epperla, N., Ye, F., Idris, A., Sakkalaek, A., Liang, H., Chyou, P.-H., . . . Yale, S. (2017). Treatment-related cardiovascular outcomes in patients with symptomatic subclavian artery stenosis. *Cureus, 9*(5), e1262.

Fortes, J. V. S., Silva, M. G. B. e, Baldez, T. E. P., Costa, M. de A. G., da Silva, L. N., Pinheiro, R. S., . . . Borges, D. L. (2016). Mortality risk after cardiac surgery: Application of Inscor in a university hospital in Brazil's northeast. *Brazilian Journal of Cardiovascular Surgery, 31*(5), 396–399.

Francis, J., Aminoff, M. J., & Wilterdink, J. L. (2018). *Delirium and acute confusional states: prevention, treatment and prognosis*. Retrieved from https://www.uptodate.com/contents/delirium-and-acute-confusional-states-prevention-treatment-and-prognosis.

Gaasch, W. H., Otto, C. M., & Yeon, S. B. (2018). *Clinical manifestations and diagnosis of chronic aortic regurgitation in adults*. Retrieved from https://www.uptodate.com/contents/clinical-manifestations-and-diagnosis-of-chronic-aortic-regurgitation-in-adults.

Gonçalves, K. K. N., Silva, J. I., Gomes, E. T., Pinheiro, L. L., Figueiredo, T. R., & Bezerra, S. M. M. (2016). Anxiety in the preoperative period of heart surgery. *Revista Brasileira de Enfermagem, 69*(2), 397–403.

Guay, J. & Ochroch, E. A. (2014). Continuing antiplatelet therapy before cardiac surgery with cardiopulmonary bypass: A meta-analysis on the need for reexploration and major outcomes. *Cardiothoracic and Vascular Anesthesia, 28*(1), 90–97.

Hearps, T., & Du Toit, E. F. (2017). An overview of the pleioptropic effects of statins and their impact on postoperative outcomes in cardiovascular surgery patients. *Journal of Cardiovascular Disorders, 4*(1), 1033.

Hulst A. H., Visscher, M. J., Godfried, M. B., Thiel, B., Gerritse, B. M., Scohy, T. V., . . . Hermanides, J. (2018). Study protocol of the randomised placebo-controlled GLOBE trial: GLP-1 for bridging of hyperglycaemia during cardiac surgery. *British Medical Journal Open, 8,* e022189. doi:10.1136/bmjopen-2018-022189

Jay, R. H., Stansby, G., Barakat, T., Seymour, R. A., Meechan, J. G., Robinson, C. M., . . . Balakrishnan, A. (2018). Dental implications of CVD. In M. Greenwood (Ed.), *Essentials of human disease in dentistry* (2nd ed, pp. 95–96). Hoboken, NJ: John Wiley & Sons.

Ko, S.-B. (2018). Perioperative stroke: Pathophysiology and management. *Korean Journal of Anesthesiology, 71*(1), 3–11.

Kouchoukos, N. T., Blackstone, E. H., Hanley, F. L., & Kirklin, J. K. (2013). Cardiac transplantation. In N. T. Kouchoukos, E. H. Blackstone, F. L. Hanley, & J. K. Kirklin (Eds.), *Kirklin/Barratt-Boyes cardiac surgery* (4th ed., pp. 809–872). Philadelphia, PA: Elsevier Saunders.

LaPar, D. J., Ghanta, R. K., Kern, J. A., Crosby, I. K., Rich, J. B., Speir, A. M., . . . Investigators for the Virginia Cardiac Surgery Quality Initiative. (2014). Hospital variation in mortality from cardiac arrest after cardiac surgery: An opportunity for improvement? *The Annals of Thoracic Surgery, 98*(2), 534–540.

Lazar, H. L, Salm, T. V, Engelman, R., Orgill, D., & Gordon, S. (2016). Prevention and management of sternal wound infections. *The Journal of Thoracic and Cardiovascular Surgery, 152*(4), 962–972.

Lazar, H. L., Wilson, C. A., & Messé, S. R. (2014). *Coronary artery bypass grafting in patients with cerebrovascular disease*. Retrieved from http://www.uptodate.com/contents/coronary-artery-bypass-grafting-in-patients-with-cerebrovascular-disease.

Leung, V., & Ragbir-Toolsie, K. (2017). Perioperative management of patients with diabetes. *Health Services Insights, 10.* doi:10.1177/1178632917735075

Lomivorotov, V. V., Efremov, S. M., Abubakirov, M. N., Belletti, A., . . . Karaskov, A. M. (2018). Perioperative management of cardiovascular medications. *Journal of Cardiothoracic and Vascular Anesthesia.* doi:10.1053/j.jvca.2018.01.018

Lomivorotov V. V., Efremov, S. M., Boboshko, V. A., Nikolaev D. A., Vedernikov, P. E., Lomivorotov, V. N., . . . Karaskov, A. M. (2013). Evaluation of nutritional screening tools for patients scheduled for cardiac surgery. *Nutrition, 29,* 436–442.

Olade, R. B., Safl, A., & Badero, O. J. (2016). *Cardiac catheterization of left heart*. Retrieved from: https://emedicine.medscape.com/article/1819224-overview

McGee, S. (2018). The heart. In S. McGee (Ed.), *Evidence-based physical diagnosis* (4th ed., pp. 301–428). Philadelphia, PA: Elsevier.

Miskovic, A., & Lumb, A. B. (2017). Postoperative pulmonary complications. *British Journal of Anaesthesia, 118*(3), 317–334.

Mohler III, E. R., & Fairman, R. M. (2014). *Carotid endarterectomy*. Retrieved from http://www.uptodate.com/contents/carotid-endarterectomy.

Montazerghaem, H., Safaie, N., & Samiei, N. V. (2014). Body mass index or serum albumin levels: Which is further prognostic following cardiac surgery? *Journal of Cardiovascular and Thoracic Research, 6*(2), 123–126.

Nadim, M. K., Forni, L. G., Bihorac, A., Hobson, C., Koyner, J. L., Shaw, A., . . . Kellum, J. A. (2018). Cardiac and vascular surgery–associated acute kidney injury: The 20th International Consensus Conference of the ADQI (Acute Disease Quality Initiative) Group. *Journal of the American Heart Association, 7*(11), e008834. doi:10.1161/JAHA.118.008834

Nishimura, R. A., Otto, C. M., Bonow, R. O., Carabello, B. A., Erwin III, J. P., Fleisher, L. A., . . ., Thompson, A. (2017). 2017 AHA/ACC focused update of the 2014 AHA/ACC guideline for the management of patients with valvular heart disease: A report of the American College of Cardiology/American Heart Association Task Force on Clinical Practice Guidelines. *Journal of the American College of Cardiology,* doi: 10.1016/j.jacc.2017.03.011

Ogawa, M., Izawa, K. P., Satomi-Kobayashi, S., Kitamura, A., Ono, R., Sakai, Y., . . . Okita, Y. (2018). Poor preoperative nutritional status is an important predictor of the retardation of rehabilitation after cardiac surgery in elderly cardiac patients. *Aging Clinical and Experimental Research, 29*(2), 283–290.

Padma, S., & Sundaram, P. S. (2014). Current practice and recommendation for presurgical cardiac evaluation in patients undergoing noncardiac surgeries. *World Journal of Nuclear Medicine, 13*(1), 6–15.

Parsonnet, V., Dean, D., & Bernstein, A. D. (1989). A method of uniform stratification of risk for evaluating the results of surgery in acquired adult heart disease. *Circulation, 79*(Suppl I), I3–I12.

Ponomarev, D., Kamenskaya, I., Klinkova, A., Loginova, I., Vedernikov, P., Kornilov, I., . . . Karaskov, A. (2017). Chronic lung disease and mortality after cardiac surgery: A prospective cohort study. *Journal of Cardiothoracic and Vascular Anesthesia, 31*(6), 1010–1026.

Powell, R., Scott, N. W., Manyande, A., Bruce, J., Vögele, C., Byrne-Davis, L. M. T., . . . Johnston, M. (2016). Psychological preparation and postoperative outcomes for adults undergoing surgery under general anaesthesia. *Cochrane Database of Systematic Reviews, 5*. Art. No.: CD008646. doi:10.1002/14651858.CD008646.pub2

Rabins, J. L., & Phipps, L. B. (2016). The use of herbs and supplements. In T. A. Touhi & K. F. Jett (Eds.), *Ebersole & Hess' toward healthy aging. Human needs and nursing response* (9th ed., pp. 115–129). Philadelphia, PA: Elsevier

Ringaitienė, D., Gineitytė, D., Vicka, V., Žvirblis, T., Šipylaitė, J., Irnius, A., . . . Ivaškevičius, J. (2016). Preoperative risk factors of malnutrition for cardiac surgery patients. *Acta Medica Lituanica, 23*(2), 99–109.

Rosiek, A., Kornatowski, T., Rosiek-Kryszewska, A., Leksowski, L., & Leksowski, K. (2016). Evaluation of stress intensity and anxiety level in preoperative period of cardiac patients. *BioMed Research International.* doi:10.1155/2016 /1248396

Ruff, C. T., & O'Gara, P. T. (2018). Preoperative evaluation for cardiac surgery. In L. H. Cohn & D. H. Adams (Eds.), *Cardiac surgery in the adult* (5th ed., 223–233). New York, NY: McGraw-Hill.

Sannakki, S., Sannakki, D., Echebarria, J. J., & Patteril, M. (2018). Preoperative assessment for cardiac surgery. *Anaesthesia & Intensive Care Medicine, 19*(7), 339–345.

Sharif, F., Moshkelgosha, F., Molazem, Z., Najafi Kalyani, M., & Vossughi, M. (2014). The effects of discharge plan on stress, anxiety and depression in patients undergoing percutaneous transluminal coronary angioplasty: A randomized controlled trial. *International Journal of Community Based Nursing and Midwifery, 2*(2), 60–68.

Shore-Lesserson, L., Baker, R. A., Ferraris, V., Greilich, P. E., Fitzgerald, D., Roman, P., & Hammon, J. (2018). STS/SCA/ AmSECT Clinical Practice Guidelines: Anticoagulation during Cardiopulmonary Bypass. *The Journal of Extra-Corporeal Technology, 50*(1), 5–18.

Silvestry, F. E. (2018). *Postoperative complications among patients undergoing cardiac surgery*. Retrieved from https:// www.uptodate.com/contents/postoperative-complications -among-patients-undergoing-cardiac-surgery.

Stoppe, C., Goetzenich, A., Whitman, G., Ohkuma, R., Brown, T., Hatzakorzian, R., . . . Heyland, D. K. (2017). Role of nutrition support in adult cardiac surgery: A consensus statement from an International Multidisciplinary Expert Group on Nutrition in Cardiac Surgery. *Critical Care, 21*, 131. doi:10.1186/s13054-017-1690-5

Sudhakaran, S., & Surani, S. R. (2015). Guidelines for perioperative management of the diabetic patient. *Surgery Research and Practice*, doi:10.1155/2015/284063

Sultan, S., Viqar, M., Ali, R., Tajik, A. J., & Jahangir, A. (2015). Essentials of herb-drug interactions in the elderly with cardiovascular disease. *Journal of Patient-Centered Research and Reviews, 2*(4). Retrieved from https:// digitalrepository.aurorahealthcare.org/cgi/viewcontent .cgi?article=1212&context=jpcrr.

Tam, D. Y., & Petsikas, D. (2014). Healthcare resource utilization after cardiac surgery: Is the follow up clinic useful? *Canadian Journal of Cardiology, 30*(10), S143–S144.

Thelwall, S., Harrington, P., Sheridan, E., & Lamagni, T. (2015). Impact of obesity on the risk of wound infection following surgery: Results from a nationwide prospective multicentre cohort study in England. *Clinical Microbiology and Infection, 21*(11), 1008, e1–e8.

Tomaras, D. (2017). Comparison of the Parsonnet score and hospital-specific models using cardiac surgery patients from Montreal (Doctoral dissertation, McGill University Libraries).

Tomoaki, S. (2018). Optimal use of arterial grafts during current coronary artery bypass surgery. *Surgery Today, 48*(3), 264–273.

Worku, B., Tortolani, A. J., Gulkarov, I., Isom, O. W., & Klein, I. (2015). Preoperative hypothyroidism is a risk factor for postoperative atrial fibrillation in cardiac surgical patients. *Journal of Cardiac Surgery, 30*(4), 307–312.

Zhan, H. T., Purcell, S. T., & Bush, R. L. (2015). Preoperative optimization of the vascular surgery patient. *Vascular Health and Risk Management, 11*, 379–385.

CHAPTER 5

Heart Valve Surgery

Tobias P. Rebmann

▶ Introduction

Heart valve surgery is performed to either repair or replace a failing valve. Cardiac valves allow for one-way, low-resistance blood flow. The opening and closing of a valve occur according to pressure gradients between each side of the valve. The valves must open widely to allow for rapid blood movement and minimal cardiac work. Conversely, they must remain tightly closed to prevent backward flow of blood, or regurgitation. Proper functioning of cardiac valves depends on normal fibroelastic tissue of the valve leaflets, proper number of cusps of the valve, ability to open and close rapidly, normal-sized ring or annulus, and proper function of chordae tendineae and papillary muscles (mitral and tricuspid) (Brzezinski, Koprivanac, Gillinov, & Mihaljevic, 2018; Fann, Ingels, & Miller, 2018). This chapter describes the various valve surgery procedures and their associated care implications.

▶ Valvular Heart Disease

Valvular heart disease (VHD) is defined according to the valve or valves affected and the type of functional alteration. Abnormality of the valve is identified as either stenosis (narrowing or constriction

that creates an abnormally high or low pressure gradient) or regurgitation (incomplete closure of the valve leaflets resulting in a backflow of blood).

Valvular heart disease may be caused by either congenital or acquired factors. Congenital factors include a bicuspid rather than tricuspid valve (except mitral valve which is normally bicuspid), and other congenital malformations. Acquired causes of valve disease include ischemic coronary artery disease (CAD), degenerative changes associated with aging, heart failure (HF), rheumatic changes, infective endocarditis (IE) from a bacterial infection, neoplasm, and thrombus (Brzezinski et al., 2018; Fann et al., 2018).

The relationship between ischemic CAD and VHD is bidirectional. Myocardial infarction (MI) due to CAD can result in ventricular remodeling (a pathologic change in the shape and size of the ventricle). Chordae tendineae, papillary muscle, and the valve annulus may be affected, leading to impaired valve function. A malfunctioning valve will cause an increase in myocardial workload and can eventually lead to ischemia as a symptom of valve disease.

Decisions about whether to pursue medical or surgical management and which type of surgical management to use are based on the goals of maximizing the life of the valve and minimizing complications of treatment (Shemin & Benharash, 2018). Often the decision to repair or replace a

Original contributions from Kristine J. Peterson

valve is made once the surgeon has an opportunity to visualize the valve. Nevertheless, patients are educated on both repair and replacement procedures.

Pros and cons exist for both mechanical and biological valves. Mechanical valves are believed to be more durable than bioprosthetic valves, but require that patients receive lifelong anticoagulation therapy with warfarin (Coumadin®). In recent years, use of bioprosthetic valves has increased significantly, while use of mechanical valves has decreased. The percentage of aortic replacement devices changed from 57% mechanical in 1995 to 84% bioprosthetic in 2010 (Kouchoukos, Blackstone, Hanley, & Kirklin, 2013). The surgeon and the patient together decide which type of valve will be used for replacement. All patients, regardless of valve prosthesis used, will require anticoagulation for some period following surgery. The American College of Cardiology/American Heart Association (ACC/AHA) provide recommendations and guidelines for anticoagulation following valve intervention.

▶ Aortic Stenosis

Aortic stenosis (AS) due to age-related calcific disease (formerly known as degenerative or senile AS) is the most common adult valve lesion in the United States. Bicuspid aortic valve disease is another cause of aortic stenosis and is believed to be present in about 1% to 2% of the population (Otto & Bonow, 2015). Given that the U.S. population is aging, the incidence of AS is increasing. Long thought to be a disease of stress and degenerative changes, the calcification of aortic stenosis is now regarded as an active proliferative and inflammatory process, similar to atherosclerosis (Brzezinski et al., 2018; Otto & Bonow, 2015).

Aortic stenosis, in which the aortic valve does not open completely, creates a left ventricular outflow tract obstruction and increases workload and afterload of the left ventricle (LV). The increase in afterload is the etiology of the signs and symptoms associated with AS (Otto & Bonow, 2015).

Factors involved in grading the severity of AS include the mean systolic gradient across the valve, blood velocity, valve area, left ventricular function, and severity of symptoms (Otto & Bonow, 2015). Normally the pressures in the LV and the aorta are virtually equal during systole, meaning there is no aortic systolic gradient. As the valve opening narrows, however, the pressure required to eject blood—and therefore the pressure in the LV—increases, creating a gradient. The normal aortic valve area is 2.6 to 3.5 cm^2 (Brzezinski et al., 2018). As the valve area narrows and the gradient increases, blood velocity increases. Mild AS is associated with a mean gradient of less than 25 mmHg, valve area less than 1.5 cm^2, and jet velocity less than 3 m/sec. Severe aortic stenosis is associated with jet velocity of more than 4 m/sec, mean systolic gradient greater than 40 mmHg, and valve area less than 1.0 cm^2 (Kouchoukos et al., 2013).

Classic signs and symptoms of AS include angina, syncope, exertional dyspnea, sudden cardiac death, and heart failure. Typically, these conditions appear only after a prolonged latent period when the disease is already severe, usually evident by age 50 to 70 for a bicuspid valve and after age 70 with age-related calcific stenosis. Heart failure symptoms are thought to be due to diastolic failure (Otto & Bonow, 2015).

Once patients become symptomatic, the outcome is poor if obstruction is not relieved (Nishimura et al., 2014; Otto & Bonow, 2015). In patients with HF, time from onset of symptoms to death is 2 years; in those with angina, time from onset of symptoms to death is 5 years (Otto & Bonow, 2015). Medical therapy may improve symptoms of heart failure but is not effective long-term therapy for AS (Nishimura et al., 2014). With the addition of transcatheter aortic valve replacement (TAVR), surgeons can choose replacement via median sternotomy, minimally invasive aortic valve replacement, or TAVR. The choice is based on patient factors, surgical risk, and surgeon/patient preference. Transcatheter aortic valve replacement is discussed in more detail in Chapter 7. **BOX 5.1** outlines the 2014 ACC/AHA recommendations for aortic valve replacement (AVR) in the presence of aortic stenosis with the 2017 focused updates. These guidelines apply to all replacement modalities.

BOX 5.1 Indications for Aortic Valve Replacement in Aortic Stenosis

Class IA

Patients who meet an indication for AVR with low or intermediate surgical risk. Indications for AVR include decreased systolic opening of aortic valve, aortic velocity of 4.0 m/sec or greater, mean pressure gradient 40 mmHg or higher, or symptoms.

1. Either surgical AVR or TAVR among *high-risk* patients with severe, symptomatic AS (stage D), after consideration by a heart valve team.

Class IB

1. Symptomatic patients with severe AS with:
   a. Decreased systolic opening of a calcified or congenitally stenotic aortic valve; and
   b. An aortic velocity 4.0 m/sec or greater or mean pressure gradient 40 mmHg or higher; and
   c. Symptoms of heart failure, syncope, exertional dyspnea, angina, or presyncope by history or on exercise testing.
2. Asymptomatic patients with severe AS and LVEF less than 50% with a decreased systolic opening, aortic velocity of 4 m/sec or greater, and mean pressure gradient of 40 mmHg or higher.
3. Severe AS when undergoing cardiac surgery for other indications when there is decreased systolic opening, aortic velocity of 4 m/sec or greater, and mean pressure gradient of 40 mmHg or higher.
4. TAVR is recommended for patients who meet an indication for AVR, have a prohibitive surgical risk, and have a predicted post-TAVR survival of more than 12 months.

Class IIaB

1. Asymptomatic patients with severe AS with:
   a. decreased systolic opening of calcified valve;
   b. an aortic velocity of 5.0 m/sec or greater or mean pressure gradient 60 mmHg or higher; and
   c. a low surgical risk.
2. Apparently asymptomatic patients with severe AS and:
   a. A calcified aortic valve;
   b. An aortic velocity of 4 to 4.9 m/sec or mean pressure gradient of 40 to 50 mmHg; and
   c. An exercise test demonstrating decreased exercise tolerance or a fall in systolic BP.
3. Symptomatic patients with low-flow/low-gradient severe AS with reduced LVEF with:
   a. Calcified aortic valve with reduced systolic opening;
   b. Resting valve area 1.0 cm^2 or less;
   c. Aortic velocity less than 4 m/sec or mean pressure gradient less than 40 mmHg;
   d. LVEF less than 50%; and
   e. A low-dose dobutamine stress study that shows an aortic velocity 4 m/sec or greater or mean pressure gradient 40 mmHg or higher with a valve area 1.0 cm^2 or less at any dobutamine dose.
4. TAVR is reasonable for patients who meet an indication for AVR and have a high or intermediate surgical risk.

Class IIaC

1. Symptomatic patients with low-flow/low-gradient severe AS with an LVEF 50% or greater, a calcified aortic valve with significantly reduced leaflet motion, and a valve area 1.0 cm^2 or less only if clinical, hemodynamic, and anatomic data support valve obstruction as the most likely cause of symptoms and data recorded when the patient is normotensive (systolic BP <140 mmHg) indicate:
   a. An aortic velocity less than 4 m/sec or mean pressure gradient less than 40 mmHg; and

(continues)

BOX 5.1 Indications for Aortic Valve Replacement in Aortic Stenosis   *(continued)*

    b.   A stroke volume index less than 35 mL/m^2; and
    c.   An indexed valve area 0.6 cm^2/m^2 or less.
  2. Patients with moderate AS (stage B) with an aortic velocity between 3.0 and 3.9 m/sec or mean pressure gradient between 20 and 39 mmHg who are undergoing cardiac surgery for other indications.

Class IIbC

  1. Asymptomatic patients with severe AS and rapid disease progression and low surgical risk.

Class IIIB

  1. TAVR not recommended for patients with comorbidities so severe they will not be able to expect to benefit from AVR.

AS, aortic stenosis; AVR, aortic valve replacement; BP, blood pressure; LVEF, left ventricular ejection fraction; TAVR, transcatheter aortic valve replacement.
Data from Nishimura et al., 2014; Nishimura et al., 2017.

As discussed in Chapter 3, the AHA classifies recommendations based on the degree of agreement, type, or amount of available evidence or any combination of these. The level of recommendation is classified as Class I, II, or III. Class I indicates that evidence, general agreement, or both exist that the intervention is effective. Class II refers to conflicting evidence, a divergence of opinion, or both exist about the efficacy. Class II is further subdivided into Class IIa and Class IIb: Class IIa indicates that evidence/opinion is in favor of efficacy, whereas Class IIb recommendations have less efficacy as established by evidence/opinion. Class III refers to evidence, general opinion, or both that an intervention is not effective or is harmful.

The strength of the level of evidence is also identified according to the type or presence of research. For example, Level of Evidence A indicates that findings from multiple randomized clinical trials or meta-analyses support the use of an intervention. Level of Evidence B indicates that a single randomized trial or nonrandomized trials support an intervention. Level of Evidence C refers to consensus opinion of experts, case studies, or standard of care (Nishimura et al., 2014).

Aortic stenosis results in development of a hypertrophied and noncompliant LV. Postoperatively, while symptoms improve rapidly, the hypertrophy and stiffness remain. Such a ventricle is dependent on adequate filling volumes. The nurse must monitor filling volumes and blood pressure closely, control heart rate, and maintain sinus rhythm. Patients may require atrioventricular (AV) pacing at rates of 90 to 100 per minute and cardioversion of atrial fibrillation (AF) to maintain adequate cardiac output (CO). In addition, the aortic valve is located very near to the AV node so some degree of AV block may occur due to edema, inflammation, hemorrhage, or suturing near the node. Epicardial pacing, implantation of a permanent pacemaker, or both may be necessary if the block fails to resolve within a few days (Jacobson, Marzlin, & Webner, 2014). More detailed discussion of postoperative nursing management for all valve surgeries is provided in later chapters.

▶ Aortic Regurgitation (Insufficiency)

When aortic regurgitation (AR) or aortic insufficiency (AI) is present, there is a reflux of blood from the aorta into the LV during diastole, because the valve leaflets fail to close completely and to remain tightly closed during diastole. Symptoms of AR depend on the acuity of onset, severity of regurgitation, and left ventricular function. Acute AR imposes a large-volume load that a normal LV cannot accommodate. The sudden increase in end-diastolic volume (preload) will result in increased left ventricular end-diastolic pressure and decreased CO. Patients with acute AR will rapidly develop hemodynamic instability and left ventricular failure. Early diagnosis and intervention are critical. Patients with concomitant CAD may develop left ventricular dilation and cardiac failure. Such patients often present with HF.

Like chronic AS, chronic AR has a slow, insidious onset and progression. Aortic regurgitation may be well tolerated for years. Because it develops slowly, the LV compensates with hypertrophy and an increase in sympathetic tone to keep the left ventricular end-diastolic pressure (LVEDP) relatively low and maintain CO. This change results in a characteristic sign of AR, a widened pulse pressure (Brzezinski et al., 2018). If left untreated, this process will lead eventually to myofibril slippage, ventricular remodeling, and irreversible changes in LV function. In chronic AR, left ventricular dilation develops over time and patients may be asymptomatic for long periods. Dyspnea on exertion, orthopnea, and paroxysmal nocturnal dyspnea will develop gradually, along with feelings of heart pounding and awareness of every heartbeat. Later in its course, angina and palpitations will develop (Otto & Bonow, 2015).

The most common causes of AR in developed countries are bicuspid valve, age-related calcific aortic valve disease, traumatic tears of the aorta, and aortic root disease (Nishimura et al., 2014; Otto & Bonow, 2015). Other causes of AR include chronic systemic hypertension, aortitis of various etiologies, and connective tissue disease such as Marfan syndrome, Reiter disease, Ehlers-Danlos syndrome, and rheumatoid arthritis (Otto & Bonow, 2015). Most commonly, AR is seen concomitantly with AS (e.g., aortic disease, rheumatoid disease, or degenerative disease) (Brzezinski et al., 2018).

Indications for Aortic Valve Replacement in Aortic Regurgitation

Surgical intervention for AR consists largely of valve replacement. Some specialized centers perform aortic valve repair; however, there is insufficient data on repair to gauge the durability of repair compared with replacement (Nishimura et al., 2014). For the purposes of this chapter, surgical intervention will consist of valve replacement. While acute AR should be treated with early valve replacement, valve replacement is not recommended for asymptomatic patients with chronic AR and good left ventricular function (Nishimura et al., 2014). Left ventricular size, as measured by left ventricular end-systolic diameter (LVESD) of greater than 50 mm, or indexed LVESD of greater than 25 mm/m^2, is a measure of the degree of LV volume overload and remodeling. It is an independent predictor of outcome (Nishimura et al., 2014; Otto & Bonow, 2015). Deteriorating left ventricular function, as indicated by an ejection fraction (EF) less than 50% to 55% and an end-diastolic dimension greater than 70 mm or an end-systolic dimension greater than 50 mm, would indicate need for surgery (Brzezinski et al., 2018). **BOX 5.2** lists the indications for surgery for AR.

Aortic regurgitation results in both volume and pressure overload for the LV. The result is a dilated LV with some degree of hypertrophy. Postoperative considerations will be similar following aortic valve replacement to those for AS, including consideration of filling volumes, heart rate, AV blocks, and maintaining sinus rhythm. Most patients will be vasodilated in the immediate postoperative period and may require vasopressor therapy (e.g., with norepinephrine or phenylephrine.

▶ Mitral Stenosis

Mitral stenosis (MS), like aortic stenosis, is a condition where the valve leaflets do not open completely, creating resistance to the forward flow of blood into the LV during diastole. Mitral stenosis is predominantly caused by rheumatic heart disease. Other causes, which are less common, include left atrial myxoma, thrombus, annular calcification, endocarditic vegetation, malignant carcinoid syndrome, and metabolic disorders (Otto & Bonow, 2015).

Most commonly, rheumatic disease is acquired in childhood; however, MS does not usually become

BOX 5.2 Indications for Aortic Valve Replacement in Aortic Regurgitation

Class IB

1. Symptomatic patients with severe AR irrespective of left ventricular function
2. Asymptomatic patients with chronic, severe AR and left ventricular systolic dysfunction (EF <50%) at rest if no other cause for systolic dysfunction is identified

Class IC

1. Chronic pure, severe AR while undergoing cardiac surgery for other reasons

Class IIaB

1. Asymptomatic patients with pure, severe AR and normal LV systolic function (LVEF >50%) but with severe left ventricular dilatation (LVESD >50 mm or indexed LVESD >25 mm/m^2)

Class IIaC

1. Patients with moderate AR while undergoing surgery on the ascending aorta
2. Patients with moderate AR while undergoing other cardiac surgery

Class IIbC

1. Asymptomatic patients with severe AR and normal left ventricular function at rest (EF ≥50%) when evidence of progressive LV dilatation (end-diastolic dimension >65 mm, decreasing exercise tolerance, or abnormal hemodynamic response to exercise if surgical risk is low)

AR, aortic regurgitation; CABG, coronary artery bypass grafting; EF, ejection fraction; LV, left ventricle; LVESD, left ventricular end-systolic diameter.
Data from Nishimura et al., 2014

symptomatic until decades later. Time from initial episode of rheumatic fever to appearance of symptoms varies from a few years to more than 20 years. The valve leaflets gradually become thickened and calcified. Often, the chordae and commissures fuse (Fann et al., 2018). Left atrial pressure rises as the disease worsens, and a progressively higher gradient develops across the mitral valve. Pulmonary artery systolic pressure increases as the valve area narrows. Defining characteristics of severe MS include a gradient of greater than 10 mmHg, LAP greater than 15 mmHg, valve area less than 1.5 cm^2, and pulmonary artery systolic pressure greater than 50 mmHg (Nishimura et al., 2014; Otto & Bonow, 2015).

Because of the resistance to the forward flow of blood, patients with MS will not develop volume overload in the LV and will likely have satisfactory left ventricular function. These individuals, however, have pulmonary hypertension, right ventricular failure, and tricuspid insufficiency. Symptoms of low CO and pulmonary venous congestion develop as left atrial and pulmonary pressures rise. At first, symptoms may occur only on exertion. As the valve area narrows, symptoms occur with less exertion, emotional stress, or atrial fibrillation (AF). Dyspnea on exertion, fatigue, and decreased exercise tolerance are the first symptoms to occur, followed by orthopnea and episodes of pulmonary edema, especially with any increase in heart rate. Once pulmonary hypertension develops, right-sided heart failure with edema, hepatomegaly, ascites, and tricuspid regurgitation (TR) are seen. Atrial fibrillation is common (Otto & Bonow, 2015).

Intervention depends on the stage of the disease, as defined by valve characteristics, hemodynamic effects, and symptoms (Nishimura et al., 2014). Close follow-up is necessary for asymptomatic patients. Anticoagulation is a class IB recommendation for patients with MS and AF, prior embolic event, or left atrial thrombus (Nishimura et al., 2014). Heart rate control, if necessary, is a class IIaB recommendation for patients in AF and a class IIbB recommendation for patients in normal sinus rhythm with exertional symptoms. Once symptoms develop, outcome is poor without intervention.

First line intervention is the percutaneous balloon mitral valvotomy (PBMV). This procedure is indicated for symptomatic patients with moderate or severe MS. This is defined as a mitral valve area less than 1 cm^2/m^2 body surface area or less than 1.5 cm^2 for a normal-sized adult (Otto & Bonow, 2015). Closed mitral commissurotomy had limited effectiveness and has been replaced by PBMV. Open commissurotomy has good results and low mortality; however, it too has mostly been replaced by the PBVM procedure. Open commissurotomy is not recommended for patients with a left atrial clot or concomitant mitral regurgitation (MR) (Otto & Bonow, 2015). Mortality and complications from PBMV are very low with acceptable improvement in hemodynamics (Kouchoukos et al., 2013). Percutaneous balloon mitral valvotomy and commissurotomy are not curative. Late mortality is usually due to thromboembolism or from complications of surgery. In general, mitral valve repair is better suited to treating MR than as a therapy for MS (Kaneko, Yammine, & Loberman, 2018). **TABLE 5.1** provides

TABLE 5.1 Indications for Interventions for Mitral Stenosis

Class	Recommendation	Level of Evidence
I	PBMV for symptomatic patients with severe MS (MVA 1.5 cm^2) and favorable valve morphology in absence of left atrial thrombus	A
I	Surgical repair or replacement for severely symptomatic patients (NYHA class III–IV) with severe MS (MVA 1.5 cm^2) who are not high risk for surgery and who are not candidates for or who have failed previous PBMV	B
I	Surgery indicated for patients with severe MS undergoing other cardiac surgery	C
IIa	PBMV for asymptomatic patients with severe MS, favorable valve morphology, and absence of contraindications	C
IIa	Surgery for severely symptomatic patients with severe MS in patients undergoing other cardiac surgery	C
IIb	PBMV for asymptomatic patients with severe MS (MVA <1.5 cm^2) and favorable valve morphology who have new onset of AF in the absence of contraindications	C
IIb	PBMV for symptomatic patients with MVA greater than 1.5 cm^2 if there is evidence of hemodynamically significant MS during exercise	C
IIb	PBMV for severely symptomatic patients (NYHA class III/IV) with severe MS (MVA <1.5 cm^2) who have suboptimal valve anatomy and are not candidates for surgery or at high risk for surgery	C
IIb	Mitral valve surgery for patients with moderate MS (MVA 1.6–2.0 cm^2) undergoing other cardiac surgery	C
IIb	Mitral valve surgery and excision of the left atrial appendage for patients with severe MS (MVA <1.5 cm^2) who have had recurrent embolic events while receiving adequate anticoagulation	C

MS, mitral stenosis; MVA, mitral valve area; NYHA, New York Heart Association; PBMV, percutaneous balloon mitral valvotomy.
Reproduced from Nishimura et al., 2014; Nishimura et al., 2017.

the 2014 ACC/AHA guideline recommendations for MS with the 2017 focused updates.

Patients with MS will have pulmonary hypertension, small LV cavity, and normal left ventricular function. Pulmonary hypertension decreases markedly in the immediate postoperative period and may continue to do so for some time. Even so, the degree of pulmonary hypertension present preoperatively will have a great effect on postoperative status. Because of pulmonary hypertension, patients will require careful monitoring of fluids, hydration status, and filling volumes to maintain CO. Ventilator times may be longer. In addition, hemodynamic support for the right ventricle (RV) is often necessary. A transesophageal echocardiogram is often used postoperatively to assist in assessing right and left ventricular function. Administration of dobutamine (Dobutrex®) or milrinone (Primacor®) in combination with norepinephrine (Levophed®) may be indicated to enhance contractility of the RV and decrease pulmonary vascular resistance (right-sided afterload). Mitral stenosis patients are frequently diuretic dependent and will require diuretics to return to their preoperative weight—another reason to carefully monitor for adequate filling volumes. Use of a right ventricular assist device may be indicated in the immediate postoperative period (Yazdchi & Rawn, 2018).

▶ Mitral Regurgitation

In mitral regurgitation, the valve leaflets do not close tightly, resulting in a backward jet of blood into the left atrium during ventricular systole. Proper function of the mitral valve depends on a complicated interaction between the mitral leaflets, annulus, chordae tendineae, papillary muscles, and left atrium and ventricle (Fann et al., 2018). The most common causes of MR include ischemic CAD, mitral valve prolapse syndrome, IE, rheumatic heart disease, mitral annular calcification, and dilated cardiomyopathy (Otto & Bonow, 2015). A sudden cause, such as ruptured papillary muscle or chordae tendineae, will result in acute and severe MR, and surgical repair is usually indicated (Nishimura et al., 2014).

Alternatively, chronic MR may progress slowly over time, with symptoms appearing only when the disease is very advanced.

Mitral regurgitation causes an increase in LVEDP because forward CO is decreased and the regurgitant flow is added to LVEDP. An enlarged left atrium is likely as well. If MR develops suddenly, CO will decrease. Patients may present with signs of severe HF and the electrocardiogram may reveal findings consistent with ischemia. Patients may also have AF and associated decrease in CO related to the enlarged left atrium. The CO achieved during exercise is the most important determinant of patient functional capacity (Otto & Bonow, 2015). The left atrium may be normal sized with decreased compliance and high atrial pressure. In long-standing MR, however, the atrium is usually significantly enlarged with only slightly elevated pressures.

The decision to perform corrective surgery is based on a number of factors. These include degree of MR, severity of symptoms, left ventricular function, feasibility of valve repair, presence of AF, presence and degree of pulmonary hypertension, and patient expectations (Kouchoukos et al., 2013). Severe MR is characterized by the following findings (Nishimura et al., 2014).

- Central jet MR greater than 40% left atrium or holosystolic eccentric jet
- Regurgitant volume 60 mL or greater
- Regurgitant fraction 50% or greater
- Effective regurgitant orifice 0.40 cm^2 or greater
- Angiographic grade 3–4+ regurgitation

Asymptomatic patients with severe MR can be safely followed for some time (Otto & Bonow, 2015).

Mitral valve repair, rather than replacement, is the preferred approach to MR because it provides better outcomes for most patients and avoids potential complications of anticoagulation and valve prostheses (Kouchoukos et al., 2013). In addition, mitral valve repair or replacement can be accomplished via minimally invasive approaches. **TABLE 5.2** provides information on the 2014 ACC/AHA guideline for surgical management of mitral regurgitation with the 2017 focused updates.

TABLE 5.2 Indications for Surgery for Mitral Regurgitation		
Class	**Recommendation**	**Level of Evidence**
I	Symptomatic patients with chronic severe primary MR and LVEF greater than 30%	B
I	Asymptomatic patients with chronic severe primary MR and LV dysfunction (LVEF 30%–60%, LVESD ≥40 mm, or both)	B
I	MV repair is recommended in preference to MVR for patients with chronic severe primary MR limited to the posterior leaflet	B
I	MV repair is recommended in preference to MVR for patients with chronic severe primary MR involving the anterior leaflet or both leaflets when a successful and durable repair can be accomplished	B
I	Repair or MVR for patients with chronic severe primary MR who are undergoing other cardiac surgery	B
IIa	MV repair for asymptomatic patients with chronic severe primary MR with preserved LV function (LVEF >60% and LVESD <40 mm) in whom the likelihood of a successful and durable repair without residual MR is greater than 95% with an expected mortality rate of less than 1% when performed at a Heart Valve Center of Excellence	B
IIa	MV repair for asymptomatic patients with chronic severe nonrheumatic primary MR and preserved LV function in whom there is a high likelihood of a successful and durable repair with (1) new onset of AF or (2) resting pulmonary hypertension (PA systolic arterial pressure >50 mmHg)	B
IIa	MV repair for patients with chronic moderate primary MR undergoing other cardiac surgery	B-R
IIa	It is reasonable to choose corral sparing mitral valve replacement over reduction annuloplasty mitral valve repair among patients operated for severe, symptomatic secondary MR	B-R
IIb	Surgery may be considered in symptomatic patients with chronic severe primary MR and LVEF less than 30%	C
IIb	Asymptomatic patients with severe primary MR with preserved left ventricular systolic function (EF >60%, end-systolic dimension 40 mm), mitral valve surgery is reasonable in setting of serial imaging studies that reveal a progressive increase in LV size or decrease in LVEF	C-LD

(continues)

Class	Recommendation	Level of Evidence
	TABLE 5.2 Indications for Surgery for Mitral Regurgitation *(continued)*	
IIb	MV repair may be considered in patients with rheumatic mitral valve disease when surgical treatment is indicated if a durable and successful repair is likely or if the reliability of long-term anticoagulation management is questionable	B
IIb	Transcatheter MV repair may be considered for severely symptomatic patients with chronic severe primary MR who have a reasonable life expectancy but a prohibitive surgical risk because of severe comorbidities	B
III	MVR should not be performed for treatment of isolated severe primary MR limited to less than one-half of the posterior leaflet unless MV repair has been attempted and was unsuccessful	B

AF, atrial fibrillation; LV, left ventricle; LVEF, left ventricular ejection fraction; LVESD, left ventricular end-systolic diameter; MR, mitral regurgitation; MV, mitral valve; MVR, mitral valve replacement; PA, pulmonary artery.
Reproduced from Nishimura et al., 2014; Nishimura et al., 2017.

A number of devices and techniques are in use or in clinical trials for percutaneous mitral valve repair. Among these are the MitraClip® (Abbott Vascular, Santa Clara, CA). This device was approved by the U.S. Food and Drug Administration in 2013 and is used in patients with very high surgical risk. The largest database to date for this registry is the ACCESS-EU study registry, which confirms that the device is safe; has a high implant success rate, low rates of mortality, and adverse events; and provides clinically meaningful functional improvement (Maisano et al., 2013).

Care in the immediate postoperative period may be challenging. Mitral regurgitation can mask LV dysfunction because of "unloading" through the regurgitant valve. Upon repair of the mitral valve for mitral regurgitation, the left atrium will no longer be receiving regurgitant blood from the LV and the patient will experience an immediate increase in afterload (systemic vascular resistance). Left ventricular dysfunction that was masked by the regurgitant valve may become apparent, requiring inotropic support or vasodilators. Further compounding the potential for cardiac dysfunction postoperatively are pulmonary hypertension and effects of myocardial

hibernation (discussed in Chapter 13) that take time to be reversed. Patients, therefore, are at risk for the development of right ventricular failure. Patients should be monitored for right ventricular failure. If they develop decreased blood pressure, decreased CO, elevated central venous pressure, decreased cardiac volumes, and variable pulmonary artery pressures, suspect right ventricular failure (Borgdorff et al., 2015).

The efficacy of medical therapy for asymptomatic MR is the topic of ongoing debate; however, diuretics, digoxin, and arterial vasodilators may be used to decrease ventricular size, regurgitant orifice size, and regurgitant volume. To date, there is a lack of data that medical therapy will improve outcomes and it is not recommended for chronic primary MR unless the patient carries a high surgical risk. Patients with AF should be anticoagulated. For MR secondary to other causes (e.g., LV dilatation) treatment of the underlying cause is sometimes effective in reducing MR. For patients with indications, biventricular pacing may improve MR as well (Otto & Bonow, 2015).

Increased mortality after mitral valve surgery has been found among perimenopausal women. The higher mortality rate is thought to be associated with a state of estrogen withdrawal that may trigger inflammatory responses (Novella, Heras, Hermenegildo, & Dantas, 2012); these responses may in turn potentiate ischemia-reperfusion injury (Schubert et al., 2016).

Choice of Valve Prosthesis

Prosthetic valves are categorized as mechanical or biologic (tissue) valves. Mechanical valves are manufactured from man-made materials such as metal alloys, pyrolite carbon, and polyethylene terephthalate (Dacron™). Biologic valves are constructed from bovine, porcine, or human cardiac tissue, although they may contain some man-made materials. Mechanical prosthetic valves are more durable and last longer than biologic valves, but they carry an increased risk of thrombotic events, necessitating long-term anticoagulation therapy. Biologic valves do not require lifelong anticoagulation therapy, but they are less durable due to their tendency toward early calcification, tissue degeneration, and stiffening of the leaflets.

Advantages and disadvantages of valve replacement with either a prosthetic or mechanical valve must be carefully weighed by the patient. Indications for either type of valve vary by patient characteristics and surgeon preference (Kouchoukos et al., 2013).

▶ Tricuspid Valve Disease

The tricuspid valve has an annular ring and three leaflets connected via chordae tendineae to papillary muscles that are integrated with the RV. It is located between the right atrium and ventricle, near the AV node, right coronary artery, and coronary sinus. Its function is to maintain forward flow of blood between the right atrium and the RV.

Tricuspid Regurgitation

The functional defects that are seen in tricuspid disease are classified as either primary or secondary. Primary valve disease is caused by conditions that affect valve anatomy (e.g., congenital abnormalities, rheumatic disease, infective endocarditis, toxicities, tumor, blunt trauma). Secondary tricuspid disease can result from right ventricular pathology, pulmonary hypertension, increased right ventricular systolic pressure (especially if >55 mmHg), mitral or aortic valve disease (that results in elevated left atrial pressure [LAP] and LVEDP), left-sided HF, dilated cardiomyopathy, tricuspid annular dilatation, or pulmonary embolism (Kouchoukos et al., 2013; Otto & Bonow, 2015). Occasionally, wires inserted through the valve such as an automatic implantable cardioverter defibrillator or pacemaker may cause TR (Shemin & Benharash, 2018). The most common cause of TR is right ventricular dilatation, causing secondary or functional TR. Other causes of TR are rheumatic disease and MR (Nishimura et al., 2014; Otto & Bonow, 2015).

If the patient does not have pulmonary hypertension, TR is generally well tolerated. Patients with pulmonary hypertension will have signs and symptoms of right ventricular failure such as reduced CO, fatigue, ascites, painful congested hepatomegaly, abnormal venous pulsations, and significant peripheral edema. Weight loss, cachexia, cyanosis, and jaundice may be present, and AF is common (Nishimura et al., 2014; Otto & Bonow, 2015).

Primary TR is generally a progressive disease, as are other valve diseases. Secondary TR is often present with mitral disease. Diuretics and therapies to reduce pulmonary vascular resistance may be used for severe TR (Nishimura et al., 2014). Because the most common cause of TR is mitral valve disease, decisions about tricuspid repair or replacement will be influenced by the degree of mitral disease. Data now indicate that TR in the presence of mitral repair or replacement should be repaired as well due to the risk of needing reoperation to repair progressive TR (Kouchoukos et al., 2013; Nishimura et al., 2014). Various repair techniques and tricuspid valve replacement are available. **TABLE 5.3** provides indications for surgery for patients with TR.

Tricuspid Stenosis

Patients with tricuspid stenosis (TS) have an obstruction to blood flow from the right atrium

TABLE 5.3 Indications for Surgery for Tricuspid Regurgitation

Class	Recommendation	Level of Evidence
I	Patients with severe TR undergoing left-sided valve surgery	C
IIa	Patients with mild, moderate, or greater functional TR at the time of left-sided valve surgery with either (1) tricuspid annular dilation or (2) prior evidence of right HF	B
IIa	Patients with symptoms due to severe primary TR that are unresponsive to medical therapy	C
IIa	Patients with moderate functional TR and pulmonary artery hypertension at the time of left-sided valve surgery	C
IIb	Asymptomatic or minimally symptomatic patients with severe primary TR, progressive degrees of moderate or greater RV dilation, systolic dysfunction, or any combination of these	C
IIb	Reoperation for isolated tricuspid valve repair or replacement may be considered for persistent symptoms due to severe TR in patients who have undergone previous left-sided valve surgery and who do not have severe pulmonary hypertension or significant RV systolic dysfunction.	C

HF, heart failure; RV, right ventricle; TR, tricuspid regurgitation.
Reproduced from Nishimura et al., 2014. 2014 AHA/ACC guideline for the management of patients with valvular heart disease: A report of the American College of Cardiology/American Heart Association Task Force on Practice Guidelines. The Journal of Thoracic and Cardiovascular Surgery, 148(1), e1–e132.

to the right ventricle. The most common etiology for TS is rheumatic heart disease, and it almost always occurs in conjunction with mitral valve disease (Otto & Bonow, 2015). Other conditions associated with TS include carcinoid syndrome, endocarditis, and intracardiac tumors. The clinical presentation of TS is logically consistent with right-sided HF: decreased CO, fatigue, anasarca, hepatomegaly, and ascites out of proportion to the degree of dyspnea (Otto & Bonow, 2015).

Surgery for Tricuspid Stenosis

Surgical options for TS include annuloplasty, bicuspidization, other repair techniques, percutaneous balloon tricuspid commissurotomy, and valve replacement. **TABLE 5.4** lists the indications for surgery for TS.

▶ Infective Valve Endocarditis

Infective valve endocarditis is a complex and serious disease with a high mortality rate even with appropriate antimicrobial therapy. In-hospital mortality is 15% to 20% and 1-year mortality is as high as 40% (Nishimura et al., 2014). The characteristic sign of IE is a vegetation. This is an amorphous mass of fibrin, platelets, microorganisms, and inflammatory cells. *Staphylococcus aureus*, streptococci, and enterococci are the causative agents in most cases (Baddour, Freeman, Suri, & Wilson, 2015). Causes of IE include hemodynamically significant mitral valve prolapse, congenital heart disease, human immunodeficiency virus, and intravenous drug abuse. Prosthetic valve

TABLE 5.4 Indications for Surgery for Tricuspid Stenosis		
Class	**Recommendation**	**Level of Evidence**
I	Patients with severe TS at the time of operation for left-sided valve disease	C
I	Patients with isolated, symptomatic severe TS	C
IIb	Percutaneous balloon tricuspid commissurotomy might be considered in patients with isolated, symptomatic severe TS without accompanying TR	C

TR, tricuspid regurgitation; TS, tricuspid stenosis.
Reproduced from Nishimura et al., 2014. 2014 AHA/ACC guideline for the management of patients with valvular heart disease: A report of the American College of Cardiology/American Heart Association Task Force on Practice Guidelines. The Journal of Thoracic and Cardiovascular Surgery, 148(1), e1–e132.

endocarditis alone accounts for as high as 30% of cases (Baddour et al., 2015). Diagnosis is made by using the Duke criteria and transesophageal echocardiogram (Nishimura et al., 2014).

Signs and symptoms are often nonspecific and may come from a complication rather than IE itself. Maintaining a high degree of suspicion is important, especially in a patient who presents with fever, a predisposing cardiac lesion, bacteremia, embolic events, new prosthetic valve dysfunction, or evidence of an active endocardial process (Baddour et al., 2015). Treatment has two arms. First, eradication of the infective organism is paramount to prevent recurrence. Second, invasive complications must be resolved. Antimicrobial therapy specific to the causative agent is critical. Complications may require surgical intervention (Baddour et al., 2015).

Indications for surgery differ (**TABLE 5.5**). Mortality has been reduced since antimicrobial

therapy has been supplemented with earlier surgical intervention (Kasner & Sexton, 2017). Early surgery is more likely to result in a successful repair and reduces the risk of infection of the prosthesis (Baddour, 2015).

▶ Complications of Heart Valve Surgery

While complications of heart valve surgery are rare, the intensive care unit nurse should be aware of the possibility of their development and implement preventive measures. Complications of heart valve surgery reported in the literature include the following conditions:

- Thromboembolism (Gaasch & Zoghbi, 2017; Misawa, 2016)
- Valve obstruction (Gaasch & Zoghbi, 2017; Hanson, 2016)
- Valve regurgitation and paravalvular leak (Gaasch & Zoghbi, 2017)
- Bleeding related to antithrombotic therapy (Gaasch & Zoghbi, 2017)
- Infective endocarditis (Gaasch & Zoghbi, 2017; Misawa, 2016)
- Hemolytic anemia (Gaasch & Zoghbi, 2017)
- Atrial dysrhythmias (Peretto, Durante, Limite, & Cianflone, 2014; Stephens & Whitman, 2015)
- Renal insufficiency (Chang et al., 2016)
- Neurologic complications, stroke, or transient ischemic attack (Waksman & Minha, 2014)
- Respiratory insufficiency (Rong, Di Franco, & Gaudino, 2016)
- AV block (Gaasch & Zoghbi, 2017)
- Myocardial infarction (Hanson, 2016)
- Sternal wound infection (Cotogni, Barbero, & Rinaldi, 2015)
- Bleeding—requiring reexploration in most cases (Misawa, 2016)
- Low cardiac output syndrome (Lehmann et al., 2015)
- Gastrointestinal complications (Aithoussa et al., 2017)

TABLE 5.5 Indications for Surgical Intervention for Infective Endocarditis

Class	Recommendation	Level of Evidence
I	Early surgery (during initial hospitalization before completion of a full course of antibiotics) for patients with IE who present with valve dysfunction resulting in symptoms of HF	B
I	Early surgery for patients with left-sided IE caused by *S. aureus,* fungal, or other highly resistant organisms	B
I	Early surgery for patients with IE complicated by heart block, annular or aortic abscess, or destructive penetrating lesions	B
I	Early surgery for patients with evidence of persistent infection as manifested by persistent bacteremia or fevers lasting longer than 5 to 7 days after onset of appropriate antimicrobial therapy	B
I	Surgery is recommended for patients with prosthetic valve endocarditis and relapsing infection (defined as recurrence of bacteremia after a complete course of appropriate antibiotics and subsequently negative blood cultures) without other identifiable source for portal of infection	C
I	Complete removal of pacemaker or defibrillator systems, including all leads and the generator, is indicated as part of the early management plan in patients with IE with documented infection of the device or leads	B
I	Complete removal of pacemaker or defibrillator systems, including all leads and the generator, is reasonable in patients with valvular IE caused by *S. aureus* or fungi, even without evidence of device or lead infection	B
IIa	Complete removal of pacemaker or defibrillator systems, including all leads and the generator, is reasonable in patients undergoing valve surgery for valvular IE	C
IIa	Early surgery for patients with IE who present with recurrent emboli and persistent vegetations despite appropriate antibiotic therapy	B
IIb	Early surgery for patients with NVE who exhibit mobile vegetations greater than 10 mm in length (with or without clinical evidence of embolic phenomenon)	B

HF, heart failure; IE, infective endocarditis; NVE, native-valve infective endocarditis.
Data from Kasner & Sexton, 2017.

▶ **Summary**
_____

Selection of a mechanical or biological prosthetic valve has lifelong implications. These patients may require lifestyle modification and medication therapy for the rest of their lives. Advances in technology in the area of heart valve surgery offer more options, facilitate less invasive techniques, and potentially improve outcomes. Vigilant postoperative nursing care is critical to help ensure a good outcome for the patient who undergoes valve surgery.

🔍 *CASE STUDY*

A 57-year-old male patient with a history of hyperlipidemia, hypertension, tobacco use, and ventricular tachycardia, which resulted in implantation of an automated implantable cardioverter-defibrillator (AICD), and chronic NYHA Class 3 systolic heart failure secondary to nonischemic cardiomyopathy is admitted. Progressive fatigue is reported as the chief complaint. Home medications include furosemide and spironolactone. Upon admission, a transesophageal echocardiogram is performed. His LVEF is 25%; and left ventricular and left atrium dilation and right ventricular enlargement, severe mitral regurgitation are noted. Upon physical exam, J. O.'s point of maximal impulse (PMI) is displaced, a holosystolic murmur is audible. No adventitious breath sounds, jugular venous distention, or edema are noted. Vitals include blood pressure 78/58, heart rate 96, respiratory rate 24. He was scheduled for mitral valve repair. His intraoperative and postoperative course were relatively uncomplicated. His immediate postoperative hemodynamic profile revealed an elevated systemic vascular resistance (SVR) and decrease in cardiac output. He was discharged from the intensive care unit on postoperative day 3 and home shortly thereafter.

Critical Thinking Questions

1. Why is there an increase in afterload following mitral valve repair?
2. What should postoperative monitoring include in this case?
3. Why may patients with mitral regurgitation develop a decrease in cardiac output?

Answers to Critical Thinking Questions

1. Upon repair of mitral regurgitation, the left atrium will no longer be receiving regurgitant blood from the left ventricle. The patient will immediately develop an increase in afterload.
2. In addition to the increase in afterload following mitral valve repair, further compounding the potential for cardiac dysfunction are pulmonary hypertension and effects of myocardial hibernation. Therefore, patients need to be monitored for right ventricular failure. If they develop decreased blood pressure, decreased cardiac output, elevated central venous pressure, and variable pulmonary artery pressures, right ventricular failure should be suspected.
3. The decrease in cardiac output is related to enlargement of the left atrium.

Self-Assessment Questions

1. Which is true regarding artificial valves?
    A. Bioprosthetic valves require the patient to remain on anticoagulant therapy throughout their lifetime.
    B. Mechanical valves are less durable.
    C. Mechanical valves are associated with decreased hemorrhagic complications.
    D. Bioprosthetic valves are associated with an increase in thromboembolic complications.

2. Which is a possible sequela of aortic stenosis?
    A. Increased systemic vascular resistance
    B. Increased oxygen delivery
    C. Decreased pulmonary vascular resistance
    D. Decreased myocardial oxygen consumption

3. Which type of murmur is associated with aortic stenosis?
    A. Continuous murmur
    B. Diastolic murmur
    C. Mid/late diastolic murmur
    D. Systolic murmur

4. A patient underwent surgery for aortic stenosis. For which should the nurse assess in the immediate postoperative period?
    A. Increased afterload
    B. Left ventricular hypertrophy
    C. Hypertension
    D. Noncompliant left ventricle

5. For which should the nurse observe when caring for a patient with left ventricular hypertrophy from aortic stenosis?
    A. Supraventricular tachycardia
    B. Second-degree AV block, Type II
    C. Ventricular fibrillation
    D. Asystole

6. Which set of hemodynamic parameters is consistent with a patient with acute aortic regurgitation?

	PAOP*	CO	HR
A.	6	3.0	120
B.	16	8.2	62
C.	5	9.7	55
D.	20	3.5	116

    *PAOP, pulmonary artery occlusion pressure

7. Following surgery to repair aortic regurgitation, the nurse should anticipate administration of which agent in the immediate postoperative period?
    A. Norepinephrine (Levophed®)
    B. Milrinone (Primacor®)
    C. Vasopressin
    D. Losartan (Cozaar®)

8. Which set of hemodynamic parameters is consistent with severe mitral stenosis?

	Left atrial pressure	Pulmonary artery systolic pressure
A.	10	40
B.	16	55
C.	12	35
D.	18	26

5. A patient has mitral stenosis. Which should the nurse anticipate being present?
    A. Left ventricular overload
    B. Right ventricular failure
    C. Aortic insufficiency
    D. Normal pulmonary artery pressure

6. A patient is admitted immediately following mitral valve repair for MR. Which hemodynamic parameter should the nurse anticipate?
    A. SVR 1600 dynes/sec/cm^{-5}
    B. Cardiac index 4.3 L/min/m^2
    C. CVP 3 mmHg
    D. HR 96

Answers to Self-Assessment Questions

1. C. **Mechanical valves are associated with decreased hemorrhagic complications.**
    Rationale: The true statement is that mechanical valves are associated with decreased hemorrhagic complications. Patients who receive mechanical valves require lifelong anticoagulant therapy, but not those with bioprosthetic valves. Mechanical valves are more durable. Bioprosthetic valves are not associated with an increase in thromboembolic events.

2. A. **increased systemic vascular resistance**
    Rationale: Aortic stenosis results in increased SVR. Aortic stenosis creates a

left ventricular outflow tract obstruction, which increases workload and afterload of the left ventricle.

3. D. **systolic murmur**
Rationale: Aortic stenosis is associated with a systolic murmur due to calcification of the aortic valve leaflets.

4. B. **left ventricular hypertrophy**
Rationale: Aortic stenosis results in development of a hypertrophied or noncompliant left ventricle. Postoperatively, while symptoms improve rapidly, the hypertrophy and stiffness remain.

5. B. **second-degree AV block, Type II**
Rationale: The aortic valve is located very near the AV node. Therefore, degree of AV block may occur due to edema, inflammation, hemorrhage, or suturing near the node.

6. D. **20/3.5/116**
Rationale: Acute aortic regurgitation imposes a large-volume load that a normal left ventricle cannot accommodate. The sudden increase in end-diastolic volume (preload) will result in an increase in left ventricular end-diastolic pressure (as reflected by PAOP) and a decrease in cardiac output.

7. A. **norepinephrine (Levophed®)**
Rationale: Most patients will be vasodilated in the immediate postoperative period and require vasopressor therapy (such as with norepinephrine).

8. B. **16/55**
Rationale: Left atrial pressure rises as disease worsens. Pulmonary artery systolic pressure increases as the valve area narrows.

9. B. **right ventricular failure**
Rationale: Because of the resistance to forward flow of blood, patients with mitral stenosis will not develop volume overload in the left ventricle and will likely have satisfactory left ventricular function. Patients will have pulmonary hypertension, right ventricular failure, and tricuspid insufficiency.

10. A. **SVR 1600 dynes/sec/cm^{-5}**
Rationale: Mitral regurgitation can mask left ventricular dysfunction because of the "unloading" through the regurgitant valve. Upon repair, the left atrium will no longer be receiving regurgitant blood from the left ventricle and the patient will experience an immediate increase in afterload.

CLINICAL INQUIRY BOX

Question: What is the mortality rate and incidence of stroke, atrial fibrillation, structural valve deterioration, and hospital length of stay of patients following aortic valve replacement with a bioprosthetic valve in patients with severe symptomatic aortic stenosis?

Reference: Foroutan, F., Guyatt, G. H., O'Brien, K., Bain, E., Stein, M., Bhagra, S., . . . Vandvik, P. O. (2016). Prognosis after surgical replacement with a bioprosthetic aortic valve in patients with severe symptomatic aortic stenosis: Systematic review of observational studies. *British Medical Journal, 354*. doi:10.1136/bmj.i5065

Objective: To determine mortality rate and incidence of stroke, atrial fibrillation, structural valve deterioration, and hospital length of stay of patients following aortic valve replacement with a bioprosthetic valve in patients with severe symptomatic aortic stenosis.

Method: Systematic review

Results: The median survival for patients who underwent aortic valve replacement with a bioprosthetic valve was 16 years in patients age 65 years or less, 12 years for patients between 65 and 75 years of age, and 7 years for patients between 75 and 85 years of age. The incidence of stroke was 0.25 per 100 patient-years. Valve deterioration was 6% at 10 years, 18.3% at 15 years, and 48% at 20 years. Length of stay was 12 days.

Conclusion: Patients with severe symptomatic aortic stenosis who undergo valve replacement with a bioprosthetic valve have slightly higher mortality rates compared with those without aortic stenosis. There is a low incidence of stroke and for up to 10 years, a low incidence of destruction of the valve. The deterioration rate of the valve increases quickly after 10 years, and more so after 15 years.

References

Aithoussa, M., Atmani, N., Moutakiallah, Y., Abdou, A., Nya, F., Bamous, M., . . . Drissi, M. (2017). Gastro-intestinal complications after open heart surgery. *Archives of Digestive Disorders, 1*(2), 8–14.

Baddour, L. M., Freeman, W. K., Suri, R. M., & Wilson, W. R. (2015). Cardiovascular infections. In R. O. Bonow, D. L. Mann, D. P. Zipes, & P. Libby (Eds.), *Braunwald's heart disease: A textbook of cardiovascular medicine* (10th ed., pp. 1524–1550). Philadelphia, PA: Elsevier.

Borgdorff, M. A., Koop, A. M., Bloks, V. W., Dickinson, M. G., Steendijk, P., Sillje, H. H., . . . Barfelds, B. (2015). Clinical symptoms of right ventricular failure in experimental chronic pressure load are associated with progressive diastolic dysfunction. *Journal of Molecular and Cellular Cardiology, 79,* 244–253.

Brzezinski, A., Koprivanac, M., Gillinov, A., & Mihaljevic, T. (2018). Pathophysiology of aortic valve disease. In L. H. Cohn & D. H. Adams (Eds.), *Cardiac surgery in the adult* (5th ed., pp. 633–648). New York, NY: McGraw-Hill Medical.

Chang, O. H., Lee, C. C., Chen, S. W., Fan, P. C., Chen, Y. C., Chang, S. W., . . . Tsai, P. C. (2016). Predicting acute kidney injury following mitral valve repair. *International Journal of Medical Science, 13*(1), 19–24.

Cotogni, P., Barbero, C., & Rinaldi, M. (2015). Deep sternal wound injury after cardiac surgery: Evidences and controversies. *World Journal of Critical Care Medicine, 4*(4), 265–273.

Fann, J. I., Ingels, N. B., & Miller, D. C. (2018). Pathophysiology of mitral valve disease. In L. H. Cohn & D. H. Adams (Eds.), *Cardiac surgery in the adult* (5th ed., pp. 761–796). New York, NY: McGraw-Hill Medical.

Gaasch, W. H., & Zoghbi, W. A. (2017). *Overview of the management of patients with prosthetic heart valves.* Retrieved from http://www.uptodate.com/contents/overview -of-the-management-of-patients-with-prosthetic-heart -valves?search=complications+of+prosthetic+heart +valve&source=search_result&selectedTitle=2%7E150.

Hanson, I. (2016*). Mitral regurgitation follow-up.* Retrieved from https://emedicine.medscape.com/article/155618-foll owup?pa=QLwvm6SYhw2hedJQ0dUD%2FHywMsjZhO fknIHO%2BeJKDftzuXZQq3fTaCqEvlYdGPye4OSVcqV 6S9mSAd9%2BSaZpiomwFHTkxqQt9fvsPApqnUY%3D.

Jacobson, C., Marzlin, K., & Webner, C. (2014). *Cardiovascular nursing practice* (2nd ed.). Burien, WA: Cardiovascular Nursing Associates.

Kaneko, T., Yammine, M., & Loberman, D. (2018). Mitral valve replacement. In L. H. Cohn & D. H. Adams (Eds.), *Cardiac surgery in the adult* (5th ed., pp. 895–923). New York, NY: McGraw-Hill Medical.

Kasner, S. E., & Sexton, D. J. (2017). *Surgery for left-sided native valve endocarditis.* Retrieved from http:// www.uptodate.com/contents/surgery-for-left-sided -native-valve-endocarditis.

Kouchoukos, N. T., Blackstone, E. H., Hanley, F. L., & Kirklin, J. K. (2013). *Kirklin/Barratt-Boyes cardiac surgery* (4th ed.). Philadelphia, PA: Elsevier.

Lehmann, S., Merk, D. R., Etz, C. D., Seeburger, J., Schroeter, T., Oberbach, A., . . . Mohr, F. W. (2015). Minimally invasive aortic valve replacement: The Leipzig experience. *Annals of Cardiothoracic Surgery, 4*(1), 49–56.

Maisano, F., Franzen, O., Baldus, S., Schäfer, U., Hausleiter, J., Butter, C., . . . Schillinger, W. (2013). Percutaneous mitral valve interventions in the real world: Early and 1-year results from the ACCESS-EU, a prospective, multicenter, nonrandomized post-approval study of the MitraClip therapy in Europe. *Journal of the American College of Cardiology, 62*(12), 1052–1061.

Misawa, Y. (2016). Valve-related complications after mechanical heart valve implantation. *Surgery Today, 45*(60), 1205–1209.

Nishimura, R. A., Otto, C. M., Bonow, R. O., Carabello, B. A., Erwin J. P., Fleisher, L. A., . . . Thompson, A. (2017). 2017 AHA/ACC focused update of the 2014 AHA/ACC guideline for the management of patients with valvular heart disease: A report of the American College of Cardiology/American Heart Association Task Force on Practice Guidelines. *The Journal of Thoracic and Cardiovascular Surgery, 70*(2), 252–289.

Nishimura, R. A., Otto, C. M., Bonow, R. O., Carabello, B. A., Erwin, J. P., Guyton, R. A., . . . Yancy, C. W. (2014). 2014 AHA/ACC guideline for the management of patients with valvular heart disease: A report of the American College of Cardiology/American Heart Association Task Force on Practice Guidelines. *The Journal of Thoracic and Cardiovascular Surgery, 148*(1), e1–e132.

Novella, S., Heras, M., Hermenegildo, C., & Dantas, A. P. (2012). Effects of estrogen on vascular inflammation: A matter of timing. *Arteriosclerosis, Thrombosis and Vascular Biology, 32,* 2035–2014.

Otto, C. M., & Bonow, R. O. (2015). Valvular heart disease. In R. O. Bonow, D. L. Mann, D. P. Zipes, & P. Libby (Eds.), *Braunwald's heart disease: A textbook of cardiovascular medicine* (10th ed., pp. 1446–1523). Philadelphia, PA: Elsevier.

Peretto, G., Durante, A., Limite, E., & Cianflone, D. (2014). Postoperative arrhythmias after cardiac surgery: Incidence, risk factors, and therapeutic management. *Cardiology Research and Practice, 2014.* Retrieved from https://www. hindawi.com/journals/crp/2014/615987/.

Rong, L. Q., Di Franco, A., & Gaudino, M. (2016). Acute respiratory distress syndrome after cardiac surgery. *Journal of Thoracic Disease, 8*(10), e1177–e1186.

Schubert, C., Raparelli, X., Westphal, C., Dworatzek, E., Petrov, G., Kararigas, G., . . . Regitz-Zagrosek, V. (2016). Reduction of apoptosis and preservation of mitochondrial injury under ischemia/reperfusion injury is mediated by estrogen receptor β. *Biology of Sex Differences, 7.* doi:10.1186/s13293-016-0104-8

Shemin, R. J., & Benharash, P. (2018). Tricuspid valve disease. In L. H. Cohn & D. H. Adams (Eds.), *Cardiac surgery in the adult* (5th ed., pp. 927–942). New York, NY: McGraw-Hill Medical.

Stephens, R. S., & Whitman, G. J. R. (2015). Postoperative critical care of the adult cardiac surgical patient. Part I: Routine postoperative care. *Critical Care Medicine, 43*(7), 1477–1497.

Waksman, R., & Minha, S. (2014). Stroke after aortic valve replacement. *Circulation, 129,* 2245–2247.

Yazdchi, F., & Rawn, J. D. (2018). Postoperative care of cardiac surgery patients. In L. H. Cohn & D. H. Adams (Eds.), *Cardiac surgery in the adult* (5th ed., pp. 405–428). New York, NY: McGraw-Hill.

Web Resources

American Association of Cardiovascular and Pulmonary Rehabilitation: http://www.aacvpr.org

American College of Cardiology: http://www.acc.org

American Heart Association: http://www.americanheart.org

Aortic Valve Stenosis: Minimally Invasive Valve Replacement Video: http://www.youtube.com/watch?v=-miuqi1iyrw

Life after Heart Valve Replacement Surgery: http://www.youtube.com/watch?v=_hUG8Np9yk8

Mended Hearts: http://www.mendedhearts.org

Mitral Valve Repair: http://www.youtube.com/watch?v=zTHPLWBNjCU

National Heart, Lung, and Blood Institute: http://www.nhlbi.nih.gov

The Society of Thoracic Surgeons: http://www.sts.org

Understanding Heart Valve Replacement Choices: What You Need to Know: http://www.youtube.com/watch?v=4xN-c8k7IPs

CHAPTER 6

Cardiopulmonary Bypass and Off-Pump Coronary Artery Bypass

Julie Miller, Shelley K. Welch, Roberta Kaplow

▶ Introduction

For years, nurses have cared for patients who have undergone traditional coronary artery bypass grafting (CABG) surgery, in which the patient is placed on a cardiopulmonary bypass (CPB) circuit. Since 1990, nurses have seen an increase in the number of patients undergoing off-pump coronary artery bypass (OPCAB) surgery, in which the surgeon sews the grafts onto the coronary arteries with the heart still beating. However, in recent years, the number of OPCAB procedures has declined in the United States (Shroyer et al., 2017). Nursing care of patients who have undergone the CABG and OPCAB procedures have a number of similarities and differences.

Care of the coronary bypass surgery patient has evolved over the years. Previously, patients spent 2 to 3 days on a ventilator, sedated, with a pulmonary artery catheter (PAC) in place and multiple vasoactive drips infusing to maintain optimal hemodynamic status. Today, a patient undergoing CABG or OPCAB may be discharged from the operating room without a PAC, extubated, and transferred from the intensive care unit (ICU) to a progressive care unit within 12 hours of surgery. Regardless of the short stay, open heart surgery is a serious and potentially complicated procedure in which patients may remain critically ill when transferred from the ICU. Nurses are often faced with the challenge of patients and families who are anxious over the potential for death throughout the course of hospitalization.

Anxiety during the preoperative and postoperative periods has been correlated with poor outcomes such as increased pain levels (Kalogianni et al., 2016) and more readmissions. Factors predictive of increased anxiety include being female, having to wait for surgery, pain prior to surgery, concerns over returning to work, prior anxiolytic or antidepressant use, and difficulty sleeping (Chocron et al., 2013).

Nurses must assess patients' anxiety levels throughout the hospitalization and seek to understand the best patient-specific approach in countering their stress. The provision of realistic information about what to expect through every step of the care delivered and effective pain management are crucial in decreasing anxiety levels. Additionally, data suggest that patients with preoperative depression may benefit from administration of antidepressant therapy (Chocron et al., 2013).

Despite the need to address anxiety levels, the hemodynamic challenges, constant observation for potential complications, and need for the astute critical care nurse remain the same. This chapter explores the similarities and differences in the care of the traditional on-pump coronary artery bypass (ONCAB or CABG) patient compared to the patient who undergoes OPCAB.

▶ Potential Complications of Bypass Surgery

Stroke, infection, bleeding, dysrhythmias, myocardial infarction (MI), gastrointestinal dysfunction, renal failure, and death are all potential complications for the bypass surgery patient, whether the procedure is performed with the on- or off-pump technique. The risk for atrioventricular heart block is present in both types of bypass procedures, and both types of patients will usually have epicardial pacing wires placed. Nursing challenges for bypass surgery patients include ensuring hemodynamic stability, monitoring for and treating cardiac dysrhythmias, balancing the need to adequately medicate for pain while guarding against oversedation and respiratory complications, and monitoring for and intervening to prevent the myriad of potential postoperative complications.

On-pump coronary artery bypass patients undergo surgery while their heart is not beating. In this procedure, through a median sternotomy incision, the heart is stopped using cardioplegia solution. Oxygen needs are met by cannulating the aorta and placing the patient on the CPB circuit. On-pump coronary artery bypass carries a higher risk of aortic dissection and embolization because

of the cannulation and cross-clamping of the aorta for bypass procedures (Moss et al., 2015).

Heparin is utilized to maintain patency of the CPB circuit and to reduce the risk of microemboli formation. Heparin-induced thrombocytopenia (HIT) and bleeding are potential complications for all patients receiving heparin. In addition, the CPB circuit can contribute to the development of systemic inflammatory response syndrome (SIRS) and microemboli (Evova et al., 2016). Moderate hypothermia is utilized during the ONCAB procedure to decrease myocardial oxygen demand. The postoperative rewarming process contributes to vasodilation and can worsen the effects of SIRS.

As part of the ONCAB procedure, the bypass grafts are sewn onto the heart and aorta while the heart is stopped. When the surgery is completed, the heart is restarted and the CPB circuit withdrawn. There is a risk that the patient will not be able to be weaned from CPB and may require an intra-aortic balloon pump (IABP) or pacemaker postoperatively. Intra-aortic balloon pump therapy is discussed in detail in Chapter 10. On rare occasions, a patient's heart does not restart following CPB.

▶ Off-Pump Coronary Artery Bypass

Off-pump coronary artery bypass is performed either through a median sternotomy incision or via a thoracotomy incision, also known as minimally invasive direct coronary artery bypass (MIDCAB). Robotic-assisted coronary artery bypass (ROBOCAB) surgery is another type of off-pump procedure that is done through a minimally invasive approach. Minimally invasive surgery is discussed in detail in Chapter 7.

In OPCAB, the surgeon sews the grafts onto the beating heart using specialized instruments to stabilize the myocardial tissue where the surgeon is sewing the graft (Lazar, 2015). These instruments, known as stabilizers, are similar in shape to the sewing foot for a sewing machine (**FIGURE 6.1**).

Off-pump coronary artery bypass techniques gained popularity in the 1990s in efforts to reduce

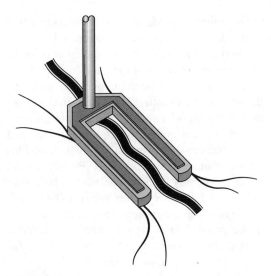

FIGURE 6.1 Stabilizer used in OPCAB.

Illustrated by James R. Perron.

the complications associated with the CPB circuit. Data suggest that OPCAP procedures have higher reocclusion rates than ONCAB and outcomes at 1 year are worse for the OPCAB than the ONCAB patients. Studies have noted that patients undergoing OPCAB receive fewer grafts than those undergoing ONCAB. This pattern may lead to a higher reintervention rate for OPCAB patients (Islam et al., 2014). The risk for postoperative aortic dissection with OPCAB has been shown to be higher than for on-pump CABG (Singh & Mehta, 2015). Patients undergoing off-pump bypass procedures may need to be converted to on-pump procedures (Borde et al., 2016). This possibility should be discussed with the patient and family during preoperative teaching.

Off-pump coronary artery bypass is performed on a patient with either mild hypothermia or normothermia. Hypothermia contributes to postoperative bleeding by causing impairment in the clotting cascade. It is theorized that less bleeding occurs with mild hypothermia as compared to the moderate hypothermia (30°–34°C) utilized in the ONCAB procedure. Mild hypothermia helps reduce myocardial oxygen demand and may be beneficial to both ONCAB and OPCAB patients. Data suggest that moderate hypothermia protects against intraoperative mortality for

on-pump patients (Greason, Kim, Suri, Wallace, & Englum, 2014). Other data from a systematic review suggest no difference in safety between normothermia and hypothermia in cardiopulmonary bypass grafting. A meta-analysis has shown that off-pump surgery is associated with fewer transfusions when compared to ONCAB (Pagano et al., 2017).

▶ Complications of On-Pump Surgery Versus Off-Pump Surgery

Off-pump coronary artery bypass grafting, also known as a beating heart procedure, was developed partly to offset the risk of postoperative alterations associated with on-pump procedures. Specifically, patients who undergo OPCAB are felt to be less likely to develop cerebral hypoperfusion, embolization, and inflammatory response associated with on-pump procedures (Islam et al., 2014). Data suggest that the cytokine and chemokine production is similar in ONCAB and OPCAB, but biomarkers such as eotaxin, macrophage inflammatory protein-1 beta (MIP-1β), and interleukin-12 (IL-12) were found to be more prevalent in the setting of ONCAB. Although more research needs to be conducted on the inflammatory response most often seen in ONCAB, OPCAB does appear to produce less of an inflammatory response. Recent studies have shown there is no difference in the endothelial response between OPCAB and ONCAB (Jongman et al., 2014).

Assessment for postoperative bleeding is essential, especially given that mediastinal reexploration rates for bypass surgery patients are as high as 6% (Fröjd & Jeppsson, 2016). Bleeding in these patients can be attributed to CPB, hypothermia, fibrinolytic agents administered during the procedure, heparin reversal, and loose anastomoses. As OPCAB was developed, concern was voiced that these patients would have more bleeding due to the risk of sewing onto the beating heart. In fact, data from randomized controlled trials suggest that OPCAB patients experience less bleeding postoperatively than ONCAB patients (Paparella et al., 2015).

In all post-bypass patients, assessment for bleeding is necessary. The mediastinal and pleural tubes must be monitored hourly for amount and quality of drainage, including assessment for clots. Monitoring for narrowing of pulse pressure is performed, as this finding could indicate cardiac tamponade in the post-bypass patient.

Heparin is utilized to maintain vessel patency and prevent thrombus formation during OPCAB, but the amount is about one-third to one-half the dose used in traditional CABG. Results of a trial using 2 or 3 mg/kg heparin for systemic heparinization did not affect the risk of postoperative bleeding in patients undergoing OPCAB (Chakravarthy et al., 2017). Because heparin is utilized in both on- and off-pump procedures, it is imperative that the nurse assess all post-bypass patients for bleeding, check lab data for presence of a coagulopathy, and assess for HIT.

Protamine is a protein that occurs in salmon sperm (DailyMed.gov, 2014). It is utilized in both on- and off-pump procedures to bind heparin and reverse its anticoagulant effect (Suelzu et.al., 2015). In one study, researchers estimated that protamine caused adverse events in approximately 2.6% of cardiac surgery patients (Lee, Cheng, & Ko, 2013). Risk factors for protamine reactions include being a patient with diabetes who uses protamine-containing insulin (most commonly NPH), previous drug reaction, and allergy to protamine or fish (Madani et al., 2014).

A minor protamine reaction may result in hypotension and an increase in pulmonary artery pressures (Lee et al., 2013). This effect is more common in patients who have diabetes, perhaps related to their use of protamine-containing insulin. Anaphylaxis has been associated with administration of protamine, and the affected patient may suffer cardiac arrest. Any adverse reaction to protamine increases the risk of mortality for both ONCAB and OPCAB patients (Shore-Lesserson et al., 2018).

The critical care nurse must be vigilant in monitoring for protamine reactions, including assessing the patient for different presentations of these reactions. Massive systemic vasodilation is manifested by hypotension, decreased systemic vascular resistance (SVR) (the amount of work the heart must do to eject blood), and increased cardiac output (CO) (the amount of blood ejected by the heart every minute). This syndrome, referred to as vasoplegia, if not responding to administration of fluid and vasopressors, may respond to an intravenous infusion of methylene blue (Hosseinian, Weiner, Levin, & Fischer, 2016). Acute pulmonary vasoconstriction will lead to an increase in pulmonary artery pressure (PAP) with subsequent right ventricular failure. The hemodynamic profile in this type of reaction will reveal bradycardia, decreased CO, elevated PAP, SVR, and pulmonary vascular resistance.

Studies suggest that a lower dose of protamine may be just as effective as the standard 1:1 ratio of protamine to heparin (Suelzu et al., 2015). Recent studies have evaluated a direct thrombin inhibitor, bivalirudin (Angiomax®), as a replacement for heparin anticoagulation for CPB and OPCAB. These studies indicate that bivalirudin can be used safely in patients with heparin allergy or increased risk for HIT (Shore-Lesserson et al., 2018). Nursing care for a patient receiving bivalirudin includes vigilant monitoring of lab data and for bleeding. Specific tests that may be used to evaluate the efficacy of bivalirudin include ecarin clotting time (ECT), activated clotting time (ACT), activated partial thromboplastin time (aPTT), international normalized ratio, and thromboelastogram (Shore-Lesserson et al., 2018).

Patients who undergo bypass procedures may develop postoperative temporary metabolic, hemodynamic, and neurohormonal changes (Kirov et al., 2017; Vukicevic et al., 2016). Hemodynamic alterations may also occur after cardiac surgery. These alterations may include a decrease in CO/cardiac index from intraoperative myocardial ischemia, tachycardia, bradycardia, increased SVR, or decreased myocardial contractility; hypotension due to decreased preload, contractility, or SVR; hypertension from a disrupted surgical anastomosis; and myocardial depression, vasoconstriction, or ventricular dysrhythmias from hypothermia (Van Diepen et al., 2017).

▶ Hemodynamic Monitoring

In the initial postoperative period for both ONCAB and OPCAB patients, the primary focus is hemodynamic stability. The first 6 hours postoperatively tend to be when the patient is the most vulnerable and unstable.

Cardiac dysfunction tends to manifest as decreased compliance and contractility from the pressure-overloaded myocardial tissue. A pressure-overloaded ventricle will have reduced compliance and be stiff, which will result in a decreased ejection fraction, CO, and contractility.

Preoperative ischemia and duration of the operative procedure contribute to instability in patients who undergo either on- or off-pump procedure. In the ONCAB patient, hemodynamic instability is related to effects from the CPB circuit and the cold potassium cardioplegia used to reduce myocardial oxygen demand. In contrast, manipulation of the beating heart for OPCAB leads to decreased compliance and contractility (Afrasiabirad, Safaie, & Montazerogoem, 2015).

A patient who has had valve replacement is typically volume overloaded (Man, 2018). In both ONCAB and OPCAB surgeries, fluid needs may be higher than expected; thus the critical care nurse will need to assess all interventions for their effect on hemodynamics to ensure adequate preload. Hemodynamic profiles of cardiac surgery patients are discussed in detail in Chapter 9.

▶ Risks of On-Pump Surgery Versus Off-Pump Surgery

A number of risks are associated with coronary artery bypass surgery, whether it is performed on an on- or off-pump basis. Specifically, stroke, atrial fibrillation (AF), acute kidney injury, acute liver failure, bleeding, infection, and death have all been associated with on- and off-pump surgeries.

The ONCAB procedure and the CPB circuit have been shown to increase the risk for development of acute kidney injury, stroke, liver failure, AF, and bleeding (Puskas et al., 2015). Use of the CPB circuit has also been associated with the development of microemboli and SIRS. SIRS occurs in OPCAB patients, albeit to a lesser degree than in ONCAB patients (Bilgin & van de Watering, 2013). Recent data suggest that OPCAB may be of greater benefit in patients who are considered high risk, such as those with chronic kidney disease (not dialysis dependent), severe aortic disease, left ventricular (LV) dysfunction, and acute coronary syndrome. Long-term survival may be higher because of better patency of the graft and higher index of revascularization. No differences between ONCAB and OPCAB in terms of patient demographics were found in this recent meta-analysis. However, choice of conduit impacted survival significantly with ONCAB having improved long-term survival after 3 years of surgery (Kirmani et al., 2016).

Off-pump coronary artery bypass grafting was developed to minimize the risks of the CPB circuit. A meta-analysis revealed a reduced incidence of stroke, AF, and infections with OPCAB as compared to ONCAB (Kowalewski et al., 2016). However, the data are not consistent. The off-pump bypass is technically more challenging than ONCAB. Critics cite this difference as a factor that complicates the process of setting up randomized controlled studies and comparing outcomes for on- and off-pump procedures. The initial ROOBY trial, conducted from February 2002 to May 2008 by the U.S. Department of Veterans Affairs, randomized 2,203 patients to either OPCAB or ONCAB using a standard median sternotomy approach. This trial showed patients in the low to moderate risk category who underwent OPCAB had higher 1-year mortality and higher arterial and saphenous vein reocclusion rates (Shroyer et al., 2009). Also, long-term survival has been shown to be better in elective CABG surgery patients undergoing ONCAB (Kim et al., 2014). In a 5-year follow-up study to the ROOBY trial, the investigators concluded that more technically difficult OPCAB may not always provide superior clinical outcomes (Shroyer et al., 2017).

Cognitive Decline

Cognitive decline has been noted in patients who have undergone coronary artery bypass. It had been theorized that this decline in function was related to the CPB circuit. In recent studies comparing ONCAB, OPCAB, and healthy patients, however, researchers determined that the rate of cognitive decline in both types of surgery was the same. Proponents of OPCAB had theorized there would be less cognitive decline without CPB. Demographic data revealed that cognitive decline was present prior to surgery in both the ONCAB and OPCAB groups at a higher level than in the healthy patients. The incidence in cognitive decline between on-pump and off-pump surgery has not shown a significant reduction in risk (Kennedy et al., 2013).

Cognitive decline in patients undergoing coronary artery bypass surgery will require more study to determine the contributing factors.

Graft Occlusion

Both on- and off-pump procedures utilize the saphenous vein and arterial conduits for grafts. Saphenous vein harvesting is accomplished endoscopically, which reduces pain and scarring associated with the historical harvest approach of an inner thigh to ankle incision (Krishnamoorthy et al., 2017). Vein grafts are implanted in a reverse direction relative to their valves and have a higher occlusion rate when compared to the left internal thoracic artery grafts (Koeola, Itoh, Fosazaki, Nakamura, & Morino, 2014). Meta-analysis on graft patency shows ONCAB significantly reduces incidents of saphenous vein graft occlusion (Zhang et al., 2014).

Arterial grafts include the left internal thoracic artery, radial artery, and, less commonly, the right internal thoracic artery. The intrathoracic arteries, formerly known as mammary arteries, are used to bypass the anterior coronary circulation and require only one anastomosis. The elimination of anastomosis to the ascending aorta may reduce emboli, which might otherwise cause stroke (Vallely, Edelman, & Wilson, 2013).

Arterial grafts have been shown to decrease the need for revascularization and reduce short- and long-term mortality; approximately 80% of these grafts are still patent 8 years after implantation (Taboulis, 2013).

The radial artery, which was first utilized as a graft in the 1970s, has regained popularity as a graft due to its long patency duration. Improved harvest techniques for radial artery grafts and the use of calcium channel blockers intraoperatively and postoperatively (e.g., diltiazem [Cardizem®]) for 6 months have produced patency rates similar to those for other arterial grafts at 5 years (Lin et al., 2013). Long-term outcomes for OPCAB show reduced graft patency and increased risk of cardiac intervention and death (Puskas et al., 2015).

Patient Assessment

Ongoing preoperative and postoperative assessments are crucial for patients undergoing radial artery harvest. In the preoperative phase, the nurse performs a detailed assessment of the patient's history, activity level, and collateral ulnar blood flow to the affected hand(s). Collateral blood flow to the hand is most commonly assessed by using the Allen test. Specifically, the Allen test is used to assess the adequacy of blood supply to the hand through the ulnar artery. **BOX 6.1**

BOX 6.1 Steps for Performing the Allen Test

Step 1: Simultaneously locate the radial and ulnar artery; palpate and compress them with three digits.

Step 2: Maintaining compression on the radial and ulnar arteries, ask the patient to clench and unclench the hand 10 times.

Step 3: Release pressure from the ulnar artery and monitor the time it takes for flushing to return to the palm, thumb, and nail beds.

Step 4: If the amount of time it takes for flushing to return is greater than 6 seconds, this means that collateral flow is impaired. The radial artery should not be used as a graft.

Data from Krishnamoorthy et al., 2017.

outlines the performance and evaluation criteria included on the Allen test. The literature varies in interpretation of an Allen test, with 5 to 9 seconds being considered a positive result (Ruzsa et al., 2014). The recommended contraindication for radial graft harvest is a positive Allen test (the red color of the palm returns) in greater than 6 seconds (Saeed, 2014). A positive Allen test has been reported to have a predictive value of 53%, which means there is a need to investigate collateral flow further.

Techniques to more closely examine collateral flow include the use of Doppler flow measurements, thumb systolic pressure, finger-pulse plethysmography, and pulse oximetry. Some sources suggest that the Allen test could give a false-negative result. Regardless of the result, it is always mandatory to have a preoperative ultrasound study if radial artery harvesting is being considered (Baikoussis, Papakonstantinou, & Apostolakis, 2014).

Patients who perform manual labor, are physically active with their hands, have suffered a stroke with upper limb involvement, have peripheral vascular disease or Raynaud's disease, or have experienced a traumatic injury to the affected side should not be considered candidates for radial artery harvest (Baikoussis, Papakonstantinou, & Apostolakis, 2014). Additionally, smoking, diabetes, hypertension, and hyperlipidemia have been associated with diminished radial artery graft patency rates. Data suggest that patients with peripheral vascular disease are more likely to have early occlusion of a radial artery graft (Cheng & Slaughter, 2013).

Baikoussis and colleagues (2014) concluded that the radial artery graft appears to be superior to saphenous vein grafts, has minimal neurologic and vascular complications related to harvest, and has an adequate length for every site. Its only negative attribute is its tendency for vasospasm.

Radial Artery Harvesting

In the early development of radial artery harvesting, it was recommended that the nondominant hand be the site of harvest owing to fear of hand ischemia. Depending on surgeon preference, the radial artery donor site may or may not have a drain placed. If a drain is placed, it is usually removed when drainage is less than 20 mL for 8 hours. The incision will be covered loosely with a sterile gauze dressing and wrapped with a compressive wrap for 24 hours (Blitz, Osterday, & Brodman, 2013).

Postoperative assessment of the affected extremity includes the amount and quality of drainage, signs and symptoms of infection, and the "six Ps" for diminished arterial blood flow (i.e., pain, pulselessness, pallor, paresthesia, paralysis, and polar [cold]). Patients should be made aware that they may experience loss of motor strength and numbness on the affected extremity. These symptoms usually resolve in most patients 6 months postoperatively.

Compartment Syndrome

The literature reports a rare occurrence of compartment syndrome in the vein donor limbs for coronary artery bypass (Te Kolste, Balm, & de Mol, 2015). Nursing assessment of the donor limb should include assessment for diminished blood flow. Like their counterparts undergoing radial artery harvesting, vein graft donors should have the six Ps assessed. Early symptoms of compartment syndrome include severe pain and tenderness on passive stretch. This assessment may be masked by the use of sedation and narcotic analgesia in the early postoperative period.

Off-pump coronary artery bypass has been associated with a reduction in cost. Factors contributing to the reduction in cost for OPCAB are shorter lengths of stay in the ICU, shorter intubation time, decreased risk of stroke, reoperations for bleeding, and use of blood products due to diminished blood loss (Brewer et al., 2014).

▶ Summary

The majority of bypass surgeries performed in the United States remain on-pump procedures, and the United States has seen a steady decline in the use of OPCAB in recent years (Shroyer, 2017).

Nursing care of both on- and off-pump coronary artery bypass patients continues to advance as evidence mounts regarding the risks and advantages of each procedure. On- and off-pump patients remain at risk for myriad complications. Patients who undergo off-pump procedures tend to experience a lower incidence of stroke, infection, and AF. A notable cost savings with the use of off-pump procedures has also been documented. As the techniques and utilization of off-pump surgery continue to evolve, so will the skill and practice of the expert cardiac surgery nurse. Care of these patients will continue to be highly challenging and rewarding.

🔍 CASE STUDY

B. L., a 65-year-old patient with a history of hypertension, diabetes mellitus, and hyperlipidemia, underwent an on-pump 3-vessel bypass procedure for the left anterior descending and right proximal coronary arteries. This was his second on-pump procedure. Postoperatively, he was transferred to the cardiovascular ICU on epinephrine, insulin, milrinone, and propofol infusions. The patient received protamine to reverse the effect of heparin used during the procedure. Immediately following the administration of protamine, the patient developed angioedema of the face and neck. His systolic blood pressure decreased from 110 mmHg to 76 mmHg. The patient received aggressive fluid resuscitation, vasopressors, and steroids. He subsequently stabilized. The remainder of his postoperative course was uncomplicated.

Critical Thinking Questions

1. What risk factors did this patient have to a protamine reaction?
2. How should the nurse distinguish between a hypersensitivity reaction and anaphylaxis?
3. Why would administration of nitric oxide be considered in a patient who developed an anaphylactic reaction to protamine?

Answers to Critical Thinking Questions

1. The patient has a history of insulin-dependent diabetes mellitus and likely was taking NPH insulin.
2. With anaphylaxis, the patient may develop hypertension (versus hypotension in this case), respiratory difficulty, nausea, vomiting, fatigue, and back pain.
3. Nitric oxide would reverse the pulmonary vasoconstriction associated with the anaphylactic reaction, if it occurred.

Self-Assessment Questions

1. For which complication is a patient more at risk when having cardiac surgery on cardiopulmonary bypass as compared to a patient having the procedure off-pump?
   A. Renal failure
   B. Embolization
   C. Infection
   D. Myocardial infarction

2. Your on-pump cardiac surgery patient has the following labs:

	On admission	Postoperative Day 1
Hgb	9.8 g/dL	9.5 g/dL
Hct	28.6%	27.5%
Platelets	140,000	70,000
PT	12.5 sec	12.8 sec
aPTT	36.5 sec	36.8 sec

Which should the nurse suspect?
A. Postoperative bleeding
B. Red blood cell hemolysis
C. Disseminated intravascular coagulation
D. Heparin-induced thrombocytopenia

3. Your patient has undergone on-pump coronary artery bypass grafting. For which set of data is the patient at risk for complications?

	HR	Temp	RR	WBC
A.	114	37.8°C (100°F)	16	10,000
B.	73	36.1°C (97°F)	14	2,000
C.	98	35.8°C (96.4°F)	22	3,000
D.	84	37.6°C (99.7°F)	18	14,000

4. Which statement by a nurse new to the cardiac surgery unit indicates that additional education is required?
A. "Patients who have off-pump procedures are more likely to need future interventions."
B. "With both on- and off-pump bypass, the heart is not beating for part of the procedure."
C. "There is less risk of aortic dissection with off-pump procedures."
D. "There is greater risk of bleeding with on-pump procedures."

5. Which patient is at greatest risk for a protamine reaction? A patient with a history of:
A. heparin-induced thrombocytopenia.
B. diabetes using NPH insulin.
C. other drug allergies.
D. asthma.

6. Which set of hemodynamic parameters is consistent with a patient experiencing a protamine reaction?

	B/P	HR	CO	PAP
A.	146/94	55	10	14/8
B.	70/52	108	3	40/28
C.	150/90	116	3.5	16.6
D.	88/50	50	9	38/25

7. Which patient is most likely to be at risk for postoperative on-pump complications? A patient with:
A. WBC 12.1/mm^3.
B. elevated cardiac markers.
C. elevated monocyte count.
D. lactate 4.2 mmol/L.

8. Your patient underwent off-pump coronary artery bypass surgery. For which is the patient at greatest risk?
A. Cognitive decline
B. Acute kidney injury
C. Stroke
D. Death

9. Which statement about an Allen test is true?
A. Prior to compressing the arteries, the patient should clench and unclench the hand 10 times.
B. If color is not restored after 5 seconds, a radial artery graft should not be done.
C. The radial and ulnar arteries are compressed in sequence and compared for time to color restoration.
D. Each artery should be kept compressed for 30 seconds and then released.

10. Which is an early sign of compartment syndrome?
A. Severe pain
B. Polar (cold)
C. Pallor
D. Paresthesia

Answers to Self-Assessment Questions

1. **B. embolization**
   Rationale: Data suggest a decreased risk of embolization in patients who undergo OPCAB. Negative effects of CPB include coagulation and microembolization.

2. **D. heparin-induced thrombocytopenia**
   Rationale: The patient's platelet count decreased by 50%. This is one of the clinical features of heparin-induced thrombocytopenia.

3.   C. **98 35.8°C (96.4°F)/22/3,000**
     Rationale: Patients undergoing ONCAB are at risk for moderate hypothermia (30°–34°C). This helps protect against intraoperative mortality.

4.   B. **"With both on- and off-pump bypass, the heart is not beating for part of the procedure."**
     Rationale: The heart is not beating with on-pump procedures only. Off-pump coronary artery bypass is also known as beating heart procedure.

5.   B. **diabetes using NPH insulin**
     Rationale: Patients with diabetes mellitus who are taking protamine (NPH) or protamine zinc insulin, those with a vasectomy, or those with an allergy to fish are at risk for a protamine reaction.

6.   D. **88/50 / 50 / 9 / 38/25**
     Rationale: Hypotension, decreased heart rate, pulmonary hypertension, shortness of breath, and temporary flushing are signs and symptoms of a hypersensitivity reaction. Patients experiencing anaphylaxis will experience hypertension, nausea, vomiting, fatigue, and back pain.

7.   D. **lactate 4.2 mmol/L**
     Rationale: Data suggest that patients who underwent OPCAB had less rise in serum lactate levels than patients who have undergone ONCAB. Both groups had elevated WBC count, neutrophils, monocytes, and cardiac markers postoperatively.

8.   D. **death**
     Rationale: Cognitive decline, development of acute kidney injury, and stroke is higher in patients who have undergone ONCAB. The mortality rate is higher in those patients who underwent OPCAB.

9.   B. **If color is not restored after 5 seconds, a radial artery graft should not be done.**
     Rationale: The patient should clench the hand 10 times. If color is not restored in 5 seconds, it indicates that the ulnar artery will not provide adequate circulation to the affected upper extremity if the radial artery is used for the procedure. The radial and ulnar arteries are compressed simultaneously, and the arteries should be compressed until the hand is clenched and unclenched 10 times.

10. A. **severe pain**
     Rationale: Early symptoms are severe pain and tenderness on passive stretch.

CLINICAL INQUIRY BOX

Question: Are there differences in the incidence of adverse events and mortality in patients undergoing on-pump versus off-pump coronary artery bypass grafting?

Reference: Shroyer, A. L., Hattler, B., Wagner, T. H., Collins, J. F., Baltz, J. H., Quin, J. A., . . . Grover, F. L. (2017). Five-year outcomes after on-pump and off-pump coronary-artery bypass. *The New England Journal of Medicine, 377*, 623–632.

Objective: To determine if there are differences in mortality and the incidence of adverse events in patients undergoing on-pump versus off-pump coronary artery bypass grafting.

Methods: Randomized controlled trial. Patients were randomized to OPCAB or ONCAB.

Results: Mortality rate was 15.2% in the OPCAB group versus 11.9% in the ONCAB group. Major adverse cardiac event rates were 31% in the OPCAB group versus 27.1% in the ONCAB group. No significant differences in nonfatal myocardial infarction, death from cardiac causes, repeat revascularization, or repeat coronary artery bypass grafting.

Conclusion: Off-pump procedures were associated with lower rates of 5-year survival and event-free survival compared to those who underwent ONCAB procedures.

References

Afrasiabirad, A., Safaie, N., & Montazerogoem, H. (2015). On-pump beating coronary artery bypass in high risk coronary patients. *Iranian Journal of Medical Sciences, 40*(1), 40–44.

Baikoussis, N. A., Papakonstantinou, N. A., & Apostolakis, E. (2014). Radial artery as graft for coronary artery bypass surgery: Advantages and disadvantages for its usage focused on structural and biological characteristics. *Journal of Cardiology, 63*(5), 321–328.

Bilgin, Y. M., & van de Watering, L. M. G. (2013). Complications after cardiac surgery due to allogeneic blood transfusions. *Journal of Clinical & Experimental Cardiology, S7.* doi:10.4172/2155-9880.S7-005. Retrieved from http://omicsonline.org/complications-after-cardiac-surgery-due-to-allogeneic-blood-transfusions-2155-9880-S7-005.php?aid=17752.

Blitz, A., Osterday, R. M., & Brodman, R. F. (2013). Harvesting the radial artery. *Annals of Cardiothoracic Surgery, 2*(4). Retrieved from http://www.annalscts.com/article/view/2418/3284.

Borde, D. P., Asegaonkar, B., Apsingekar, P., Khade, S., Futane, S., Khodve, B., . . . Joshi, S. (2016). Intraoperative conversion to on-pump coronary artery bypass grafting is independently associated with higher mortality in patients undergoing off-pump coronary artery bypass grafting: A propensity-matched analysis. *Annals of Cardiac Anaesthesia, 19*(3), 475–480.

Brewer, R., Theurer, P. F., Cogan, C. M., Bell, G. F., Prager, R. L., . . . Paone, G. (2014). Morbidity but not mortality is decreased after off-pump coronary artery bypass surgery. *Annals of Thoracic Surgery, 97*(3), 831–836.

Chakravarthy, M., Prabhakumar, D., Thimmannagowda, P., Krishnamoorthy, J., George, A., & Jawali, V. (2017). Comparison of two doses of heparin on outcome in off-pump coronary artery bypass surgery patients: A prospective randomized control study. *European Journal of Cardio-Thoracic Surgery, 53*(1), 79–111.

Cheng, A., & Slaughter, M. S. (2013). How I choose conduits and configure grafts for my patients—rationales and practices. *Annals of Cardiothoracic Surgery, 2*(4). Retrieved from http://www.annalscts.com/article/view/2417/3283.

Chocron, S., Vandel, P., Durst, C., Laluc, F., Kaili, D., Chocron, M., . . . Etievent, J-P. (2013). Antidepressant therapy in patients undergoing coronary artery bypass grafting: The MOTIV-CABG Trial. *The Annals of Thoracic Surgery, 95*(5), 1609–1618.

Evova, P. R. B., Bottura, C., Arcênciu, L., Sumarelli, A. A., Évova, P. M., & Rodrigues, A. J. (2016). Key points in curbing cardiopulmonary bypass inflammation. *Acta Cirugica Brasileira, 31*(Suppl 1). doi:10.1590/S0102-8650 2016001300010

Fröjd, V., & Jeppsson, A. (2016). Reexploration for bleeding and its association with mortality after cardiac surgery. *Annals of Thoracic Surgery, 102*(1), 109–117.

Greason, K. L., Kim, S., Suri, R. M., Wallace, A. S., & Englum, B. R. (2014). Hypothermia and operative mortality during on-pump coronary artery bypass grafting. *The Journal of Thoracic and Cardiovascular Surgery, 148*(6), 2712–2718.

Hosseinian, L., Weiner, M., Levin, M. A., & Fischer, G. W. (2016). Methylene blue: Magic bullet for vasoplegia? *Anesthesia & Analgesia, 122*(1), 194–201.

Hu, X., & Zhao, Q. (2011). Systematic comparison of the effectiveness of radial artery and saphenous vein or right internal thoracic artery coronary bypass grafts in non-left anterior descending coronary arteries. *Journal of Zhejiang University Science, 12*(4), 273–279.

Islam, M. Y., Ahmed, M. U., Khan, M. U., Bawany, F. I., Khan, F., & Arshad, M. H. (2014). On pump coronary artery bypass graft surgery versus off pump coronary artery bypass graft surgery: A review. *Global Journal of Health Science, 6*(3), 186–193.

Jongman, R. M., Zijlstra, J. G., Kok, W. F., van Harten, A. E., Mariani, M. A., Moser, J., . . . van Meurs, M. (2014). Off-pump CABG surgery reduces systemic inflammation compared with on-pump surgery but does not change systemic endothelial responses: A prospective randomized study. *Shock, 42*(2), 121–128.

Kalogianni, A., Almpani, P., Vastardis, L., Baltopoulos, G., Charitos, C. & Brokalaki, H. (2015). Can nurse-led preoperative education reduce anxiety and postoperative complications of patients undergoing cardiac surgery? *European Journal of Cardiovascular Nursing, 15*(6), 447–458.

Kennedy, E., Choy, K., Alston, R. P., Chen, S., Farhan-Alanie, M., Anderson, J., . . . Sykes, R. (2013). Cognitive outcomes after on- and off-pump coronary artery bypass grafting surgery: A systematic review and meta-analysis. *Journal of Cardiothoracic and Vascular Anesthesia, 27*, 253–265.

Kim, J. B., Yun, S. C., Lim, J. W., Hwang, S. K., Jung, S. H., Song, H., . . . Choo, S. J. (2014). Long-term survival following coronary artery bypass grafting off-pump versus on-pump strategies. *Journal of the American College of Cardiology, 63*(21), 2280–2288.

Kirmani, B. H., Brazier, A., Sriskandarajah, S., Alshawabkeh, Z., Gurung, L., Azzam, R., . . . Abunasra, H. (2016). Long-term survival after off-pump coronary artery bypass grafting. *Annals of Thoracic Surgery, 102*(1), 22–27.

Kirov, H., Schwarzer, M., Neugelbauer, S., Faerber, G., Diab, M., & Doenst, T. (2017). Metabolomic profiling in patients undergoing off-pump or on-pump coronary artery bypass surgery. *BMC Cardiovascular Disorders.* doi:10.1186/s12872-017-1710518-1

Koeola, Y., Itoh, T., Fusazaki, T., Nakamura, M., & Morino, Y. (2014). A unique stenosis in saphenous vein graft visualized by optical coherence tomography. *Heart and Vessels, 29*(2), 278–281.

Kowalewski, M., Pawliszak, W., Malvindi, P. G., Bokszanski, M. P., Perlinski, D., Raffa, G. M., . . . Anisimowicz, L. (2016). Off-pump coronary artery bypass grafting improves short-term outcomes in high-risk patients compared with on-pump coronary artery bypass grafting: Meta-analysis. *Journal of Thoracic and Cardiovascular Surgery, 151*(1), 60–77.

Krishnamoorthy, B., Critchley, W. R., Thompson, A. J., Payne, K., Morris, J., Venkateswaren, R. V., . . . Yonan, N. (2017). Study comparing vein integrity and clinical outcomes in open vein harvesting and 2 types of endoscopic vein harvesting for coronary artery bypass grafting: The VICO randomized clinical trial (Vein Integrity and Clinical Outcomes). *Circulation, 136*(18), 1688–1702.

Lazar, H. L. (2015). Off-pump coronary artery bypass: Past, present and future of a controversial technology. *Current Opinion in Cardiology 30*(6), 629–635.

Lee, C.-H., Cheng, H.-C., & Ko, L. W. (2013). Successful treatment of anaphylactic shock after protamine administration. Report of a case. *Emergency Medicine, 3.* doi:10.4172/2165-7548.1000157

Lin, J., Cheng, W., Czer, L. S., De Robertis, M. A., Mirocha, J., Ruzza, A., . . .Trento, A. (2013). Coronary artery bypass graft surgery using the radial artery as a secondary conduit improves patient survival. *Journal of the American Heart Association, 2*(4), e000266. doi:10.1161/JAHA.113.000266

Madani, H., Sadiki, E. O., Bouziane, M., Amaarouch, S., Madini, M., & Khalou, E. M. (2014). Anaphylaxis to protamine during cardiovascular surgery. *Annales Pharmaceutiques, Francaises, 72*(3), 143–145.

Man, A. (2018). Cardiac surgery: Aftercare. *The Pharmaceutical Journal.* Retrieved from https://www.pharmaceutical-journal.com/learning/learning-article/cardiac-surgery-caring-for-a-patient-and-managing-complications/2006681.article.

Moss, E., Puskas, J., Thourani, V., Kilgo, P., Chen, E., Leshnower, B., . . . Halkos, M. (2015). Avoiding aortic clamping during coronary artery bypass grafting reduces postoperative stroke. *Journal of Thoracic and Cardiovascular Surgery, 149*(1), 175–180.

Pagano, D., Milojevic, M., Meesters, M., Umberto, B., Bolliger, D., von Heymann, C., . . . Boer, C. (2017). 2017 EACTS/EACTA guidelines on patient blood management for adult cardiac surgery. *European Journal of Cardio-Thoracic Surgery, 53*(1), 79–111.

Paparella, D., Guida, P., Scrascia, G., Fanelli, V., Contini, M., Zaccaria, S., . . . Mazzei, V. (2015). On-pump versus off-pump coronary artery bypass surgery in patients with preoperative anemia. *Cardiovascular Surgery, 149*(4), 1018–1026.

Perrotti, A., Mariet, A., Durst, C., Monaco, F., Vandel, P., Monnet, E., . . . Chocron, S. (2016). Relationship between depression and health-related quality of life in patients undergoing coronary artery bypass grafting: a MOTIV-CABG substudy. *Quality of Life Research: An International Journal of Quality of Life Aspects of Treatment, Care and Rehabilitation, 25*(6), 1433–1440.

Puskas, J., Martin, J., Cheng, D., Benussi, S., Bonatti, J., Diegeler, A., . . . Zamvar, V. (2015). ISMICS consensus conference and statements of randomized controlled trials of off-pump versus conventional coronary artery bypass surgery. *Innovations, 10*(4), 219–229.

Ruzsa, Z., Tóth, K., Berta, B., Koncz, I., Szabo, G., Jambrik, Z., . . . Nemes, A. (2014). Allen's test in patients with peripheral artery disease. *European Journal of Medicine, 9*(1), 34–39.

Saeed, G. (2014). Radial artery: A valuable conduit for coronary artery bypass grafting with precise indications, contraindications, and surgical strategy. *Journal of the Saudi Heart Association, 26*(2), 127–128.

Shore-Lesserson, L., Baker, R. A., Ferraris, V. A., Greilich, P. E., Fitzgerald, D., Roman, P., . . . Hammon, J. W. (2018). The Society of Thoracic Surgeons, the Society of Cardiovascular Anesthesiologists, and the American Society of ExtraCorporeal Technology: Clinical practice guidelines—anticoagulation during cardiopulmonary bypass. *Annals of Thoracic Surgery, 105*(2), 650–662.

Shroyer, A. L., Grover, F. L., Hattler, B., Collins, J. F., McDonald, G. O., Kozora, E., . . . Novitzky, D. (2009). On-pump versus off-pump coronary-artery bypass surgery. *New England Journal of Medicine, 361,* 1827–1837.

Shroyer, A. L., Hattler, B., Wagner, T. H., Collins, J. F., Baltz, J. H., Quin, J. A., . . . Grover, F. L. (2017). Five-year outcomes after on-pump and off-pump coronary-artery bypass. *New England Journal of Medicine, 377,* 623–632.

Singh, A., & Mehta, Y. (2015). Intraoperative aortic dissection. *Annals of Cardiac Anaesthesia, 18,* 537–542.

Suelzu, S., Cossu, A., Pala, G., Portoghese, M., Columbanu, V., Sales, G., . . . Brazzi, L. (2015). Impact of different dosage of protamine on heparin reversal during off-pump coronary artery bypass: A clinical study. *Heart, Lung and Vessels, 7*(3), 238–245.

Taboulis, N. (2013). Total arterial coronary revascularization-patient selection, stenosis, conduits, targets. *Annals of Cardiothoracic Surgery, 2*(4). Retrieved from http://www.annalscts.com/article/view/2414/3280.

Te Kolste, H. J., Balm, R., & de Mol, B. (2015). Acute compartment syndrome of the lower leg after coronary artery bypass grafting: A silent but dangerous complication. *The Thoracic and Cardiovascular Surgeon, 63*(4), 300–306.

Vallely, M. P., Edelman, J. B., & Wilson, M. K. (2013). Bilateral internal mammary arteries: Evidence and technical considerations. *Annals of Cardiothoracic Surgery, 2*(4). Retrieved from http://www.annalscts.com/article/view/2423/3289.

Van Diepen, S., Katz, J., Albert, N., Henry, T. D., Jacobs, A. K., Kapur, N. K., . . . Cohen, M. (2017). Contemporary management of cardiogenic shock: A scientific statement from the American Heart Association. *Circulation, 137*(7), e1–e37.

Vukicevic, P., Mikic, N., Korur-Stevuljevic, J., Bogavac-Stanojevic, N., Milic, N., & Martinovic, J. (2016). Oxidative stress and platelet activation during on-pump and off-pump coronary artery bypass grafting in patients with double grafted vessels. *Biotechnological Equipment, 30,* 1132–1141.

Zhang, B., Zhou, J., Li, H., Liu, Z., Chen, A., & Zhao, Q. (2014). Comparison of graft patency between off-pump and on-pump coronary artery bypass grafting: An updated meta-analysis. *Annals of Thoracic Surgery, 97*(4), 1335–1341.

Web Resources

CABG 3-D video:

http://www.yourpracticeonline.com.au/cabg-surgery-3dvideo.html

Off-Pump Videos:

http://www.cts.usc.edu/videos-mpeg-offpumpcoronaryarterybypassgrafting.html

http://www.yourpracticeonline.com.au/opcab-surgery-3dvideo.html

CHAPTER 7

Minimally Invasive Cardiac Surgery

Alison Yam, Becky Dean, Kari Hatfield

▶ Introduction

After almost a decade of laparoscopic procedures being performed for gastrointestinal and gynecologic surgeries, cardiac surgeons began to accept the concept of minimally invasive cardiac surgery (MICS) in the mid-1990s (Doenst, Diab, Sponholz, Bauer, & Färber, 2017). While no official definition of MICS has been established, it is often defined as cardiac surgery without the use of cardiopulmonary bypass (CPB), without a median sternotomy, or both. Since the late 1990s, MICS has become much more popular. Like other surgical specialties, advances in minimally invasive procedures have been largely driven by the desire to reduce pain, surgical healing time, postoperative complications, and hospital length of stay (LOS). In cardiac surgical operations, the desire to minimize or avoid the use of CPB and all of the potential complications associated with it has been a primary endpoint. In addition, reducing the potential for both respiratory dysfunction and the morbidity associated with deep sternal wound infection prompted the use of alternative surgical incisions to avoid the use of a median sternotomy.

Improvements in MICS have progressed to such a degree that it has become common to perform coronary artery bypass grafting (CABG) without the use of CPB. However, since the early 2000s, perhaps the greatest advances in MICS have been appreciated in the area of valve repair/replacement surgery. This chapter describes a variety of MICS procedures for coronary revascularization, valve repair/replacement, and atrial fibrillation (AF) surgery. In addition, the relatively new procedure for percutaneous valve repair/replacement is discussed.

▶ Minimally Invasive Coronary Revascularization

Since the 1960s, traditional CABG surgery has entailed creating a median sternotomy incision,

Original contributions from Tamara S. Goda, Brianna Gee

aortic cross-clamping, and being connected to a bypass machine to maintain oxygenation and perfusion during cardiac standstill (Dieberg, Smart, & King, 2016). Cardiopulmonary bypass refers to the temporary rerouting of blood from the right atrium to the aorta via an oxygenator (bypass machine), such that blood flow is circumvented around the heart and lungs during the surgical procedure (Sarkar & Prabhu, 2017). During a CABG, a bypass conduit is harvested, and new avenues for oxygenated blood are created from the aorta to the targeted blood vessel, "bypassing" the diseased segment of coronary artery.

Traditional CABG surgery is associated with a prolonged ventilation time (initially days; now 8–12 hours), prolonged intensive care unit (ICU) stay (initially 1 week; now 24 hours if the case is uncomplicated), prolonged hospitalization (initially several weeks; now 1 week), a prolonged rehabilitation phase (now 8–12 weeks), and potential sternal wound infection (SWI). Other complications associated with traditional CABG and their associated etiologies are listed in **TABLE 7.1**. These and other complications associated with CABG provided the impetus to develop procedures to perform CABG in a less invasive way.

TABLE 7.1 Pathophysiologic Changes Associated with a Traditional CABG Procedure and CPB	
Pathophysiologic Change	**Etiology**
Bleeding and thrombotic complications: disseminated intravascular coagulation, heparin-induced thrombocytopenia, and thrombosis	■ Activation of platelets and plasma proteins ■ Patients are heparinized and given supplementary doses during bypass, titrated against clotting studies ■ Bleeding times after full reversal of heparin do not become normalized for as long as 12 hours after bypass
Considerable interstitial fluid shifts	■ Increased systemic venous pressure ■ Volume loading ■ Decreased plasma protein concentration (secondary to dilution and absorption onto the bypass circuit, and the inflammatory response increasing capillary permeability)
Increased levels of cortisol, epinephrine, and norepinephrine (remain elevated for at least 24 hours)	■ Stress of surgery ■ Hypothermia ■ Cardiopulmonary bypass ■ Nonpulsatile flow
Hyperglycemia	■ Stress of surgery ■ Hypothermia ■ Cardiopulmonary bypass ■ Nonpulsatile flow
Decreased circulating triiodothyronine (T3)	■ Stress of surgery ■ Hypothermia ■ Cardiopulmonary bypass ■ Nonpulsatile flow

Pathophysiologic Change	Etiology
Decreased myocardial compliance and contractility	■ Myocardial stunning ■ Ischemia ■ Edema ■ Cardiac handling during surgery ■ Direct injury to the myocardium
Decreased myocardial function related to cardioplegia and surgical arrest (for 6–8 hours postoperatively)	■ Ischemia-reperfusion injury ■ Inflammatory injury due to cardiopulmonary bypass
Progressive need for volume resuscitation	■ Vasodilation ■ Capillary leak ■ Anemia ■ Hypovolemic shock
Pulmonary edema	■ Activation of complement system ■ Sequestration of neutrophils in pulmonary vasculature (can mediate increase in capillary permeability, which is compounded by fluid shifts)
Pulmonary dysfunction	■ Cardiopulmonary bypass decreases the effect of surfactant ■ General anesthesia ■ Median sternotomy ■ Cardiopulmonary bypass increases shunts, decreases compliance and functional residual volume, and can cause acute lung injury
Ischemic stroke	■ Emboli released during the cannulation and clamping of the aorta
Hemorrhagic stroke	■ Anticoagulation necessary for bypass
Impaired renal function	■ Hemodilution ■ Microemboli ■ Catecholamines ■ Low perfusion pressure ■ Diuretics ■ Hypothermia ■ Hemolysis
Peptic ulceration	■ Stress response
Endotoxin translocation, adding to the inflammatory response	■ Greater permeability of gut mucosa

Data from Adamik, B., Kubler, A., Gozdzik, A., & Gozdzik, W., 2017; Grosset-Janin, Barth, Bertrand, Detante, 2015; Lomivorotov, Efremov, Kirov, Fominskiy, & Karaskov, 2017; Mao et al., 2015; Saito et al., 2015; Sarkar & Prabhu, 2017; Chikwe, Donaldson, & Wood, 2006; Sinan, 2015; Sugita & Fujiu, 2018; Pickering, James & Palmer, 2015; Theile, Isbell & Rosner, 2015; Theissen, Vanhorebeek, & Van den Berghe, 2015; Thielmann et al., 2017.

Several different MICS procedures for coronary revascularization have been developed, each of which has its own patient selection criteria. Two approaches that can be used for these procedures are anterior mini-thoracotomy incisions and an endoscopic approach. The major types of MICS procedures that are currently performed include off-pump coronary artery bypass (OPCAB), minimally invasive direct coronary artery bypass (MIDCAB), or totally endoscopic or robot-assisted coronary artery bypass (TECAB). Both MIDCAB and TECAB can be performed with or without the use of CPB support. A number of alternative names for these various MICS procedures appear in the literature.

Off-Pump Coronary Artery Bypass

Coronary artery bypass grafting done without the use of CPB—"off pump"—is also known as beating heart surgery, and is commonly and routinely utilized for full coronary revascularization. One or both of the internal thoracic arteries (ITA), the saphenous vein, or radial arteries, harvested in typical fashion, can be utilized for this procedure. However, an endoscopic vein harvest approach is noninferior to an open harvest, which reduces wound-related complications and increases overall patient satisfaction. The endoscopic approach has also been shown to reduce major adverse cardiac events (Halkos et al., 2014).

Off-pump coronary artery bypass is often performed using the median sternotomy incision to gain full access for all vessels, including those on the back of the heart, for revascularization. Special equipment has been developed that allows the surgeon to position the heart to isolate the diseased vessel and stabilize the localized region of epicardium for anastomosis without cardioplegic arrest—while the heart is beating. The stabilizer (see Chapter 6) provides a direct view, dampens the movement of the epicardium, and permits a nontraumatic grip on the beating heart (Yanagawa & Puskas, 2016). In addition to specific surgeon skill, OPCAB surgery requires meticulous attention by cardiac anesthesia as heart rate and blood pressure are extremely labile with manipulation of the beating heart (Alston, 2015).

The International Society of Minimally Invasive Cardiac Surgery (ISMICS) reviewed over 100 randomized controlled studies to assess short- and long-term outcomes of OPCAB and conventional coronary artery bypass (CCAB). The ISMICS recommended short-term outcomes of OPCAB, which may include reduced risk of stroke, AF, wound infection, blood transfusion, ventilation time, and hospital LOS. Additionally, patients particularly at high risk because of renal disease, cirrhosis of the liver, and calcific disease of the ascending aorta may benefit from avoidance of aortic cross-clamping and exposure to CPB. However, long-term outcomes may include reduced graft patency, increased risk of cardiac reintervention, and increased mortality (Puskas et al., 2015). Additional information regarding OPCAB is covered in detail in Chapter 6.

Minimally Invasive Direct Coronary Artery Bypass

Minimally invasive direct coronary artery bypass, which is an alternative approach to traditional CABG, has been performed since the 1990s (Melly, Torregrossa, Lee, Jansens, & Puskas, 2018). In lieu of a median sternotomy, a left lateral thoracotomy incision is made. There are a variety of incision sizes and variations, but most typically a 5- to 6-cm incision is created along the fourth intercostal space. Rib spreaders are used to spread and elevate the rib cage to provide ample space to dissect the ITA. The left mini-thoracotomy approach provides direct visualization of the left anterior descending (LAD) artery and the anastomotic site when a left internal thoracic artery (LITA) to the LAD is being performed (Ling, Bao, Yang, Chen, & Gao, 2016). Off-pump coronary artery bypass can be applied to a MIDCAB approach (Alston, 2015).

Minimally invasive direct coronary artery bypass surgery is now utilized for full multivessel revascularization; however, patient selection criteria and surgeon expertise play into the equation when MIDCAB is being considered as a surgical option. Differences between MIDCAB and traditional CABG are primarily related to the incision size and associated surgical trauma. During this procedure, the patient is intubated with a double-lumen endotracheal tube, thereby allowing for ventilation of the right lung and deflation of the left lung, providing more room to manipulate the heart. In addition to the incision size being much smaller, a left lateral incision 4 to 6 inches in length is made between the ribs, thereby avoiding a full sternotomy. Importantly, because MIDCAB is typically a beating heart procedure, no cardioplegia or CPB is utilized, thereby avoiding the issues related to the pump and myocardial arrest (Raja et al., 2018; Tekin & Arslan, 2017).

Documented advantages of MIDCAB include decreased pain secondary to a less invasive surgical approach, earlier mobilization secondary to decreased pain, shorter ICU and hospital LOS, decreased infection rates especially with SWIs, earlier return to baseline physical activities, and reduced transfusion requirements. Most importantly, preliminary data on the long-term patency of MIDCAB grafts show that it appears to be comparable to traditional CABG (Dieberg et al., 2016; Zhang et al., 2015).

TABLE 7.2 lists additional advantages and disadvantages of the MIDCAB approach.

TABLE 7.2 Advantages and Disadvantages of the MIDCAB Approach

Advantages	Disadvantages
Faster recovery/return to routine ADLs	Limited access and exposure to the operative area
Long-term graft patency appears to be similar to that of traditional CABG	Technical difficulty with beating heart
No risk of SWI	Steep learning curve; need experienced surgeon to perform
LITA/RITA more resistant to atherosclerosis/increased longevity of patency	Increased risk of incomplete revascularization
No adverse effects related to CPB	Unable to access/visualize posterior heart for revascularization
Cosmetic results; no sternotomy	MIDCAB limits target vessels
Shorter hospital stay	Acute graft occlusion and incomplete revascularization risk increased
Decreased blood loss and transfusion requirements	Thoracotomy incision can be painful
Shorter postoperative ventilation time	Decreased exposure to coronary vasculature
No aortic manipulation	Less choice of vessels that can be grafted (usually only the internal thoracic artery to the LAD)
Capable of revascularization of multivessel lesions	More trauma to costal cartilage
Decreased risk of musculoskeletal injury	
Can be used for primary or redo procedures	
No risk of SIRS, coagulopathies, thromboembolic events, endothelial dysfunction, dysrhythmias, or MODS associated with CPB	
No risk of aortic dissection or neurologic consequences associated with aortic cross-clamping	
Decreased risk of stroke	
Decreased OR time	
Decreased incidence of AF	

ADLs, activities of daily living; AF, atrial fibrillation; CABG, coronary artery bypass grafting; CPB, cardiopulmonary bypass; LAD, left anterior descending; LITA, left internal thoracic artery; MIDCAB, minimally invasive direct coronary artery bypass; MODS, multiple organ dysfunction syndrome; OR, operating room; RITA, right internal thoracic artery; SWI, sternal wound infection; SIRS, systemic inflammatory response syndrome.
Data from Bojar, 2011; Dieberg et al. 2016; Iribarne et al., 2011; Ling et al., 2016; Pike, 2015; Raja et al., 2018; Tekin & Arslan, 2017; Zhang et al., 2015.

Robotic Assisted or Totally Endoscopic Coronary Artery Bypass Grafting

There has been a growing body of research around the use of robotics in coronary artery revascularization surgery since the introduction of surgical robotics in the 1990s (Melly et al., 2018). Minimally invasive equipment had reached its limits; the two-dimensional (2-D) endoscopic camera impaired visualization and challenged precise manipulation by surgeons. Historically, surgical interventions were innovated such as the Automated Endoscopic System for Optimal Positioning (AESOP) and ZEUS Robotic Surgical System. Modern equipment has evolved for robotic surgical intervention to the current and only clinically available da Vinci® Surgical System (Intuitive Surgical, Inc.) (**FIGURE 7.1**).

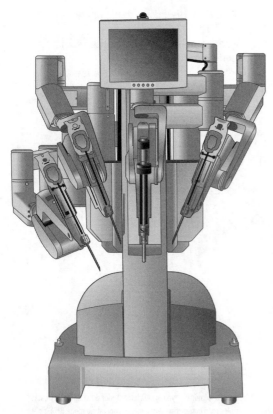

FIGURE 7.1 da Vinci® Surgical System.
Courtesy of Intuitive Surgical System

The first robotically assisted CABG was performed in 1998 using the da Vinci surgical robot. The da Vinci surgical system allows the surgeon to access the heart through 4, half-inch incisions made in the intercostal spaces; these incisions are used to introduce instruments and a videoscope. Micro-instruments receive digital instructions from an interfaced computer. The (real-life) surgeon stays seated at a computer console with a 3-dimensional (3-D) display and acts as the "driver" of the computer. The surgeon initiates the digital instructions by controlling the hand grips. By using the hand grips, the surgeon's hand movements at the console are then duplicated by the robot, with software filtering out physiologic hand tremors (Gao, 2014).

Totally endoscopic coronary artery bypass grafting procedures are performed entirely through trocar accesses without surgical incision, the majority of which are performed robotically (Leonard et al., 2018). These procedures are primarily selected when the LITA is harvested and used to graft a diseased LAD graft. Through a series of instrument exchanges, the LITA can be harvested, the pericardium opened, the LAD identified and stabilized, and the LITA to LAD anastomosis performed. Multivessel bypass grafting can also be performed by robotically assisted takedown of the LITA followed by a MIDCAB. This can be accomplished using either remote access perfusion or endoballoon aortic occlusion on the beating or arrested heart. Despite successful reports of TECAB, this operation has not become widely accepted mainly because of the increased time and personnel requirements of the surgical robot; and a traditional approach is easier when multiple grafts are needed, although MIDCAB and TECAB perform equally in terms of perioperative results—yocardial infarction and stroke—and midterm follow-up (Kofler et al., 2017).

▶ Hybrid Coronary Revascularization

Hybrid coronary revascularization (HCR) is a newer approach to treating multivessel coronary artery disease (CAD). Clinical trials ASCERT,

FREEDOM, and SYNTAX comparing survival rates of CABG to percutaneous coronary intervention (PCI) patients have supported superior long-term survival with CABG. The LITA to LAD bypass graft is thought to be a contributor, as most of the left ventricular blood supply comes from the left main coronary artery. Hybrid coronary revascularization combines the survival benefits of the LITA to LAD bypass graft with a minimally invasive technique, and other diseased vessels are treated with PCI. Currently this procedure has been reserved for those patients who are too high risk for more traditional procedures because of the high rate of reintervention that is required following PCI. However, as drug eluting stent technology evolves and the need for reintervention becomes less, HCR may quickly become a viable option for many patients with multivessel CAD who desire a less invasive procedure. Cardiothoracic surgeons and interventional cardiologists have worked together as pioneers of this procedure, and it is possible that their roles may merge in the future (Melly et al., 2018). Among elderly patients with a Class 1 indication for CABG who were randomized to receiving PCI or CABG, those who received PCI had shorter hospital stays and fewer discharges to rehabilitation facilities but had higher rates of repeat revascularization (Barsoum et al., 2016).

Minimally invasive CABG with the usage of either single or bilateral internal thoracic arteries (SITA/BITA) is another approach that may provide an additional option for patients who might not otherwise be a candidate for a traditional CABG procedure. Using this approach, there were no significant differences in major complications—deaths, stroke, or new-onset renal failure requiring temporary dialysis. Additionally, there was no need for conversion to a sternotomy, there was no need to convert to using bypass, nor were there any major complications while harvesting the vessels (Kikuchi, Chen, Mori, Kurata, & Tao, 2017).

The ITA graft is the gold standard with a patency rate of approximately 90%. This is superior to the saphenous vein (SV), which has a patency rate of 50% to 60% (Baikoussis, Papakonstantinou, & Apostolakis, 2014). However,

endoscopic technology can be used to harvest the greater saphenous vein. Instead of a long incision spanning the thigh to the lower leg, or both legs, the vein can be dissected out using the endoscope and various instruments that may also cut or burn branches of the vein while it is still in the leg. This technology has also been adopted and applied to assist with removal of the radial artery from the forearm (Ferdinand et al., 2017; Tribble & Urencio, 2015). Utilization of additional arterial conduits—bilateral ITAs, radial arteries (RAs), the right gastroepiploic artery (GEA), and the inferior epigastric artery (IEA)—has been recommended to improve long-term graft patency and outcomes. An Allen test (see Chapter 6) or modified Allen test (using pulse oximeter) must be performed prior to radial artery removal to guarantee adequate collateral circulation in the extremity. However, this test has a high false-positive rate, and supplementary assessment techniques such as digital plethysmography and Doppler ultrasonography have been used (Baikoussis et al., 2014).

Endoscopic vein harvest (EVH) for saphenous vein and endoscopic radial artery harvest (ERAH) are performed through much smaller incisions. Compared with open harvest, these procedures reduce surgical trauma, postoperative LOS, wound resource utilization and increase patient satisfaction. The ISMICS has issued recommendations (Class 1, Level B) that endoscopic saphenous vein and radial artery harvesting should be the standard if these conduits are required for coronary revascularization. Although endoscopic conduit harvest is more widely used, highly skilled operators and a standardized harvesting technique are necessary to maintain quality of the conduit and to avoid neurologic or infectious complications (Ferdinand et al., 2017).

The most recent literature suggests that HCR is appropriate and safe particularly for patients who are elderly, have CAD that is stable, favorable anatomy as evidenced by preoperative computed tomography (CT) angiogram—which reduces the need for prior diagnostic cardiac catheterization (Doenst et al., 2017)—preserved or mildly reduced ejection fraction, and intermediate risk and SYNTAX scores. Hybrid coronary revascularization additionally provides a number of short-term advantages, including lower perioperative complications, fewer blood transfusions, no SWI, reduced postoperative AF, shorter ventilatory time, shorter hospital LOS, increased patient satisfaction with the procedure, aesthetic appearance and minimal scarring, and earlier return to society (Panoulas, Colombo, Margonato, & Maisano, 2015; Rosenblum et al., 2016).

▶ Minimally Invasive Valve Surgery

Perhaps the greatest advances in MICS have been realized in the area of valve repair and replacement procedures. With the advent of new surgical instrumentation, including robotics, MICS has become widely accepted for certain surgical conditions, specifically valve repair/replacement (mitral, aortic, pulmonic, or tricuspid), pulmonary vein isolation and the Maze procedure to treat AF, congenital cardiac defects (e.g., atrial septal defects), and descending thoracic aortic aneurysm disease treatment (Appoo et al., 2014; Gregory et al., 2018; Jung & Kim, 2016; Lancaster, Melby, & Damiano, 2016). Unlike coronary revascularization, aortic and mitral valve surgeries always require CPB and cardioplegia; however, various alternate approaches have allowed for these procedures to be performed minimally invasively (Algarni, Suri, & Schaff, 2015).

Minimally Invasive Mitral Valve Surgery (MIMVS)

Mitral regurgitation is associated with severe left ventricular dysfunction as a result of CAD or idiopathic myocardial disease. The large, dilated left ventricle causes papillary muscle displacement, which results in leaflet tethering and associated annular dilation, preventing adequate leaflet coaptation (Nishimura et al., 2017). The first MIMVS was performed in the mid-1990s though a parasternal incision. Since then, various pioneers—including Drs. Cosgrove, Carpentier,

and Chitwood—developed and refined procedures that allowed for port access, video assistance and direction, transthoracic aortic cross-clamping, and retrograde cardioplegia. There is some evidence, however, that antegrade perfusion is better and more physiological, and is associated with lower incidence of neurologic complications, and prevents wound dehiscence and pseudoaneurysm complications related to femoral cannulation (Glauber et al., 2015a).

In 1996, the first minimally invasive mitral valve repair was performed using the da Vinci surgical system (Algarni et al., 2015). Currently many institutions are performing MIMVS. Although robotically assisted mitral valve surgery is being performed at various centers of excellence throughout the country and around the world, it has been limited by the rigorous training of the surgeon and the financial backing of the institution in terms of the cost of a dedicated robotic surgical system.

Various incisions can be utilized for MIMVS, such as the mini-sternotomy, the parasternal incision, the port-access technique, and the right mini-thoracotomy (Van Praet et al., 2018). The most common approach is a right anterior mini-thoracotomy incision. This approach allows the surgeon to gain access to the mitral valve through the left atrium. The valve can either be repaired or replaced. During a repair, the valve leaflets are brought back together and the annulus reinforced with a ring to prevent further dilatation. During a replacement, the native valve is removed and fully replaced with either a bioprosthetic or mechanical implant (Glauber et al., 2015a). The least invasive approach is the robotic-assisted MIMVS, which is performed through 1- to 2-cm robotic access port incisions without a thoracotomy or rib spreading (Algarni et al., 2015).

During robotic-assisted procedures, the surgeon sits at the control and looks through two lenses (like a microscope) that display the image from the camera. The computer generates a 3-D image of the surgical site. As the surgeon moves, the robotic arms mimic the multidirectional movements that may be even more precise than the surgeon's natural hand movement (Gao, 2014). Various instruments are utilized and exchanged

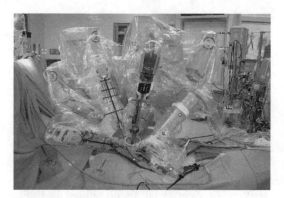

FIGURE 7.2 da Vinci Surgical System®.
Courtesy of East Carolina Heart Institute

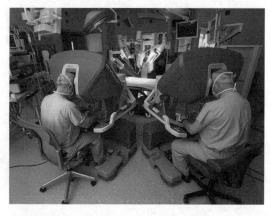

FIGURE 7.3 da Vinci Surgical System®.
Courtesy of East Carolina Heart Institute

through the access ports to allow the surgeon to repair or replace the valve. Additionally, specially designed titanium clips (the Cor-Knot™) are used to secure the valve sutures rather than tying knots. See **FIGURES 7.2** and **7.3**.

Various access techniques have been developed for cannulation and the institution of CPB to assist with MIMVS. Typical cannulation for minimal MIMVS involves cannulation of the femoral vasculature. However, central cannulation using the superior/inferior vena cava and the aorta can also be utilized in MIMVS to avoid the potential complications associated with lower extremity cannulation (Pope & Ailawadi, 2014). Improvements in both CPB equipment and technique now allow for percutaneous cannulation of the lower extremities, making femoral cannulation less risky.

Regardless of the approach, the primary benefit of MIMVS is the avoidance of a median sternotomy. In some cases, even though a minimally invasive approach is intended, some patients may need to be converted to a full sternotomy due to bleeding, adhesions, or dissection. Decreased hospital LOS and reduced pain and potential for complications, combined with increased patient satisfaction and earlier return to full activity, have propelled MIMVS to popularity (Glauber et al., 2015a). In many centers, MIMVS has shown equivalent or superior outcomes of in-hospital mortality, stroke rates, repairability index of mitral valve, long-term durability of valve, and less blood transfusion compared with traditional valve surgery (Algarni et al., 2015).

The various incisions utilized for mitral valve surgery are shown in **FIGURE 7.4**.

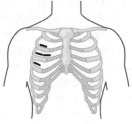

Robotic-Assisted
Heart Surgery
(Closed Surgery)

Less than 2 inch incision and
four (4) robotic ports

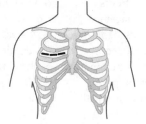

Right Thoracotomy

3–4 inch incision on side of chest

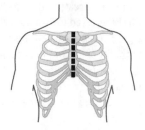

Median Sternotomy
(Open Surgery)

6–8 inch incision in
middle of chest

FIGURE 7.4 Mitral valve repair surgical comparison.

BOX 7.1 Robotic Surgery Procedures

- Single-vessel and multivessel CABG
- Mitral valve repair and replacement
- Aortic valve repair and replacement
- ASD repair
- VSD repair
- Removal of cardiac tumors
- Ablation for treatment of atrial fibrillation (Maze procedure)

ASD, atrial septal defect; CABG, coronary artery bypass grafting; VSD, ventricular septal defect.

Endoscopic procedures have another benefit: They assist in making reentry into the sternum safer. Using this approach, the surgeon can readily visualize structures behind the sternum. Adhesions can form between the heart and the sternum, which can cause damage to the heart if reentry is required. Now the adhesions can be cut with the assistance of the scope prior to a second sternotomy, thereby reducing the risk of damaging the heart.

BOX 7.1 outlines procedures that can be performed with robotic assistance.

Minimally Invasive Tricuspid Valve Surgery

Tricuspid valve (TV) disease has traditionally been considered less clinically important than mitral or aortic valve disease, and effective management and treatment is controversial. Patients are rarely referred for isolated TV repair/replacement, with most procedures done simultaneously with other planned cardiac surgery procedures. Tricuspid regurgitation (TR) can lead to functional impairment and has an adverse impact on perioperative outcomes, functional class, and survival. Tricuspid regurgitation is generally well tolerated, but in the presence of pulmonary hypertension, cardiac output declines and right heart failure worsens. Despite improved actuarial survival in patients undergoing TV annuloplasty at the time of mitral valve (MV) surgery, TR remains frequently undertreated.

Tricuspid regurgitation may be classified as primary, accounting for 25% of cases, or secondary "functional" TR. Primary cases are caused by a leaflet abnormality due to a congenital cause—Ebstein's anomaly, valve tethering due to ventricular septal aneurysm or defect—or an acquired cause, such as endocarditis, rheumatic fever, toxins, or trauma. Secondary causes include left heart disease (including mitral valve disease); right ventricular dysfunction due to cardiomyopathy, ischemia, or volume overload; pulmonary hypertension; or right atrial abnormalities, including AF (Rodés-Cabau et al., 2016).

Determining the etiology of secondary TR is crucial, and a right heart catheterization will assist with this determination. It is important to rule out the presence of precapillary pulmonary hypertension, both the degree and origin, which will guide treatment and help determine whether or not to treat severe TR. Because TR can vary according to the preload, afterload, and right ventricular function, the assessments of leaflet morphology, annular dimension (from the middle part of the septal annulus to the middle part of the anterior annulus), and pulmonary artery pressure are particularly important for determining management. Further imaging with a transthoracic echocardiogram (TTE) and a transesophageal echocardiogram (TEE) may be performed. There is some debate regarding the utility of a TTE due to the variability of the imaging planes as well as technical difficulty in performing due to body habitus of the patient, but it can be helpful in the initial diagnosis of TR. A TEE provides a more thorough and comprehensive view of the TV and should include mid-esophageal, deep-esophageal, and transgastric views. Other imaging modalities include 3-D echocardiography, multidetector computed tomography (MDCT), and cardiac magnetic resonance (CMR), but there are limitations and challenges to using these (Rodés-Cabau et al., 2016).

Tricuspid annulus diameter greater than 40 mm or 21 mm/m^2 measured in the 4-chamber view should indicate the need for TV repair, which should be prioritized in patients with preoperative AF. Management guidelines indicate a move toward more aggressive treatment of TR. For patients undergoing left-sided valve surgery,

TV repair or replacement is universally recommended in the presence of severe TR or tricuspid annular dilatation because it does not resolve spontaneously after correction of MV disease as once believed (Ricci et al., 2014).

Like other cardiac surgeries, a median sternotomy has been the standard of care for tricuspid valve repair. This is especially risky because of the position of the right heart in relation to the sternum due to right ventricular dilation. Preserving the integrity of the ventricle may prevent further dilation after repair or replacement and further progression of right heart failure (Misfeld et al., 2017).

Minimally invasive TR repair is a novel treatment option with great potential. In ex vivo porcine models, the MitraClip (Abbott Vascular), which has been approved for mitral valve procedures, was used off label in simulated TR conditions. One or two clips were placed along the valve leaflets and immediate postprocedural hemodynamic measurements were obtained, with immediate improvement in the right heart cardiac output (Vismara et al., 2016). Minol and colleagues (2014) and Ricci and colleagues (2014) describe using a mini-thoracotomy for isolated TV repair with promising results. In-hospital mortality was previously reported as 13% to 26% for isolated TV surgery. In the Minol cohort, in-hospital mortality was 4%, with a 1-year mortality of 20%. The Ricci cohort reported hospital mortality of 7.8%, with 5-year survival between 81.3% and 94.1%.

There are a number of devices and procedures in development with promising results. Campelo-Parada and colleagues (2015) used the FORMA Repair System (Edwards Lifesciences), which is an innovative transcatheter treatment approach for patients with severe TR and who are considered to be at high or prohibitive risk for surgery. The device is intended to reduce severe TR by occupying the regurgitant area and providing a surface for leaflet coaptation. The procedure is done via the left axillary vein with fluoroscopy to ensure adequate device positioning. Patients in this study were without major intraoperative or postoperative complications. There were also no complications related to the access site or the device at 30 days postprocedure, and all patients experienced a reduction in their TR symptoms

and improvement in their functional status (Campelo-Parada et al., 2015).

The SCOUT trial was a small, multicenter trial utilizing the Trialign System (Mitralign Inc.). In this study, a guidewire was inserted in the right coronary artery (RCA) to assist with identifying the position relative to the tricuspid annulus (TA). Two 14-French gauge sheaths were introduced into the right jugular vein for delivery of the device. A guide catheter was introduced to position a wire delivery catheter beneath the TA, in the posteroseptal position. Before crossing the TA, TEE imaging is used to visualize the wire delivery catheter and confirm (1) annular depth 2 to 4 mm from the base of the leaflet, (2) distance from the RCA, and (3) direction (into the right atrium). Sutures are then deployed to repair the valve leaflets by reducing the annular dimensions and regurgitant orifice. There was a 93% procedural success rate, with no procedural mortality, no emergency reintervention, no 30-day mortality, and improved New York Heart Association (NYHA) functional class in all patients (Hahn et al., 2017).

Tricuspid surgery is evolving and there are a number of devices in development, including the TriCinch System™ (4Tech) and the SAPIEN XT valve (Edwards Lifesciences). Most of the data regarding tricuspid surgery are limited to small trials with fewer than 75 patients, but the results are promising. Tricuspid valve surgery may now be an option for people who have been previously denied surgical intervention and managed medically. As surgeons advance and become more comfortable with tricuspid surgical interventions, TV surgery may be utilized more frequently, even in patients who are considered to be high risk.

Minimally Invasive Aortic Valve Replacement

The first minimally invasive aortic valve replacement (MIAVR) was described in 1996. Since that time, there has been significant evolution and acceptance of this procedure. The most commonly seen incision for MIAVR is a partial upper mini-sternotomy; a right anterior mini-thoracotomy can also be utilized. Both of these approaches allow the surgeon to gain access while maintaining the stability of the rib cage. In addition to the smaller incision, several cannulation methods for institution of CPB have also been described for MIAVR. Cannulation by ascending aorta may avoid wound infection, pseudoaneurysms, and neurologic complications associated with peripheral cannulation (Glauber, Ferrarini, & Miceli, 2015b). Minimally invasive aortic valve replacement improved patient satisfaction, LOS, and ventilation time (despite a longer operative time) compared to traditional aortic valve replacement (Pope & Ailawadi, 2014).

Transcatheter Aortic Valve Replacement

One of the most recent breakthroughs in MICS is that of transcatheter aortic valve replacement (TAVR). The first TAVR performed on an adult occurred in Europe in early 2002 by the French interventional cardiologist Alain G. Cribier. The driving force behind this innovation was the need to provide a suitable and effective alternative to surgical aortic valve replacement (SAVR) in select patients with severe aortic stenosis for whom a surgical intervention was deemed to be too high risk. Since then, minimally invasive valve replacement methods have rapidly evolved. Transcatheter aortic valve replacements have been performed in the United States since 2007 as part of clinical trials, most notably the PARTNER (Placement of AoRTic TraNscathetER) trial utilizing the Edwards Lifesciences SAPIEN bioprosthetic stent heart valve (**FIGURE 7.5**) that received U.S. Food and Drug Administration approval for commercial use in nonsurgical candidates in 2011. Today, new-generation transcatheter heart valves (THVs), such as the Edwards Lifesciences SAPIEN XT and Medtronic CoreValve™, are available to both high-risk nonsurgical and surgical candidates alike. Previously, TAVR procedures were mostly confined to the high-risk surgical population who had been refused SAVR. However, this patient selection is shifting toward lower risk patients, and their outcomes are being

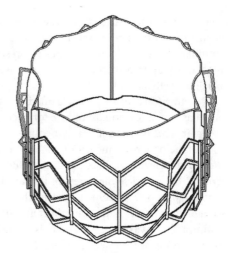

FIGURE 7.5 The SAPIEN transcatheter heart valve.
Illustrated by James R. Perron

investigated in PARTNER II and SURTAVI trials. Surgical risk algorithms such as EuroSCORE II and Society of Thoracic Surgeons (STS) are meant to provide a more accurate mortality rate for high-risk patients (Rozeik, Wheatley, & Gourlay, 2014).

Access routes for TAVRs include transfemoral (TF), transapical (TA), transaortic, transaxillary/trans-subclavian, transcaval, transcarotid, and transeptal. Determination of the best access route is made based on a multitude of factors, including vessel size and integrity, previous sternotomies, comorbid conditions, ejection fraction, and suitability for other approaches. The TF route is the most common and preferred access site for TAVR. The TF-TAVR is contraindicated in patients who have small vessel diameter and highly calcified or tortuous vessels (Greenbaum et al., 2017; Pascural et al., 2017; Rozeik et al., 2014). In these cases, alternative entry sites are chosen. Transcatheter aortic valve replacements can be performed either totally percutaneously or via a small right anterior thoracotomy incision. In the TF approach, a delivery catheter is threaded up the femoral artery via an introducer sheath and reaches the aortic valve in a retrograde fashion by way of the descending and ascending aortae. Older generation THVs required sheaths as large as 24-French, which could lead to major vascular complications. Newer generation THVs reduce this risk with smaller sheath sizes, which vary from 16- to 18-French. The THV is guided into position under echocardiography and fluoroscopy, and once in place, the new valve is deployed against the orifice of the native valve. A transvenous pacer lead wire is placed in the right ventricle via the right femoral vein. A 6- or 7-French venous sheath is typically used for this purpose. Pacing may be required should conduction problems occur during the procedure. Also, depending on the type of valve being placed (SAPIEN versus CoreValve), deployment of the valve is done during rapid ventricular pacing (RVP), which is necessary when using balloon devices to reduce forward blood flow and pulse pressure. This prevents migration of the valve and provides for optimal stability during expansion and deployment (Rozeik et al., 2014).

The TA approach requires a mini-thoracotomy. The aortic valve is accessed through the apex of the left ventricle. The transaortic access is achieved with either a mini-sternotomy or right thoracotomy and the aortic valve is reached through the ascending aorta. Axillary or subclavian TAVRs also provide for a shorter and more direct pathway to the aortic valve. However, certain considerations must be made prior to selecting the trans-subclavian method to avoid complications associated with an occluded or damaged subclavian artery.

Transcaval access is relatively new and provides access options for patients whose anatomy leaves no other options for arterial access (Pascual et al., 2017). The catheter is introduced via the inferior vena cava through the femoral vein and crosses over to the abdominal aorta to reach the heart valve in a retrograde fashion. The catheter is then removed via the reverse route and the aortic puncture site is closed by deploying an occluder against the aortic wall (Greenbaum et al., 2017). Other access sites, such as with transcarotid or transseptal, are options for select patients who are not candidates for other TAVR methods (Pascual et al., 2017; Rozeik et al., 2014).

The traditional SAVR remains the standard of care for patients with severe aortic stenosis if they are good surgical candidates. However, because aortic stenosis is a disease that occurs more

frequently in the aging population, a large number of these patients are inoperable due not only to advanced age but also frailty and other comorbid conditions. Patients with severe aortic stenosis are evaluated using specific criteria: an aortic valve area of less than 1.0 cm^2 and either a mean gradient greater than 40 mmHg or a jet velocity of greater than 4 meters/second (Nishimura et al., 2014). Furthermore, patients being evaluated for TAVR must be seen by two cardiac surgeons, both agreeing that TAVR is a better option than SAVR.

Transcatheter aortic valve replacement centers nationwide perform these procedures in a hybrid operating room (OR) or specially outfitted catheterization lab where CPB is readily available if and when it is needed. However, increasingly more TAVR centers in the United States are performing TF TAVRs in the catheterization lab using moderate sedation. In all procedural areas, TAVRs are performed in collaboration with a dedicated heart valve/structural heart team that includes, but is not limited to, cardiac surgeons, interventional cardiologists, heart valve coordinators, echocardiographers, and a multitude of other highly specialized staff members. These practitioners help with everything from the initial evaluation to postprocedure care. Most TAVR centers also have a valve clinic dedicated to the evaluation and workup of these patients. Once a patient is determined to be a potential candidate for TAVR, multiple preoperative studies are obtained to rule out contraindications to the procedure, accurately size the aortic annulus, and evaluate access vessels to determine the approach for the procedure. Frailty parameters are also obtained as is a 5-meter walk test and a quality of life questionnaire (most commonly used is the Kansas City Cardiomyopathy Questionnaire).

The TAVR procedure is done most commonly using either the TF or TA approach. It can also be deployed directly via the transaortic approach (**FIGURE 7.6**). Traditionally the procedure is done under general anesthesia with CPB standby should the patient need that level of support during the procedure. Currently, transcatheter valves are approved only for use in the aortic position; however, mitral valve stents and tricuspid valve devices for treatment of MV and TV regurgitation are being investigated and trialed in the United States

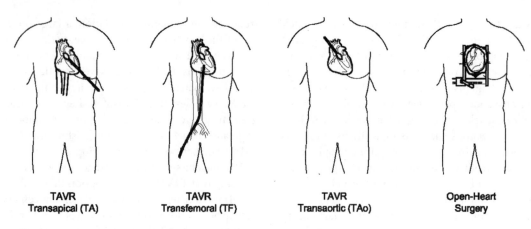

| TAVR | TAVR | TAVR | Open-Heart |
| Transapical (TA) | Transfemoral (TF) | Transaortic (TAo) | Surgery |

FIGURE 7.6 Transcatheter aortic valve replacement.
Illustrated by James R. Perron

(Dai et al., 2017; Moore et al., 2017; Ramlawi & Gammie, 2016; Rodés-Cabau et al., 2016)

Postprocedure Nursing Care

Postprocedure nursing care varies depending on the access route of the intervention. Patients receiving general anesthesia, experiencing significant intraoperative complications, or both are recovered in the postanesthesia care unit and then transferred to a coronary care unit or ICU. Barring any postprocedure complications, the patient is stepped down from the ICU on postoperative day (POD) 2 to an intermediate-care telemetry nursing floor before being discharged to home on POD 3. The LOS varies among TAVR centers and ranges from 3 to 8 days.

Postprocedure Complications

Transcatheter aortic valve replacement complications of particular concern to nursing staff during the postprocedure period include stroke, arrhythmias, and bleeding. Discussion of vascular complications is more extensively presented under "General Nursing Care" later in the chapter.

Stroke. Stroke in post-TAVR patients is commonly related to athero, calcific, device, or air emboli and may be more common depending on the access method used. Thus post-TAVR

nursing care involves conducting frequent neurologic checks, recognizing signs and symptoms of stroke, and initiating and escalating treatment in the event of a stroke diagnosis.

Dysrhythmias. New-onset AF and heart block are two of the most common dysrhythmias seen in post-TAVR patients. Heart block can occur as a result of the atrioventricular conduction system and intermodal branches being inadvertently manipulated and compressed during balloon valvuloplasty and subsequent valve implantation. Valve type and shape also affect the development of heart block. Temporary or permanent pacemaker placement may be required in these patients.

New-onset AF is a common post-TAVR complication. This significantly increases the risk of cardioembolic stroke. In some cases, AF may spontaneously resolve. For persistent cases, treatment goals include rate and rhythm control with antiarrhythmic medication or synchronized cardioversion.

Other dysrhythmias that develop are bradycardia and junctional rhythms. Temporary pacing may be required to stabilize the patient. With persistent bradyarrhythmias, permanent pacemaker placement may be required.

Bleeding. Bleeding is a complication of any surgical intervention. A TAVR patient is at high risk for postprocedure bleeding mostly related to vascular access with large-diameter catheters. Arterial sheaths are generally 14- to 20-French. Even though the arterial incision is closed via a vascular closure device, once the sheath is removed, oozing or failure of the closure site is not uncommon (Pascual et al., 2017). Frequent assessment of the incision site is necessary to monitor for oozing, bleeding, and hematoma formation.

Retroperitoneal hemorrhage is a life-threatening complication related to vascular injury during the procedure, but may not present until after the sheath has been removed and the patient has been transferred to the unit or floor. A sudden drop in blood pressure and intractable back or flank pain are telltale signs of a retroperitoneal bleed. Fluid resuscitation should be started immediately, emergent CT scan should be performed to confirm the bleed, and the patient should be transferred back to the OR or catheterization lab for surgical or percutaneous repair.

General Nursing Care

Postprocedural care varies among TAVR centers. In all cases, TAVR patients are cared for in specially designated units where the nursing staff is well trained and highly skilled in providing care for this patient population.

Post-TAVR care includes the following:

1. Patients who have had general anesthesia are extubated either immediately in the procedure area or within a few hours after arriving to the ICU. Many of these patients have a history of chronic obstructive pulmonary disease (COPD). Combined with immobility and pain, they are at high risk for developing respiratory complications. This can be avoided with good pulmonary toileting, including the regular use of an incentive spirometer, coughing, deep breathing, and frequent turning.

2. Pain management is important for patient comfort and safety. For TF TAVRs, a low-dose oral narcotic analgesic may suffice to achieve good pain control. With any TAVR necessitating a mini-thoracotomy or vascular cutdown, more aggressive pain management regimens with higher potency narcotics that are given more frequently are required to manage the incisional pain and the pain related to chest tube placement, drainage, and removal. Chest tubes are removed when drainage output is less than 150 mL in a 24-hour period, there is no air leak, and the patient is ambulatory.

3. Vital signs are monitored every 30 minutes for the first 2 hours postprocedure and then either hourly in the ICU or every 4 hours thereafter on the intermediate-care telemetry floor. In addition, all TAVR patients require 24-hour telemetry monitoring as dysrhythmias frequently develop 24 to 48 hours postprocedure. Early recognition and appropriate treatment of any dysrhythmias are part of the standard post-TAVR nursing care.

4. Optimal blood pressure control should be maintained and hypertensive/hypotensive states must be avoided. Significantly elevated systolic blood pressure can stress the new valve and increase the risk of bleeding. Hypertension can be controlled with oral or intravenous (IV) antihypertensive medications as needed (Gaasch, Brecker, & Aldea, 2014). Hypotension can be related to decreased volume status, intraoperative and postoperative bleeding, or any combination of these. Patients who are volume depleted generally respond well to IV fluid administration. If hypotension is related to bleeding, the source must be investigated and quickly remedied. In severe cases, blood transfusions may be necessary to stabilize the patient.

5. Indwelling urinary catheters are removed POD 1. Urine output and daily serum creatinine levels should be closely monitored for indications of renal stress or injury.

6. Surgical sites must be assessed for appropriate healing and possible infection. Dressings stay in place through POD 2 unless saturated with blood or drainage, or are otherwise soiled or not intact. On assessment, surgical incisions should be well approximated and free of unusual swelling, erythema, and purulent and malodorous discharge.

7. Transfemoral TAVRs will have at least two groin punctures (one arterial and one venous) and in some cases three (one arterial and two venous). The large sheaths are pulled in the procedure area, but patients may arrive to the unit with a smaller venous sheath still in place. This smaller sheath is pulled by the nurse according to specific coagulation parameters. Patients must lie supine with both legs kept straight until the sheath is removed and hemostasis is achieved. Afterward, the patient remains on bed rest in the same position for at least 4 hours. Should complications arise in the groin site after sheath removal, such as bleeding or hematoma formation, bed rest may be extended. Groin sites must be assessed for oozing, bleeding, hematoma, and new bruit. In addition, pedal and tibial pulses must be monitored and confirmed either by palpation or Doppler. Absent pulses indicate blood flow problems and must be reported to the provider immediately.

8. Preoperative medications should be resumed as soon as the patient is hemodynamically stable, alert and responsive, and able to tolerate oral intake. Mechanical venous thromboembolism prophylaxis should be initiated within the first 24 hours post-TAVR. Any subcutaneously administered low-molecular-weight heparin is avoided within the first 48 hours after the procedure. Typically, dual antiplatelet therapy is initiated with aspirin and clopidogrel (Plavix®) prior to discharge if the patient is not already on anticoagulation therapy.

9. Antibiotic prophylaxis is started preoperatively and should be continued postoperatively as ordered. Avoiding infection is paramount. Diligent monitoring for changes in temperature, relevant labs such as white blood cell and platelet counts, and signs and symptoms of inflammation are required after TAVR. Focusing care on early mobility, toileting, and nutrition (Harris, Dean, Babaliaros, & Keegan, 2014) plays an important part in boosting an already compromised immune system and averting secondary infections from other nonsurgical sources.

10. On POD 2, the patient is typically stable enough to transfer to a step-down telemetry floor if not already there. Prior to transfer out of the ICU, central lines are removed and a peripheral IV is placed. The patient may be transferred to the floor with the chest tube in place if criteria for removing it have not been met but the patient is otherwise stable. Continuous cardiac monitoring will continue until discharge. Once on the floor, the emphasis is on ambulation, toileting, and nutrition (Harris et al., 2014). Although patients are transitioned to a solid-food diet once the sheath is removed on POD 1, eating may be hampered by bed rest and other factors while in the ICU. Early ambulation is prognostic for uncomplicated recovery so patients are ambulated once bed rest is complete at the earliest or by POD 2 at the latest. Lack of movement and food as well as narcotic pain medication can result in constipation. Conversely, early ambulation and eating help support elimination. Stool softeners or laxatives may be indicated if normal bowel function is not restored by POD 2.

Discharge

Patients are instructed to follow up with their heart valve/structural heart team provider at 30 days, 6 months, and 1 year post-TAVR and annually thereafter. Dual antiplatelet therapy is initiated in the hospital and continued for up to 6 months following the procedure with aspirin continuing for life (Gaasch et al., 2014). Otherwise, discharge instructions and patient education are center specific. In general, all TAVR patients should be educated on what problems to report and what precautions to take should problems arise; how to care for wounds and incisions; activity and exercise limitations, if any; self-care requirements; and any equipment, supplies, or safety aids that might be needed for home recovery.

Innovation in Nursing Practice

As centers nationwide continue to hone their processes, patients are benefiting from both the technological advancements with TAVR and care innovations being made at these facilities. One TAVR center has shown that patients undergoing TF TAVR can be successfully and safely managed on an intermediate-care cardiac floor postprocedure. This is possible due to (1) careful patient selection preprocedure, (2) the experience level of the center and structural heart team, (3) the procedural technique used and the use of moderate sedation for select TF cases, (4) optimal staffing ratios of the floor, and (5) the skill level of the nursing staff with sheath management and femoral access patients (Harris et al., 2014). Avoiding the ICU when possible and nursing care that focuses on early ambulation, good nutrition, effective toileting and bowel management, and family involvement have provided the model upon which standards of nursing care for TF TAVRs have been developed at TAVR centers. As such, an innovation in nursing practice has emerged by putting into place new clinical guidelines for postprocedure care of TAVR patients. By following these guidelines, nursing staff have contributed significantly to positive patient outcomes that include shortened recovery times and LOS (Harris et al., 2014). Lastly, the financial impact of recovering TF TAVR patients on the cardiac inpatient floor

rather than the ICU cannot be ignored, because a floor bed is less costly than an ICU bed.

Ongoing developments in TAVR will have implications for nurses caring for TAVR patients. New frontiers in valve replacement procedures are occurring at lightning speed. Transcatheter aortic valve replacements are still being perfected and new-generation THVs are enabling implants through increasingly smaller delivery systems. This has provided the groundwork for ongoing developments and research with valve replacement procedures and new-generation bioprosthetic heart valves. Nurses are ideally positioned to significantly impact the future of transcatheter valve replacement by standardizing patient care that is linked to evidence-based outcomes. This will pave the way for other centers seeking to take advantage of the benefits that highly skilled nurses can provide to these patients.

MitraClip. Although percutaneous mitral valves are being trialed in the United States, there is a catheter-based therapy available for those patients who are ineligible for traditional mitral valve surgery. The MitraClip (Abbott Vascular) was developed to treat patients with symptomatic degenerative mitral regurgitation (MR) of grade 3+ or greater who are too high risk for surgery. Approved for commercial use in the United States in October 2013, the MitraClip delivery system is introduced via a transvenous, transseptal approach by the femoral vein. Once deployed, the MitraClip approximates the valve leaflet edges, mimicking a surgical mitral valve repair (Kothandan, Kian, Keong, & Chih, 2014; Suradi, Kavinsky, & Hijazi, 2016). Although these patients still have residual MR postprocedure, recent data reveal patients have symptomatic relief of symptoms, fewer hospitalizations, and improved quality of life (D'ascenzo et al., 2015; Deuschl, Schofer, Lubos, Blankenberg, & Schäfer, 2016). Similar to TAVR, a heart team approach is essential to the evaluation and management of these critically ill patients. These patients are most often in heart failure and have multiple comorbid conditions. The MitraClip will not be successful without aggressive heart failure medical management prior to and following the procedure. MitraClip patients also require close follow-up in the valve clinic, with regularly scheduled postprocedure echocardiograms and outpatient visits.

Minimally Invasive Pulmonic Valve Replacement

The first report of an experimental transcatheter pulmonic valve replacement (tPVR) was performed by Bonhoeffer and colleagues in 2000 (Chatterjee et al., 2017) on a patient who had undergone a prior implantation of a conduit for pulmonary atresia. A second, compassionate use case was performed in 2005 on a patient with severe congenital aortic stenosis who had previously undergone a Ross operation. Since then, it is difficult to discern the exact number of cases that have been performed, but tPVR has emerged as a newer therapy assisted by novel devices, innovative surgical techniques, and careful patient selection (Hijazi et al., 2015).

Currently, there are only two valves available for tPVR—the Melody™ valve by Medtronic and the SAPIEN valve from Edwards Lifesciences. There are a number of other options in development and several clinical trials underway. Patients who meet criteria and are suffering from pulmonary insufficiency—either symptomatic or diagnosed by magnetic resonance imaging (MRI) or echocardiogram—are eligible for the procedure. Many patients have had prior surgical procedures to correct congenital cardiac defects, most often reconstruction of the right ventricular outflow tract or placement of a bioprosthetic valve. Over time, the reconstruction may lead to pulmonic stenosis or regurgitation, leading to right ventricular dysfunction. Patients may require numerous surgical procedures in their lifetime, thus a minimally invasive tPVR is a viable alternative.

The tPVR procedure has many of the same benefits previously outlined, including shorter hospital LOS. Performance and longevity of the valves are comparable to surgically implanted bioprosthetic valves (DeGiovanni, 2017). The Melody Valve Investigational Device Exemption Trial found that tPVR provided excellent hemodynamic and clinical outcomes up to 7 years after implant,

with a median time to follow-up of 4.5 years. Primary valve failure was rare. The primary cause of tPVR dysfunction was stenosis related to implanted stent fracture, which was virtually eliminated once prestenting of the previously established conduit became more widely adopted partway through the trial (Cheatham et al., 2015). There is not, however, any established or validated operative risk calculator for this procedure, so the final decision is based on surgeon preference and ability. This procedure is still in its infancy and thus expert guidelines have not been established as of yet. However, tPVR offers hope to patients who were either deemed "untreatable" or where the only option was traditional open heart surgery (Hijazi et al., 2015). The procedure is generally considered to be safe, but vascular injury, stent/valve displacement, conduit rupture, tricuspid damage, or valve malfunction are all potential complications (DeGiovanni, 2017).

▶ Minimally Invasive Atrial Fibrillation Ablation

Atrial fibrillation is the most common dysrhythmia reported. Worldwide, it is estimated that AF affects 33.5 million (Chugh et al., 2014). In the United States, there are more than 750,000 hospitalizations and an estimated 130,000 deaths each year due to AF, with the death rate rising every year (Craig et al., 2014). Atrial fibrillation costs the United States about $6 billion each year (Mozaffarian et al., 2015). The complications of AF—embolic stroke and anticoagulation-associated hemorrhage—make it a very morbid condition, particularly for the elderly who are often the affected (Katritsis & Katritsis, 2017). For these reasons, surgery for AF (covered in Chapter 3) has become increasingly popular. With three decades of clinical evolution, the Cox-Maze procedure has been established as a gold standard for the surgical treatment of AF. The Cox-Maze IV (CMIV) procedure is performed through a minimally invasive right mini-thoracotomy approach on CPB. A majority of the time, the Maze procedure is being performed in conjunction with another cardiac procedure (e.g., tricuspid or mitral valve surgery). As a standalone procedure, several methods have emerged to assist in this minimally invasive approach—extended left atrial sets, video-assisted pulmonary vein isolation, and a hybrid approach. The complete Maze operation involves isolation of both the left and right pulmonary veins. Because the left atrium is typically the focus of AF reentry, a left-sided Maze is the most commonly performed procedure. Bipolar radiofrequency and cryothermal ablation are used to create the lesions (i.e., myocardial scars), which block the micro reentrant circuits causing AF (Ad, Holmes, Lamont, & Shuman, 2017; Lancaster et al., 2016).

In addition to ablation, the basic Maze procedure also involves ligation of the left atrial appendage to remove the thromboembolic source in AF patients. Because the procedure is performed on a beating heart, atrial function can be monitored during treatment. Patients may convert to normal sinus rhythm during the procedure or it may take up to 12 weeks. The minimally invasive or robotic Maze procedure is associated with less postoperative pain due to smaller incisions and results in fewer complications, because CPB is not required.

Left Atrial Appendage Procedure

Nonpharmacologic treatment for stroke prevention is an unmet need, leading to the development of alternatives to pharmacologic therapies. Several approaches to left atrial appendage (LAA) occlusion have evolved, including surgical suturing, endovascular occlusion, amputation, and stapling. The WATCHMAN™ device (Atritech) was approved by the Food and Drug Administration in 2015 for patients who have nonvalvular AF (NVAF). There are other devices available, either in international markets or off label, such as the AMPLATZER™ Cardiac Plug (St. Jude Medical) and the Lariat® (SentreHEART Inc.) (Tzikas et al., 2016).

The PROTECT AF (2009) and the PREVAIL trials (2014) were conducted to determine the safety and efficacy of the WATCHMAN device and to establish whether patients could be offered a nonpharmacologic treatment option for their NVAF. The device is implanted via a trans-septal puncture by use of a catheter-based delivery system, which is meant to seal the ostium of the LAA. The device implantation is guided by fluoroscopy and TEE to verify proper stability and positioning. After device implantation, patients were treated with warfarin (Coumadin®) for 45 days to facilitate device attachment to the endothelium. Serial TEE imaging was done at 45 days, 6 months, and 1 year to assess for any residual peridevice flow from the LAA and to check device position and stability. Patients were able to discontinue warfarin if the 45-day TEE showed either complete closure of the LAA or minimal residual peridevice flow. After stopping warfarin, once daily clopidogrel (Plavix®, 75 mg) and aspirin (81–325 mg) were prescribed until the 6-month follow-up, from which point aspirin alone was continued indefinitely.

There were some initial safety concerns with using the WATCHMAN device. Some patients in the intervention group who received the device experienced pericardial effusions and air emboli; there was no permanent disability or mortality. Hemorrhagic stroke, however, was significantly reduced in the intervention group, with 0.2% of patients having hemorrhagic stroke compared to 2.5% of patients in the control group. Complications in the intervention group were mainly a result of periprocedural complications, and the thought was that these complications would decline with further training and experience using the device, which was validated in the PREVAIL trial (Holmes et al., 2014). A patient-level meta-analysis further confirmed that the WATCHMAN device is noninferior to anticoagulation therapy and provides additional reductions in major bleeding (especially disabling hemorrhagic strokes) and mortality (Reddy et al., 2017).

▶ Nursing Care and Special Considerations for MICS

Preoperative teaching should be provided to all patients and families prior to cardiac surgery. However, any time a minimally invasive procedure is being planned, there may be unforeseen circumstances in which MICS may turn into a traditional CABG. Teaching should include the participation of not only the patient, but also any caregivers, because unforeseen activity restrictions may result from the need for a full sternotomy. Patients may be fearful of having their chest "cracked open," but this may be avoidable with the MICS procedure. Preoperative teaching for the intended procedure should also include a review of the potential complications associated with CPB and the standard of care employed by the facility.

Although emphasis should be placed on the decreased amount of postoperative pain experienced with MICS, patients should be encouraged to report pain levels honestly to help avoid complications and improve patient satisfaction. Specifically, patients should be encouraged to volunteer information regarding pain level and efficacy of treatment. Pain control can improve pulmonary function, increase patient satisfaction, and decrease delirium after cardiac surgery (Dieberg et al., 2016; Glowacki, 2015; Stephens & Whitman, 2015a). The value of aggressive pulmonary toileting and early ambulation cannot be overemphasized despite a minimally invasive approach. Expectations for coughing and deep breathing as well as the use of incentive spirometry should be taught in the preoperative period similar to that of traditional cardiac procedures.

Immediate postoperative care of patients who have undergone MICS will, for the most part, follow the same path as care for those who required a sternotomy; however, there are a few specific issues that warrant discussion. Approximately 1 hour prior to the patient's arrival to the ICU, the OR nurse usually calls in a report to the admitting ICU nurse. After receiving the initial brief report, the patient's family should be updated. Early contact establishes a rapport with family and provides time to obtain information for the admission assessment and emergency contact names and numbers. The family should be notified where they will be contacted and the anticipated time until visitation after the patient arrives in the ICU. If the patient was not in the hospital prior to surgery and did not receive preoperative education, family members should be prepared for what to expect with the ICU environment to help reduce their stress level. Questions should be addressed, and any anticipated resources (e.g., pastoral care) may be provided at this time.

Admission to the ICU: The First 15 Minutes

Patients who are intubated will be sedated. The intraoperative paralytics are often reversed to assist with early extubation. Depending on the facility, the anesthesia provider will start a sedation infusion to promote comfort, decrease myocardial oxygen consumption, and enhance tolerance to the ventilator until weaning commences. A formal handover with surgical and anesthesia teams will provide a more in-depth report. Standardized handover protocols can decrease critical omissions and improve caregiver teamwork. This should include, but not be limited to, the patient's past medical history, allergies, intraoperative course, last set of pertinent lab results, IV fluid administration, antibiotics administered and times, urinary output, and, if CPB was required, length of time on bypass and length of time the aorta was cross-clamped (Stephens & Whitman, 2015a).

While settling the patient after surgery, maintaining hemodynamic stability is essential. Baseline vital signs should be obtained and all pressure lines zeroed and leveled to the phlebostatic axis (Jacq et al., 2015) (**FIGURE 7.7**). In addition to vital signs, an initial hemodynamic assessment should include a review of IV access, current medications, cardiac rhythm, and central venous pressure (CVP). If the patient has a pulmonary artery (PA) catheter in place, pulmonary artery pressure (PAP) and pulmonary artery occlusive pressure (PAOP) should be measured. However, routine placement of a PA catheter is not necessary or helpful except in high-risk patients. Alternatives such as esophageal Doppler monitoring, pulse contour analysis, and transpulmonary thermodilution are also available. The Fick principle can be used to obtain cardiac output (CO) and venous oxygen saturation (SvO_2). Fluid and medication infusion rates should be titrated to maintain hemodynamic stability, and may utilize "goal-directed therapy" (GDT) protocol to optimize CO.

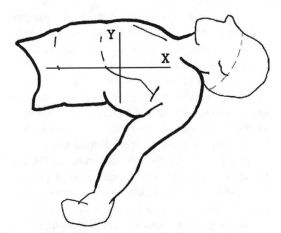

FIGURE 7.7 The phlebostatic axis (intersection of the X and Y reference lines).

Illustrated by James R. Perron

Among patients who did not have CPB, hypothermia is uncommon. A temperature less than 35°C (95°F) is considered hypothermic; in such a case, warming techniques should be implemented. Patients who have undergone MICS are routinely hypovolemic and have labile blood pressure, requiring volume repletion to achieve hemodynamic stability. Hypothermia can occur from open body cavities, cold pericardial irrigation, and administration of blood products or fluids. This can result in dysrhythmias, impaired coagulation, decreased CO, and longer ventilation times. The frequency with which vital signs and a hemodynamic profile are obtained depends on the facility guidelines and the patient's condition.

The patient's height and weight should be entered into the monitoring system database to ensure accurate calculations based on body surface area (e.g., cardiac index [CI]). If the patient is hypothermic, CI values will be skewed and reflect "cold numbers." A true hemodynamic picture will not be reflected until the patient is normothermic.

Laboratory specimens should be collected as prescribed by unit protocol or as indicated by the patient's clinical status. Baseline postoperative labs will likely include an arterial blood gas (ABG), ionized calcium, serum chemistries, coagulation profile, and a complete blood count (CBC). If the patient is bleeding, a fibrinogen level may be obtained as well. The patient should also have a portable chest radiograph and an electrocardiogram (ECG) performed.

An ECG after MICS is imperative because of the potential complications related to myocardial ischemia and graft patency. Early graft closure and arterial graft spasm may be manifested the same way as in traditional cardiac surgery, ST segment elevation, T-wave inversion, and Q waves present in the leads, which is reflective of the revascularized myocardium.

Placement of chest tubes may be less than ideal because of the limited exposure in MICS. Chest tubes are typically left in place to drain the mediastinum and the pleural space similar to that in traditional cardiac surgery. All chest drains, regardless of type, should be connected to wall suction and should be assessed regularly for amount and type of drainage, patency, and presence of clots. If a patient's blood pressure permits, the head of the bed should be elevated to facilitate chest tube drainage. Risk factors for excessive bleeding include urgent or complicated procedures, age, male gender, use of an ITA, long CPB time, anemia, decreased cardiac function, and preoperative dual antiplatelet therapy. As long as there is no air leak, chest drains are removed once output reaches acceptable volume (e.g., <100 mL/ 8 hours).

Secondary Assessment: The Next 15 Minutes

After initial stabilization of the MICS patient is achieved and a preliminary patient assessment for clinically significant issues (e.g., bleeding, hypotension, hypertension, agitation, dysrhythmias) is performed, a more focused head-to-toe assessment is completed. The neurologic assessment is ongoing and more complete as the patient emerges from anesthesia. Skin is assessed for temperature, color, and location of incisions (procedure based).

Pain should be anticipated, and can be significant with MICS due to the rib retraction required for exposure. Pain level should be assessed with a scale appropriate for the cognitive status of the patient. Measures to relieve the incisional pain should be implemented immediately. In the initial postoperative period, patients will primarily receive opioid analgesics or patient-controlled analgesia. Patients should also be premedicated prior to potentially painful procedures (e.g., chest tube removal). As discussed in Chapter 14, inadequate analgesia can result in tachycardia, increased peripheral vascular resistance, imbalance between oxygen supply and demand, hypoxemia, pneumonia, and atelectasis. Lower levels of pain are typically encountered with a minimally invasive procedure; chest tubes are frequently a source of pain regardless of the minimally invasive nature of the procedure. Nonpharmacologic methods of pain management, such as music therapy, may also be effective during rehabilitation (Stephens & Whitman, 2015a, 2015b).

Although many MICS procedures are done without the use of CPB, many procedures continue to require bypass; therefore, alternative cannulation sites are utilized. Minimally invasive mitral valve surgery performed with or without robotic assistance frequently utilizes both femoral artery and vein. Because of the high incidence of concomitant aortoiliac and femoral disease, it is absolutely essential that distal perfusion of those extremities be assessed at the conclusion of the procedure and frequently in the ICU. The highest risk for peripheral vascular injury and embolization may be related to peripheral cannulation with retrograde perfusion (Algarni et al., 2015). Establishing a baseline for the presence of warm, strong peripheral pulses is critical to recognition of the development of extremity vascular and motor function complications.

Hemodynamic Monitoring

Successful hemodynamic monitoring begins with knowing the normal range for hemodynamic values. "Normal" in this case is a relative term, because normal values are based on healthy individuals with healthy hearts. The values most commonly monitored are identical to those utilized for traditional cardiac surgery patients; they are covered in detail in Chapter 9.

In the early postoperative period, most patients have myocardial dysfunction and decreased ventricular compliance secondary to intravascular hypovolemia and vasodilation. Managing a patient's hemodynamic profile entails evaluating the patient's clinical condition and past medical and surgical histories so the correct decision is made about how to optimize preload, afterload, and contractility. Depending on comorbidities, hemodynamic values may be skewed (Stephens & Whitman, 2015a). For example, a patient with pulmonary hypertension may have elevated pulmonary artery pressures and CVP secondary to lung disease. A valuable source for a patient's baseline hemodynamic values is the cardiac catheterization lab report. Trying to maintain a patient with underlying disease within the standard norms is unrealistic and can even be detrimental to the patient. For example, a patient with hypertension may not have adequate kidney perfusion with a mean arterial pressure (MAP) of 80 mmHg, but instead may need a slightly higher MAP of 90 to 95 mmHg to maintain end-organ perfusion.

The key to hemodynamic stability starts with maintaining and normalizing heart rate and stroke volume. This goal may be accomplished through the administration and titration of fluids and medications. Stroke volume is affected by preload, afterload, and contractility (Mehta & Arora, 2014). These variables are described further in Chapter 9.

Some of the more common etiologies of hemodynamic compromise are myocardial ischemia, hypothermia, and postoperative dysrhythmias. These are discussed in detail in Chapters 13 and 15. The goal of therapy is optimal end-organ perfusion with hemodynamic stability. Although hemodynamic parameter goals should be individualized, suggested minimum values for most patients will likely include an SvO_2 greater than 60%, a MAP of 60 to 90, and CI greater than 2.2 to 2.5 L/min/m^2 (Stephens & Whitman, 2015a).

Postoperative Complications

Postoperative complications of cardiac surgery in general are discussed in detail in Chapter 13. It is essential for the ICU nurse to monitor patients who have undergone MICS procedures for development of complications, intervene to prevent them from occurring, and promptly recognize and treat any complications that develop.

MICS-Specific Complications

Some of the complications related to MICS specifically are felt to be related to the more technically challenging nature of these procedures and to procedure-related stress on the heart. Because there is a learning curve associated with these operations, CPB time is often prolonged—more than 4 hours. All of the complications discussed in Chapter 13 apply to MICS, with the primary offending factor being nonpulsatile blood flow for those procedures requiring CPB. Single-lung ventilation is often required for these procedures, and can result in atelectasis (Stephens & Whitman, 2015a).

Dysrhythmias

Dysrhythmias are a common occurrence following cardiac surgery, especially with patients undergoing TAVR procedures. Conduction disturbances most commonly occur the first 3 days postoperatively, and up to 20% of these patients will require permanent pacemakers.

Atrial fibrillation can occur in patients with no prior history from electrolyte imbalances, volume overload, surgical manipulation, or acid–base imbalance. Patients undergoing minimally invasive Maze procedures may be loaded with IV amiodarone coming out of the OR to obtain or maintain normal sinus rhythm. There is a 3-month threshold or "blanking period" after ablation in which rhythm disturbances are expected (Lawrance, Henn, & Damiano, 2015).

Lethal arrhythmias, such as ventricular tachycardia or ventricular fibrillation (VF), can also occur in the immediate postoperative period of MICS. Electrolyte imbalance, cardiac irritability from the surgery, and acidosis may be contributing factors to their development. Resuscitation of these dysrhythmias should follow the American Heart Association recommendations. Development of VF may require opening the patient's chest at the bedside. Postoperative dysrhythmias are discussed in more detail in Chapter 15.

Bleeding

Postoperative bleeding is a risk with any cardiac surgery, including MICS. However, less bleeding is associated with MICS—especially robotic procedures. The risk increases if the procedure is performed on CPB, as higher doses of heparin are administered. As with traditional cardiac surgery, hemodilution, fibrinolysis, and hypothermia are risk factors for postoperative bleeding (Stephens & Whitman, 2015a). As previously stated, chest tube patency and evaluation of chest radiograph are very important, because chest tube placement and drainage of the pleural cavity can be challenging when working via limited incisions. Vascular access points should be assessed for hematoma, especially with concomitant hypotension (Stephens & Whitman, 2015b). Postoperative bleeding is discussed in more detail in Chapter 13.

Postoperative Ventilatory Support

Patients who undergo MICS may be extubated in the OR, or soon after arrival to the ICU (within 6 hours). Patients may be weaned from mechanical ventilation when certain criteria, which may vary among facilities, are met. In general, these conditions may include the patient being awake and cooperative, dissipation of neuromuscular blocking agent effects (usually manifested with a sustained head lift), hemodynamic stability, absence of dysrhythmias, ABG values within physiologic range, normal chest radiograph findings, normothermia, chest tube drainage less than 100 mL/hour, and urine output more than 1 mL/kg/hr. A spontaneous breathing trial (SBT) can be used to assess readiness for extubation. In addition, other factors should be considered while weaning the patient off ventilatory support, such as patient age, comorbidities, length of time in the OR, and intraoperative course (Stephens & Whitman, 2015a, 2015b). Weaning from mechanical ventilation following cardiac surgery is discussed in detail in Chapter 11.

Acute Kidney Injury

Hemodynamic instability, pharmacologic agents, mechanical trauma, cardiopulmonary bypass, intravenous fluids, hypoxia, nephrotoxic agents, and inflammation are some of the factors associated with acute kidney injury (AKI) after cardiac surgery. There are no pharmacologic agents known to reduce the risk of AKI (Thiele, Isbell, & Rosner, 2015), but attempts should be made to avoid those that increase the risk if possible. Angiotensin-converting enzyme (ACE) inhibitors, inotropes, and nonsteroidal anti-inflammatory drugs (NSAIDs) have all been linked to AKI. In addition, intravascular contrast utilized to guide valve placement or percutaneous intervention in transcatheter procedures can also contribute to acute kidney injury. Other complications such as bleeding or hypotension can further aggravate this issue. Renal function and urinary output should be closely monitored, as half of all patients will have a reduction in renal function (25% increase in serum creatinine). AKI increases mortality, and length of ICU and hospital stay.

Recovery from MICS

Patients who undergo MICS procedures traditionally have a quicker and less complicated recovery than patients who undergo conventional surgical procedures. Minimally invasive direct coronary artery bypass and OPCAB procedures are both typically performed on the beating heart, without CPB, and have reduced risk of sternal wound infection and musculoskeletal injury. They can be performed primarily or as a reoperation, and avoid systemic inflammatory response associated with CPB. These patients typically return to the ICU hemodynamically stable, but often require inotrope or pressor support intraoperatively during the cardiac positioning necessary for OPCAB.

Minimally invasive cardiac surgery patients, like all cardiac surgery patients, should have an ECG immediately upon return from the OR.

Procedures performed through small incisions are often limited by full surgical exposure of the heart. Because of this lack of direct visualization and the lack of full revascularization, graft patency and ischemia may be an issue postoperatively. The ICU nurse plays a key role in detection of ECG changes that may be an early sign of a problem with an anastomosis. There should be a low threshold for these patients to have additional testing—echocardiogram to assess for wall motion abnormalities and coronary angiography if postoperative ischemia is suspected (Stephens & Whitman, 2015b).

As previously stated, the lack of traditional epicardial pacing wires following MIDCAB and MIMVS may pose problems in the early postoperative period. Patients may return to the ICU with a right ventricular pacing lead as part of a special pulmonary artery catheter, which means catheter position may be a factor in pacing wire capture. Additionally, external pacing may be required, which is often less than optimal if the patient is awake.

Postoperative pain management is crucial for patients who have undergone rib-spreading procedures. The American Pain Society recommends using neuraxial analgesia for significant thoracic and abdominal procedures in patients at high risk for pulmonary or cardiac complications (Chou et al., 2016). One advantage of epidural analgesia is that it can be given via patient-controlled analgesia (PCA) pump, which evidence suggests demonstrates greater effectiveness and patient satisfaction (McNicol, Ferguson, & Hudcova, 2015). In addition to epidural and intercostal analgesia, use of nonnarcotic medications can be helpful in preventing pulmonary complications following thoracotomy procedures. Ketorolac (Toradol®) and IV acetaminophen (Tylenol®) have both been used as adjunctive therapy to narcotics to accomplish early extubation.

Despite specific concerns related to the recovery of patients undergoing MICS, these patients often require less time in the ICU and overall LOS. In a cost analysis, MIMVS was associated with a lower total hospital cost compared with conventional mitral valve surgery (Algarni et al., 2015).

▶ # Summary

Minimally invasive cardiac surgery, with all of its benefits, provides a viable option for the patient who meets the criteria established for this type of procedure. The major benefits of MICS are faster recovery and early mobilization (Dieberg et al., 2016). Additionally, decreased incidence of postoperative complications related to CPB and aortic cross-clamping, intraoperative anticoagulation, cardioplegia, and sternal wound infections have been documented. Cardiac surgery centers

of excellence with teams who have mastered the learning curve for MIMVS have achieved equivalent morbidity and mortality when compared to standard mitral valve surgery (Algarni et al., 2015). The cardiac surgery ICU nurse is a part of that important multidisciplinary team, taking on many roles when caring for this type of patient: educator, advocate for the patient and family, and collaborator with the multidisciplinary team. While MICS is not an innovative new treatment for cardiac disease, it is certainly an attractive approach to a traditional procedure.

⌕ CASE STUDY

A. L. is a 78-year-old patient who presented to the emergency department (ED) with reports of progressive dyspnea. He had a 2-vessel CABG with sternotomy 5 years ago. His past medical history is also significant for hypertension, COPD, NYHA Class III, and aortic stenosis. His home medications include a statin, hydrochlorothiazide, and an ACE inhibitor. An echocardiogram performed in the ED revealed preserved left ventricle (LV) function and an ejection fraction of 45%.

The patient was admitted and taken for a TAVR. He had a stable procedural course. On POD 1, he had his sheath removed but developed decreased LV function. He also experienced a sudden decrease in systolic blood pressure, abdominal pain, and severe pain to his back. Echocardiogram revealed a left ventricular ejection fraction (LVEF) of 35%.

The patient otherwise had a stable postoperative course and was discharged on POD 4.

Critical Thinking Questions

1. Why was a TAVR performed?
2. Why was a TAVR the correct procedure to be performed on this patient?
3. What should the nurses suspect as a source of the patient's decrease in blood pressure?

Answers to Critical Thinking Questions

1. A TAVR was performed to eradicate the patient's outflow obstruction.
2. A TAVR was the appropriate procedure for this patient as he was considered high risk for surgical aortic valve replacement due to his previous sternotomy.
3. The nurse should suspect retroperitoneal bleeding following removal of the sheath.

Self-Assessment Questions

1. The family of a patient who just returned from the OR for a coronary artery bypass grafting procedure asked why the patient's heart is not functioning as well as it should be. The nurse's best response is:

A. "It is related to the decrease in body temperature in the operating room."
B. "Some of the body fluid is leaking from his vessels."
C. "The patient received anticoagulants for the procedure."
D. "Ischemia-reperfusion injury can occur."

2. Hemorrhagic stroke can occur after traditional coronary artery bypass grafting due to which of the following?
   A. Hypothermia
   B. Anticoagulants
   C. Red blood cell hemolysis
   D. Clamping of the aorta

3. The family of a patient who just returned from the OR for a coronary artery bypass grafting procedure asked why the patient's blood sugar is elevated. The nurse's best response is:
   A. "It could be related to the steroids given during surgery."
   B. "He might have had a fever in the operating room; I will check."
   C. "You can get higher blood sugars from being on bypass."
   D. "During surgery, there is activation of the complement system."

4. A patient is told that minimally invasive cardiac surgery was not feasible and that traditional cardiac surgery would be required. Which of the following conditions does this patient likely have?
   A. Atrial septal defect
   B. Multivessel coronary artery disease
   C. Aortic stenosis
   D. Atrial fibrillation

5. A nurse is asked to explain minimally invasive direct coronary artery bypass. Which of the following statements demonstrates an understanding of the procedure?
   A. "There is minimal to no pain associated with this procedure."
   B. "Patients with 3 or more vessel disease can be treated with this procedure."
   C. "There is minimal time spent on cardiopulmonary bypass."
   D. "There are smaller but more incisions than with traditional CABG."

6. Which of the following is true during minimally invasive direct coronary artery bypass?
   A. The heart's movement is limited throughout the procedure.
   B. It is only used in patients requiring single-vessel bypass.

   C. The left lung is deflated during the procedure.
   D. Because of the multiple lesions, early mobility is more challenging than with traditional bypass.

7. Which of the following is an advantage of minimally invasive direct coronary artery bypass?
   A. Decreased risk of atelectasis
   B. Aortic manipulation
   C. Cardioplegia
   D. Decreased blood loss

8. Which of the following is a difference between minimally invasive direct coronary artery bypass and off-pump bypass?
   A. Number of vessels repaired
   B. Amount of cardioplegia instilled
   C. Time the heart is not beating during the procedure
   D. Degree of postoperative inflammatory response

9. Which of the following is true regarding a minimally invasive direct view procedure?
   A. It entails the use of robotics.
   B. It can be used for tricuspid valve replacement.
   C. It cannot be performed on a patient who has had a median sternotomy in the past.
   D. The patient will have an 8-cm incision.

10. Which of the following patients will likely be excluded from having a minimally invasive direct coronary artery bypass procedure? A patient with a(n):
    A. HbA_{1c} 8%.
    B. BMI 41 kg/m^2.
    C. troponin 0.4 ng/mL.
    D. serum creatinine 1.5 mg/dL.

Answers to Self-Assessment Questions

1. D. "**Ischemia-reperfusion injury can occur.**" Rationale: Ischemia-reperfusion injury is the reciprocal damage to the myocardium from a STEMI. If the blocked coronary

artery or arteries are not rapidly reperfused and no collateral circulation is present, most of the area at risk becomes necrotic. Early reperfusion has been shown to help prevent this injury from occurring.

2. B. **anticoagulants**

   Rationale: Anticoagulation use can increase risk for hemorrhagic stroke, and some patients may have additional risk factors. Both thromboembolic and bleeding risks should be assessed prior to procedure. Timing of the last direct oral anticoagulants (DOAC) before an invasive procedure, the bleeding risk of the procedure, and the elimination half-life of the DOAC are all important considerations. Patients with atrial fibrillation may be treated with alternative procedures such as left atrial appendage occlusion or ligation to avoid the risks of anticoagulation.

3. C. **"You can get higher blood sugars from being on bypass."**

   Rationale: Use of cardiopulmonary bypass disturbs glucose homeostasis and aggravates the hyperglycemic response.

4. B. **multivessel coronary artery disease**

   Rationale: Advantages of traditional cardiac surgery in patients with multivessel disease include a reduction in repeat revascularization, myocardial infarction, and long-term all-cause mortality. Atrial septal defect can be used in MICS or traditional cardiac surgery. Outcomes for these procedures were equivalent for mortality and morbidity. Aortic stenosis and atrial fibrillation are also treatable with minimally invasive techniques.

5. D. **"There are smaller but more incisions than with traditional CABG."**

   Rationale: There is a significant amount of pain associated with minimally invasive procedures secondary to rib retraction and involvement of intercostal nerves. Three or more vessel disease, or more commonly referred to as multivessel disease, is often treated with traditional cardiac surgery. The patient usually spends more time on cardiopulmonary

bypass with MICS than a traditional CABG. Smaller incisions are made with minimally invasive direct coronary artery bypass, decreasing the risk of sternal trauma.

6. C. **The left lung is deflated during the procedure.**

   Rationale: A MIDCAB is typically a beating heart procedure. It is primarily used in patients with isolated LAD lesions, but has been used to treat multivessel disease. The left lung is deflated during the procedure. Mobility is improved with MIDCAB procedure secondary to reduced surgical trauma and rapid healing.

7. D. **decreased blood loss**

   Rationale: Minimally invasive cardiac surgery, especially robotics, is associated with less blood loss. However, there should be a lower threshold set for bleeding with MICS procedure because of the decreased risk. There is an increased risk of atelectasis secondary to single lung deflation during the procedure. Aortic manipulation and CPB (utilizing cardioplegia) are generally avoided for this procedure.

8. A. **number of vessels repaired**

   Rationale: MIDCAB is done through a lateral thoracotomy on a beating heart. The initial indication for MIDCAB was single vessel disease not amenable to percutaneous transluminal coronary angioplasty (PTCA) and wanting to avoid CPB. The off-pump coronary artery bypass procedure goal is to repair one or more vessels on a beating heart versus median sternotomy.

9. D. **The patient will have an 8-cm incision.**

   Rationale: For MIDCAB procedure, the patient is intubated with a double-way endotracheal tube, an 8-cm submammary incision is made, pleural space entered, and left lung deflated for the procedure.

10. B. **BMI 41 kg/m^2**

    Rationale: In patients undergoing median sternotomy, obesity (BMI >30 kg/m^2) is a known preoperative risk factor for sternal dehiscence and sternal wound infection, most notably mediastinitis.

CLINICAL INQUIRY BOX

Question: What is the most recent evidence regarding minimally invasive cardiac surgery?

Reference: Doenst, T., Diab, M., Sponbholz, C., Bauier, M., & Färher, G. (2017). The opportunities and limitations of minimally invasive cardiac surgery. *Deutsches Ärzteblatt International, 114*(46), 777–784.

Objective: To determine the present evidence on minimally invasive cardiac surgery.

Method: A review of current evidence (randomized controlled trials [RCTs]) on minimally invasive cardiac surgery. Seven RCTs were found on aortic valve replacement. Three RCTs were found on mitral valve replacement surgery.

Results: Minimally invasive cardiac surgery is associated with fewer wound infections and faster mobilization. There are no differences in survival between minimally invasive cardiac surgery and open procedures. Minimally invasive cardiac surgical procedures are technically demanding and have certain anatomical prerequisites (e.g., coronary morphology for multiple bypass procedures).

Conclusion: Minimally invasive cardiac surgery procedures yield results that are at least as good as classic open heart surgery.

References

Ad, N., Holmes, S. D., Lamont, D., & Shuman, D. J. (2017). Left-sided surgical ablation for patients with atrial fibrillation who are undergoing concomitant surgical procedures. *Annals of Thoracic Surgery, 103,* 58–65.

Adamik, B., Kubler, A., Gozdzik, A., & Gozdzik, W. (2017). Prolonged cardiopulmonary bypass is a risk factor for intestinal ischeamic damage and endotoxaemia. *Heart, Lung, and Circulation, 26,* 717–723.

Algarni, K. D., Suri, R. M., & Schaff, H. (2015). Minimally invasive mitral valve surgery: Does it make a difference? *Trends in Cardiovascular Medicine, 25,* 456–465.

Alston, R. P. (2015). Anaesthesia for off-pump coronary artery bypass grafting surgery. *Anaesthesia and Intensive Care Medicine, 16*(10), 524–527.

Appoo, J. J., Tse, L. W., Pozeg, Z. I., Wong, J. K., Hutchison, S. J., Gregory, A. J., . . . Herget, E. J. (2014). Thoracic aortic frontier: Review of current applications and directions of thoracic endovascular aortic repair (TEVAR). *Canadian Journal of Cardiology, 30,* 52–63.

Baikoussis, N. G., Papakonstantinou, N. A., & Apostolakis, E. (2014). Radial artery as graft for coronary artery bypass surgery: Advantages and disadvantages for its usage focused on structural and biological characteristics. *Journal of Cardiology, 63,* 321–328.

Barsoum, E. A., Azab, B., Patel, N., Spagnola, J., Shariff, M. A., Kaleem, U., . . . McCord, D. A. (2016). Long-term outcome after percutaneous coronary intervention compared with minimally invasive coronary artery bypass surgery in the elderly. *The Open Cardiovascular Medicine Journal, 10,* 11. doi:10.2174/1874192401610010011

Campelo-Parada, F., Perlman, G., Philippon, F., Ye, J., Thompson, C., Bédard, E., . . . Dvir, D. (2015). First-in-man experience of a novel transcatheter repair system for treating severe tricuspid regurgitation. *Journal of the American College of Cardiology, 66*(22), 2475–2483.

Chatterjee, A., Bajaj, N. S., McMahon, W. S., Cribbs, M. G., White, J. S., Mukherjee, A., . . . Law, M. (2017). Transcatheter pulmonary valve implantation: A comprehensive systematic review and meta-analyses of observational studies. *Journal of the American Heart Association, 6*(8), e006432. Retrieved from https://www.ncbi.nlm.nih.gov/pmc/articles/PMC5586471/.

Cheatham, J. P., Hellenbrand, W. E., Zahn, E. M., Jones, T. K., Berman, D. P., Vincent, J. A., . . . McElhinney, D. B. (2015). Clinical and hemodynamic outcomes up to 7 years after transcatheter pulmonary valve replacement in the US melody valve investigational device exemption trial. *Circulation, 131*(22), 1960–1970.

Cheung, A., & Lichtenstein, M. (2012). Illustrated techniques for transapical aortic valve implantation. *Annals of Cardiothoracic Surgery, 1*(2), 231–239.

Chou, R., Gordon, D. B., de Leon-Casasola, O. A., Rosenberg, J. M., Bickler, S., Brennan, T., . . . Griffith, S. (2016). Management of postoperative pain: A clinical practice guideline from the American Pain Society, the American Society of Regional Anesthesia and Pain Medicine, and the American Society of Anesthesiologists' committee on regional anesthesia, executive committee, and administrative council. *The Journal of Pain, 17*(2), 131–157.

Chugh, S. S., Havmoeller, R., Narayanan, K., Singh, D., Rienstra, M., Benjamin, E. J., . . . Murray, C. J. (2014). Worldwide epidemiology of atrial fibrillation: A global burden of disease 2010 study. *Circulation, 129*(8), 837–847.

Craig, T., January, C. T., Wann, L. S., Alpert J. S., Calkins, H., Cigarroa, J. E., . . . Yancy, C. W. (2014). AHA/ACC/HRS guideline for the management of patients with atrial fibrillation. *Journal of the American College of Cardiology, 64*(21), 2246–2280.

Dai, H., Huenges, K., Pokorny, S., Fischer, G., Cremer, J., Metzner, A., . . . Lutter, G. (2017). Transcatheter mitral valve implantation: A percutaneous transapical system. *Interactive Cardiovascular Thoracic Surgery, 24*(4), 527–533.

D'ascenzo, F., Moretti, C., Marra, W. G., Montefusco, A., Omede, P., Taha, S., . . . Gaita, F. (2015). Meta-analysis of the usefulness of Mitraclip in patients with functional mitral regurgitation. *American Journal of Cardiology, 116*(2), 325–331.

DeGiovanni, J. (2017). Transcatheter pulmonary valve replacement. The Edwards Sapien valve. *Journal of Structural Heart Disease, 3*(3), 62–72.

Deuschl, F., Schofer, N., Lubos, E., Blankenberg, S., & Schäfer, U. (2016). Critical evaluation of the MitraClip system in the management of mitral regurgitation. *Vascular Health and Risk Management, 12*, 1–8.

Dieberg, G., Smart., N. A., & King, N. (2016). Minimally invasive cardiac surgery: A systematic review and meta-analysis. *International Journal of Cardiology, 223*, 554–560.

Doenst, T., Diab, M., Sponholz, C., Bauer, M., & Färber, G. (2017). The opportunities and limitations of minimally invasive cardiac surgery. *Deutsches Ärzteblatt International, 114*(46), 777–784.

Ferdinand, F. D., MacDonald, J. K., Balkhy, H. H., Bisleri, G., Hwang, H. Y., Northrup, P., . . . Kiaii, B. B. (2017). Endoscopic conduit harvest in coronary artery bypass grafting surgery: An ISMICS systematic review and consensus conference statements. *Innovations: Technology and Techniques in Cardiothoracic and Vascular Surgery, 12*(5), 301–319.

Gaasch, W. H., Brecker, S. J. D., & Aldea, G. S. (2014). *Transcatheter aortic valve replacement.* Retrieved from http://www.uptodate.com/contents/transcatheter-aortic-valve-replacement.

Gao C. (2014). Overview of robotic cardiac surgery. In C. Gao (Ed.), *Robotic cardiac surgery* (pp. 1–14). Dordrecht, Netherlands: Springer.

Glauber, M., Miceli, A., Canarutto, D., Lio, A., Murzi, M., Gilmanov, D., . . . Solinas, M. (2015a). Early and long-term outcomes of minimally invasive mitral valve surgery through right minithoracotomy: A 10-year experience in 1604 patients. *Journal of Cardiothoracic Surgery, 10*(181), 1–9.

Glauber, M., Ferrarini, M., & Miceli, A. (2015b). Minimally invasive aortic valve surgery: State of the art and future directions. *Annals of Cardiothoracic Surgery, 4*(1), 26–31.

Glowacki, D. (2015). Effective pain management and improvements in patients' outcomes and satisfaction. *Critical Care Nurse, 35*(3), 33–41.

Greenbaum, A. B., Babaliaros, V. C., Chen, M. Y., Stine, A. M., Rogers, T., O'Neill, W. W., . . . Lederman, R. J. (2017). Transcaval access and closure for transcatheter aortic valve replacement: A prospective investigation. *Journal of the American College of Cardiology, 69*(5), 511–521.

Gregory, S. H., Sodhi, N., Zoller, J. K., Quader, N., Ridley, C. H., Maniar, H. S., . . . Zajarias, A. (2018). Anesthetic considerations for the transcatheter management of mitral valve disease. *Journal of Cardiothoracic and Vascular Anesthesia.* Retrieved from https://www.jcvaonline.com/article/S1053-0770(18)30387-2/pdf

Grosset-Janin, D., Barth, E., Bertrand, B., & Detante, O. (2015). Percutaneous left atrial appendage occlusion for stroke prevention in patients with atrial fibrillation and contraindication for anticoagulation. *Revue Neurologique, 171*, 426–432.

Guyton, R. A., Block, P. C., Thourani, V., Lerakis, S., & Babaliaros, V. (2013). Carotid artery access for transcatheter aortic valve replacement. *Catheterization and Cardiovascular Interventions, 82*, e583–e586.

Hahn, R. T., Meduri, C. U., Davidson, C. J., Lim, S., Nazif, T. M., Ricciardi, M. J., . . . Fowler, D. (2017). Early feasibility study of a transcatheter tricuspid valve annuloplasty: SCOUT trial 30-day results. *Journal of the American College of Cardiology, 69*(14), 1795–1806.

Halkos, M., Liberman, H., Devireddy, C., Walker, P., Finn, A., Jaber, W., . . . Puskas, J. D. (2014). Early clinical and angiographic outcomes after robotic-assisted coronary artery bypass surgery. *The Journal of Thoracic and Cardiovascular Surgery, 147*(1), 179–185.

Harris, A., Dean, A., Babaliaros, V., & Keegan, P. (2014). TAVR patients on an intermediate care unit: Direct from the cath lab to the floor. Poster session presented at the 10th annual conference of the American Association of Heart Failure Nurses, Los Angeles, CA.

Hijazi, Z. M., Ruiz, C. E., Zahn, E., Ringel, R., Aldea, G. S., Bacha, E. A., . . . Feldman, T. (2015). SCAI/AATS/ACC/STS operator and institutional requirements for transcatheter valve repair and replacement, part III: Pulmonic valve. *The Journal of Thoracic and Cardiovascular Surgery, 149*(5), e71–e78.

Holmes, D. R., Kar, S., Price, M. J., Whisenant, B., Sievert, H., Doshi, S. K., . . . Reddy, V. Y. (2014). Prospective randomized evaluation of the Watchman left atrial appendage closure device in patients with atrial fibrillation versus long-term warfarin therapy: The PREVAIL trial. *Journal of the American College of Cardiology, 64*(1), 1–8.

Jacq, G., Gritti, K., Carré, C., Fleury, N., Lang, A., Courau-Courtois, J., . . . Legriel, S. (2015). Modalities of invasive arterial pressure monitoring in critically ill patients: A prospective observational study. *Medicine, 94*(39), 1–6.

Jung, J. C., & Kim, K.-H. (2016). Minimally invasive cardiac surgery versus conventional median sternotomy for atrial septal defect closure. *The Korean Journal of Thoracic and Cardiovascular Surgery, 49*, 421–426.

Katritsis, G. D., & Katritsis, D. G. (2017). Management of complications in anticoagulated patients with atrial fibrillation. *Arrhythmia & Electrophysiology Review, 6*(4), 167–178.

Kikuchi, K., Chen, X., Mori, M., Kurata, A., & Tao, L. (2017). Perioperative outcomes of off-pump minimally invasive coronary artery bypass grafting with bilateral internal thoracic arteries under direct vision. *Interactive Cardiovascular and Thoracic Surgery, 24*(5), 696–701.

Kofler, M., Schachner, T., Reinstadler, S. J., Stastny, L., Dumfarth, J., Wiedemann, D., . . . Bonaros, N. (2017).

Comparative analysis of perioperative and mid-term results of TECAB and MIDCAB for revascularization of anterior wall. *Innovations: Technology and Techniques in Cardiothoracic and Vascular Surgery, 12*(3), 207–213.

Kothandan, H., Kian, H. V., Keong, Y. K., & Chih, H. N. (2014). Anesthesia management for MitraClip device implantation. *Annals of Cardiac Anesthesia, 17*(1), 17–22.

Lancaster, T. S., Melby, S. J., & Damiano, R. J. (2016). Minimally invasive surgery for atrial fibrillation. *Trends in Cardiovascular Medicine, 26*, 268–277.

Lawrance, C. P., Henn, M. C., & Damiano, R. J. (2015). Surgery for atrial fibrillation. *Cardiology Clinics, 32*(4), 563–571.

Leonard, J. R., Rahouma, M., Abouarab, A. A., Schwann, A. N., Scuderi, G., Lau, C., . . . Gaudino, M. (2018). Totally endoscopic coronary artery bypass surgery: A meta-analysis of the current evidence. *International Journal of Cardiology, 261*, 42–46.

Ling, Y., Bao, L., Yang, W., Chen, Y., & Gao, Q. (2016). Minimally invasive direct coronary artery bypass grafting with an improved rib spreader and a new-shaped cardiac stabilizer: Results of 200 consecutive cases in a single institution. *BMC Cardiovascular Disorders, 16*(42), 1–6.

Lomivorotov, V. V., Efremov, S. M., Kirov, M. Y., Fominskiy, E. V., & Karaskov, A. M. (2017). Low-cardiac output syndrome after cardiac surgery. *Journal of Cardiothoracic and Vascular Anesthesia 31*, 291–308.

Mao, Z., Zhong, X., Yin, J., Zhao, Z., Hu, X., & Hackett, M. L. (2015). Predictors associated with stroke after coronary artery bypass grafting: A systematic review. *Journal of the Neurological Sciences, 357*, 1–7.

McNicol, E. D., Ferguson, M. C., & Hudcova, J. (2015). Patient controlled opioid analgesia versus non-patient controlled opioid analgesia for postoperative pain. *Cochrane Database of Systematic Reviews 2015*, (6). doi:10.1002/14651858. CD003348.pub3

Mehta, Y., & Arora, D. (2014). Newer methods of cardiac output monitoring. *World Journal of Cardiology, 6*(9), 1022–1029.

Melly, L., Torregrossa, G., Lee, T., Jansens, J.- L., & Puskas, J. D. (2018). Fifty years of coronary artery bypass grafting. *Journal of Thoracic Disease, 10*(3), 1960–1967.

Minol, J. P., Boeken, U., Weinreich, T., Heimann, M., Gramsch-Zabel, H., Akhyari, P., . . . Lichtenberg, A. (2015). Isolated tricuspid valve surgery: A single institutional experience with the technique of minimally invasive surgery via right minithoracotomy. *The Thoracic and Cardiovascular Surgeon, 65*(8), 606–611.

Misfeld, M., Davierwala, P., Banusch, J., Ender, J., Mohr, F. W., & Pfannmüller, B. (2017). Minimally invasive, beating heart tricuspid valve surgery in a redo case. *Annals of Cardiothoracic Surgery, 6*(3), 290–293.

Moore, B. M., Bernard, H. K., Naoum, C., Simmons, L., Cartwright, B. L., Wilson, M. K., . . . Ng, M. (2017). Transcatheter mitral valve replacement with a novel dual stent bioprosthesis. *Circulation: Cardiovascular Interventions, 10*(6). doi:10.1161/CIRCINTERVENTIONS.116.004841

Mozaffarian, D., Benjamin, E. J., Go, A. S., Arnett, D. K., Blaha, M. J., Cushman, M., . . . Turner, M. B. (2015). Heart disease and stroke statistics—2015 update: A report from the American Heart Association. *Circulation, 131*(4), e29–e322.

Nishimura, R. A., Otto, C. M., Bonow, R. O., Carabello, B. A., Erwin, J. P., Fleisher, L.A., . . . Thompson,, A. (2017). 2017 AHA/ACC focused update of 2014 AHA/ACC guideline for the management of patients with valvular heart disease: A report of the American College of Cardiology/American Heart Association Task Force on Clinical Practice Guidelines. *Circulation, 135*(25), e1159–e1195.

Panoulas, V. F., Colombo, A., Margonato, A., & Maisano, F. (2015). Hybrid coronary revascularization: Promising, but yet to take off. *Journal of the American College of Cardiology, 65*(1), 85–97.

Pascual, I., Carro, A., Avanzas, P., Hernández-Vaquero, D., Diaz, R., Rozado, J., . . . Moris, C. (2017). Vascular approaches for transcatheter aortic valve implantation. *Journal of Thoracic Disease, 9*, S478–S487.

Pike, R. D. B. (2015). Off pump coronary artery bypass and minimally invasive direct coronary artery bypass. In M. J. Murray, R. A. Harrison, J. T. Mueller, S. H. Rose, C. T. Wass, & D. J. Wedel (Eds.), *Faust's anesthesiology review* (4th ed., pp. 341–342). Philadelphia, PA: Elsevier Saunders.

Pope, N. H., & Ailawadi, G. (2014). Minimally invasive valve surgery. *Journal of Cardiovascular Translational Research, 7*(4), 387–394.

Puskas, J. D., Martin, J., Cheng, D. C. H., Benussi, S., Bonatti, J. O., Diegeler, A., . . . Zamvar, V. (2015). ISMICS consensus conference and statements of randomized controlled trials of off-pump versus conventional coronary artery bypass surgery. *Innovations, 10*(4), 219–229.

Raja, S. G., Garg, S., Rochon, M., Daley, S., De Robertis, F., & Bahrami, T. (2018). Short-term clinical outcomes and long-term survival of minimally invasive direct coronary bypass grafting. *Annals of Cardiothoracic Surgery.* Retrieved from http://www.annalscts.com/article/view/16504.

Ramlawi, B., & Gammie, J. S. (2016). Mitral valve surgery: Current minimally invasive and transcatheter options. *Methodist Debakey Cardiovascular Journal, 12*(1). doi: 10.14797/mdcj-12-1-1

Reddy, V.Y., Doshi, S. K., Kar, S., Gibson, D. N., Price, M. J., Huber, K., . . . Holmes, D.R. (2017). 5-Year Outcomes After Left Atrial Appendage Closure: From the PREVAIL and PROTECT AF trials. *Journal of the American College of Cardiology, 70*(24), 2964–2975.

Ricci, D., Boffini, M., Barbero, C., El Qarra, S., Marchetto, G., & Rinaldi, M. (2014). Minimally invasive tricuspid valve surgery in patients at high risk. *The Journal of Thoracic and Cardiovascular Surgery, 147*(3), 996–1001.

Rodés-Cabau, J., Hahn, R. T., Latib, A., Laule, M., Lauten, A., Maisano, F., . . . Vahanian, A. (2016). Transcatheter therapies for treating tricuspid regurgitation. *Journal of the American College of Cardiology, 67*(15), 1829–1845.

Rosenblum, J. M., Harskamp, R. E., Hoedemaker, N., Walker, P., Liberman, H. A., de Winter, R. J., . . . Halkos, M. E. (2016). Hybrid coronary revascularization versus coronary artery bypass surgery with bilateral or single internal mammary artery grafts. *Journal of Thoracic and Cardiovascular Surgery, 151*(4), 1081–1089.

Rozeik, M. M., Wheatley, D. J., & Gourlay, T. (2014). Percutaneous heart valves: Past, present and future. *Perfusion, 29*(5), 397–410.

Saito, K., Toyama, H., Ejima, Y., Kurotaki, K., Yamauchi, M., & Kurosawa, S. (2015). Anticoagulant managements of left ventricular assist device implantation in two patients with heparin-induced thrombocytopenia (HIT): Use of argatroban as an anticoagulant for cardiopulmonary bypass. *Anesthesia & Clinical Research, 6*(4), 1–5.

Sarkar, M., & Prabhu, V. (2017). Basics of cardiopulmonary bypass. *Indian Journal of Anaesthesia, 61*(9), 760–767.

Sinan, U. Y. (2015). The cardiac related thrombocytopenia. *Journal of Hematology & Thromboembolic Diseases, 3*(4), 1–4.

Stephens, R. S., & Whitman, G. J. R. (2015a). Postoperative critical care of the adult cardiac surgical patient. Part I: Routine postoperative care. *Critical Care Medicine, 43*(7), 1477–1497.

Stephens, R. S., & Whitman, G. J. R. (2015b). Postoperative critical care of the adult cardiac surgical patient. Part II: Procedure-specific considerations, management of complications, and quality improvement. *Critical Care Medicine, 43*(9), 1995–2014.

Sugita, J., & Fujiu, K. (2018). Systemic inflammatory stress response during cardiac surgery. *International Heart Journal 59*, 457–459.

Suradi, H. S., Kavinsky, C. J., & Hijazi, Z. M. (2016). Percutaneous mitral valve repair: The MitraClip device. *Global Cardiology Science & Practice, 2*, 1–12.

Tekin, A. I., & Arslan, U. (2017). Perioperative outcomes in minimally invasive direct coronary artery bypass versus off-pump coronary artery bypass with sternotomy. *Videosurgery and Other Miniinvasive Techniques, 12*(3), 285–290.

Theissen, S., Vanhorebeek, I., & Van den Berghe, G. (2015). Glycemic control and outcome related to cardiopulmonary bypass. *Best Practice & Research Clinical Anaesthesiology, 29*(2), 177–187.

Thiele, R. H., Isbell, J. M., & Rosner, M. H. (2015). AKI associated with cardiac surgery. *Clinical Journal American Society of Nephrology, 10*(3), 500–514.

Thielmann, M., Sharma, V., Al-Attar, N., Bulluck, H., Bisleri, G., Bunge, J., . . . Holfeld, J. (2017). ESC Joint Working Groups on Cardiovascular Surgery and the Cellular Biology of the Heart Position Paper: Perioperative myocardial injury and infarction in patients undergoing coronary artery bypass graft surgery. *European Heart Journal, 38*(31), 2392–2407.

Thourani, V. N., Gunter, R. L., Neravetla, S., Block, P., Guyton, R. A., Kilgo, P., . . . Babaliaros, V. (2013). Use of transaortic, transapical, and transcarotid transcatheter aortic valve replacement in inoperable patients. *Annals of Thoracic Surgery, 96,* 1349–1357.

Tribble, C., & Urencio, M. (2015). Open saphenous vein harvest. *Journal of the American College of Surgeons, 220*(3), e35–e39.

Tzikas, A., Shakir, S., Gafoor, S., Omran, H., Berti, S., Santoro, G., . . . Park, J-W. (2016). Left atrial appendage occlusion for stroke prevention in atrial fibrillation: Multicenter experience with the AMPLATZER cardiac plug. *EuroIntervention, 11*(10), 1170–1179.

Van Praet, K. M., Stamm, C., Sündermann, S. H., Meyer, A., Unbehaun, A., Montagner, M., . . . Kempfert, J. (2018). Minimally invasive surgical mitral valve repair: State of the art review. *Interventional Cardiology Review, 13*(1), 14–19.

Vismara, R., Gelpi, G., Prabhu, S., Romitelli, P., Troxler, L. G., Mangini, A., . . . Jaworek, M. (2016). Transcatheter edge-to-edge treatment of functional tricuspid regurgitation in an ex vivo pulsatile heart model. *Journal of the American College of Cardiology, 68*(10), 1024–1033.

Yanagawa, B., & Puskas, J. D. (2016). Off-pump coronary artery bypass grafting. *Operative Techniques in Thoracic and Cardiovascular Surgery, 21*, 2–19.

Zellinger, M. (2007). Cardiac surgery and heart transplant. In R. Kaplow & S. R. Hardin (Eds.), *Critical care nursing: Synergy for optimal outcomes* (pp. 229–242). Sudbury, MA: Jones and Bartlett.

Zhang, L., Cui, Z., Song, Z., Yang, H., Fu, Y., Gong, Y., & Ling, Y. (2015). Minimally invasive direct coronary bypass for left anterior descending artery revascularization—analysis of 300 cases. *Videosurgery and Other Miniinvasive Techniques, 10*(4), 548–554.

Web Resources

Aortic Stenosis: Minimally Invasive: http://www.youtube.com/watch?v=-miuqi1iyrw

Hybrid Maze Procedure: http://www.youtube.com/watch?v=XRGLCmkSqso

Minimally Invasive Direct Coronary Artery Bypass (MIDCAB): http://www.youtube.com/watch?v=Iq4HXtDYxS8

Robotically Assisted Single-Vessel Coronary Artery Bypass Surgery: http://www.youtube.com/watch?v=YIRP3vS4zV0

CHAPTER 8

Recovery from Anesthesia

Roberta Kaplow

▶ Introduction

It is estimated that between 2016 and 2027, 18.73 million cardiovascular procedures will be performed worldwide. This reflects an average annual increase of 3.7% in both surgical and interventional cardiovascular procedure volume growth. In the United States, approximately 2,300 patients undergo heart transplantation annually despite a shortage of donors (Texas Heart Institute, 2016). Thanks to advances in surgical techniques, anesthetic agents, and postoperative medications, thousands of cardiac surgery patients have enjoyed speedy recovery times. More importantly, improvements in anesthetic techniques have allowed patients to transition quickly from the immediate postoperative period at the intensive care unit (ICU) to a cardiac surgery unit and then home in increasingly shorter periods of time. Given these trends, ICU nurses must be assiduous in the care of these patients. This chapter focuses on care in the immediate postoperative period.

▶ Hand-off Communication or Situation-Background-Assessment-Recommendation (SBAR)

Postoperative care begins immediately after the patient is transferred from the operating room (OR). Following cardiac surgery, patients are typically transferred to the ICU for monitoring, hemodynamic stabilization, assessment for complications, and possibly extubation. Vital information is exchanged in the hand-off communication between the anesthesia provider and the ICU nurse. Data should include pertinent information regarding the surgical procedure, any intraoperative complications or events, hemodynamic and ventilatory status, cardiopulmonary bypass (CPB) time, recent laboratory data, type and amount of intravenous (IV) fluids and blood products

Original contributions from Toni Patricia Johnson

administered, reversal of anticoagulants, pertinent medical and surgical history, preoperative status, location of intravenous lines and invasive catheters, vasopressor and inotropic agents used, and current infusion rates. Additional information includes use of mechanical cardiac assist devices, presence of pacing wires, length of surgery, estimated blood loss, intraoperative intake and output, patient position on the OR table, location of drains and dressings, and anesthetic and reversal agents administered. **TABLE 8.1** lists the more common anesthetic agents used.

In addition to the information provided by the anesthesia provider, an extensive preoperative evaluation is conducted prior to cardiac surgery. Details of this evaluation are described in Chapter 4. Information about existing comorbidities, cardiac disease, tobacco use, nutritional status, medication history, preoperative cardiac status, and any optimizing that might have taken place prior to surgery will help the ICU nurse anticipate the patient's immediate postoperative course and potentially required interventions. By way of illustration, as discussed in Chapter 5, the hemodynamic profile and resultant interventions indicated for patients who undergo cardiac surgery for valvular disease will vary with the pathophysiology of each respective disorder.

A patient's comorbidities may also help the ICU nurse anticipate problems in the immediate postoperative period. For example, patients with a history of conditions such as valvular disease, recent myocardial infarction (MI), arterial hypertension, diabetes, previous cardiac surgery, chronic peripheral vascular disease, involvement of three or more vessels, elevated serum creatinine, ejection fraction less than 40%, chronic kidney disease, endocarditis, or chronic obstructive pulmonary disease (COPD) are more likely to require prolonged mechanical ventilation (Gutsche et al., 2014; Totonch, Baazm, Chitsazan, Seifi, & Chitsazan, 2014). Data specific to patients who underwent coronary artery bypass graft (CABG) procedure reveal risk factors of advanced New York Heart Association (NYHA) class, chronic renal dysfunction, and longer perfusion times (Gumus et al., 2015).

If the patient underwent CPB, the potential for a systemic inflammatory response with associated hemodynamic effects should be anticipated. As described in Chapter 13, the inflammatory response may be related to the surface of the CPB circuit being in contact with blood or reperfusion injury associated with aortic cross-clamping (Gil-Gomez et al., 2014). Other intraoperative risk factors include type of surgery, operative and pump times, and intraoperative transfusions.

TABLE 8.1 Anesthetic Agents/Adjuncts Commonly Used in Cardiac Surgery

Intravenous Induction Agents	Neuromuscular Blocking Agents	Analgesics/ Sedatives	Inhalation Agents
Propofol (Diprivan®) Etomidate (Amidate®) Thiopental sodium (Pentothal®)	Rocuronium (Zemuron®) Vecuronium (Norcuron®) Succinylcholine (Anectine®) Atracurium besylate (Tracrium®) Mivacurium chloride (Mivacron®) Cisatracurium (Nimbex®) Doxacurium (Raplon®) Pancuronium (Pavulon®) Tubocurarine Metocurine	Fentanyl (Sublimaze®) Sufentanil (Sufenta®) Alfentanil (Alfenta®) Remifentanil (Ultiva®) Morphine sulfate Midazolam (Versed®) Lorazepam (Ativan®) Dexmedetomidine (Precedex®)	Isoflurane (Forane®) Desflurane (Suprane®) Sevoflurane (Ultane®) Enflurane (Ethrane®) Halothane (Fluothane®)

Data from Faulk, Fleisher, Jones & Nussmeier, 2014; Landoni et al., 2013; Shahani, 2017.

Postoperative risk factors include the presence of bleeding and dependency on inotropes (Totonch et al., 2014). Specific to postoperative CABG patients, higher body mass index, lower ejection fraction, and use of cardiopulmonary bypass were risk factors (Wise et al., 2017).

▶ Immediate Postoperative Care

The foremost objectives when caring for a cardiac surgery patient in the immediate postoperative period are maintenance of cardiac perfusion and maximization of tissue perfusion (Yazdchi & Rawn, 2018). Goals of the first hour of care include stabilization of hemodynamic, oxygenation, and thermoregulatory status. Postoperative care requires assessment of physiologic parameters and hemodynamic monitoring, as well as assessment, prompt recognition, and treatment of potential complications related to either patient comorbidities, effects of anesthesia, or the surgical procedure itself.

Control of the cardiac surgery patient's blood pressure in the immediate postoperative period is important. In fact, variability in perioperative blood pressure is associated with an increase in 30-day mortality. The ICU nurse should monitor for hypertension to avoid associated complications such as bleeding, myocardial ischemia, dysrhythmias, stroke, or graft dehiscence. Initial management of hypertension may entail administration of opioids, sedatives, or both. However, infusion of a vasodilator may be required if initial therapies are not effective in controlling hypertension (Silvestry, 2017).

▶ Assessment

The nurse performs a detailed physical assessment. Electrocardiogram (ECG) monitoring of heart rate and rhythm is performed. The patient's hemodynamic profile (e.g., blood pressure, pulmonary artery pressures, pulmonary artery occlusive pressure [PAOP], central venous pressure [CVP], cardiac output [CO]/cardiac index [CI], systemic vascular resistance [SVR]), temperature, and pulse oximetry are evaluated. Additional invasive monitoring (e.g., mixed venous oxygen saturation) may be performed as well. The ICU nurse can then correlate these data with an assessment of peripheral perfusion. If temporary pacing wires are present, they should be checked to ensure proper function for emergent temporary pacing. A baseline postoperative ECG should be attained to determine presence of ischemia, infarction, conduction abnormalities, or graft spasm (Silvestry, 2017).

Assessment of neurologic status typically includes level of consciousness, degree of orientation, pupil size and reaction, and ability to move extremities. A more in-depth neurologic assessment may follow later in the postoperative period. Inherent in a neurologic assessment is an initial and ongoing assessment of pain. If the patient is able to self-report the level of pain, that would be the most reliable indicator. If the patient is cognitively impaired and cannot self-report, a valid and reliable behavioral pain rating scale should be used. The ICU nurse should differentiate incisional pain from anginal pain. Management of pain in the postoperative cardiac surgery patient is discussed in detail in Chapter 14.

An initial respiratory assessment typically includes auscultation of breath sounds; oxygen delivery mode; presence of symmetrical chest expansion; and respiratory rate, depth, effort, and rhythm. If the patient remains on mechanical ventilation, assessment of tube placement by the markings on the endotracheal tube should be noted, and ventilator settings (e.g., mode, fractional inspired oxygen [FiO_2], rate, tidal volume, positive end-expiratory pressure [PEEP], pressure support, alarm settings) should be verified as applicable. Typical ventilator settings in the immediate postoperative period following cardiac surgery are discussed in Chapter 11. Once these data are obtained, the patient's respiratory status can be correlated with pulse oximetry, end-tidal carbon dioxide ($ETCO_2$) level, and arterial blood gas (ABG) results. A baseline chest radiograph should be obtained to verify placement of the endotracheal tube (2–3 cm above the carina), catheters, wires, or any other devices that were inserted in the OR. The presence of any postoperative atelectasis, pneumothorax, or other common respiratory complication following cardiac surgery can also be determined (Silvestry, 2017).

Types and number of drainage catheters will vary based on the operative procedure and approach used. If a minimally invasive approach is used, a small-diameter catheter will be noted. If the patient had a sternotomy but the pleural space is not opened, the patient will have a mediastinal chest tube, or a chest tube in the mediastinal and pleural spaces (Andreasen et al., 2016).

Tubes are connected to −20 cm of wall suction. The ICU nurse should assess the amount, color, and viscosity of initial operative and subsequent drainage. Patency of the catheters must be maintained at all times. Volume repletion, treatment of the underlying cause (if possible), and monitoring of the patient's coagulation profile are indicated if the patient is experiencing bleeding (Colson et al., 2016; Najafi & Faraoni, 2014). As discussed in Chapter 13, there are variable definitions of excessive bleeding following cardiac surgery. These include 200 mL/hour or 1,500 mL/8 hours (Stephens & Whitman, 2015). General guidelines for excessive mediastinal bleeding are characterized by continuous chest tube output of greater than 200 mL/hour for 2 hours.

If a mediastinal chest tube becomes clotted, cardiac tamponade may ensue. Signs and symptoms may include sudden decrease or cessation of mediastinal bleeding, dyspnea, decreased CO and hypotension, tachycardia, low-voltage QRS on ECG, increased CVP, altered mental status, cyanosis or pallor, and anxiety (Kaplow & Iyere, 2017). Other signs and symptoms are described in Chapter 13.

Preventive measures include positioning the patient on the side with the head of the bed elevated 30 degrees to facilitate catheter drainage. Until the condition is treated, the ICU nurse should administer volume to help counteract the decrease in preload from the associated decrease in diastolic filling pressures of the tamponade. Administration of afterload reducers (i.e., vasodilators) may help promote contractility (Silvestry, 2017). Cardiac tamponade management is discussed in detail in Chapter 13.

An initial assessment of the patient's fluid and electrolyte status should be performed upon admission to the ICU. In addition to the output from drains, a correlation between the patient's hemodynamic status and the intraoperative intake and output of fluids should be made. The ICU nurse should anticipate third spacing of fluid in the immediate postoperative period (Kayiloglu et al., 2015). Evaluation of serum electrolytes should be included in the initial assessment, as imbalances may be anticipated. Anticipated alterations and management of fluid and electrolytes in the postoperative cardiac surgery patient are discussed in detail in Chapter 17.

▶ Anesthetic Agents

Balanced anesthesia or "fast-tracking" is generally employed to facilitate early extubation of the cardiac surgery patient while concomitantly decreasing anxiety, pain, length of ICU stay, and complications; minimizing mechanical ventilation time; and promoting a quicker, uneventful recovery from anesthesia. Typically, shorter acting agents—although more costly—result in earlier extubation and reduced postoperative stays (Kianfar et al., 2015). It is important for the ICU nurse to recognize signs and symptoms, multisystem effects, and postoperative nursing implications of commonly used anesthetic agents administered during surgery.

Induction Agents

Combinations of intravenous agents are administered to augment the effects of inhalation agents. Classifications of these agents include barbiturates (e.g., thiopental sodium), nonbarbiturates (e.g., etomidate, propofol), and tranquilizers (e.g., midazolam, lorazepam) (Faulk, Fleisher, Jones, & Nussmeier, 2014).

Barbiturates depress the central nervous system (CNS). Thiopental sodium, for example, causes cardiovascular depression and negative inotropy, resulting in hypotension, decreased CO, and peripheral vascular resistance. Barbiturates also cause respiratory depression, which puts the patient at risk for apnea, airway obstruction, and, at higher doses, loss of laryngeal reflexes; the latter effect puts the patient at risk for aspiration (Lafferty, 2017). Other side effects may include headache, emergence agitation, prolonged somnolence, and nausea. Nursing considerations include monitoring for the prolonged effects of thiopental, which could persist for as long as 36 hours (Tembelopoulos, Carr, & Tressy-Murphy, 2012).

Etomidate is a hypnotic agent with no analgesic effects. It is considered the agent of choice in patients with cardiovascular instability. When this agent is used, it is less likely to cause hypotension. Heart rate, contractility, and CO remain stable, and negative inotropic effects are negligible with etomidate (Wagner et al., 2014). Some patients may develop postoperative nausea and vomiting (PONV), hiccoughs, involuntary tremors, or suppressed adrenal function following administration of etomidate (DeJong & Jaber, 2014).

Propofol (Diprivan) is a sedative that is primarily used as an induction agent. Compared with barbiturates, it causes less myocardial depression. Hypotension seen following propofol administration is felt to be related to arterial and venous dilation, which decreases venous return to the heart and CI (Kakazu & Lippmann, 2015). An infusion of propofol is generally initiated en route to the ICU and discontinued 10 to 15 minutes prior to ventilator weaning. The maintenance infusion rate is 50 to 150 mcg/kg/min. Propofol has a low incidence of postoperative side effects and is less likely to cause PONV than etomidate. It allows the patient to quickly regain consciousness with minimal residual CNS effects, allowing for early extubation. Because propofol has no analgesic properties, postoperative analgesics will be required (Orlewicz, 2017).

Benzodiazepines are used as adjuncts to induction agents prior to cardiac surgery. Midazolam (Versed®) may also be used postoperatively for sedation in the patient who remains intubated. This agent can cause respiratory depression, bradycardia, and mild vasodilation, but it minimizes PONV (Nishiyama, 2016). Nursing considerations include monitoring of vital signs and oxygen saturation. If severe, respiratory depression may be reversed by administering flumazenil (Romazicon®). The initial dose of flumazenil may be administered as 0.2-mg IV doses over 15 seconds. If the initial dose is not effective, additional 0.2-mg doses may be administered over 1 minute. Additional doses may be administered over 1 minute after waiting 45 seconds to determine if the drug is effective. The maximum amount of flumazenil that may be administered is 1 mg (Frandsen & Pennington, 2014).

Inhalation Agents

Inhalation agents cause circulatory depression and hypotension as a result of vasodilation and decreased contractility (Neubert & Sinha, 2015). They may be administered either alone or in combination with intravenous anesthetics. Nursing considerations include monitoring for ventricular ectopy, fibrillation, and tachycardia, which generally manifest during the immediate postoperative period. Inhalation agents typically do not possess analgesic properties. They are eliminated through the lungs; the amount of time it takes depends on the patient's CO. Patients will require oxygen therapy and encouragement to cough and deep breathe. Hemodynamic monitoring is essential given the sensitization to catecholamines associated with many of these inhalation agents.

Because some of the inhalation agents are fat soluble and are absorbed into adipose tissue, elimination and recovery times are longer when these agents are given. Further, patients with higher percentages of body fat will have a longer recovery time when administered fat-soluble inhalation agents. Prompt management of pain and PONV are other vital ICU nursing responsibilities at this time.

Sevoflurane and halothane have depressant effects on the respiratory system. Additionally, smooth bronchial muscles and laryngeal and pharyngeal reflexes are blunted by these agents, placing the patient at risk for aspiration. Sevoflurane and halothane side effects may include decreased responsiveness to oxygenation and ventilation, and elevated carbon dioxide (CO_2) levels. Halothane decreases mucociliary function for as long as 6 hours, which increases the patient's risk for atelectasis and pneumonia. Its cardiovascular effects include myocardial depression and peripheral vasodilation. Two benefits of halothane are the associated low incidence of PONV and its bronchodilator properties, making this agent useful in patients with pulmonary disease. Sevoflurane does not appear to irritate the respiratory system or sensitize the heart to catecholamines, although it may cause hypotension by decreasing afterload (Tsikas, Jordan, & Engelis, 2015).

Enflurane and isoflurane may cause laryngospasm, coughing, and breath holding. These side effects predispose the patient to noncardiogenic pulmonary edema. Attributes of isoflurane include that it is not associated with increased cardiac sensitization to catecholamines, it stabilizes the cardiovascular system, and it has the least related increase in cerebral blood flow (Walters, n.d.).

Enflurane has residual CNS depressant effects, which manifest during the postoperative period. Other effects include decreased blood pressure, stroke volume, and SVR, and increased heart rate; this medication also sensitizes the heart to catecholamines. Enflurane causes mild coronary vasodilation (Lenzarini, Di Lascio, Shea, Kusmic, & Faita, 2016). A benefit of enflurane is the low associated incidence of PONV (Feinleib, Kwan, & Yamani, 2017). Nursing considerations include anticipation of delayed awakening and extubation.

Isoflurane augments the effects of nondepolarizing muscle relaxants. It is a coronary artery vasodilator that is associated with increased coronary perfusion (Gustafson & Brown, 2017).

Neuromuscular Blocking Agents

Neuromuscular blocking agents (NMBAs) are used as adjuncts to inhalation agents to provide relaxation of skeletal muscles, facilitate intubation, and decrease shivering (Gustafson & Brown, 2017). These agents are classified as either depolarizing or nondepolarizing agents. Neuromuscular blocking agents that are commonly administered during cardiac surgery include rocuronium, vecuronium, and succinylcholine. Succinylcholine is an example of a depolarizing NMBA; rocuronium and vecuronium are examples of nondepolarizing agents. They are short- to medium-acting agents, respectively. Rocuronium, cisatracurium, doxacurium, and vecuronium have no cardiovascular side effects

and, therefore, are useful in cardiac surgery. These agents are eliminated by the hepatic system, as opposed to the renal system (Lee, Athanassoglou, & Pandit, 2016). As a consequence, their effects will be prolonged in patients with severe liver disease.

Return paralysis can occur during the early postoperative period. The ICU nurse should observe for a descending trend in minute ventilation, which can be caused by inadequate reversal of the NMBA. Nondepolarizing agents are reversed with anticholinesterase drugs (e.g., neostigmine [Prostigmin®]). Depolarizing NMBAs cannot be pharmacologically reversed because they are metabolized by pseudocholinesterase, an endogenous enzyme.

It is essential that the ICU nurse realize NMBAs have no amnestic or analgesic properties, nor do they cause a loss of consciousness. Analgesics must be administered to the postoperative cardiac surgery patient despite the patient's inability to quantify pain levels. Medications to achieve decreased levels of consciousness or amnesia must similarly be administered if those effects are desired in the postoperative cardiac surgery patient.

Opioids

Intravenous opioids are used as analgesics or as induction agents. When administered, these medications decrease the response and perception to pain. The most frequently used opioid in cardiac surgery is fentanyl. Nursing considerations include monitoring for bradycardia, which may be treated with atropine or glycopyrrolate (Robinul®). Postoperative nausea and vomiting are common side effects of opioids and of clinical concern.

▶ Postoperative Care

Hemodynamic Management

The primary goal of care for the cardiac surgery patient in the immediate postoperative period is optimization of hemodynamic status to help achieve a balance between oxygen supply and demand. This goal can best be accomplished by maintaining an adequate CO.

As described in Chapter 9, CO is affected by a patient's preload, afterload, and contractility. Preload refers to the heart's filling pressures, reflected as the amount of volume returning to the right and left sides of the heart. It is evaluated by measuring CVP and PAOP, respectively. Afterload refers to the amount of work the heart must do to eject blood. Typically, left-sided afterload (i.e., SVR) is evaluated most often. These two parameters can be evaluated and manipulated by the ICU nurse to optimize a patient's hemodynamic profile.

Causes of alterations in preload in the postoperative cardiac surgery patient include vasodilation from a systemic inflammatory response associated with CPB procedures, medications, loss of vasomotor tone, vasodilation from rewarming, bleeding, third spacing from increased capillary permeability, and increased urinary output from hypothermia. Further, compliance of the left ventricle is often decreased following cardiac surgery from postischemic injury and myocardial stunning (Silvestry, 2017). Volume repletion is indicated for patients with decreased preload. The decision of whether to use crystalloids or colloids for fluid resuscitation remains unresolved given the pros and cons of each option. If volume resuscitation alone is inadequate to maintain filling pressures and CO in a patient who has adequate pump function and vasodilation, consideration should be given to adding an infusion of a vasopressor (e.g., phenylephrine [Neo-Synephrine®], vasopressin, methylene blue) (Silvestry, 2017). Methylene blue is an inhibitor of nitric oxide, which is released in large quantities in patients following CPB. Nitric oxide produces profound vasodilation and vasoplegia (hypotension with normal or high CO, low CVP, low PAOP, and low peripheral vascular resistance) (Zhao, Vanhoutte, & Leung, 2015). Methylene blue is not U.S. Food and Drug Administration approved for the indication, but is frequently used in the treatment of vasodilatory shock or vasoplegic syndrome in the immediate postoperative CPB period (Hosseinian, Weiner, Levin, & Fischer, 2016). Chapter 12 discusses vasopressor therapy in more detail.

An increase in afterload may be related to postoperative hypertension, use of medications that cause vasoconstriction, hypothermia, pain, anxiety, hypovolemia, or postoperative pump failure. Infusion of a vasodilator (e.g., sodium nitroprusside [Nipride®], clevidipine [Cleviprex®], nitroglycerin [Tridil®], esmolol [Brevibloc®], or nicardipine [Cardene®]) is indicated for patients who are hypertensive or who have inadequate pump function but with individual-specific normal blood pressure (Mastropietro & Uribe, 2015). Increased afterload may result in decreased stroke volume and cardiac output and increased myocardial oxygen demand (Silvestry, 2017). Vasodilator therapy is discussed in more detail in Chapter 12. A decrease in afterload may be caused by vasodilation from the CPB-associated systemic inflammatory response, administration of medications that cause vasodilation, or fever (Silvestry, 2017).

Once a patient's preload and afterload have been optimized, if CO is inadequate, administration of an inotropic agent may be considered to augment contractility. Agents such as milrinone (Primacor®) or dobutamine (Dobutrex®) increase CO by augmenting contractility and decrease afterload by causing vasodilation (Silvestry, 2017). Chapter 12 discusses inotropic agents in more detail.

As described in Chapter 13, although acceptable postoperative hemodynamic values will vary with the patient's cardiac history, optimal hemodynamic parameters in a postoperative cardiac surgery patient include a CI of more than 2 L/min/m^2, PAOP of approximately 15 mmHg, CVP 5 to 15 mmHg, mean arterial pressure (MAP) 60 to 90 mmHg, systolic blood pressure (SBP) in the range of 90 to 140 mmHg, PAOP 10 to 15 mmHg, and systemic vascular resistance index in the range of 1,400 to 2,800 dyne/sec/cm^{-5}/m^2 (Silvestry, 2017).

Alterations in Heart Rate and Rhythm

Postoperative dysrhythmias can be anticipated in the postoperative cardiac surgery patient. The most common dysrhythmias are atrial in origin; ventricular dysrhythmias and bradycardic rhythms are possible as well. Dysrhythmias may or may not manifest in the initial postoperative period. If present, however, dysrhythmias may cause hemodynamic instability. If the patient has a clinically significant dysrhythmia, then pharmacologic control of rate, rhythm, or both may be indicated. Management of alterations in heart rate and rhythm is discussed in detail in Chapter 15.

Postoperative Nausea and Vomiting

Postoperative nausea and vomiting are common occurrences in the immediate postoperative period, primarily due to the medications administered intraoperatively. Both increase the risk of pulmonary aspiration, disrupt surgical repairs secondary to retching, increase postoperative bleeding, and cause electrolyte disturbances (e.g., hypokalemia, hyponatremia, hypochloremia), dehydration, and esophageal rupture and tears (Weismann, Kranke, & Eberhart, 2015). Postoperative nausea and vomiting can be minimized by assessing for risk factors (e.g., age, gender, history of PONV or motion sickness, and use of volatile anesthetics and opioids) in the preoperative phase and by implementing preventive strategies utilizing a multimodal approach (**BOX 8.1**).

Administering prophylactic antiemetics that affect different receptor sites in the brain has been shown to decrease the incidence of PONV. Medications that may be used to treat PONV include

---

BOX 8.1 Multimodal Management of Postoperative Nausea and Vomiting

Glucocorticoids (e.g., dexamethasone [Decadron®])
5-HT3 receptor antagonists (e.g., ondansetron [Zofran®], granisetron [Granisol®], dolasetron [Anzemet®], palonosetron [Aloxi®])
Anticholinergics (e.g., scopolamine patch)
Butyrophenones (e.g., droperidol [Inapsine®], haloperidol [Haldol®])
Antihistamines (e.g., diphenhydramine [Benadryl®], dimenhydrinate [Dramamine®])
NK1 antagonists (e.g., aprepitant [Emend®], fosaprepitant [Emend IV®], rolapitant [Varubi®])
Hydration
Pain and comfort management

Data from Feinleib, Kawn, & Yamani, 2017; Weismann, Kranke, & Eberhart, 2015

---

ondansetron (Zofran®), promethazine (Phenergan®), and prochlorperazine (Compazine®). If PONV is not relieved following two doses of antiemetics, it should be reported to the anesthesia provider. If it is not contraindicated or if the cause of PONV is hypotension, hydration may also be effective in reducing the occurrence of PONV (Feinleib et al., 2017). Patients who are vomiting should be positioned to prevent aspiration. Conscious patients should be positioned in the semirecumbent position; patients who are unconscious should be positioned in the lateral position (Wayne, 2016).

Thermoregulation (Hypothermia)

Postoperative nursing considerations related to promoting normothermia include the identification of patients at risk for hypothermia and application of passive and active warming devices (e.g., bonnet, cotton blankets, socks, forced air warming device). Patients are considered hypothermic if they have a temperature of less than 36°C (96.8°F) (Levin, Wright, Pecoraro, & Kopec, 2016). Factors affecting the development of hypothermia include patient age, health status, surgical procedure, exposed body areas, duration of anesthesia or surgery, ambient room temperature, prepping and irrigation solutions, administration of cool IV fluids, and peripheral vascular disease (O'Brien, 2013).

The postoperative cardiac surgery patient should be monitored consistently until normothermia is achieved.

Attaining and maintaining postoperative normothermia is vital, because inadvertent postoperative hypothermia has been linked to adverse effects. Overall, postoperative patients admitted from the OR with a core temperature less than 36°C have prolonged mechanical ventilation, shivering, and increasing oxygen consumption. Hemodynamic effects of hypothermia include increased SVR and greater likelihood of developing dysrhythmias, hypertension, tachycardia, decreased preload, impaired contractility, or coronary graft spasm (Nearman, Klick, Eisenberg, & Pesa, 2014). They are also at risk for development of ventricular dysrhythmias, coagulopathy, platelet dysfunction, wound infection and impaired healing, increased need for blood transfusions, myocardial infarction, thermal discomfort, and death (Levin et al., 2016; Saad & Aladawy, 2013).

Hypothermia alters drug metabolism, causing delays in patients' emergence from anesthesia. It also causes a disruption of the coagulation pathway, increasing the need for blood transfusions. Hypothermia leads to delays in wound healing, which increases susceptibility to surgical site infections, and shivering, which increases myocardial oxygen demand and consumption (Nearman et al., 2014). Shivering increases oxygen consumption and carbon dioxide production. It increases sympathetic activity, which can lead to development of dysrhythmias. Shivering also can cause splanchnic vasoconstriction, which can result in renal and mesenteric ischemia (Stephens & Whitman, 2015)

Postoperative Respiratory Management

In addition to managing a patient's hemodynamic status, respiratory management is another pivotal role of the ICU nurse in the immediate postoperative cardiac surgery period. Unless the patient was "fast-tracked" and extubated in the OR, short-term mechanical ventilation is employed until anesthetic agents have been eliminated. Early extubation should be a goal for all patients.

Weaning and extubation protocols vary among facilities. Nevertheless, these processes are generally based on adequate muscle strength, pulmonary function, and hemodynamic stability (Barbosa e Silva et al., 2015). As discussed in Chapter 11, extubation criteria typically include presence of a heart rate less than 140, respiratory rate less than 25, normothermia, and absence of ischemia and infusion of vasoactive agents. The patient should be alert and cooperative (i.e., able to respond to commands). Presence of a cough and gag reflex is important, because the patient must be able to maintain a patent airway following extubation. The patient must also demonstrate adequate muscle strength by sustaining a head lift for at least 5 seconds. Other weaning criteria include ability to breathe spontaneously

and adequately while maintaining adequate oxygen saturation and ABG values. Physiologic parameters that may be measured to assess potential readiness for extubation include a negative inspiratory force (NIF) of at least 20–25 cm H_2O, minute volume no greater than 10 L/min, and vital capacity 10–15 mL/kg (Bauman & Hyzy, 2014). Barbosa e Silva and colleagues (2015) have reported predictive indices for weaning to include respiratory frequency to tidal volume (f/Vt) less than 105 cycles/min/L, integrative weaning index of at least 25 mL/cmH_2O/cycles/min/L, respiratory rate less than 30, partial pressure of oxygen (PaO_2)/FiO_2 greater than 255 mmHg, static compliance at least 30 cmH_2O/L/min, and tidal volume at least 315 mL. Bainbridge and Cheng (2015) recommend patients being awake, hemodynamically stable, and having a vital capacity of at least 25 mL/kg. Typically, cardiac surgery patients are extubated within 12 hours of their arrival to the ICU from the OR (Badhwar et al., 2014).

Upon determination that the patient is ready for extubation, the patient's mouth should be suctioned and the tube-securing device removed. The cuff on the endotracheal tube is deflated with a syringe. The presence of an air leak should then be ascertained; such a leak may be either heard or felt. The patient is instructed to take a deep breath and cough, with the tube being removed toward the end of the cough. Supplemental humidified oxygen is applied (Bainbridge & Cheng, 2015). Placement on low-flow oxygen such as nasal cannula is common practice.

Stir-up Regimen

Cardiac surgery patients who received an inhalation agent as part of their anesthesia will require the stir-up regimen in the immediate postoperative period, because such agents cause respiratory depression and are eliminated with ventilation. The stir-up regimen is accomplished by elevating the head of the bed and encouraging deep breathing and coughing at regular intervals. This practice facilitates movement of the inhalation agent from an area of higher concentration (the patient's lungs) to an area of lower concentration (room air), and thereby eliminating it (Ochampaugh, 2015).

Complications Related to Extubation

Complications following extubation are fairly uncommon but may include laryngospasm, non-cardiogenic pulmonary edema, bronchospasm, hypoventilation, and hypoxia.

Laryngospasm and Noncardiogenic Pulmonary Edema

Laryngospasm is a partial or total obstruction of air flow in and out of the lungs owing to spasms of the vocal cord (Al Ghofaily, Simmons, Chen, & Liu, 2013). Causes include aspiration, suctioning, and histamine release associated with some medications. Signs of laryngospasm include "rocking" respirations, wheezing, stridor, dyspnea, use of accessory muscles, and tachypnea. The patient should be encouraged to cough, as this action may be effective in eradicating a partial obstruction (O'Brien, 2013).

Patients can have laryngospasm during extubation, which can trigger noncardiogenic pulmonary edema. Noncardiogenic pulmonary edema occurs following an acute airway obstruction, such as when the patient forcefully inspires against a closed glottis, thereby creating an increase in intrathoracic pressure and resulting in pulmonary edema (Al Ghofaily et al., 2013). Protein and fluid accumulate and extravasate into the alveoli without an associated increase in PAOP (Nearman et al., 2014). Symptoms of this condition, which typically have a rapid onset, include agitation, tachypnea, tachycardia, decreased oxygen saturation, and pink, frothy sputum. Crackles will be audible.

Prompt recognition and treatment of both laryngospasm and noncardiogenic pulmonary edema are crucial; indeed, the patient may require reintubation until these problems resolve. Treatment of laryngospasm generally involves positive-pressure breathing with a bag-valve-mask device with 100% oxygen and mandibular support. If these measures prove ineffective, succinylcholine can be administered intravenously. Lidocaine may be effective in preventing a laryngospasm.

Noncardiogenic pulmonary edema management involves maintenance of a patent airway,

supplemental oxygen, and administration of a diuretic. Mechanical ventilation with PEEP may be required in severe cases. Chest radiograph may reveal findings consistent with pulmonary edema. Treatment of noncardiogenic pulmonary edema includes supplemental oxygen, respiratory support, and diuretics unless ventilatory support is required (Skalická & Bělohlávek, 2015).

Bronchospasm

Bronchospasm can occur as a result of constriction of bronchial smooth muscles after extubation. However, it resolves quickly after airway irritants are eliminated. Symptoms include wheezing, dyspnea, and tachypnea. Treatment involves administration of a bronchodilator and humidified oxygen. In severe cases, muscle relaxants, lidocaine, epinephrine, or hydrocortisone may be administered to relax the airway (O'Brien, 2013).

Hypoventilation and Hypoxia

Hypoventilation is common in the immediate postoperative period. It may result from the anesthetic agents administered or the surgical procedure itself. Treatment entails eradicating the underlying cause. If the underlying cause is related to opioid administration, then treatment may include administration of naloxone (Narcan®) for patients with shallow or slow respirations. Institutional policy varies regarding use of opioid antagonists (O'Brien, 2013).

Hypoxemia is defined as an oxygen saturation less than 90%. Hypoxemia can have numerous undesired sequelae, including cardiac dysrhythmias and myocardial ischemia. Signs and symptoms may include cyanosis, agitation, somnolence, tachycardia, bradycardia, hypertension, and hypotension. Depending on the severity of the symptoms or hypoxemia, reintubation and mechanical ventilation may be required (O'Brien, 2013).

Inadequate reversal of NMBAs' effects can cause hypoventilation and hypoxia after extubation. Extubation of a patient who is partially paralyzed increases the individual's risk of developing postoperative complications. Residual respiratory muscle weakness can cause airway obstruction, hypoventilation, and an impaired response to hypoxia. Cardiac surgery patients are at increased risk if they receive a long-acting NMBA whose action is inadequately reversed with anticholinesterase agents. Reparalysis can occur when an NMBA has a longer half-life than the reversal agents. If this problem occurs, the patient will demonstrate weak, shallow respirations and poor chest rise; anxiety and restlessness may become apparent as well. Treatment involves administration of additional doses of a reversal agent, respiratory support, and temporary reintubation until muscle strength is regained.

During weaning and extubation, opioids should be used judiciously. Opioids decrease respiratory effort, oxygen saturation, and respiratory rate and depth. Pain management is of concern; however, small doses of short-acting analgesics (e.g., dexmedetomidine [Precedex™]) may be recommended (Chorney, Gooch, Oberdier, Keating, & Stahl, 2013). Complications that arise after extubation can be minimized by recognizing and treating respiratory emergencies and by adhering to weaning and extubation criteria.

▶ Potential Postoperative Complications

The ICU nurse plays a pivotal role in preventing or promptly identifying and treating postoperative complications. Among the more common complications seen in the immediate postoperative period are hemodynamic compromise, respiratory insufficiency, neurologic issues, and hematologic problems. Some complications are related to patient comorbidities; others are related to the surgical procedure itself. These complications and the associated ICU nursing responsibilities are discussed in detail in Chapters 13 and 16. Potential complications related to effects of anesthesia are addressed in this section. One unique complication related to the surgical procedure is covered here as well.

Malignant Hyperthermia

Malignant hyperthermia (MH) is a genetic, life-threatening disorder that is triggered by certain anesthetic agents, depolarizing skeletal muscle relaxants, and stress. With this condition, a defect in the sarcoplasmic reticulum leads to a buildup of excess calcium in the mycoplasma. This results in sustained skeletal muscle contraction that is intense and prolonged, leading to a hypermetabolic state of heat production.

The onset of MH usually occurs during induction of anesthetic agents. Halothane, enflurane, isoflurane, desflurane, and succinylcholine are the most common triggering agents. The triggering of events is characterized by muscle rigidity of the jaw (masseter rigidity), tachypnea, tachycardia, elevated CO_2 level, cyanosis, respiratory and metabolic acidosis, elevated serum creatine phosphokinase (CPK), and hyperkalemia. Late signs include temperature elevation, bleeding from venipuncture sites, and rhabdomyolysis. MH typically manifests in the OR but it can develop within 24 hours postoperatively (O'Brien, 2013).

Treatment of MH includes discontinuation of triggering agents and immediate intravenous administration of dantrolene sodium (Dantrium®) 2.5 mg/kg (up to a maximum dose of 10 mg/kg). Dantrolene inhibits the release of calcium. Once the loading dose is administered, dantrolene is infused at a dose of 1 mg/kg every 4 hours for at least 48 hours (Chapin, 2017).

Hyperventilation, administration of 100% oxygen, body surface area cooling, administration of sodium bicarbonate, maintenance of fluid and electrolyte balance, and treatment of associated conditions (e.g., hypertension, dysrhythmias) are also essential interventions in the setting of MH. Lab data that may be obtained include ABG, serum electrolytes, liver enzymes, renal function studies, blood counts, and coagulation profile (Hooper, 2013; Kaplow, 2013; O'Brien, 2013). Effective management involves prompt recognition, guidance of the multidisciplinary team, and expert direction from the Malignant Hyperthermia Association of the United States (MHAUS).

Pseudocholinesterase Deficiency

Prolonged mechanical ventilation after cardiac surgery may be caused by a deficiency in pseudocholinesterase. A small percentage of patients lack this enzyme, which is responsible for metabolizing medications such as succinylcholine. Patients with pseudocholinesterase deficiency exhibit prolonged responses to these medications when given, and can have sustained skeletal muscle paralysis, and apnea lasting up to 48 hours after administration. Management involves emotional support and mechanical ventilation until the effects of the medication are completely eliminated (Kaplow, 2013).

Protamine Sulfate Allergic Reactions

Protamine sulfate is administered as a reversal agent for heparin. If it is given too rapidly, severe hypotension and anaphylactic reactions may result. Consequently, caution should be used when administering protamine sulfate to patients who may be at increased risk of allergic reaction—specifically, individuals who have previously undergone procedures such as coronary angioplasty or CPB, diabetics who have been treated with protamine insulin, patients who are allergic to fish, and men who have had a vasectomy or are infertile and may have antibodies to protamine. Patients undergoing prolonged procedures involving repeated doses of protamine should be subject to careful monitoring of clotting parameters. Protamine sulfate reactions are discussed in more detail in Chapter 12.

▶ Summary

Although much progress has been made with respect to the postoperative care of the cardiac surgery patient, critical thinking and caring practices of the ICU nurse are primary determinants of positive outcomes. The initial hours following cardiac surgery are tenuous. The patient's preoperative status, the intraoperative course, and the effects of anesthesia all contribute to the complexity of the patient's profile.

⌕ CASE STUDY

A 62-year-old patient, underwent mitral valve replacement under cardiopulmonary bypass. The patient's history is significant for insulin-dependent diabetes mellitus and the patient takes protamine zinc insulin. The patient reports an allergy to fish. The patient was heparinized for the procedure to maintain an activated clotting time of 450 seconds and received protamine sulfate at the end of the procedure. The intraoperative course was uneventful. Immediate postoperative vital signs were: BP 116/78, HR 78, left atrial pressure (LAP) 6 mmHg. Thirty minutes following administration of the protamine sulfate, the patient developed hypotension and bronchospasm. At that time, vital signs were BP 72/48, HR 110, LAP 0 mmHg. The patient was treated with aggressive fluid resuscitation, diphenhydramine 25 mg, dopamine at 20 mcg/kg/min, methylprednisolone 2 g, epinephrine at 10 mcg/kg/min, and furosemide 200 mg.

Critical Thinking Questions

1. Why was protamine sulfate required in this case?
2. What patient's risk factors were present for a protamine allergy?
3. What is the rationale for the treatment provided?

Answers to Critical Thinking Questions

1. The protamine was used to neutralize the heparin required for CPB.
2. The patient has insulin-dependent diabetes and is taking NPH insulin. The patient also has a fish allergy.
3. The patient had hypotension, which required an alpha-adrenergic agonist. The patient needed volume expansion due to increased third spacing of fluid from the allergic reaction. The antihistamine was given to combat the increased histamine concentration; histamine increases capillary permeability and third spacing of fluid.

Self-Assessment Questions

1. The nurse should anticipate need for prolonged mechanical ventilation after cardiac surgery in a patient with a history of:
   A. hypotension.
   B. unstable angina.
   C. two-vessel disease.
   D. ejection fraction 30%.
2. A postoperative cardiac surgery patient develops the following vital signs: BP 78/50, HR 118, CVP 18 mmHg, CO 3.2 L/min. A low-voltage QRS complex is noted on the cardiac monitor. The drainage from the mediastinal chest tube has dramatically decreased in the past hour. Which should the nurse suspect?
   A. Unstable angina
   B. Hypovolemia
   C. Cardiac tamponade
   D. Cardiogenic shock
3. A patient develops cardiac tamponade following cardiac surgery. Which should the nurse initially anticipate?
   A. Administration of fluids
   B. Preparation for pericardiocentesis
   C. Titration of vasopressors
   D. Performing a 12-lead ECG
4. A cardiac surgery patient received etomidate while in the OR. Which should the ICU anticipate?
   A. Emergence delirium
   B. Decreased cardiac output
   C. Involuntary tremors
   D. Increased adrenal function
5. A cardiac surgery patient received isoflurane in the OR. For which should the nurse observe?
   A. Noncardiogenic pulmonary edema
   B. Increased sensitization to catecholamines
   C. Hypercarbia
   D. Bronchodilation
6. Patients who receive midazolam in the OR should be observed for:
   A. tachycardia.
   B. respiratory depression.
   C. vasoconstriction.
   D. postoperative nausea and vomiting.

7. A cardiac surgery patient is admitted directly from the OR. Initial temperature was 35.8°C (96.4°F). Which should the nurse anticipate?
   A. SVR 900 dyne/sec/cm^{-5}
   B. BP 88/50
   C. CVP 9 mmHg
   D. HR 120
8. Which is a potential effect of postoperative hypothermia?
   A. Decreased myocardial consumption
   B. Increased infection risk
   C. Increased clot formation
   D. Decreased need for transfusions
9. Postextubation, a patient develops "rocking" respirations, tachypnea, stridor, and use of accessory muscles. The initial nursing intervention should be to:
   A. prepare for reintubation.
   B. suction the oropharynx.
   C. encourage the patient to cough.
   D. administer a short-acting neuromuscular blocking agent.
10. A patient received halothane as part of induction to anesthesia. Upon admission to the ICU, the patient has a temperature of 39°C (102.2°F). Which should the ICU nurse perform initially?
    A. Begin cooling the patient
    B. Administer dantrolene sodium
    C. Hyperventilate with 100% oxygen
    D. Treat associated dysrhythmias

Answers to Self-Assessment Questions

1. D. **ejection fraction 30%**
   Rationale: A patient with an ejection fraction is at risk for requiring prolonged mechanical ventilation following cardiac surgery. Other patients at risk are those with a history of hypertension, myocardial infarction, and three or more vessel disease.
2. C. **cardiac tamponade**
   Rationale: These are signs and symptoms of cardiac tamponade. Patients with hypovolemia and cardiogenic shock will not manifest with low-voltage QRS complexes.

3. A. **administration of fluids**
Rationale: Fluids are needed to help counteract the decrease in preload from the associated decrease in diastolic filling pressures associated with cardiac tamponade.

4. C. **involuntary tremors**
Rationale: Involuntary tremors are associated with administration of etomidate. Cardiac output remains stable with etomidate administration and there is suppressed adrenal function with this agent. Emergence delirium does not occur after etomidate administration.

5. A. **noncardiogenic pulmonary edema**
Rationale: Isoflurane may lead to development of laryngospasm, which may predispose the patient to noncardiogenic pulmonary edema. Isoflurane is not associated with increased sensitization to catecholamines but may cause laryngospasm.

6. B. **respiratory depression**
Rationale: Midazolam can cause respiratory depression. It also can cause bradycardia and vasodilation, and it minimizes development of postoperative nausea and vomiting.

7. D. **HR 120**
Rationale: Tachycardia is associated with hypothermia as is an increase in SVR, hypertension, and a decrease in preload.

8. B. **increased infection risk**
Rationale: There is an increased risk of infection with hypothermia as well as an associated increase in myocardial oxygen consumption, disruption of the coagulation pathway, and an increased need for transfusions.

9. C. **encourage the patient to cough**
Rationale: Coughing may eradicate the patient's partial airway obstruction. Intubation is not the initial intervention that is indicated and may not be able to be accomplished due to the narrowing of the upper airway. Suctioning will not correct the patient's problem. A short-acting neuromuscular blocking agent may ultimately be required, but is not the initial intervention indicated.

10. C. **hyperventilate with 100% oxygen**
Rationale: This patient has developed malignant hyperthermia. Hyperventilating with 100% oxygen is initially indicated. Temperature elevation is typically a later sign of MH. Cooling will need to be conducted but is not the initial priority. Treatment of associated dysrhythmias is not the first priority. Hyperventilating with 100% oxygen may prevent or eradicate the dysrhythmias. Dantrolene administration is required but its reconstitution takes time. Preparation of this medication can begin to take place once hyperventilation has begun.

CLINICAL INQUIRY BOX

Question: What are the risk factors for postoperative nausea and vomiting following cardiac surgery and what is the role of betamethasone with or without droperidol for its prevention?

Reference: Champion, S., Zieger, L., & Hemery, C. (2018). Prophylaxis of postoperative nausea and vomiting after cardiac surgery in high-risk patients: A randomized controlled study. *Annals of Cardiac Anesthesia, 21*, 8–14.

Objective: To determine the risk factors for postoperative nausea and vomiting following cardiac surgery and the role of betamethasone with or without droperidol for its prevention.

Method: Randomized open-label controlled trial. Those randomized to the intervention arm received betamethasone with or without droperidol. Those randomized to the control arm received routine hospital practices.

Results: Postoperative nausea and vomiting occurred less frequently in those in the intervention arm (45.5% versus 54%). Use of a visual analog scale to quantify degree of nausea revealed 10 mm versus

15.3 mm, respectively. There was an increased risk of postoperative nausea and vomiting in those of female gender, history of postoperative nausea and vomiting, and migraines. Motion sickness, tobacco use, and volatile anesthesia were not risk factors of postoperative nausea and vomiting. No side effects related to the intervention arm were reported.

Conclusion: Betamethasone with or without droperidol decreased the incidence of postoperative nausea and vomiting in high-risk cardiac surgery patients without adverse events.

References

Al Ghofaily, L., Simmons, C., Chen, L., & Liu, R. (2013). Negative pressure pulmonary edema after laryngospasm: A revisit with a case report. *Journal of Anesthesia & Clinical Research, 3*(10), 252.

Andreasen, J. J., Sorensen, G. V., Abrahamsen, E. R., Hansen-Nard, E., Bundgaard, K., Bendtsen, M. D., . . . Troelsen, P. (2016). Early chest tube removal following cardiac surgery is associated with pleural and/or pericardial effusions requiring invasive treatment. *European Journal of Cardio-Thoracic Surgery, 49*(1), 288–292.

Badhwar, V., Esper, S., Brooks, M., Mulukutla, S., Hardison, R., Mallios, D., . . . Subramaniam, K. (2014). Extubating in the operating room following adult cardiac surgery safely improves outcomes and lowers costs. *The Journal of Thoracic and Cardiovascular Surgery, 148*(6), 3103–1309.

Bainbridge, D., & Cheng, D. C. (2015). Early extubation and fast-track management of off-pump cardiac patients in the intensive care unit. *Seminars in Cardiovascular and Vascular Anesthesia, 19*(2), 163–168.

Barbosa e Silva, M. G., Borges, D. L., Costa, M de A., Baldez, T. E., da Silva, L. N., Oliveira, R. L., . . . Albuquerque, R. A. (2015). Application of mechanical ventilation weaning predictors after elective cardiac surgery. *Brazilian Journal of Cardiovascular Surgery, 30*(6), 605–609.

Bauman, K., & Hyzy, R. (2014). *Extubation management.* Retrieved from http://www.uptodate.com/contents/extubation-management?source=machineLearning&search=extubation+cardiac+surgery&selectedTitle=1%7E150&sectionRank=2&anchor=H2#H2.

Chapin, J. W. (2017). *Malignant hyperthermia treatment and management.* Retrieved from https://emedicine.medscape.com/article/2231150-treatment.

Chorney, S. R., Gooch, M. E., Oberdier, M. T., Keating, D., & Stahl, R. F. (2013). The safety and efficacy of dexmedetomidine for postoperative sedation in the cardiac surgery intensive care unit. *HSR Proceedings in Intensive Care & Cardiovascular Anesthesia, 5*(1), 17–24.

Colson, P. H., Gaudard, P., Fellah, J.-L., Bertet, H., Faucanie, M., Amour, J., . . . ARCOTHOVA Group. (2016). Active bleeding after cardiac surgery: A prospective observational multicenter study. *PLoS ONE, 11*(9), e0162396. doi:10.137/journal.pone.0162396

DeJong, A., & Jaber, S. (2014). Etomidate for anesthesia induction. Friend or foe in major cardiac surgery? *Critical Care, 18*(5). doi:10.1186/s13054-014-0560-7

Faulk, S. A., Fleisher, L. A., Jones, S. B., & Nussmeier, N. A. (2014). *Overview of anesthesia and anesthetic choices.* Retrieved from http://www.uptodate.com/contents/overview-of-anesthesia-and-anesthetic-choices?source=machineLearning&search=anesthetic+agents&selectedTitle=1%7E150&sectionRank=1&anchor=H6#H28.

Feinlieb, J., Kwan, L. H., & Yamani, A. (2017). *Postoperative nausea and vomiting.* Retrieved from https://www.uptodate.com/contents/postoperative-nausea-and-vomiting.

Frandsen, G., & Pennington, S. S. (2014). Drug therapy with general anesthetics. In G. Frandsen & S. S. Pennington (Eds.), *Abrams' clinical drug therapy: Rationales for nursing practice* (10th ed., pp. 915–933). Philadelphia, PA: Lippincott Williams & Wilkins.

Gil-Gomez, R., Blasco-Alonso, J., Reyes, J., Gonzalez-Correa, J., De La Cruz, J., & Milano, G. (2014). Post-operative systemic inflammatory response after cardiac surgery using extracorporeal circulation in children. *Experimental & Clinical Cardiology, 20*(6), 3906–3919.

Gumus, F., Polat, A., Yektas, A., Totoz, T., Bagco, M., Erentug, V., . . . Alagol, A. (2015). Prolonged mechanical ventilation after CABG: Risk factor analysis. *Journal of Cardiothoracic and Vascular Anesthesia, 29*(1), 52–58.

Gustafson, K. A., & Brown, A. S. (2017). Neuromuscular blocking agents: Use and controversy in the hospital setting. *U.S. Pharmacist.* Retrieved from https://www.uspharmacist/com/article/neuromuscular-blocking-agents.

Gutsche, J. T., Erickson, L., Ghadimi, K., Augoustides, J. G., Dimartino, J., Szeto, W. Y., . . . Ochroch, E. A. (2014). Advancing extubation time for cardiac surgery patients using lean work design. *Journal of Cardiothoracic and Vascular Anesthesia, 8*(6), 1490–1496.

Hooper, V. D. (2013). Care of the patient with thermal imbalance. In J. Odom-Forren (Ed.), *Drain's perianesthesia nursing: A critical care approach* (6th ed., pp. 740–750). St. Louis, MO: Elsevier Saunders.

Hosseinian, L., Weiner, M., Levin, M. A., & Fischer, G. W. (2016). Methylene blue: Magic bullet for vasoplegia? *Anesthesia & Analgesia, 122*(1), 194–201.

Kakazu, C. Z., & Lippmann, M. (2015). Playing with fire: Debate about propofol-induced hypotension. *British Journal of Anaesthesia, 114*(1), 164–165.

Kaplow, R. (2013). Safety of patients transferred from the operating room to the intensive care unit. *Critical Care Nurse, 33*(1), 68–70.

Kaplow, R., & Iyere, K. (2017). When cardiac tamponade puts the pressure on. *Nursing, 47*(2), 24–30.

Kayiloglu, S. I., Dinc, T., Sozen, I., Bostanoglu, A., Cete, M., & Coskun, F. (2015). Postoperative fluid management. *World Journal of Critical Care Medicine, 4*(3), 192–201.

Kianfar, A. A., Ahmadi, Z. H., Mirhossein, S. M., Jamaati, H., Kashani, B. S., Mohajerani, S. A., . . . Hashemian, S. M. (2015). Ultra fast-track extubation in heart transplant surgery patients. *International Journal of Critical Illness and Injury Science, 5*(2), 89–92.

Lafferty, K. A. (2017). *Barbiturate toxicity*. Retrieved from https://emedicine.medscape/article/813155-overview.

Landoni, G., Greco, T., Biondi-Zoccai, G., Neto, C. N., Febres, D., Pintaudi, M., . . . Zangrillo, A. (2013). Anaesthetic drugs and survival: A Bayesian network meta-analysis of randomized trials in cardiac surgery. *British Journal of Anaesthesia, 111*(6), 886–896.

Lee, L. A., Athanassoglou, V., & Pandit, J. J. (2016). Neuromuscular blockade in the elderly patient. *Journal of Pain Research, 9*, 437–444.

Lenzarini, F., Di Lascio, N., Shea, F., Kusmic, C., & Faita, F. (2016). Time course of isoflurane-induced vasodilation: A doppler ultrasound study of the left coronary artery in mice. *Ultrasound Medicine and Biology, 42*(4), 999–1009.

Levin, R. F., Wright, F., Pecoraro, K., & Kopec, W. (2016). Maintaining perioperative normothermia: Sustaining an evidence-based practice improvement project. *AORN Journal, 103*(2), 213e1–213e13.

Mastropietro, C. W., & Uribe, D. A. (2015). Nicardipine for hypertension following aortic coarctectomy or superior cavopulmonary anastomosis. *World Journal for Pediatric and Congenital Heart Surgery*. Retrieved from http://journals.sagepub.com/doi/full/10.1177/2150135115608815

Najafi, M., & Faraoni, D. (2014). Updates on coagulation management in cardiac surgery. *The Journal of Tehran Heart Center, 9*(3), 99–103.

Nearman, H., Klick, J. C., Eisenberg, P., & Pesa, N. (2014). Perioperative complications of cardiac surgery and postoperative care. *Critical Care Clinics, 30*(3), 527–555.

Neubert, L., & Sinha, A. (2015). Inhalational anesthetics. In P. Sinha, S. Beaman, & J. Street (Eds.), *Basic clinical anesthesia* (pp. 123–130). New York, NY: Springer.

Nishiyama, T. (2016). Effects of sedation with midazolam or propofol infusion on stress hormone and heart rate variability in spinal anesthesia. *Anaesthesia, Pain & Intensive Care, 20*(2), 159–164.

O'Brien, D. (2013). Postanesthesia care complications. In J. Odom-Forren (Ed.), *Drain's perianesthesia nursing: A critical care approach* (6th ed., pp. 394–414). St. Louis, MO: Elsevier Saunders.

Ochampaugh, B. (2015). Back to basics: Stir-up regimen. *Newsletter of the New York State PeriAnesthesia Nurses Association, 37*(1), 1.

Orlewicz, M. S. (2017). *Procedural sedation*. Retrieved from https://emedicine.medscape.com/article/109695-overview.

Saad, H., & Aladawy, M. (2013). Temperature management in cardiac surgery. *Global Cardiology Science & Practice, 2013*(1), 44–62.

Shahani, R. (2017). *Coronary artery bypass grafting medication*. Retrieved from https://emedicine.medscape.com/article/1893992-medication.

Silvestry, F. E. (2017). *Postoperative complications among patients undergoing cardiac surgery*. Retrieved from http://www.uptodate.com/contents/postoperative-complications-among-patients-undergoing-cardiac-surgery?source=search_result&search=cardiac+surgery&selectedTitle=1%7E150.

Skalická, H., & Bělohlávek, J. (2015). Non-cardiogenic pulmonary edema, acute respiratory distress syndrome. *Ceskych lekaru Ceskych, 154*(6), 273–279 (abstract).

Stephens, R. S., & Whitman, G. (2015). Postoperative critical care of the adult cardiac surgery patient: Part I: Routine postoperative care. *Critical Care Medicine, 43*(7), 1477–1497.

Tembelopoulos, K., Carr, J., & Tressy-Murphy, C. (2012). Emergence agitation: What it is and what can we do? *Journal of PeriAnesthesia Nursing, 27*(3), e24.

Texas Heart Institute. (2016). *A heart surgery overview*. Retrieved from www.texasheart.org.

Totonch, Z., Baazm, F., Chitsazan, M., Seifi, S., & Chitsazan, M. (2014). Predictors of prolonged mechanical ventilation after open heart surgery. *Journal of Cardiovascular and Thoracic Research, 6*(4), 211–216.

Tsikas, D., Jordan, J., & Engelis, (2015). Blood pressure-lowering effects on propofol or sevoflurane anaesthesia are not due to enhanced nitric oxide formation or bioavailability. *British Journal of Clinical Pharmacology, 79*(6), 1030–1033.

Wagner, C. E., Bick, J. S., Johnson, D., Ahmad, R., Han, X., Ehrenfeld, J. M., . . . Pretorius, M. (2014). Etomidate use and postoperative outcomes among cardiac surgery patients. *Anesthesiology, 20*(3), 579–589.

Walters, F. J. (n.d.). Neuropharmacology—intracranial pressure and cerebral blood flow. *Update in Anesthesia*. Retrieved from http://e-safe-anaesthesia.org/e_library/06/Neuropharmacology_intracranial_pressure_and_cerebral_blood_f.pdf.

Wayne, G. (2016). *Risk for aspiration*. Retrieved from https://nurselabs.com/risk-for-aspiration.

Weismann, T., Kranke, P., & Eberhart, L. (2015). Postoperative nausea and vomiting-a narrative review of pathophysiology, pharmacology and clinical management strategies. *Expert Opinion in Pharmacology, 7*, 1069–1077.

Wise, E. S., Stonko, D. P., Glaser, Z. A., Garcia, K. L., Huang, L. J., Kim, J. S., . . . Eagle, S. S. (2017). Predication of prolonged ventilation after coronary artery bypass grafting: Data from an artificial neural network. *Heart Journal Forum,* *20*(1). doi:10.1532/hsf.1566

Yazdchi, F., & Rawn, J. D. (2018). Postoperative care of the cardiac surgery patient. In L. H. Cohn & D. H. Adams (Eds.), *Cardiac surgery in the adult* (5th ed., pp. 405–428). New York, NY: McGraw Hill.

Zhao, Y., Vanhoutte, P. M., & Leung, W. S. (2015). Vascular nitric oxide: Beyond eNOS. *Journal of Pharmacological Sciences, 129*(2), 83–94.

Web Resources

Cardiac tamponade: https://www.youtube.com/watch?v=C87TgEAMVOs

Dr. Bernadine Healy takes a tour of the hospital. The operating room is a virtual beehive during heart surgery and afterward in the intensive care unit: https://www.youtube.com/watch?v=9xx8PX77fOY

Postoperative complications of cardiac surgery: https://www.youtube.com/watch?v=cUuFrd3iz88

CHAPTER 9

Hemodynamic Monitoring

Mary Zellinger

▶ Introduction

Hemodynamic monitoring of the patient after cardiac surgery is a routine part of the immediate postoperative care. Data obtained during this period guide the clinician in initiating the optimal intervention to ensure a smooth recovery. Hemodynamics, or the study of the dynamics of blood circulation, can be assessed through both invasive and noninvasive mechanisms; the ultimate goal is to determine the adequacy of cardiac output (CO) (the amount of blood ejected by the heart each minute). This chapter reviews the essentials of hemodynamic monitoring in the patient who has undergone cardiac surgery. Both basic and newer technologies are discussed.

▶ Essentials of Hemodynamic Monitoring

Monitoring assists in determining changes in fluid status and cardiac performance at the earliest possible time so that fluctuations in three factors that affect cardiac output (i.e., preload, afterload, and contractility) (**BOX 9.1**) can be quickly addressed with appropriate or targeted treatment.

New monitoring devices and techniques are introduced annually to the critical care arena, each of which has the goal of increasing accuracy and decreasing invasive monitoring. It is imperative for the clinician to incorporate data from a variety of sources when assessing the hemodynamic picture, not relying on a single and potentially misleading parameter.

BOX 9.1 Hemodynamic Monitoring Terms and Definitions

Preload: The stretch on the sarcomeres just prior to systole (i.e., contraction). Preload is quantified with CVP and PAOP to reflect pressure on the right and left sides of the heart, respectively.

Afterload: The force against which the ventricle must contract, to eject blood.

Contractility: The intrinsic strength of the ventricle independent of loading conditions. It is affected intrinsically by circulating catecholamines.

CVP, central venous pressure; PAOP, pulmonary artery occlusive pressure.
Data from Dhonnchú, (2015).

▶ Initial Postoperative Assessment

Following cardiac surgery, the intensive care unit (ICU) nurse or anesthesia technician will connect the patient to the bedside monitor upon receipt from the operating room (OR). The electrocardiogram (ECG) leads are connected to the bedside monitor from the transport monitor, and heart rate and rhythm are assessed. The pulse oximetry probe is connected to the finger, earlobe, or forehead. Pulse oximetry is a simple, noninvasive method of monitoring the percentage of hemoglobin that is saturated with oxygen. The target oxygen saturation (SpO_2) is 95% or greater in a patient without a history of chronic obstructive pulmonary disease (COPD).

Preparing Hemodynamic Equipment

After elevating the head of the bed (HOB), the transducers are leveled at the phlebostatic axis, which is located at the fourth intercostal space, midpoint of the anterior–posterior diameter (see Figure 7.7). The transducers are then zero-balanced, establishing atmospheric pressure as zero. Leveling at the phlebostatic axis is performed to eradicate the effects of hydrostatic forces on the hemodynamic pressures (Barros et al., 2016). Cardiac pressures may be accurately obtained with the HOB elevated up to 60 degrees if the patient's legs are parallel to the floor (Barros et al., 2016). A square wave test is performed to ensure responsiveness (**BOX 9.2**; see Figure 9.1). Proper setup and functioning of the monitoring

---

BOX 9.2   Square Wave Test

A square wave test (also referred to as a fast flush or dynamic response test) is performed to ensure the waveforms that appear on the monitoring screen accurately reflect pulmonary artery pressures (Barros et al., 2016). It is accomplished by pulling and releasing the pigtail or squeezing the button of the flush device so that the flow through the tubing is increased (from 3 mL/hr obtained with a pressure bag inflated to 300 mmHg). This causes a sudden rise in pressure in the system, such that a square wave is generated on the monitor oscilloscope. An acceptable response is the pressure waveform reverting to baseline within one to two oscillations. If the response is lacking in shape, amplitude, or time to return to baseline, the ICU nurse should troubleshoot the system until an acceptable response is achieved (Barros et al., 2016). If an underdamped or overdamped waveform is present, hemodynamic measurements will not be accurate. It is recommended that a square wave test (**FIGURE 9.1**) be performed when the system is being initially set up, at least once a shift, after opening the catheter system (e.g., for rezeroing, blood sampling, or changing tubing), and whenever, after ensuring there is no air in the line, the pressure waveform appears to be damped or distorted (Barros et al., 2016).

An overdamped waveform is sluggish and has an exaggerated or falsely widened and blunt tracing. It will cause the patient's systolic blood pressure (SBP) to be recorded as falsely low and the diastolic blood pressure (DBP) to be recorded as falsely high. Causes of an overdamped waveform include the presence of large

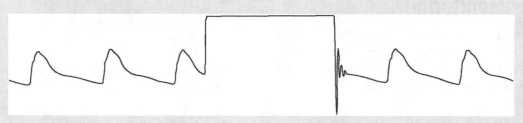

FIGURE 9.1 Square wave test.

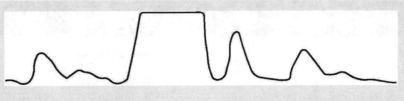

FIGURE 9.2 Overdamped waveform.

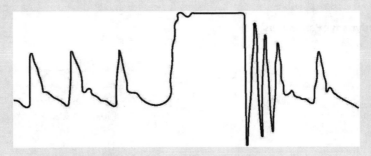

FIGURE 9.3 Underdamped waveform.

bubbles in the system, loose connections, no or low fluid in the flush bag, low pressure of the flush solution pressure bag, or a kink in the catheter (Yartsev, 2018) (**FIGURE 9.2**).

An underdamped waveform consists of an overresponse, which is seen as an exaggerated, narrow, artificially peaked tracing. In this case, the waveform overestimates the patient's SBP and underestimates the DBP. Causes of an underdamped waveform include the presence of small bubbles in the system, long pressure tubing, or a defective transducer (Yartsev, 2018) (**FIGURE 9.3**).

DBP, diastolic blood pressure; ICU, intensive care unit; SBP, systolic blood pressure.

system itself are essential to obtain accurate values, regardless of the specific parameter being measured. A number of variables (e.g., number of stopcocks, length of the tubing, responsiveness of the tubing, and presence of air bubbles) can influence accuracy of the readings.

Vital Signs and Hemodynamic Assessment

An initial assessment of vital signs and hemodynamic parameters (**BOX 9.3**) is obtained, ensuring that the latter are assessed at end expiration. Readings are obtained at this point in the respiratory cycle to eliminate the effects of changes in intrathoracic pressure that occur with breathing (Arora,

Singh, Goudra, & Sinha, 2014). The frequency of obtaining subsequent sets of vital signs and hemodynamic parameters varies by facility and according to the patient's clinical status. It is imperative to obtain the patient's baseline and hemodynamic status from the OR during hand-off report, which includes the cardiac surgeon/resident, cardiac anesthesiologist, ICU medical provider, respiratory therapist, and bedside registered nurse (RN). Knowing the trends and status of the hemodynamics from the past several hours will help guide management in the ICU.

Depending on unit-specific protocols, health care provider orders, and baseline hemodynamic values, cardiac output/index may be measured. From cardiac output/index and invasive pressure data, several hemodynamic calculations can be

---

BOX 9.3 Hemodynamic Parameters and Normal Values

Parameters	Normal Values
Systolic and diastolic blood pressure	100–130/60–90 mmHg
Mean arterial pressure	70–105 mmHg
Right atrial pressure (central venous pressure)	0–8 mmHg
Right ventricular pressure	25–30/0–8 mmHg
Pulmonary artery pressure	15–30/6–12 mmHg
Pulmonary artery occlusive pressure	4–12 mmHg

Derived Hemodynamic Parameters

Cardiac output/cardiac index	4–8 L/min/2.5–4.2 L/min/m^2
Systemic vascular resistance	770–1,500 dynes/sec/cm^{-5}
Pulmonary vascular resistance	20–120 dynes/sec/cm^{-5}
Systemic vascular resistance index	1,680–2,580 dynes/sec/cm^{-5}
Pulmonary vascular resistance index	69–177 dynes/sec/cm^{-5}
Stroke volume/index	60–130 mL/beat/30–65 mL/beat/m^2
Right ventricular stroke work	8–16 g-m/beat
Right ventricular stroke work index	5–10 g-m/m^2/beat
Left ventricular stroke work	58–104 g-m/beat
Left ventricular stroke work index	50–62 g-m/m^2/beat

Oxygenation Parameters

Arterial oxygen saturation	95%–100%
Mixed venous oxygen saturation	60%–80%
Arterial oxygen content	17–20 mL/dL
Venous oxygen content	12–15 mL/dL
Oxygen delivery	900–1150 mL/min
Oxygen consumption	200–290 mL/min
Oxygen extraction ratio	22%–30%

Data from McCleaster & Heuer, 2010; Rodriguez, 2016.

performed, yielding valuable information about cardiac performance.

The ICU nurse will check the vasoactive drips and other fluids infusing to verify their type, concentration, infusion status, and dosages. The relationships among the amount of volume infused and lost in the OR, baseline postoperative vital signs, and hemodynamic status are assessed. Setting monitor alarm limits specific to the patient's baseline profile and ensuring these alarms are activated are crucial at this stage.

Patient Assessment

A complete baseline physical assessment is then completed. While the primary nurse is performing the baseline assessment, a number of concomitant essential activities related to the patient's hemodynamic status are performed. These activities are listed in **BOX 9.4**.

A comprehensive head-to-toe assessment will enable the nurse to evaluate several indices to determine the overall adequacy of perfusion. A complete neurologic assessment may prove challenging if the patient has not been reversed from general anesthesia or is receiving a continuous infusion of an anesthetic agent or sedation. Some hospital protocols require the anesthetic agent or sedation infusion be weaned and temporarily discontinued in the immediate postoperative period so that appropriate neurologic function can be confirmed. If the baseline neurologic status is met, the infusion can then be restarted until the ventilator weaning process begins. If not, the patient should have a neurologic assessment every 2 hours until the baseline is achieved. An awake and alert patient is one indicator of adequacy of CO. More often now, most hospital protocols encourage lighter sedation so that the patient is comfortable but arousable. If the patient is receiving a sedative, it is one that has little to no impact on respiratory effort so that continuous assessment for ventilator weaning is possible. If a heavier sedative is ordered, it is most often because of the patient having an open chest or other physiologic processes occurring that are increasing myocardial oxygen consumption (MVO_2). In these situations, the patient may require heavier sedation to decrease MVO_2.

Extremity movement, warm skin, and palpable pulses indicate acceptable perfusion, unless obstructive peripheral vascular disease is present and limits perfusion to the distal extremities.

Assessment of heart sounds provides additional information about cardiac function and any valve dysfunction. The presence of extra heart sounds, although normal in certain situations, warrants further investigation. An S3 or S4 heart sound may be a sign of decreased ventricular compliance. The presence or sudden absence of murmurs may indicate changes in native or prosthetic valve function. Placing the HOB between 30 and 45 degrees and observing for jugular vein distention will reinforce other findings of right-sided heart failure or fluid overload.

Breath sounds should be auscultated in all fields, noting any areas that are diminished or abnormal. Pulmonary congestion may be indicative of pulmonary dysfunction from the surgical process, be the effect of complications from mechanical ventilation, or occur as a result of cardiac dysfunction. In addition, transfusion-related acute lung injury (TRALI) from numerous intraoperative transfusions may develop.

Urinary output is another indication of adequacy of cardiac output, although it may sometimes misrepresent the adequacy of perfusion to the kidneys. Postoperatively, cardiac surgery patients should be evaluated for renal insufficiency if urinary output is less than 0.5 mL/kg/hr for 2 to 3 consecutive hours and serum creatinine levels are increasing (Shin, Kim, Kim, Shin, & Sohn, 2016). Given that cardiac surgery patients may exhibit a relative diuresis of 200 to 400 mL/hr owing to the effects of hemodilution and osmotic agents sometimes administered during cardiopulmonary bypass (CPB) as well as elevated levels of atrial natriuretic peptide (Moriyama et al., 2017), urinary output may not be indicative of perfusion for the first several hours after surgery. Following the initial few hours postoperatively, urinary output should be at least 0.5 mL/kg/hr.

▶ Blood Pressure Monitoring

In the immediate postoperative period, maintaining hemodynamic stability is the priority. Intra-arterial pressure monitoring provides for the direct measurement of arterial blood pressure, and in many clinical situations (e.g., vasoconstrictive states), it is more accurate than the measurement with auscultation. Variables such as cuff size may underestimate SBP greater than 95 mmHg and overestimate systolic blood pressure less than 95 mmHg (Lakhal et al., 2015). This difference occurs because of the Korotkoff sounds produced by blood flow. As blood flow diminishes, the sound becomes less audible to the point that the faint early sounds may be missed. Indirect measurement of blood pressure, whether obtained manually or with a noninvasive automated pump, provides the best estimate of SBP but underestimates DBP when the patient is at rest (Jahangir, 2013).

Intra-arterial monitoring is indicated in situations when the patient's condition necessitates close hemodynamic observation. Patients who undergo mechanical manipulation of the heart, as in cardiac surgery, those who receive vasoactive drug therapy, and those in whom an intra-aortic balloon pump (IABP; discussed in Chapter 10) is used will all require frequent assessment of arterial pressure postoperatively. An intra-arterial line will also assist in assessing perfusion associated with dysrhythmias. When an intra-arterial catheter is in place in a peripheral artery, the SBP readings may be falsely elevated because of the amplitude of the waveform. However, mean arterial pressure (MAP) and DBP data are accurate (Koyfman, 2017).

Mean arterial pressure is the driving force for peripheral blood flow, the best assessment of coronary perfusion pressure, and the preferred pressure to be evaluated in unstable patients. On the monitor screen, it appears as a digital readout adjacent to the displayed blood pressure, usually in parentheses. Mean arterial pressure can also be calculated by the nurse using the formula given in **BOX 9.5**. Mean arterial pressure readings do not change as the pressure waveform moves distally along the arterial tree. This pressure is measured electronically by first integrating the area under the arterial pressure waveform and then dividing by the duration of the cardiac cycle. Many clinical conditions may be reflected by changes in the arterial waveform.

Pulsus alternans (**FIGURE 9.4**) is believed to be a sign of decreased myocardial contractility.

BOX 9.5 Mean Arterial Pressure Calculation

$$MAP = \frac{\text{Systolic blood pressure} + (\text{Diastolic blood pressure} \times 2)}{3}$$

For example, if the patient's blood pressure is 120/80, the MAP can be calculated as follows:

$$\frac{120 + (80 \times 2)}{3} = \frac{120 + 160}{3} \quad \text{or} \quad \frac{280}{3} = 93 \text{ mmHg}$$

MAP, mean arterial pressure.

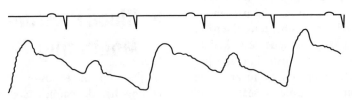

FIGURE 9.4 Pulsus alternans.

A paradoxical pulse is an exaggeration of the normal variation in the pulse during the inspiratory phase of respiration, in which the pulse becomes weaker as the person inhales and stronger as the person exhales. Pulsus alternans is an indicator of the presence of severe ventricular systolic failure (Chinyere, Moukabary, Goldman, & Juneman, 2017) and can be a sign of several conditions, including cardiac tamponade, which is a concern following cardiac surgery.

Complications associated with an intra-arterial catheter include ischemia or thrombosis of the affected extremity, infection, and bleeding. Prolonged hyperextension of the wrist can cause nerve conduction deficits. Close assessment for proper positioning and for signs of any complications related to indwelling intra-arterial catheters (e.g., presence of paresthesias, redness, extremity temperature and color) is an essential nursing responsibility and should be included in routine assessments (Koyfman, 2017). An arm board is frequently used to stabilize the catheter position, because excessive movement may cause the catheter to perforate the intima of the artery, which can lead to a hematoma or exsanguination if it also perforates the skin.

▶ Central Venous Pressure Monitoring

Because of the lack of supportive data on current use of pulmonary artery catheters (PACs), CVP catheters are being used more often in the cardiac surgical population. In one study, researchers compared low-risk patients undergoing coronary artery bypass grafting (CABG) with CVP with patients undergoing the same procedure with a PAC. Patients who had surgery with a PAC in place had higher weight gain and longer intubation time. Further, it is also speculated that the PAC may be associated with increased morbidity and resource utilization (Magder, 2015; Sotomi et al., 2014; Whitener, Konoske, & Mark, 2014). Circumstances in which a PAC may be used include patients with pulmonary hypertension, low CO, predicted postoperative hemodynamic instability following cardiac surgery, and when assessing the hemodynamic response to therapies (Whitener et al., 2014).

It can be anticipated that patients will manifest a decrease in blood and plasma volume within the first 24 hours following cardiac surgery. Patients who undergo CPB will often experience a systemic inflammatory response, which causes fluid to leak from the vessels to the interstitium. Vasodilation also occurs during rewarming and secondary to use of vasodilator therapy. Diuretic use in the postoperative period further contributes to hypovolemia (Hugyh, Peeters, Bernards, & Malbrain, 2016; Weinhouse, 2017). Other etiologic factors for a decrease in plasma and blood volume include the patient's underlying cardiac disease, medications (preoperative, anesthesia, and vasoactive agents), procedure-induced hypothermia, rewarming, and bleeding. There is no reported agreement on which data should be used to guide fluid therapy in these patients. Filling pressures (e.g., CVP and pulmonary artery diastolic [PAD]) are often misleading as signs of optimal left ventricular (LV) filling, especially in patients with alterations in ventricular compliance (Marx et al., 2016). In a landmark study, significant variations were reported in hemodynamic data following cardiac surgery. Because hemodynamic reference data had not been previously reported and great variability existed among the participants in this study, it remains difficult to use hemodynamic data as the sole basis for treatment decisions. Indeed, using acceptable values to guide treatment may result in overtreatment of some patients (Jakobsen, 2014). Rather, correlating hemodynamic data with the patient's clinical presentation may be the most advantageous course of action.

Causes of elevated CVP readings may include hypervolemia, increased venous tone, right ventricular (RV) or LV dysfunction, valve disease (mitral, tricuspid, aortic), pulmonary hypertension and other pulmonary problems such as fibrosis or embolism, atrial fibrillation, high pericardial pressures (such as seen in tamponade), high intrathoracic pressure (such as seen in pneumothorax or with positive pressure ventilation), and high intra-abdominal pressure. A low CVP value is most often indicative of hypovolemia or a decrease in cardiac output (Magder, 2017). Volume repletion with a crystalloid, colloid, blood, or blood product, along with identifying and treating the source of fluid loss, will resolve the problem. The most common sources of hypovolemia are warming, third spacing, hemorrhage, and overzealous diuresis, but causes may also include diaphoresis and vasodilation. Central venous pressure readings are influenced by the relationships among intravascular volume status, ventricular compliance, and intrathoracic pressure. As a consequence, trending data and correlating them with the patient's clinical status prior to treatment is more likely to optimize the patient's hemodynamic status than evaluating and treating just one isolated numeric value.

To further help ensure the accuracy of CVP readings, pressure waveforms are read at end expiration. Reading the tracing at this point minimizes the influence of intrathoracic pressure on the values.

In addition to aligning the transducer to the phlebostatic axis and interpreting the waveforms at end expiration, analysis of waveform morphology is essential when the nurse is collecting hemodynamic data. A typical CVP tracing consists of three waves and two descents. An "a" wave represents contraction of the right atrium and corresponds with the P wave on an ECG tracing. An "a" wave will not be seen in patients with tricuspid stenosis, RV hypertrophy, pulmonary hypertension, pulmonary stenosis, or atrial fibrillation (AF). Giant "a" waves may be visible if the right atrium is attempting to eject blood into the RV through a closed or partially closed tricuspid valve, as occurs in tricuspid stenosis (Nicolescu, 2017a). Pericardial constriction may be reflected by a prominent "a" wave.

A "c" wave is produced with bulging of the tricuspid valve into the right atrium at the start of ventricular systole. It corresponds with the start of the QRS complex on an ECG tracing (Nicolescu, 2017a). A large "v" wave may be present in patients who have tricuspid regurgitation.

The "X descent" represents atrial relaxation and corresponding displacement of the tricuspid valve during ventricular systole (Nicolescu, 2017a). Absence of the "X descent" may be present in patients who have tricuspid regurgitation.

A "v" wave represents filling of the right atrium with a closed tricuspid valve. It corresponds to the area immediately following the T wave on an ECG tracing. A giant "v" wave may be seen where an acute increase in pressure in the RV occurs (Nicolescu, 2017a), as is seen in patients who have tricuspid regurgitation. Pericardial constriction may be reflected by a prominent "v" wave.

Finally, a "Y descent" represents opening of the tricuspid valve. At this time, blood is flowing from the right atrium (causing an associated decrease in right atrial pressure) into the RV (Nicolescu, 2017a) (**FIGURE 9.5**). An attenuated "Y descent" may be seen in tricuspid stenosis, reflecting obstruction to right atrial emptying.

The nurse must keep in mind that alterations in waveforms may result in inaccurate numeric displays and that analysis of the waveforms is essential to obtain accurate hemodynamic data. Hemodynamic monitors assess the height and depth of the waveforms and translate this into a numerical value. If there is air in the line or a clot at the tip of

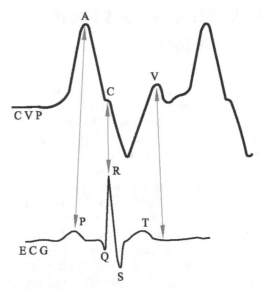

FIGURE 9.5 CVP waveform.

multidisciplinary rounds (Chan, Chang, Chiu, Huang, & Wang, 2015; Tang et al., 2014). Many hospitals use central line dressing teams so that a designated person changes the central line dressings on all patients on one set day of the week. The decrease in variability having one person change the lines may improve central line–associated bloodstream infection rates.

Finally, staff should keep in mind that an excellent maneuver to reinforce or validate CVP findings is by performing the passive leg raise (PLR). The PLR is easily performed at the bedside by keeping the patient in the supine position and raising the patient's legs to 45 degrees for at least 1 minute. This action will draw blood from the venous compartments in the abdomen and lower limbs and return to the heart, therefore allowing the clinician to determine if the patient is volume depleted. It is easily reversible, and may be performed quickly and at any time (Monnet, Marik, & Teboul, 2016) (**FIGURE 9.6**).

BOX 9.6 Complications Associated with CVP Catheters

Pneumothorax (usually occurs during catheter placement)
Thrombus
Infection
Air embolism
Adjacent vessel perforation
Catheter shearing and embolization
Thrombophlebitis
Extravasation of fluid or medication into the mediastinum, pericardium, retroperitoneum, or pleural cavity
Hemothorax
Vascular injuries (e.g., local hematoma, arterial laceration, perforation of the superior vena cava, pericardial perforation)
Arterial puncture
Subpleural hematoma
Uncontrolled venous bleeding

Data from Haider, Aziz, & Ahmed 2016; Kornbau, Lee, Hughes, & Firstenberg, 2015; Gerhardt & Skeehan, 2007; Roe, 2012; Young, 2014.

---

the catheter, the waveform will be damped and the numerical value displayed will be inaccurate.

BOX 9.6 lists complications associated with use of a CVP catheter. Some of these complications are site dependent—for example, pneumothorax is associated with internal jugular or subclavian insertion sites but not external jugular or femoral site use.

The risk of vascular injuries may be reduced with use of real-time ultrasound imaging during catheter insertion. Infectious complications may be minimized when steps to prevent infection are taken, and such steps should be part of every hospital's protocol. Preventive strategies include hand hygiene, maximal barrier precautions, chlorhexidine skin antisepsis, optimal catheter site selection, and use of antibiotic-impregnated catheters. These components are all part of the "call to order" that should be performed by the medical provider and RN prior to catheter insertion. A daily review of catheter necessity must be performed during change-of-shift report and during

Patient in semi-recumbent position

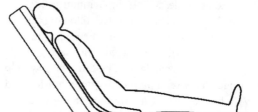

Patient supine with legs elevated to 45 degrees

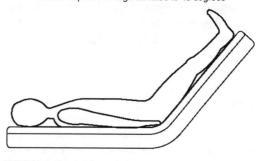

FIGURE 9.6 Passive leg raise.

▶ Monitoring Using a Pulmonary Artery Catheter

A PAC may be used to assess cardiac function, cardiac output/index, and intracardiac pressures (Magder, 2015). Achieving a cardiac index in the range of 2.5 to 4.2 L/min/m^2 is a goal for most postoperative cardiac surgery patients. Obtaining these hemodynamic data directly from the left ventricle would be ideal. Unfortunately, because of the potential for both damage to the LV wall and dysrhythmias, it is not possible to directly monitor these pressures on a continuous basis. Some indications for using a PAC may include patients undergoing CABG who have poor LV performance; those undergoing LV aneurysmectomy; those who recently had a myocardial infarction; those who have pulmonary hypertension, diastolic dysfunction, or acute ventricular septal rupture; or those having an LV assist device inserted, extracorporeal membrane oxygenation (ECMO), or heart transplantation (Nicolescu, 2017b; Weinhouse, 2017).

A PAC may also be inserted following cardiac surgery if signs of RV failure are present. Ideally, capacity for continuous mixed venous oxygen saturation (SvO$_2$) is available. The catheter may help distinguish between pulmonary hypertension and RV ischemia so that appropriate therapy can be initiated. Other indications for pulmonary artery catheter insertion include unstable hemodynamic status, low cardiac output syndrome, or hypovolemia (Weinhouse, 2017).

A change in left atrial pressure is the earliest indicator of a change in LV preload if no obstruction to flow is present (e.g., mitral stenosis). A left atrial catheter may be placed during cardiac surgery to directly reflect left atrial pressures, and may be used for direct vasoactive medication infusion when the drug administered may be deleterious if routed through the pulmonary system before reaching the left heart. However, because the possibility of tamponade with catheter removal and entry of air or catheter dislodgement exists while the catheter is in place, a left atrial pressure line is not a routine choice for most clinicians.

A PAC may be the next choice because it sits in the pulmonary artery and would provide an earlier indication of changes in the LV than a CVP catheter. With no obstruction to flow, pulmonary artery pressure (PAP) will indirectly reflect left atrial pressure and approximate value of LV end-diastolic pressure (left-sided preload). Values obtained with a PAC include pulmonary artery systolic (PAS), PAD, pulmonary artery mean (PAM), and PAOP:

- The PAS reflects pressure measured from the tricuspid to the mitral valve and is a good overall indicator of PAP. Conditions such as COPD, acute respiratory distress syndrome, and pulmonary hypertension are likely to increase PAS pressure.
- The PAD reflects pressure in the area between the pulmonic and aortic valves. If there is no obstruction to blood flow, the PAD is a good indicator of LV function.
- The pressure in the pulmonary artery is dynamic; it increases when blood is ejected from the right ventricle and then decreases until the next ejection of blood. The mean PAP (PAM) is the continuous average of the pressure in the pulmonary artery during one complete cardiac cycle (from the start of ejection of blood to the next) (Chemla, Humbert, Sitbon, Montani, & Hervé, 2015).
- The PAOP, obtained by inflating the PAC balloon, reflects the pressure between the tip of the PAC and the aortic valve. Because it assesses less surface area, the PAOP is more reflective of LV function than is the PAD. In most circumstances, the PAOP is thought to closely equate to left atrial pressure and LV end-diastolic pressure (LVEDP) or LV preload.

Fluid therapy and titration of vasoactive agents are based on these data. In some conditions, the PAOP is reported as greater than LVEDP (e.g., in mitral valve disease, increased pulmonary vascular resistance, use of positive-pressure ventilation with associated increase in intrathoracic pressure, tachycardia, and COPD). In other conditions, the PAOP is reported as less than LVEDP (e.g., in the presence of aortic regurgitation, a noncompliant left ventricle, or pulmonary embolism). There are data suggesting that during revascularization procedures, patients may have an elevated PAOP while having a low-volume status (Kassick, 2014).

Normally, the PAD is slightly higher than the PAOP, and the normal correlation is less than 5 mmHg (Kassick, 2014). To obtain the PAOP, the balloon must be inflated, which increases the potential risk of pulmonary artery rupture, pulmonary infarction, pulmonary thrombosis or embolism, and pulmonary artery hemorrhage. Obtaining PAOP readings may not be performed routinely but may be done if an acute change in the patient's clinical status or PAD occurs, or if no correlation between the PAD and PAOP exists. Unit-specific protocols for obtaining hemodynamic data should be followed.

When obtaining PAOP readings, balloon inflation time should be minimized to two to three respiratory cycles or 10 to 15 sec. During balloon inflation, blood flow to the lung is decreased and pulmonary infarction may result. The balloon should be inflated slowly to avoid migration of the catheter into a smaller pulmonary artery or vessel rupture. The balloon should be left deflated at all other times (Weinhouse, 2017).

▶ Cardiac Output Measurement

The PAC also allows measurement of CO via thermodilution or the assumed Fick method. A bolus of either normal saline or D_5W is injected into the right atrium (proximal) port. The fluid mixes with the blood as it travels past the tricuspid valve, through the right ventricle past the pulmonic valve and into the pulmonary artery. The overall temperature of the mixed blood and injectate is measured by the thermistor (a temperature-sensing device) at the tip of the catheter. The amount of time it takes the cooler blood to pass the thermistor is used to calculate CO. The longer it takes for the cooler blood to pass, the lower the CO. An electronic display of the time–temperature curve and calculated numerical CO value are displayed on the monitor.

Several variables must be assessed to ensure the accuracy of the CO displayed. Accuracy of CO results is essential, because many of the hemodynamic calculations listed earlier and subsequent therapeutic modalities are based on accurate CO determination (Whitener et al., 2014). Intracardiac shunts produce shunting of cold injectate into the left heart, which decreases pulmonary artery cooling and lowers the peak of the time–temperature curve, as seen with a right-to-left shunt; this condition also results in an underestimation of CO. Tricuspid regurgitation causes underestimation of the CO, because the injectate will reflux back into the right atrium and prevent adequate mixing.

In patients with a left-to-right shunt, increased right heart volume dilutes the injectate, resulting in an overestimation of CO. Temperature of the injectate, injectate technique, minimal manipulation of the injectate-filled syringe, time between measurements, and lack of obstruction to a smooth injection must be confirmed and the patient's body position assessed to ensure accuracy of measurements. The monitor must be preset with the gauge of the PAC in place and the amount of injectate to be infused (5 mL or 10 mL). In addition, forward flow, so that adequate mixing occurs, is important. Dysrhythmias, such as AF, will prevent thorough mixing. Thus the trend in CO values obtained is extremely important to monitor.

Continuous Cardiac Output

Potential causes of errors in obtaining intermittent measurements of CO have been discussed. Continuous cardiac output (CCO) catheters use a tracer that is not cool but warm; a 10-cm thermal filament is placed on the outside of the catheter at the level of the right ventricle. The filament warms the catheter every 30 to 60 seconds, with low levels of heat energy being transferred to the blood that is adjacent to the filament. The same process is used to determine CO as with the intermittent injectate method. The only difference is that with this technology CO is calculated based on the amount of time it takes the warmed blood to pass the thermistor instead of cooled blood. The CO value is averaged over 3 to 6 minutes, and a numeric display of the calculated value appears on the monitor screen (Hugyh et al., 2016; Mehta & Arora, 2014).

Benefits of contour CO include avoidance of individual variations in the volume and speed of infusion of the tracer bolus, and the fact that CO is based on a time-weighted average versus a single instantaneous measurement. Drawbacks include the expense and delayed response time after changes in CO (Hugyh et al., 2016; Mehta & Arora, 2014). Light sedation and the initiation of early mobility are essential for any ICU patient to prevent delirium; therefore, frequent assessment of the need and potential ability to remove the PAC must be discussed at every opportunity. Although mobilization of a patient with a PAC is certainly possible without complications (Fields, Trotsky, Fernandez, & Smith, 2015), logistically it is easier for the patient and staff without the burden of excessive monitoring lines.

Alternative Methods to Determine Cardiac Output

Even as the incorporation of goal-directed therapy using CO or similar parameters to guide intravenous fluid and inotropic therapy continues to increase, other less invasive options for monitoring CO are being adopted in many practices. Minimally invasive CO monitoring devices use one of four main principles to measure CO: pulse contour analysis, pulsed Doppler technology, applied Fick principle, and bioimpedance/bioreactance (Mehta & Arora, 2014). Technologies that are based on arterial pressure can provide CO determinations and measure other clinically important variables, such as stroke volume variation (SVV), pulse pressure variation (PPV), and systolic pressure variation (SPV). Clinical use of these parameters is emerging as a means for determining the patient's ability to respond to changes in fluid levels. Stroke volume variation occurs due to changes in intrathoracic pressure during spontaneous breathing; blood pressure decreases during inhalation and increases during exhalation. The opposite changes are observed when a patient is receiving positive pressure ventilation.

Arterial Pulse Contour CCO

Arterial pulse contour CCO monitoring estimates CO based on pulse contour analysis; it is an indirect method based on analysis of the arterial pressure pulsation waveform. This technology relies on the concept that the contour of the arterial pressure waveform is proportional to stroke volume. The arterial pressure waveform is used to calculate CO, stroke volume variance, intrathoracic volumes, and extravascular lung water. These data are then used to predict response to fluid therapy (Mehta & Arora, 2014). The arterial waveform is typically recorded from an intra-arterial catheter, although noninvasive recordings have also been used. The efficacy of arterial pulse contour–based CO technology has been demonstrated in some patients who underwent CABG procedures (Hendy & Bubenek, 2016). Despite prior exclusion of well-known confounding factors, PPV has also been shown to be of poor clinical utility globally to predict fluid responsiveness, and digital pleth variability index is not discriminant for routine practice in the conventional cardiac surgery setting (Fischer et al., 2013). Three of the currently available pulse contour CO systems use intra-arterial waveform analysis. The Pulse index Continuous Cardiac Output (PiCCO) system uses thermodilution for calibration and requires femoral or axillary arterial catheterization. It incorporates use of a catheter with a thermistor on the tip. The catheter records aortic pressure waveforms, and CO is then calculated using a formula based on the area under the systolic portion of the waveform (Hugyh et al., 2016; Mehta & Arora 2014). The PiCCO system uses an algorithm based on the analysis of the arterial pulse contour so that it is possible to continuously monitor CO and stroke volume, allowing assessment of beat-to-beat variations of stroke volume and CO in changing preload conditions. SVV and PPV may help guide fluid loading in critical care settings. The system also allows the measurement of global end-diastolic volume (GEDV), intrathoracic blood volume (ITBV), and extravascular lung water (EVLW). The PiCCO provides a true continuous CO and rapidly available measurements allowing the assessment of fluid responsiveness (Huygh et al., 2016).

The second pulse contour CO system available is LiDCO®, which uses lithium dilution for calibration and arterial pulse wave analysis from PulseCO®. The radial or brachial artery is used as the access site. With this technique, a small dose of intravenous lithium chloride is administered. Cardia output is then determined by a dilution curve made by a lithium-sensitive electrode that is attached to the intra-arterial catheter (Hugyh et al., 2016; Mehta & Arora, 2014).

FloTrac™/Vigileo™, the third method of pulse contour analysis, does not employ a calibration process to improve monitor precision, but instead uses a formula or algorithm to continually update a constant that is used to determine CO (Mehta & Arora, 2014). The FloTrac sensor and Vigileo monitor together constitute the FloTrac system. As with the other pulse contour CO systems, SVV may be calculated. Data used to calculate SVV include the patient's blood pressure, age, gender, and body surface area. The patient's CO is determined from the stroke volume and heart rate. An accurate arterial pressure waveform is essential for accurate contour CO determination. Any factor that may alter the tracing (e.g., dysrhythmias, hypotension, equipment issues) may affect the results.

Data suggest that each of the three methods for pulse contour CO is comparable to using a PAC with the intermittent injectate method (Cho, Koo, Kim, Hong, & Jeon 2016; Hendy & Bubenek, 2016).

Stroke Volume Variation

Stroke volume variation produces data on changes in preload that occur with mechanical ventilation. It is "the difference between the maximum and minimum stroke volume during one mechanical breath relative to the mean stroke volume" (Berkenstadt et al., 2005, p. 721). Stroke volume variation monitoring can provide data that suggest whether a patient's stroke volume will improve with volume repletion (Kang, Kim, Woo, & Yoon, 2014).

There are conflicting data regarding the ability of SVV to predict response to fluid therapy. Some data suggest that SVV predicted preload responsiveness in cardiac surgery patients.

Conversely, other data reported that SVV did not predict fluid responsiveness in cardiac surgery patients (Piccioni, Bernasconi, Tramontano, & Langer, 2017). Possible explanations for the discrepancies in results include differences in tidal volumes used and differences in the cardiac stability of the two groups of patients (Hendy & Bubenek, 2016).

Pulse Pressure Variation

Pulse pressure variation is "the difference between the maximum and minimum values of the arterial pulse pressure during one mechanical breath divided by the mean of the two values" (Berkenstadt et al., 2005, p. 721). The variation of PPV induced by mechanical ventilation is known to be a very accurate predictor of fluid responsiveness (Soloman, Samir, Neggar, & Dehely, 2015). Reports suggest that variations in PPV can accurately predict response to fluid therapy in patients with shock and in surgical procedures. Upon evaluating the Frank-Starling curve, an increase in preload is associated with a decrease in PPV; conversely, a decrease in preload is associated with an increase in PPV and contractility. It has been suggested that PPV is more accurate in predicting fluid response than CVP and PAOP, SPV, and SVV (Michard, Chemia, & Teboul, 2015; Rathore, Singh, Lamsal, Taank, & Paul, 2017).

Systolic Pressure Variation

Systolic pressure variation is "the difference between the maximum and minimum systolic blood pressure during one mechanical breath" (Berkenstadt et al., 2005, p. 721). It can reportedly indicate decreases in CO from blood loss and predict a patient's response to volume repletion. This parameter is used to estimate circulating volume (Perel, Pizov, & Cotev, 2014).

In a study of patients in the ICU who underwent CABG, researchers determined that PPV and SPV were both able to predict whether a patient would respond to volume repletion with an increase in CO. While PPV was demonstrated to be superior to SPV at predicting response to fluid therapy, the researchers concluded that both

PPV and SPV were far superior to CVP and PAOP data (Michard et al., 2015; Rathore et al., 2017).

Doppler Methods

Doppler-based methods use ultrasound and the Doppler effect to determine CO. When ultrasound waves strike moving objects, the waves are reflected back to their source at a different frequency, which is directly related to the velocity of the moving objects and the angle at which the ultrasound beam strikes these objects. Proper probe placement is essential when using these methods to monitor CO. Several different Doppler-based methods may be used to measure CO, each of which uses a slightly different site in the body for measuring blood flow. Data comparing ultrasound determination of CO with data from a PAC have conflicting results (Thiele, Bartels, & Gan, 2015).

The esophageal Doppler technique is another method to measure blood flow velocity in the descending aorta by means of a Doppler transducer placed at the tip of a flexible probe. The probe is introduced into the esophagus of sedated, mechanically ventilated patients and then rotated so the transducer faces the descending aorta and a characteristic aortic velocity signal is obtained. The CO is calculated based on the diameter of the aorta (measured or estimated), the distribution of the CO to the descending aorta, and the measured flow velocity of blood in the aorta (Mehta & Arora, 2014).

Electrical Bioimpedance

Electrical bioimpedance is a noninvasive method to determine CO. Using this technology, CO is measured based on changes in impedance that occur as blood is ejected from the left ventricle into the aorta and is calculated from changes in thoracic impedance. With this method, changes in thoracic blood volume during the cardiac cycle can be used to calculate CO. This technique is a successful method of monitoring CO because the algorithm eliminates the impedance due to body tissue and lung volume changes, instead using only the change in thoracic blood volume for CO determination. An alternative approach uses a specially designed endotracheal tube to measure electrical impedance changes in the ascending aorta (Huygh et al., 2016; Mehta & Arora, 2014).

▶ Assessment of Oxygenation Parameters

Venous Oxygen Saturation

In addition to direct pressure measurements and CO assessment, other hemodynamic data may assess a patient's condition following cardiac surgery. Another type of PAC provides for continuous monitoring of SvO_2. A patient's SvO_2 reveals the association between oxygen delivery (the amount of oxygen that is carried to the tissues each minute) and oxygen consumption (the amount of oxygen used by the tissues) or tissue oxygen balance (Howard & Christie, 2016).

Mixed venous blood represents the amount of oxygen in the systemic circulation after the blood's passage through the tissues. Venous oxygen saturation data reflect tissue oxygenation and cardiopulmonary function and can be used to discover whether a patient is clinically deteriorating. Normal SvO_2 is in the range of 60% to 80%. Trends and changes in oxygen delivery, oxygen consumption, or tissue oxygenation may be identified by reviewing data related to venous oxygen saturation. These data can also be used to determine the efficacy of interventions implemented to optimize these variables as well as procedures performed by the ICU nurse while caring for a postoperative cardiac surgery patient (Reyer, 2013). With continuous digital readout of SvO_2 measurements, early recognition and prompt intervention to eradicate effects of poor tissue oxygenation can be implemented by the ICU nurse. Causes of changes in SvO_2 are many and include most variables affecting preload, afterload, and contractility. Although not specific to any one factor, any change in SvO_2 alerts the ICU nurse to quickly investigate.

Central Venous Oxygen Saturation

Catheters that allow for assessment of central venous oxygen saturation ($ScvO_2$) are being used in some cardiac surgical programs as the transition away from PACs continues. With this monitoring approach, a blood sample is obtained from a central venous catheter and is analyzed. A normal ScvO$_2$ is 70% or greater. If the value is less than 70%, it indicates that the tissues are extracting more oxygen than is normal and that the tissues do not perceive that their oxygen needs are being met; this is an indicator of a bad outcome (Dirks, 2017; Reyer 2013).

One of the newest noninvasive CO monitors is the Nexfin®. Rather than a minimally invasive monitor, it is a completely noninvasive method of determining the patient's hemodynamic parameters, as the need for an invasive arterial catheter or a central line is obviated. The monitor is connected to the patient by wrapping an inflatable cuff around the middle phalanx of the finger. The pulsating finger artery is "clamped" to a constant volume by applying a varying counterpressure equivalent to the arterial pressure, resulting in a pressure waveform. The finger arterial pressure is then reconstructed into brachial arterial pressure waveform using a transfer function and a level correction based on a vast clinical database. The resulting brachial pressure waveform serves as the basis for determining continuous CO (Saugel, Cecconi, Wagner, & Reuter, 2015). However, Nexfin does not provide consistent results at this time (Maass, Roekaerts, & Lancé, 2014).

Postoperative Hemodynamic Assessment

Some of the initial goals for patients in the immediate postoperative period following cardiac surgery include promoting satisfactory oxygen levels and ventilation, repleting intravascular volume, and augmenting perfusion by stabilizing blood pressure and CO (Nicholas, 2014). The ICU nurse caring for a postoperative cardiac surgery patient must be aware of both normal and baseline parameter values so that any clinical deterioration or improvement in the patient may be promptly noted. Some patients, because of their comorbidities or their disease process (such as valve disease), may require higher filling pressures postoperatively to maintain an adequate cardiac output/index.

An adequate cardiac index in the range of 2.5 to 4.2 L/min/m^2 will be sustained by normalizing heart rate and stroke volume as soon as possible. Many variables may affect heart rate and rhythm in the postoperative period. The most common causes in the postoperative cardiac surgery patient include hypovolemia and pain, both of which should be addressed promptly. Despite sedation, the nurse should assess for other signs and symptoms that indicate the presence of pain. Pain assessment and management are discussed in detail in Chapter 14.

Dysrhythmias that may be seen in the postoperative period include AF, premature ventricular contractions, and ventricular tachycardia; the latter two dysrhythmias may occur due to electrolyte imbalance. All of the dysrhythmias may arise as a result of cardiac irritability from operative manipulation. Ventricular fibrillation, although rare, may also occur. The presence of any dysrhythmia may affect a patient's hemodynamic status and requires rapid intervention. The etiology and management of postoperative dysrhythmias are discussed in detail in Chapter 15.

After assessing heart rate, an adequate stroke volume should be ensured. Variables that influence stroke volume (i.e., preload, afterload, and contractility) often are affected in the intraoperative and postoperative periods. For example, preload may be decreased as the patient undergoes the rewarming process, which may lead to vasodilation. Bleeding from chest tubes or third spacing that results from the inflammatory process may also decrease preload, resulting in a decrease in CO. Postoperative bleeding is always a concern for the cardiac surgical patient. Blood loss will decrease the oxygen-carrying capacity to vital organs and tissues (Joshi, de Witt, & Mosier, 2014). Logically, decreased circulating volume will decrease preload, stroke volume, and CO.

The causes of postoperative bleeding are many. For instance, the CPB circuit may cause platelet destruction as the blood circulates through it, in addition to decreasing levels of clotting factors. Inadequate hemostasis from incomplete heparin reversal or excessive protamine administration is another potential cause of altered hemostasis, as is a surgical bleed from a suture site.

If chest tube drainage exceeds 100 mL/hour for more than 3 hours, 200 mL/hour for 3 hours, or 300 mL in the first hour following surgery, the surgeon should be notified. Transfusion of blood or blood products may be ordered if the coagulation studies are outside the normal range or if the patient's hematocrit level is low. If the patient is hypertensive, the blood pressure must be decreased to prevent stress on the suture sites, which may cause further bleeding. The patient may need to undergo surgical reexploration. Decreases in blood pressure, cardiac filling pressures, and urinary output are signs of hypovolemia that must be evaluated. Adjustments to volume administration are frequently necessary as well. Volume repletion is accomplished by administration of isotonic crystalloids (e.g., lactated Ringer's, PlasmaLyte, or normal saline) or colloids (e.g., albumin, blood, or blood products) as determined by the patient's hemodynamic status and lab results. Conversely, if preload indices are too high, holding further volume administration, diuretics, or vasodilators (e.g., nitroglycerin) may be used.

An increased afterload may result from severe LV dysfunction, hypovolemia, vasoconstriction, hypothermia, or increased catecholamine stimulation from the surgical procedure. Along with volume-related interventions and use of a warming blanket, arterial vasodilator administration may be beneficial in such cases. A decreased afterload may be the result of significant vasodilation from warming; this condition may be treated with administration of an agent that causes vasoconstriction.

Decreased contractility in the postoperative period may be the result of an increase or decrease in preload, an increase in afterload, or factors that affect myocardial contractility directly (e.g., ischemia, RV or LV failure, and aneurysms). Electrolyte imbalance and tamponade may also alter contractility. In such a scenario, preload and afterload are optimized while other interventions to treat the underlying cause are completed. If indicated, administration of positive inotropic agents is initiated. If further afterload reduction is needed after the use of vasodilators, an IABP may be added. The IABP can increase CO by as much

as 1 L and may be necessary to support the patient through an acute event. Intra-aorta balloon pump therapy is discussed in detail in Chapter 10. Lactate levels are also helpful in determining altered tissue perfusion and response to therapy (Vincent, Quintairos e Silva, Couto, & Taccone, 2016). The use of biventricular pacing has also been reported to improve contractility following bypass procedures (Gielgens et al., 2017).

If blood builds up inside the mediastinum, cardiac tamponade may occur, resulting in physical compression of the heart, limitation of diastolic filling time, and a decrease in CO. In addition to a plateau of filling pressures and a narrowed pulse pressure, waveform changes are helpful in assessing for this state. Cardiac tamponade and several other postoperative complications are discussed in detail in Chapter 13.

▶ Summary

The number of cardiac surgical patients with PACs has decreased worldwide. Although little published evidence exists to associate use of patient monitoring with improved clinical outcomes, this lack of evidence does not necessarily equate to a lack of benefit. Thus catheters will still be used, albeit with caution.

ICU nurses play a pivotal role in monitoring the postoperative hemodynamic status of patients following cardiac surgery. They must obtain accurate data, integrate those monitoring data with information gained by assessing the patient's clinical status, and use clinical judgment to select the best interventions to optimize the patient's status given the patient's current condition and past medical history. Having expertise helps to ensure that obtained parameters are not reflecting nonphysiologic events such as patient turning, artifact, and inaccurate leveling and that values are assessed at end expiration. The ICU nurse with high levels of critical judgment and clinical inquiry competencies will use accurate information and evidence-based guidelines to determine when activities can be clustered or when oxygen consumption is too high to do so.

By definition, the cardiac surgical patient always has underlying cardiac pathology that will have a major impact on postoperative recovery. Monitoring that incorporates a clinical evaluation, review of physiology, and expected responses relative to the type of cardiac surgery performed is essential. Invasive catheters may be used to augment but not replace monitoring for subtle changes. The expert ICU nurse validates signs and intervenes quickly. Each of these competencies is essential to achieve an optimal patient outcome following cardiac surgery.

🔍 CASE STUDY

A 68-year-old male patient with a history of having undergone percutaneous coronary intervention (PCI), is admitted from the emergency department with reports of palpitations, weakness, fatigue, nausea, and dizziness. Upon examination, the patient is found to be cold, clammy, and diaphoretic. Vital signs are BP 82/60, Mean (67), HR 168, RR 28, T 37°C (98.6°F), SpO$_2$ 92% on room air. Upon connection to the cardiac monitor, ventricular tachycardia is noted. While setting up for synchronized cardioversion, the patient becomes unresponsive, apneic, and pulseless. Ventricular fibrillation is noted. The patient was defibrillated with 120 joules and has a return of spontaneous circulation. Postresuscitation ECG reveals ST segment elevation myocardial infarction (STEMI) in leads V2 to V6, I, and aVL. The patient is transported to the catheterization lab for emergent PCI. Cardiac catheterization reveals 95% left main occlusion. The patient remained hypotensive in the catheterization lab; a pulmonary artery catheter was inserted and IABP therapy was started. Initial hemodynamic findings were PAP 45/25 (38), CVP 12 mmHg, PAOP 23 mmHg, SVR 2500 dynes/sec/cm^{-5}, and cardiac index (CI) 1.7 L/min/m^2. The patient is seen by a cardiac surgeon and was taken to the OR for emergent 3-vessel CABG surgery. The IABP timing was adjusted and the patient's CI increased to 1.9 L/min/m^2. Postoperatively, the patient was admitted to the CVICU on a milrinone (Primacor®) infusion at 0.5 mcg/kg/min. The IABP was set at 1:1. Vital signs upon admission are BP 80/52 (61), HR 98 (normal sinus rhythm), RR 20, PAP 40/22 (28), CVP 12 mmHg, and PAOP 20 mmHg.

Critical Thinking Questions

1. What is the etiology of the patient's hemodynamic parameters when the pulmonary artery catheter was inserted in the catheterization lab?
2. Why did the patient require IABP therapy?
3. For which parameters should the nurse evaluate to help determine if the milrinone infusion can be titrated off?

Answers to Critical Thinking Questions

1. The patient had an anterolateral STEMI and developed cardiogenic shock. This was caused by occlusion of the left main coronary artery (as reflected by leads V2 to V6, I, and aVL).
2. The patient needed afterload reduction as the SVR was 2,500 dynes/sec/cm^{-5} and cardiac index was 1.9 L/min/m^2. These data are consistent with a patient with cardiogenic shock.
3. As milrinone is an arterial and venous vasodilator, the nurse should monitor the patient's blood pressure, pulmonary artery pressures, CVP, PAOP, and cardiac index.

Self-Assessment Questions

1. The nurse notices an overdamped waveform on the arterial line tracing. Which should the nurse suspect?
   A. Small bubbles in the system
   B. Pressure tubing too long
   C. Defective transducer
   D. Low pressure in the flush bag

2. A cause of an underdamped waveform may include:
   A. large bubbles in the system.
   B. loose connections.
   C. low pressure in the flush solution pressure bag.
   D. pressure tubing too long.

3. Placement of the transducer below the phlebostatic axis will result in:
   A. small air bubbles gathering in the pressure tubing.
   B. falsely elevated pressure readings.
   C. decreased perfusion to the area of insertion.
   D. an overdamped waveform.

4. Presence of pulsus alternans following cardiac surgery may indicate:
   A. diastolic failure.
   B. loose connections of the pressure bag.
   C. increasing pleural effusion.
   D. decreased myocardial contractility.

5. Which hemodynamic parameter should the nurse anticipate in the first 24 hours after cardiac surgery?
   A. Systolic BP greater than 140 mmHg
   B. Pulmonary artery pressure 35/20
   C. Central venous pressure 1 mmHg
   D. Cardiac index 4 L/min/m^2

6. Which may cause an elevated CVP reading following cardiac surgery?
   A. Decreased pulmonary artery pressures
   B. Atrial fibrillation
   C. Pulmonic valve disease
   D. Pleural effusion

7. You are caring for a patient following cardiac surgery. The patient has not been reversed. The following CVP tracing is seen on the monitor. What CVP reading should be documented?

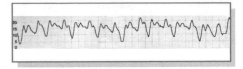

   A. 25 mmHg
   B. 3 mmHg
   C. 5 mmHg
   D. 10 mmHg

8. Which is true about a "v" wave?
   A. It represents atrial relaxation.
   B. It corresponds with the QRS complex of the ECG tracing.
   C. It will not be seen in patients with pulmonary hypertension.
   D. If prominent, it may indicate pericardial constriction.

9. Pulmonary artery systolic pressure:
   A. represents left-sided preload.
   B. is a good indicator of left ventricular function.
   C. may be decreased in patients with acute respiratory distress syndrome.
   D. reflects pressure measured from the tricuspid to mitral valve.

10. When observing PAOP readings:
    A. balloon inflation should not exceed 3 L.
    B. balloon inflation should occur in 1 sec to avoid catheter migration.
    C. values should be obtained hourly and compared to PAD values.
    D. the balloon should remain inflated for no more than 3 sec.

Answers to Self-Assessment Questions

1. D. **low pressure in the flush bag**
   Rationale: An overdamped waveform is sluggish and has an exaggerated or falsely widened and blunt tracing. It will cause the patient's SBP to be recorded as falsely low and the DBP to be recorded as falsely high.

2. D. **pressure tubing too long**
   Rationale: An underdamped waveform consists of an overresponse, which is seen as an exaggerated, narrow, artificially peaked tracing. In this case, the waveform overestimates the patient's SBP and underestimates the DBP.

3. B. **falsely elevated pressure readings**
   Rationale: Transducers are zero balanced, establishing atmospheric pressure as zero. Leveling at the phlebostatic axis is performed to eradicate the effects of hydrostatic forces on the hemodynamic pressures. If the transducer is placed lower than the phlebostatic axis, the pressures will be falsely elevated. The opposite is true if the transducer is placed higher than the phlebostatic axis.

4. D. **decreased myocardial contractility**
   Rationale: Pulsus alternans is believed to be a sign of decreased myocardial contractility. A paradoxical pulse is an exaggeration of the normal variation in the pulse during the inspiratory phase of respiration, in which the pulse becomes weaker as the person inhales and stronger as the person exhales. Pulsus alternans is an indicator of the presence of severe ventricular systolic failure.

5. C. **central venous pressure 1 mmHg**
   Rationale: It can be anticipated that patients will manifest a decrease in blood and plasma volume within the first 24 hours following cardiac surgery. Patients who undergo CPB often will experience a systemic inflammatory response, which causes fluid to leak from the vessels to the interstitium. Vasodilation also occurs during rewarming and secondary to use of vasodilator therapy.

Diuretic use in the postoperative period further contributes to hypovolemia.

6. B. **atrial fibrillation**
   Rationale: Causes of elevated CVP readings may include hypervolemia, increased venous tone, RV or LV dysfunction, valve disease (mitral, tricuspid, aortic), pulmonary hypertension and other pulmonary problems such as fibrosis or embolism, atrial fibrillation, high pericardial pressures (such as seen in tamponade), high intrathoracic pressure (such as seen in pneumothorax or with positive pressure ventilation), and high intra-abdominal pressure.

7. D. **10 mmHg**
   Rationale: Hemodynamic tracings are read at end expiration to avoid effects of changes in intrathoracic pressure.

8. D. **If prominent, it may indicate pericardial constriction.**
   Rationale: A "v" wave represents filling of the right atrium with a closed tricuspid valve. It corresponds to the area immediately following the T wave on an ECG tracing.

9. D. **reflects pressure measured from the tricuspid to mitral valve**
   Rationale: The pulmonary artery systolic value reflects pressure measured from the tricuspid to the mitral valve and is a good overall indicator of PAP

10. D. **the balloon should remain inflated for no more than 3 sec.**
    Rationale: To obtain the PAOP, the balloon must be inflated, which increases the potential risk of pulmonary artery rupture, pulmonary infarction, pulmonary thrombosis or embolism, and pulmonary artery hemorrhage. When obtaining PAOP readings, balloon inflation time should be minimized, inflated for two to three respiratory cycles or 10 to 15 seconds. During balloon inflation, blood flow to the lung is decreased and pulmonary infarction may result. The balloon should be left deflated at all other times.

CLINICAL INQUIRY BOX

Question: Does omega-3 polyunsaturated fatty acid infusion reduce the incidence of postoperative atrial fibrillation in patients following coronary artery bypass grafting?

Reference: Lomivorotov, V. V., Efremov, S. M., Pokushalov, E. A., Romanov, A. B., Ponomarev, D. N., Chermiavsky, A. M., . . . Lomivorotov, V. N. (2014). Randomized trial of fish oil infusion to prevent atrial fibrillation after cardiac surgery: Data from an implantable continuous cardiac monitor. *Journal of Cardiothoracic & Vascular Anesthesia, 28*(5), 1278–1284.

Objective: To determine if omega-3 polyunsaturated fatty acid infusion reduces the incidence of postoperative atrial fibrillation in patients following CABG using an implantable continuous cardiac monitor.

Method: Prospective, randomized, double-blind, placebo-controlled trial.

Results: At 10-day follow-up, POAF occurred in 19% of patients in the control group and 27.8% of patients developed POAF in the experimental group. After 2 years, 27.8% of patients in the control group and 35.3% in the experimental group developed atrial fibrillation.

Conclusion: Infusion of omega-3 polyunsaturated fatty acids did not prevent development of postoperative atrial fibrillation in patients 2 years following CABG surgery.

References

Arora, S., Singh, P. M., Goudra, B. G., & Sinha, A. C. (2014). Changing trends of hemodynamic monitoring in ICU— from invasive to non-invasive methods: Are we there yet? *International Journal of Critical Illness and Injury Science, 4*(2), 168–177.

Barros, L., Bridges, E., Cockerham, M., Greco, S., Herrera, F., & Solvang, N. (2016). Pulmonary artery/central venous pressure monitoring in adults. *Critical Care Nurse, 36*(4), e12–e18.

Berkenstadt, H., Friedman, Z., Preisman, S., Keidan, I., Livingstone, D., & Perel, A. (2005). Pulse pressure and stroke volume variations during severe haemorrhage in ventilated dogs. *British Journal of Anaesthesia, 94*(6), 721–726.

Chan, M., Chang, C., Chiu, Y., Huang, T., & Wang, C. (2015). Effectiveness analysis of cross-functional team to implement central venous catheter care bundle. *Journal of Microbiology, Immunology, and Infection, 48*(2, suppl 1), S90. doi:10.1016/j.jmii.2015.02.317

Chemla, D., Humbert, M., Sitbon, O., Montani, D., & Hervé, P. (2015). Systolic and mean pulmonary artery pressures: Are they interchangeable in patients with pulmonary hypertension? *Chest, 147*(4), 943–950,

Chinyere, I., Moukabary, T., Goldman, S., & Juneman, E. (2017). Electrical and mechanical alterations during ventricular tachycardia with moderate chronic heart failure. *Journal of Electrocardiology, 51*(1), 33–37.

Cho, Y. J., Koo, C., Kim, T. K., Hong, D. M., & Jeon, Y. (2016). Comparison of cardiac output measures by transpulmonary thermodilution, pulse contour analysis, and pulmonary artery thermodilution during off-pump coronary artery bypass surgery: A subgroup analysis of the cardiovascular anaesthesia registry at a single tertiary centre. *Journal of Clinical Monitoring and Computing, 30*(6), 771–782.

Dirks, J. L. (2017). Continuous venous oxygen saturation monitoring. In D. L. Wiegand (Ed.), *AACN procedure manual for high acuity, progressive, and critical care* (7th ed., 116–122). St. Louis, MO: Elsevier.

Dhonnchú, T., Gough, A., & Walcot, N. (2015). Postoperative care of adult cardiac surgery patients. *Surgery (Oxford), 33*(2), 57–61.

Fields, C., Trotsky, A., Fernandez, N., & Smith, B. A. (2015). Mobility and ambulation for patients with pulmonary artery catheters: A retrospective descriptive study. *Journal of Acute Care Physical Therapy, 6*(2), 64–70.

Fischer, M., Pelissier A., Bohadana D., Gérard, J. L., Hanouz, J. L., . . . Fellahi, J. L. (2013). Prediction of responsiveness to an intravenous fluid challenge in patients after cardiac surgery with cardiopulmonary bypass: A comparison between arterial pulse pressure variation and digital plethysmographic variability index. *Journal of Cardiothoracic and Vascular Anesthesia, 27*(6), 1087–1093.

Gielgens, R. C., Herold, I. H., van Straten, A. H., van Gelder, B. M., Bracke, F. A., Korsten, H. H., . . . Bouwman, R. A. (2017). The hemodynamic effects of different pacing modalities after cardiopulmonary bypass in patients with reduced left ventricular function. *Journal of Cardiothoracic and Vascular Anesthesia, 32*(1), 259–266.

Hendy, A., & Bubenek, S. (2016). Pulse waveform hemodynamic monitoring devices: Recent advances and the place in goal-directed therapy in cardiac surgical patients. *Romanian Journal of Anaesthesia and Intensive Care, 23*(1), 55–65.

Howard, B. M., & Christie, D. B. (2016). Hemodynamic monitoring in surgical critical care. In N. Martin & L. Kaplan (Eds.), *Principles of adult surgical critical care.* Cham, Switzerland: Springer International Publishing.

Huygh, J., Peeters, Y., Bernards, J., & Malbrain, M. L. N. (2016). Hemodynamic monitoring in the critically ill: An overview of current cardiac output monitoring methods. *F1000Research.* doi:10.12688/f1000research.8991.1

Jahangir, E. (2013). *Blood pressure assessment.* Retrieved from http://emedicine.medscape.com/article/1948157-overview.

Jakobsen, C. (2014). Transfusion strategy: Impact of haemodynamics and the challenge of haemodilution. *Journal of Blood Transfusion, 2014.* doi:10.1155/2014/627141

Joshi, R., de Witt, B., & Mosier, J. M. (2014). Optimizing oxygen delivery in the critically ill: The utility of lactate and central venous oxygen saturation (ScvO2) as a roadmap of resuscitation in shock. *Journal of Emergency Medicine, 47*(4), 493–500.

Kang, W., Kim, J. Y., Woo, N. S., & Yoon, T. G. (2014). The influence of different mechanical ventilator settings of peak inspiratory pressure on stroke volume variation in pediatric cardiac surgery patients. *Korean Journal of Anesthesiology, 66*(5), 358–363.

Kassick, M. A. (2014). Clinical monitoring: Cardiovascular system. In J. J. Nagelhout & K. L. Plaus (Eds.), *Nurse anesthesia* (5th ed., pp. 292–312). St. Louis, MO: Elsevier Saunders.

Kornbau, C., Lee, K. C., Hughes, G. D., & Firstenberg, M. S. (2015). Central line complications. *International Journal of Critical Illness & Injury Science, 5*(3), 170–178.

Koyfman, A. (2017). *Arterial line placement.* Retrieved from https://emedicine.medscape.com.

Lakhal, K., Ehrmann, S., Martin, M., Faiz, S., Reminiac, F., Cinotti, R., . . . Boulain, T. (2015). Blood pressure monitoring during arrhythmia: agreement between automated brachial cuff and intra-arterial measurements. *British Journal of Anaethesia, 115*(4), 540–549.

Maass, S. W., Roekaerts, P. M., & Lancé, M. D. (2014). Cardiac output measurement by bioimpedance and noninvasive pulse contour analysis compared with the continuous pulmonary artery thermodilution technique. *Journal of Cardiothoracic and Vascular Anesthesia 28*(3), 534–539.

Magder, S. (2015). Invasive hemodynamic monitoring. *Critical Care Clinic, 31,* 67–87.

Magder, S. (2017). Right atrial pressure in the critically ill: How to measure, what is the value, what are the limitations? *Chest, 151*(4), 908–916.

Marx, G., Schindler, A. W., Mosch, C., Albers, J., Bauer, M., Gnass, I., . . . Eikermann, M. (2016). Intravascular volume therapy in adults: Guidelines from the Association of the Scientific Medical Societies in Germany. *European Journal of Anaesthesiology, 33*(7), 488–521.

McCleaster, S., & Heuer, A. J. (2010). Review existing data in patient's record. In C. L. Scanlan, A. J. Heuer, & L. M. Sinopoli (Eds.), *Certified respiratory therapist exam: Review guide* (pp. 43–60). Sudbury, MA: Jones and Bartlett Publishers.

Mehta, Y., & Arora, D. (2014). Newer methods of cardiac output monitoring. *World Journal of Cardiology, 6*(9), 1022–1029. doi:10.4330/wjc.v6.i9:1022

Michard, F., Chemla, D., & Teboul, J. (2015). Applicability of pulse pressure variation: How many shades of grey? *Critical Care, 19*(1). doi:10.1186/s13054-015-0869-x

Monnet, X., Marik, P., & Teboul, J. (2016). Passive leg raising for predicting fluid responsiveness: A systematic review and meta-analysis. *Intensive Care Medicine, 42*(12), 1935–1947.

Moriyama, T., Hagihara, S., Shiramomo, T., Nagaoka, M., Iwakawa, S., & Kanmura, Y. (2017). The protective effect of human atrial natriuretic peptide on renal damage during cardiac surgery. *Journal of Anesthesia, 31*(2), 163–169.

Nicholas, J. A. (2014). Management of postoperative complications: Cardiovascular disease and volume management. *Clinics in Geriatric Medicine, 30*(2), 293–301.

Nicolescu, T. (2017a). CVP. In T. D. Raj (Ed.), *Data interpretation in anesthesia: A clinical guide* (pp. 3–6). Cham, Switzerland: Springer International Publishing.

Nicolescu, T. (2017b). Pulmonary artery catheters. In T. D. Raj (Ed.), *Data interpretation in anesthesia: A clinical guide* (pp. 7–12). Cham, Switzerland: Springer International Publishing.

Perel, A., Pizov, R., & Cotev, S. (2014). Respiratory variations in the arterial pressure during mechanical ventilation reflect volume status and fluid responsiveness. *Intensive Care Medicine, 40*(6), 798–807.

Piccioni, F., Bernasconi, F., Tramontano, G. T., & Langer, M. (2017). A systematic review of pulse pressure variation and stroke volume variation to predict fluid responsiveness during cardiac and thoracic surgery. *Journal of Clinical Monitoring and Computing, 31*(4), 677–684.

Rathore, A., Singh, S., Lamsal, R., Taank, P., & Paul, D. (2017). Validation of pulse pressure variation (PPV) Compared with stroke volume variation (SVV) in predicting fluid responsiveness. *Turkish Journal of Anaesthesiology and Reanimation, 45*(4), 210–217.

Reyer, E. (2013). *White paper: The hemodynamic and physiological relevance of continuous central venous oxygenation monitoring: It's not just for sepsis.* Retrieved from http://www.icumed.com/media/402627/m1-1430-reyer-scvo2-oximetry-white-paper-rev02-web.pdf.

Rodriguez, M. E. (2016). Cardiopulmonary anatomy and physiology. In R. Knapp (Ed.), *Hemodynamic monitoring made incredibly visual* (3rd ed., pp. 1–18). Philadelphia, PA: Lippincott Williams & Wilkins.

Saugel, B., Cecconi, M., Wagner, J. Y., & Reuter, D. A. (2015). Noninvasive continuous cardiac output monitoring in perioperative and intensive care medicine. *British Journal of Anaesthesia, 114*(4), 562–575.

Shin, S. R., Kim, W. H., Kim, D. J., Shin, I., & Sohn, J. (2016). Prediction and prevention of acute kidney injury after cardiac surgery. *Biomed Research International, 2016,* 1–10. doi:10.1155/2016/2985148

Soloman, R., Samir, S., Neggar, A., & Dehely, K. (2015). Stroke volume variation compared with pulse pressure variation and cardiac index changes for prediction of fluid responsiveness in mechanically ventilated patients. *The Egyptian Journal of Critical Care Medicine, 3*(1), 9–16.

Sotomi, Y., Sato, N., Kaimoto, K., Sakata, Y., Mizuno, M., Minami, Y., . . . Takano, T. (2014). Impact of pulmonary artery catheter on outcome in patients with acute heart failure syndromes with hypotension or receiving inotropes: From the ATTEND Registry. *International Journal of Cardiology, 172*(1), 165–172.

Tang, H., Lin, H., Lin, Y., Leung, P., Chang, Y., & Lai, C. (2014). The impact of central line insertion bundle on central line-associated bloodstream infection. *BMC Infectious Diseases, 14*(356). doi:10.1186/1471-2334-14-356

Thiele, R., Bartels, K., & Gan, T. (2015). Cardiac output monitoring: A contemporary assessment and review. *Critical Care Medicine, 43*(1), 177–185.

Vincent, J.-L., Quintairos e Silva, A., Couto, L., & Taccone, F. S. (2016). The value of blood lactate kinetics in critically ill patients: A systematic review. *Critical Care, 20*(1). doi:10.1186/s13054-016-1403-5

Weinhouse, G. L. (2017). *Pulmonary artery catheterization: Indications, contraindications, and complications in adults.* Retrieved from https://www.uptodate.com/contents /pulmonary-artery-catheterization-interpretation-of -hemodynamic-values-and-waveforms-in-adults.

Whitener, S., Konoske, R., & Mark, J. B. (2014). Pulmonary artery catheter. *Best Practice & Research Clinical Anaesthesiology, 28*(4), 323–335.

Yartsev, A. (2018). *Arterial line dynamic response testing.* Retrieved from http://www.derangedphysiology.com/main /cicm-primary-exam/required-reading/cardiovascular -system/Chapter%207.5.9/arterial-line-dynamic-response -testing.

Young, M. P. (2014). Complications of central venous catheters and their prevention. Retrieved from http://www.uptodate .com/contents/complications-of-central-venous-catheters -and-their-prevention.

Web Resource

NTI 2010 Hemodynamic Boot Camp: http://www.cardionursing .com/pdfs/Boot-Camp-Hemodynamic-Monitoring.pdf

CHAPTER 10

Intra-Aortic Balloon Pump

Antonia Ash

▶ Introduction

The intra-aortic balloon pump (IABP) is a mechanical device that is temporarily used to improve cardiac function. In many situations, the IABP is life saving in its ability to stabilize patients as they await procedures such as heart transplant, coronary artery bypass grafting (CABG), or percutaneous coronary interventions (PCI) such as percutaneous transluminal coronary angioplasty/stent placement (Chen, Yin, Ling, & Krucoff, 2014; Hatch & Baklanov, 2014; Parissis et al., 2016; Van Nunen et al., 2016).

An IABP may be further indicated in the management of cardiogenic shock (Haddad, 2015; Parissis et al., 2016; Van Nunen et al., 2016). Medications such as vasodilators and inotropes are used initially to improve cardiac function. If they are not effective, the IABP may be used alone or with pharmacotherapy to assist left ventricular (LV) function and improve cardiac output (CO) (Hatch & Baklanov, 2014).

Since its introduction in the late 1960s, IABP has become a widely used device in preoperative, intraoperative, and postoperative cardiac surgery (Townsley, 2018; White & Ruygrok, 2015). In the United States, it is estimated that more than 70,000 IABP catheters are inserted annually (Grieshaber et al., 2018). A description of how an IABP improves cardiac function is provided in **BOX 10.1**.

▶ Components of an IABP

The IABP consists of two main parts: (1) a double-lumen catheter with an inflatable balloon attached to the distal end, and (2) a console that regulates the inflation and deflation of the balloon. One lumen of the balloon catheter is attached to a pressure-transducer device that monitors the patient's arterial aortic pressure; the other lumen (with the balloon) is attached to a gas reservoir. The console allows for appropriate timing of balloon inflation and houses the helium tanks. The tanks contain the helium gas that will be used to inflate the balloon during therapy. Additionally, the console has a monitor that displays the arterial waveforms, electrocardiogram (ECG), and balloon-pressure waveforms. Waveforms assist practitioners in determining whether the timing of balloon inflation/deflation is appropriate and allow for any necessary adjustments to be made (Goldich, 2014; Webb, Weyker, & Flynn, 2015).

Original contributions from Barbara Hutton-Borghardt

BOX 10.1 Goals of IABP Therapy

The IABP achieves its goals of stabilizing cardiac function by several mechanisms:

- It improves cardiac function (i.e., CO) by decreasing LV end-diastolic volume (preload) and by decreasing afterload.
- It improves myocardial oxygen supply by increasing blood flow to the coronary arteries.
- It decreases myocardial oxygen demand by decreasing LV wall tension.
- It stabilizes cardiac function in patients with dysrhythmias and myocardial ischemia.

CO, cardiac output; IABP, intra-aortic balloon pump; LV, left ventricular.
Data from Ihdayhid, Chopra, & Rankin, 2014; Parissis et al., 2016; Van Nunen et al., 2016; White & Ruygrok, 2015.

Physiology of Balloon Function

The IABP is timed to inflate and deflate in opposition to the cardiac cycle. The goal of inflation of the IABP balloon is to enhance perfusion. The balloon inflates at the beginning of diastole and deflates before ventricular systole, a process known as counterpulsation (Van Nunen et al., 2016; White & Ruygrok, 2015). To correlate the inflation and deflation to the ECG, the balloon begins to inflate in the middle of the T wave and to deflate before the end of the QRS complex (Parissis et al., 2016).

Inflation of the balloon at the beginning of diastole displaces blood upward toward the aortic root and augments the diastolic pressure between the balloon and the aortic origin. The increase in diastolic pressure, which is known as diastolic augmentation, forces blood back into the coronary arteries, which are normally perfused during diastole (DeWaha et al., 2014). Consequently, blood flow to the coronary arteries is increased, with a resultant improvement in myocardial oxygen supply. IABP inflation further causes a decrease in afterload and enhances LV function. Ischemia of the myocardial muscle is diminished or relieved with the ensuing improved CO (Murks & Juricek, 2016). During inflation, blood is also pushed forward to the periphery. In this way, blood flow is increased below the inflated balloon, which may enhance perfusion of the renal arteries and systemic blood vessels (Ihdayhid, Chopra, & Rankin, 2014; Webb et al., 2015).

Deflation of the balloon immediately before systole occurs pulls blood forward away from the left ventricle, allowing for more complete emptying. This enhanced LV emptying decreases preload (or end-diastolic volume) and myocardial oxygen demand. The tension caused by the pressure of blood on the left ventricle as it ejects blood (afterload) is diminished as well, further decreasing myocardial oxygen demand and increasing CO and ejection fraction (EF). Systolic blood pressure is noted to be lower with the reduction in afterload (DeWaha et al., 2014; Murks & Juricek, 2016).

Secondary effects of the IABP placement result from the improvement in cardiac function as well. Pulmonary artery diastolic, pulmonary artery occlusive pressures (PAOP), and systemic vascular resistance (SVR) are decreased; mean arterial pressure (MAP), CO, cardiac index (CI), and perfusion to vital organs such as the brain and kidneys are increased (Murks & Juricek, 2016; Ternus, Jentzer, Joyce, Stulak, & Barsness, 2016).

▶ Indications for IABP Therapy

The IABP is used in a variety of clinical situations; initially, however, it was used for patients in cardiogenic shock. Although still used for this purpose, the recently completed IAPB-SHOCK II trial, which studied the effect of the use of the IABP for 600 patients in cardiogenic shock after an acute myocardial infarction (AMI), did not demonstrate a significant improvement in the mortality rates of patients who received therapy with the IABP as compared with those who did not (White & Ruygrok, 2015). Cardiogenic shock is a complication in approximately 6% to 10% of patients with an AMI and carries a historically high mortality rate in the range of 50% to 80%. Early revascularization with angioplasty, fibrinolysis, or bypass surgery is initiated to improve mortality in such circumstances (Hochman & Reyentovich, 2014). In the case of the patient with cardiogenic shock, the IABP may be used to reduce myocardial ischemia and improve cardiac function, especially as the patient is prepared for a revascularization procedure (Van Nunen et al., 2016; Xiushui, 2014). In post-MI patients, data suggest that persistent ischemia and reinfarction may also be prevented through use of an IABP (Chen et al., 2014).

For patients with unstable angina who are receiving maximum medical therapy but who still experience chest pain/discomfort, the IABP has been successful in reducing or entirely eliminating symptoms. The patient's condition can be stabilized in preparation for surgery or revascularization procedure (Parissis et al., 2016).

In post-MI patients, structural damage such as a ventriculoseptal defect (VSD) or mitral regurgitation may occur. The IABP can help hemodynamically stabilize these patients until surgical repair can be performed (Ihdayhid et al., 2014). With a VSD, there is an abnormal opening between the right and left ventricles. Because pressure is higher in the left ventricle than in the right ventricle (RV), blood is shunted into the RV, resulting in a lower CO and right ventricular failure. The decrease in afterload produced by the IABP decreases the shunt (Jones et al., 2014; Kaneko, Isoda, Maksuki, Yamazaki, & Masuda, 2017; Parissis et al., 2016; Sari, Kahveci, Kilicgedik, Ayturk, & Pala, 2018).

Mitral regurgitation in post-MI patients is often due to papillary muscle dysfunction or rupture. The papillary muscles, which are located in the middle to lower ventricles, are connected to the valve leaflets by the stringlike chordae tendineae. When LV systole occurs, the papillary muscles contract and pull on the chordae. This action prevents the mitral valve leaflets from inverting. In the setting of papillary muscle dysfunction, the mitral valve becomes incompetent and regurgitant blood flow occurs. Blood is then forced back up into the left atrium during ventricular

systole, increasing the pressure in that chamber. The increased left atrial pressure is transmitted into the pulmonary vasculature, causing pulmonary congestion and edema. Use of the IABP to decrease afterload can diminish this regurgitant blood flow, thereby relieving pulmonary congestion as the patient awaits surgical repair (Ihdayhid et al., 2014; Parissis et al., 2016).

The IABP may be essential to assist cardiac function in patients with end-stage cardiac disease or damage while they are awaiting transplant (i.e., as a bridge to transplant) (Murks & Juricek, 2016; Nwaejike, Son, Milano, & Daneshmand, 2017). Insertion of the IABP into the subclavian artery may enable these patients to ambulate as they await transplant. The IABP may be used on a longer basis (12–70 days) in these instances (Murks & Juricek, 2016; Nwaejike et al., 2017).

Refractory ventricular dysrhythmias may also be responsive to IABP therapy. Poor LV function, coupled with an increase in afterload and increased myocardial oxygen demand, will produce ventricular stretching. Ventricular stretching increases irritability, resulting in difficult-to-treat dysrhythmias. The use of the IABP improves coronary blood flow, thereby helping to reduce irritability. Additionally, because the IABP decreases preload and afterload, the ventricle will be less distended, which further decreases irritability and arrhythmogenicity (Ihdayhid et al., 2014).

It is often difficult to wean postoperative on-pump cardiac surgery patients from cardiopulmonary bypass (CPB) due to preexisting poor cardiac function and the effects of CPB itself (White & Ruygrok, 2015). Placing patients on CPB involves stopping the heart, usually with the use of a cold electrolyte solution (cardioplegia), and inducing a controlled state of ischemia. In the postoperative period, the myocardial muscle is stunned and may need assistance to function effectively (Lomivorotov, Efremov, Kirov, Fominskiy, & Karaskov, 2017; Van Nunen et al., 2016). The IABP stabilizes the hemodynamic profile of these cardiac surgery patients and allows them to be weaned more slowly with less risk of organ damage from a failing heart. Myocardial stunning is discussed in detail in Chapter 13.

Preoperative use of the IABP in patients who are considered at high risk for cardiac surgery has been shown to lower the postoperative mortality rate and shorten intensive care recovery (Deppe et al., 2017; Hatch & Baklanov, 2014). High-risk patients include those with two of the following characteristics: poor LV function (EF <30%), unstable angina, left main coronary artery stenosis of greater than 70%, multivessel disease, cardiomyopathy, and hemodynamic instability (Deppe et al., 2017; Hatch & Baklanov, 2014; White & Ruygrok, 2015).

In a worldwide study known as the Benchmark Registry, the largest study to date, nearly 17,000 patients who had undergone IABP support were evaluated. The most common indications for initiating IABP therapy were to provide hemodynamic support during or after a cardiac catheterization procedure, cardiogenic shock, postoperative cardiac surgery in which CPB was used, preoperative cardiac support in high-risk patients, and unstable angina refractory to medical therapy (White & Ruygrok, 2015).

▶ Contraindications to IABP Therapy

Contraindications to the use of the IABP are few and can be divided into two subsets: absolute and relative. Absolute contraindications are those in which the patient should not receive IABP therapy; they include abdominal aortic aneurysm, aortic dissection, and aortic insufficiency (Haddad, 2015; Webb et al., 2015; White & Ruygrok, 2015). Relative contraindications are those in which the potential risk of using the IABP must be weighed against the potential benefit; they include patients with peripheral vascular disease, coagulopathies or thrombocytopenia (Bridgewater & Soon, 2014; Haddad, 2015; White & Ruygrok, 2015), terminal diseases, uncontrolled sepsis, and end-stage cardiomyopathies that are not suitable for transplant (Webb et al., 2015).

▶ Insertion of an IABP

Insertion of an IABP catheter may be performed at the bedside in the intensive care unit (ICU), in

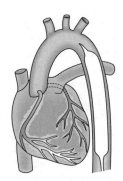

FIGURE 10.1 Inflated balloon catheter in descending aorta.
Illustrated by James R. Perron

the catheterization lab, or in the operating room (OR). Generally, institutional policy requires an informed consent to be signed and reviewed for completeness prior to insertion.

After preparation of the area and administration of a local anesthetic, the balloon catheter is inserted into either the right or left femoral artery. It is threaded up into the descending aorta so that the tip of the catheter is located 1 to 2 cm below the subclavian branch of the aortic arch and above the branches of the renal arteries (Hatch & Baklanov, 2014; Webb et al., 2015) (**FIGURE 10.1**). In bridge-to-transplant patients, the catheter may be inserted in the axillary/subclavian fossa, with the distal end being located above the renal arteries (Murks & Juricek, 2016; Nwaejike et al., 2017).

Traditionally, the balloon catheter is inserted through an introducer sheath, although many newer catheters are designed to be sheathless. The latter design results in a smaller diameter catheter in the femoral artery, decreasing the chance of ischemic complications to the lower extremity (De Jong et al., 2018).

The catheter may be inserted under fluoroscopy, which facilitates direct visualization—a key consideration in ensuring proper placement of the catheter. If fluoroscopy is not used, a radiograph film will be checked immediately following the procedure (Haddad, 2015). When viewed, the tip of the catheter should be located at the second or third intercostal space. Proper positioning is essential, because a catheter placed too high will obstruct blood flow to the subclavian artery, which supplies the head and upper extremities. A catheter placed too low can obstruct blood flow to the renal arteries (Goldich, 2014; Webb et al., 2015).

After the catheter is secured in place, a sterile dressing is applied to the insertion site. The patient's ECG tracing is displayed on the console's monitor; review of the ECG is important to maintain proper triggering of the pump. The central lumen of the balloon catheter is attached to a pressure-monitoring device with continuous flush to monitor the arterial pressure waveform. The balloon lumen is attached to the gas reservoir of the IABP console. A heparin drip, which prevents thrombus formation on the catheter, is usually started after a bolus infusion. The goal is to maintain an activated partial thromboplastin time (aPTT) of 60 to 80 sec (Haddad, 2015; Harper, 2017).

Upon its initial setup and every hour thereafter, the balloon will be inflated with a syringe or by the autofill function on some consoles, with the appropriate volume of helium. Helium, which has replaced carbon dioxide (CO_2) on most pump systems, is beneficial, especially with faster heart rates, because it is lighter in density than CO_2 and can travel at a faster speed in and out of the balloon circuit. Balloon volume size varies from 25 or 34 mL for a smaller adult to 40 or 50 mL for a larger adult. Most balloons used are 40 mL in size (Haddad, 2015; Parissis et al., 2016).

▶ Timing

Correct timing of balloon inflation and deflation is imperative to achieve the optimal benefit (Haddad, 2015). Usually, the ECG is used to trigger the pump. The pump identifies the R wave to signify ventricular systole. Other triggers, such as an arterial pressure waveform or pacer spikes, may also be used (Grieshaber et al., 2018; Webb et al., 2015). If the designated trigger is not noted, the pump will not initiate inflation and deflation of the balloon. In such a case, the trigger must be restored or a different trigger selected for the pump to work.

The arterial waveform displayed on the console's monitor is used to identify whether the timing of inflation and deflation is accurate. Balloon inflation should start at the beginning of diastole; deflation occurs just before systole or at the onset of systole. Initially, the inflation frequency is set at 1:2 (every other beat assisted) so that the unassisted and assisted waveforms can be compared. Later, the frequency may be switched to 1:1 (every beat assisted) if the patient's status requires this timing. As the patient's condition improves, the frequency may be weaned to 1:2, 1:3, 1:4, or 1:8 before IABP therapy is discontinued, usually over several hours (Harper, 2017; Webb et al., 2015).

To confirm that the timing of inflation and deflation is correct, specific characteristics are observed on the arterial waveform. First, it is necessary to become familiar with the normal arterial waveform, noting the dicrotic notch (**FIGURE 10.2**). Next, the arterial waveform of a patient receiving IABP therapy is observed. The unassisted systole, the dicrotic notch signifying closure of the aortic valve, and the unassisted aortic end-diastolic pressure should be identified (**FIGURE 10.3**). Following

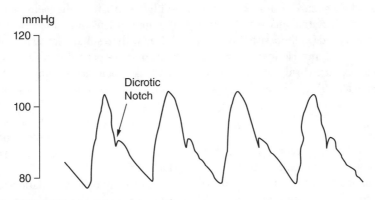

FIGURE 10.2 Normal arterial waveform.

Illustrated by James R. Perron

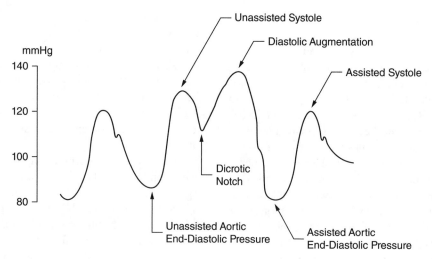

FIGURE 10.3 Arterial waveform of IABP patient, 1:2 counterpulsation.

Illustrated by James R. Perron

the dicrotic notch of an assisted beat will be diastolic augmentation. The dicrotic notch should form a distinct V shape between the unassisted systole and the augmented diastolic, indicating that pressure increased in the aortic root during balloon inflation (Webb et al., 2015). Following the augmented diastolic is the assisted end-diastolic pressure, which is lower than the unassisted diastolic pressure because deflation of the balloon results in lower aortic pressure.

Balloon inflation is optimal when (1) a sharp V is noted at the dicrotic notch, and (2) following the dicrotic notch, the augmented diastolic is as high as or higher than the previous systolic blood pressure. Balloon deflation is optimal when (1) the assisted end-diastolic pressure is lower, usually by 5 to 10 mmHg, than the unassisted aortic end-diastolic pressure, and (2) the assisted systolic blood pressure is 5 to 10 mmHg lower than the unassisted systolic pressure (Bridgewater & Soon, 2014; Van Nunen et al., 2016; Webb et al., 2015).

Timing Errors

Although most IABPs have automatic timing, it is essential that continuous monitoring be maintained. Often, manual adjustments to optimize timing are needed. With timing errors, not only

are patients not receiving optimal benefit, but they may also suffer deleterious consequences, especially when inflation is not timed correctly (Webb et al., 2015).

Timing errors occur when there is early or late inflation or early or late deflation of the balloon. With early balloon inflation, the balloon inflates before closure of the aortic valve. This action forces the valve to close early, resulting in aortic regurgitation and subsequent reduction in stroke volume, as well as increases in end-diastolic volume and myocardial oxygen demand (Haddad, 2015; Harper, 2017; Webb et al., 2015). In such a case, the arterial waveform will lose its characteristic V shape before diastolic augmentation (**FIGURE 10.4**). With late inflation, the balloon inflates later than the appropriate time after closure of the aortic valve, with resultant lower augmented diastolic and coronary perfusion pressures. As a result, the IABP's key benefit—improving blood and oxygen supply to the coronary arteries—is lost or reduced (Haddad, 2015; Harper, 2017). On the waveform, the peak of the augmented diastolic will be farther away from the dicrotic notch and will be lower, instead of higher, than the unassisted systolic (**FIGURE 10.5**).

Normally, balloon deflation occurs just before the beginning of systole. If it occurs too far before

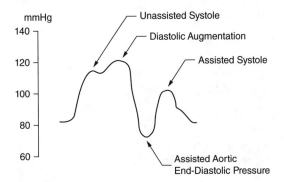

FIGURE 10.4 Arterial waveform with early balloon inflation.

Illustrated by James R. Perron

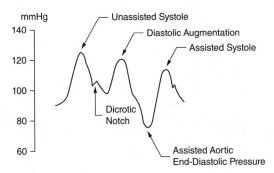

FIGURE 10.5 Arterial waveform with late balloon inflation.

Illustrated by James R. Perron

the onset of systole (early balloon deflation), however, the patient's diastolic pressure will rise, leading to increases in afterload and myocardial oxygen demand. The arterial waveform reveals a sharp drop-off in the augmented diastolic curve, followed by a U-shaped curve before the next systolic upstroke (**FIGURE 10.6**). When the balloon deflates later than the optimal time (late balloon deflation), its volume decreases *as* the aortic valve opens instead of before it opens. This results in the loss of the afterload reduction benefit; it may also increase afterload (and myocardial oxygen demand) as the inflated balloon impedes the ejection of blood from the left ventricle. The waveform will reveal a widened augmented diastolic wave and a slow rise of the next assisted systole (Harper, 2017; Webb et al., 2015) (**FIGURE 10.7**).

Most IABP consoles have a display for the balloon pressure waveform. This waveform represents the pressure as gas is propelled in and out of the balloon catheter. Monitoring this waveform is beneficial as it will assist the ICU nurse in determining whether the balloon is functioning effectively (Harper, 2017; Webb et al., 2015) (**FIGURE 10.8**). Caregivers may find it necessary to follow the specific manufacturer's directions for many settings on such devices, because consoles offered by different companies may have unique properties.

Refer to **BOX 10.2** for definitions related to IABP therapy.

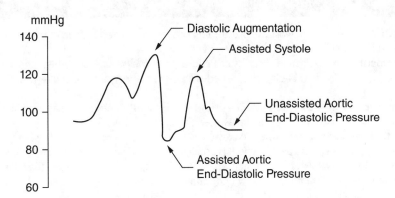

FIGURE 10.6 Arterial waveform with early balloon deflation.

Illustrated by James R. Perron

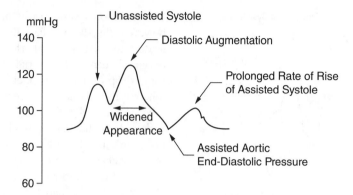

FIGURE 10.7   Arterial waveform with late balloon deflation.
Illustrated by James R. Perron

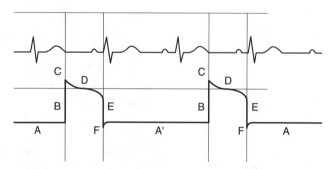

FIGURE 10.8   IABP waveform.
A = balloon pressure baseline; B = rapid inflation; C = peak inflation artifact; D = balloon pressure plateau (balloon is
completely inflated); E = rapid deflation; F = balloon deflation artifact; A' = return to baseline (balloon completely deflated).
Illustrated by James R. Perron

BOX 10.2   IABP Therapy Waveform Definitions

Dicrotic notch: An area on the downstroke of the arterial waveform that results from the slight pressure increase created by closure of the aortic valve.

Diastolic augmentation: The increase in pressure in the aorta above the balloon catheter that results with balloon inflation during diastole. It increases perfusion in the coronary arteries and myocardial oxygen supply.

Unassisted aortic end-diastolic pressure: The pressure in the aorta at the end of diastole when counterpulsation via the balloon pump has not assisted that cardiac cycle.

Assisted aortic end-diastolic pressure: The pressure in the aorta at the end of diastole when counterpulsation has assisted the cardiac cycle. It is usually lower than the unassisted end-diastolic pressure.

Unassisted systole: The systolic aortic pressure when counterpulsation has not assisted the cycle.

Assisted systole: The systolic aortic pressure when counterpulsation has assisted the cardiac cycle. It is usually lower than the unassisted systole due to the action of balloon deflation.

Data from Goldich, 2014; Harper, 2017; Ihdayhid et al., 2014; Webb et al., 2015.

▶ Complications of IABP Therapy

Although the mortality rate directly associated with the use of the IABP is low, the rate of major complications is reported to be at 2.6%; 4.2% of patients experienced minor complications (Haddad, 2015).

The most prevalent complications are vascular in nature, with the most common being lower-limb ischemia below the insertion site. Fortunately, catheter sizes are becoming smaller and many do not require a sheath for placement. Over the years, smaller catheter size and sheathless introducers have helped to reduce complication rates (Webb et al., 2015). Some patients, however, are more prone to limb ischemia. Especially vulnerable populations include the elderly, diabetics, females, obese patients, and individuals with peripheral vascular disease (De Jong et al., 2018; Webb et al., 2015; White & Ruygrok, 2015). Limb ischemia can occur while the catheter is in place or within hours of its removal and is related to presence of a clot at the catheter site. Thrombectomy is usually required to treat this complication (De Jong et al., 2018; Goldich, 2014; Parissis et al., 2016).

Other vascular complications include bleeding or hemorrhage from the insertion site, perforation of the femoral artery, superficial or deep vein thrombosis, stroke, aortic dissection or perforation, and compartment syndrome (DeWaha et al., 2014; Parissis et al., 2016; Webb et al., 2015). Vascular complications can result in severe consequences, to the point that the patient may require an amputation, thrombectomy, blood transfusions, or vascular surgery (De Jong et al., 2018).

Balloon-related complications can occur as well. Balloon rupture will result in the release of a helium bolus into the bloodstream, because the gas will no longer be contained within the balloon circuit. Blood noted within the gas tubing, inability to maintain augmentation, and low pressure/gas alarms are indicators of possible balloon rupture. Balloon rupture is more likely to occur in patients with atherosclerosis, in whom the balloon will be inflating against rough calcium deposits in the aorta (Bhamidipaty, Mees, & Wagner, 2016; Goldich, 2014; Parissis et al., 2016).

Balloon migration within the aorta is also possible. If the balloon migrates upward, blood supply to the upper extremities and head may be compromised. If the balloon migrates downward, blood supply to the renal and visceral arteries may be impaired (Murks & Juricek, 2016; Webb et al., 2015).

The ICU nurse should monitor for a variety of other complications when an IABP is used. Infection at the insertion site or in the systemic circulation may occur due to the presence of an indwelling catheter; red blood cell hemolysis and thrombocytopenia are possible due to the action of the balloon on blood components as they pass through the aorta (DeWaha et al., 2014; Haddad, 2015). Other complications include spinal cord ischemia, visceral ischemia, renal failure, and peripheral neuropathy (Webb et al., 2015).

▶ Weaning from IABP Therapy

The IABP is a temporary device that is usually discontinued postoperatively. Occasionally, some patients who are awaiting cardiac transplant may have it in place longer. Others may have IABP therapy discontinued intraoperatively if it was used to stabilize the patient's condition in the preoperative period. Unless complications occur, the IABP is removed after a period of weaning. Weaning will depend on the improvement in the patient's cardiac function and on a decrease in dependence on inotropes/vasoactive medications (Harper, 2017). The ICU nurse, while monitoring the patient on an ongoing basis, is often the first to assess readiness for weaning. Although the orders for weaning will be instituted by a medical or midlevel provider, the ICU nurse is responsible for determining the patient's tolerance to the weaning process. Some parameters that may suggest readiness for weaning are listed in **BOX 10.3**.

- Stable hemodynamic parameters (stable on low doses of vasoactive medications)
- No unstable dysrhythmias (Heart rate should be normal or near normal without dysrhythmias that compromise hemodynamic parameters.)
- Low or normal serum lactate levels
- Normal electrolyte levels
- Acceptable hemoglobin/hematocrit levels
- No chest pain/discomfort or dyspnea
- No mental status changes indicative of poor cerebral perfusion
- Urine output greater than 0.5 mL/kg/hr

Data from Goldich, 2014; Harper, 2017; Webb et al., 2015.

Weaning from the IABP involves decreasing the frequency of assisted beats, decreasing the volume in the balloon over time, or both. Frequency weaning involves switching from 1:1 (every beat assisted by IABP) to 1:2 (every other beat assisted). Switching from a 1:1 to 1:2 ratio provides the most marked decrease in blood flow to the coronary arteries—more than switching from 1:2 to 1:3 or 1:4, or from 1:4 to 1:8 (Harper, 2017; Webb et al., 2015). As a consequence, the patient who is weaned in this manner will require frequent monitoring, especially during the first stage of weaning.

Anticoagulation used during IABP therapy should be tapered and ultimately discontinued prior to catheter removal. Frequency of balloon inflation can be set to 1:8 while the heparin effect, if used, is allowed to wear off (Goldich, 2014; Harper, 2017; Webb et al., 2015).

Once the catheter is removed, pressure should be applied to the site for 30 to 45 minutes, followed by application of a sterile pressure bandage for 2 to 4 hours (Harper, 2017; Webb et al., 2015). After placement of the pressure bandage, the patient should be checked for bleeding every 30 minutes for 2 to 4 hours, then every 2 hours for 24 hours. Monitoring should confirm that a hematoma is not developing under the bandage, because hematomas can be a significant source

of blood loss. The patient should be instructed to keep the head of the bed at 30 degrees or less, with no flexion of the hip for at least 8 hours following IABP catheter removal (Harper, 2017; Webb et al., 2015). Institutional policies and protocols should be followed with regard to patient positioning following catheter removal.

▶ Troubleshooting the IABP

With the IABP, as with any mechanical device, problems may occur that need to be addressed promptly. Often it is best to refer to the manufacturer's troubleshooting guide, because it contains a complete reference of problems likely to be encountered. A few of the most common problems are discussed in this section.

Low Diastolic Augmentation

Low diastolic augmentation is noted when the pressure in the aortic root (above the balloon) does not rise enough after balloon inflation to sufficiently perfuse the coronary arteries. Potential causes of low diastolic augmentation include incorrect balloon timing, dysrhythmias that result in low stroke volume, hypotension or low vascular resistance, balloon leak or rupture, incorrect balloon catheter placement or balloon migration, inappropriate balloon size, and balloon not fully opened.

If the balloon or balloon catheter is found to be faulty, it should be removed as soon as possible (within 30 minutes) to avoid thrombus development on an idle catheter (Harper, 2017). Most consoles have an alarm system that warns providers of a gas leak or a rapid loss of gas. Slow leaks may be the result of a hole in the balloon or a loose connection in the gas tubing. A rapid loss of gas, in contrast, is usually the result of balloon rupture or a disconnected gas circuit. In this scenario, the gas line should be clamped off immediately. If blood is noted in the balloon catheter or gas circuit, it is recommended that the pump be stopped immediately because the balloon or catheter has a leak. Continuing to pump will introduce gas into the bloodstream, producing an air embolus (Harper, 2017; Webb et al., 2015).

Faulty Trigger

On occasion, the ECG trigger may not function properly. Common causes of a faulty trigger include poor electrode placement, low ECG voltage, faulty electrode pads or cables, dysrhythmias, and other equipment's interference with the ECG signal (Webb et al., 2015). If the problem cannot be easily rectified, switching to the arterial pressure trigger will be necessary until the problem can be resolved.

Autofill Failure

The autofill feature on the IABP maintains the volume of gas within the balloon. Should this feature not function, an autofill alarm will sound. The cause of this problem could be an insufficient amount of gas in the tank or occlusion of the gas outlet. The amount of gas in the tank should be checked and the tank replaced as needed. Also,

the provider should assess for and correct any kinks or leaks in the tubing and ensure that the valve on the tank is in the open position (Webb et al., 2015).

In the event of pump failure or if pumping needs to be stopped, the IABP balloon should be manually inflated with a syringe every 5 min. The syringe should be filled with a volume of gas that is 10 mL less than balloon capacity to prevent thrombus formation (Harper, 2017).

ICU nurses caring for a patient receiving IABP therapy must be knowledgeable about the potential complications that can occur during catheter/balloon insertion and removal and during therapy. They must equally be aware of management strategies and preventive measures to implement to avoid or minimize associated morbidity. Patients receiving IABP therapy need to have continuous monitoring, and the nurse-to-patient ratio is encouraged to be 1:1. Often these patients are critically ill and have complex problems related to their condition as well as the difficulties experienced by dependence, even for a few days, on highly specialized equipment. **BOX 10.4** lists nursing interventions required by the patient who is receiving IABP therapy.

BOX 10.4 Nursing Interventions for the Patient Receiving IABP Therapy

Preinsertion Interventions

- Perform a two-person identification verification and time-out to ensure the correct patient for the procedure.
- Provide as calm an environment as possible because the patient will likely be overwhelmed.
- Provide reassurance that the IABP therapy is temporary.
- Explain the procedure and the steps to help ensure safety (as time permits).
- Allow families to participate in discussions and to express concerns.
- Ascertain that consent is signed and complete if required.
- Obtain a 12-lead ECG; insert a urinary catheter.
- Assist with the insertion of invasive lines such as an arterial line and a pulmonary artery catheter.
- Obtain baseline hemodynamic readings: HR, RR, BP, MAP, PAP, PAOP, CVP, CO or CI, SVR, and urine output.
- Obtain baseline blood work: ABG, mixed venous blood gas, chemistries with BUN/creatinine, CBC with platelets and differential, coagulation profile, and type and crossmatch.
- Perform a peripheral vascular assessment, including checking ankle-brachial index,* skin temperature, presence and strength of pulses, and capillary refill in lower extremities.
- Monitor for the presence of a left radial pulse. Inform the health care provider if the pulse is lost so that the catheter can be repositioned.

(continues)

BOX 10.4 Nursing Interventions for the Patient Receiving IABP Therapy *(continued)*

Postinsertion Interventions

- Monitor and record hemodynamic measurements every 15 to 30 minutes until the patient is stable, then hourly and PRN.
- Obtain an ECG and chest radiograph daily and PRN.
- Titrate vasopressors/inotropic agents as required to desired hemodynamic parameters. Hemodynamic stability is essential to maintain optimal perfusion to the limb.
- Maintain IV fluid therapy as ordered to maintain an acceptable preload.
- Assess for pain/discomfort, anxiety, and mental status changes hourly.
- Document IABP settings hourly; include the assisted and unassisted pressures.
- Print and document the arterial waveform tracing every 12 hours and PRN with changes.
- Assess for presence and strength of distal pulses, indices of adequate limb perfusion, and sensorimotor function of both lower extremities every 15 minutes for 1 hour, then 30 minutes for 1 hour, and then hourly or according to unit protocol.
- Assess the ankle-brachial index every 4 hours.
- Monitor for the presence of a left radial pulse. Loss of pulse indicates that the catheter has migrated upward, is occluding the left subclavian artery, and requires repositioning.
- Maintain and titrate the heparin infusion to desired anticoagulation as ordered. Obtain coagulation studies 6 hours after dosage changes or follow the facility protocol.
- Obtain daily blood work: chemistries, CBC with platelets, coagulation profile, ABG, lactate level, and mixed venous blood gas.
- Monitor respiratory status: Assess breath sounds every 4 hours. Maintain oxygen, ventilator therapy, or both. Encourage coughing and deep breathing/incentive spirometry every 2 hours. Keep the head of the bed at a 15- to 30-degree angle to prevent aspiration. Perform chest physiotherapy when the patient is logrolled.
- Maintain NPO or clear liquids as tolerated. If tolerated, maintain tube feedings via feeding tube. Check residual every 4 hours and notify the physician if it is greater than 200 mL.
- Prevent skin breakdown related to immobility. Maintain the patient on bedrest, with sedation if needed. Encourage the patient not to flex the hip on the affected side. Use a leg immobilizer if necessary. If tolerated, logroll the patient every 4 hours; perform meticulous skin care. Provide passive range-of-motion exercises for the lower extremity without a catheter and for upper extremities every 4 hours.

*To check ankle-brachial index:
- With patient supine and at rest, apply blood pressure cuff around both ankles and arms.
- Inflate blood pressure cuffs above the patient's normal SBP.
- Deflate blood pressure cuffs. Obtain blood pressure readings using a Doppler and record SBP measurements from the arms and ankles.
- Divide ankle systolic pressure by the highest arm pressure; this will yield an ABI value for each leg.

An index value of 0.9 to 1.3 is considered normal. Values greater than the normal range indicate the presence of some degree of peripheral vascular disease. Presence of mild, moderate, or severe peripheral vascular disease warrants reevaluation of vein selection for cardiac surgery.

ABG, arterial blood gas; ABI, ankle-brachial index; BP, blood pressure; BUN, blood urea nitrogen; CBC, complete blood count; CI, cardiac index; CO, cardiac output; CVP, central venous pressure; ECG, electrocardiogram; HR, heart rate; IABP, intra-aortic balloon pump; IV, intravenous; MAP, mean arterial pressure; NPO, nothing by mouth; PAOP, pulmonary artery occlusive pressure; PAP, pulmonary artery pressure; PRN, as needed; RR, respiratory rate; SBP, systolic blood pressure; SVR, systemic vascular resistance (afterload).

Data from Goldich, 2014; Harper, 2017; Webb, Weyker, & Flynn, 2015.

▶ Monitoring for Complications of IABP Therapy

There are a number of potential complications associated with having an IABP in place. There are several complications that are vascular in nature (de Jong et al., 2018) and occur more often with individuals presenting with risk factors such as diabetes, hypertension, peripheral vascular disease, and smoking.

- *Limb ischemia.* Perform peripheral vascular checks, including pulses, capillary refill time, skin color, and temperature of lower extremities. After discontinuation of therapy, distal pulses should be checked every hour for 2 hours, then at least every 4 hours until the patient is discharged. Patients should be instructed to notify the nurse if they note any changes in circulation (Harper, 2017).
- *Bleeding at the insertion site.* Check the dressing and under the patient's thigh for bleeding every 2 hours. Check for hematoma development under dressing.
- *Anemia and thrombocytopenia.* Obtain a daily complete blood count (CBC). Transfuse platelets and red blood cells as indicated.
- *Infection.* Monitor for signs and symptoms of infection: greater than temperature 38.8°C (101.8°F), white blood cell count greater than 10,000 cells/mm^3, chills, or mental status changes. If infection is suspected, send specimens for peripheral blood, urine, and sputum cultures. Culture the IABP port as well. Change the insertion site dressing according to facility policy and examine the skin around the site for redness, increased temperature, or purulent drainage. Institute antibiotics promptly as prescribed. Infection can occur at the insertion site or systemically, and the risk increases as the length of time the catheter is left in the patient increases (DeWaha et al., 2014; Harper, 2017; Parissis et al., 2016).
- *Catheter migration.* Monitor the patient's pulses, skin color, and temperature; assess for altered sensation in the left upper extremity every 1 to 2 hours. Report urine output of less than 0.5 mL/kg/hr, increasing blood urea nitrogen (BUN)/creatinine, or flank pain. Assess the patient for increased abdominal girth or discomfort with absent bowel sounds. Monitor the level of consciousness and evaluate the patient for unilateral neurologic impairment. Obtain a chest radiograph and anticipate repositioning or reinsertion of the catheter if migration is suspected (Harper, 2017; Murks & Juricek, 2016).
- *Aortic dissection.* This complication occurs very rarely in IABP insertions. Assess the patient for abdominal, back, intrascapular, or shoulder pain, usually of sudden onset. The pain may be described as "tearing." Other symptoms include increased abdominal girth and absent or unequal peripheral pulses with concomitant decreased blood pressure and urine output. Obtain a computed tomography (CT) scan or magnetic resonance imaging (MRI) if dissection is suspected. Treatment consists of prompt surgical repair (Bridgewater & Soon, 2014; Murks & Juricek, 2016).

▶ Summary

Care of the patient receiving IABP therapy is complex and challenging. Patients require prompt intervention for problems and empathy for their critical illness. For the ICU nurse, additional instruction both in theory and in hands-on experience is required to maintain and troubleshoot the complex IABP apparatus. Management of this device is accomplished while balancing evidence-based care that involves critical thinking and decision making, preventing and detecting complications, and providing emotional support to patients and families who are experiencing one of the most vulnerable times in their lives.

○ CASE STUDY

T. J. is a 69-year-old male who was recently hospitalized with pulmonary edema and was diagnosed with heart failure. He had not seen his primary care physician in 8 years, and is an active 50-pack/year smoker with hypertension and hyperlipidemia. One month after discharge, the patient returned with chest pain. Cardiac catheterization revealed occlusions of the left anterior descending, obtuse marginal, and ramus intermedius; EF was 20%. Percutaneous coronary intervention failed and the patient was consented for surgery. An IABP was placed intraoperatively prior to incision via the femoral artery. Placement was guided by ultrasound and transesophageal echocardiogram. T. J. underwent coronary artery bypass grafting for three vessels and was taken to the ICU postoperatively.

Dexmedetomidine was used for sedation while the patient remained intubated and on mechanical ventilation. In the ICU, infusions of epinephrine at 0.1 mcg/kg/min, milrinone at 0.375 mcg/kg/min, and norepinephrine at 0.07 mcg/kg/min were used. On postoperative day (POD) 1, weaning trials of the IABP (1:1, 1:2, and 1:3 over a 2-hour period) were unsuccessful; cardiac index was 2.0 and the patient continued to require vasopressor and inotropic support. T. J. was extubated on POD 1 and ultimately weaned off the norepinephrine and dexmedetomidine. He tolerated decreasing doses of epinephrine and milrinone. Weaning trials from the IABP were successful on POD 2 and the catheter was removed; his cardiac index was 3.0 on low-dose milrinone 4 hours following IABP removal. The patient was transferred to a stepdown unit on POD 4 and was discharged home 4 days later.

Critical Thinking Questions

1. What was the indication for IABP therapy for T. J.?
2. What nursing care should be provided to a patient receiving IABP therapy?
3. What criteria should be used to determine readiness to wean from IABP therapy?

Answers to Critical Thinking Questions

1. The IABP was placed due to risk factors of recent pulmonary edema, diagnosis of heart failure, failed PCI attempt, ejection fraction of 20%, and history of hypertension. The IABP assisted with T. J.'s coming off of cardiopulmonary bypass.
2. An occlusive sterile dressing with a chlorhexidine patch over the insertion site should be applied and maintained. Titration of drips within prescribed parameters, establishment of a reliable trigger for the IABP (e.g., ECG, arterial waveform) and for IABP timing, and comparison between assisted and unassisted arterial waveforms for optimization of timing for inflation and deflation of the balloon are essential. Other nursing care includes checking of peripheral pulses and monitoring of laboratory data, monitoring for complications of IABP therapy, and troubleshooting as indicated.
3. Parameters that should be assessed to determine readiness to wean from IABP therapy include presence of stable hemodynamic parameters, no unstable dysrhythmias, normal or below normal serum lactate level, normal electrolyte and CBC results, no chest pain or discomfort, no dyspnea, no mental status changes, and urinary output of at least 0.5 mL/kg/hr.

Self-Assessment Questions

1. Intra-aortic balloon pump inflation should correspond with which part of the ECG?
   A. On the R wave
   B. Middle of the T wave
   C. Just before the P wave
   D. In the PR interval

2. Intra-aortic balloon pump deflation should correspond with which part of the ECG?
   A. Before end of the T wave
   B. At the beginning of the P wave
   C. Before the end of the QRS
   D. In the middle of the PR interval

3. Intra-aortic balloon pump inflation causes:

	Coronary perfusion	SVR	LV function
A.	decreased	increased	decreased
B.	decreased	increased	increased
C.	increased	decreased	decreased
D.	increased	decreased	increased

4. Deflation of the intra-aortic balloon pump balloon results in:
   A. increased blood flow to the coronary arteries.
   B. increased myocardial oxygen delivery.
   C. decreased heart rate.
   D. decreased myocardial oxygen demand.

5. Inflation of the intra-aortic balloon pump balloon results in:
   A. decreased myocardial oxygen demand.
   B. increased coronary perfusion pressure.
   C. increased ejection fraction.
   D. decreased systolic blood pressure.

6. Patients with which rhythm may benefit from intra-aortic balloon pump therapy?
   A. Atrial fibrillation
   B. Supraventricular tachycardia
   C. Second-degree AV block, Type II
   D. Refractory ventricular dysrhythmias

7. Which is an absolute contraindication for intra-aortic balloon pump therapy?
   A. Peripheral vascular disease
   B. Thrombocytopenia
   C. End-stage cardiomyopathy
   D. Aortic insufficiency

8. Early balloon inflation results in:
   A. aortic regurgitation.
   B. decreased PAOP.
   C. decreased myocardial oxygen demand.
   D. mitral regurgitation.

9. Early intra-aortic balloon pump deflation will result in:
   A. increased diastolic blood pressure.
   B. decreased afterload.
   C. decreased myocardial oxygen demand.
   D. increased coronary artery perfusion.

10. You are caring for a patient with an intra-aortic balloon pump in place and note blood within the gas tubing. Which should the nurse suspect?
    A. Red blood cell hemolysis
    B. Balloon migration

C. Thrombocytopenia
D. Balloon rupture

Answers to Self-Assessment Questions

1. **B. middle of the T wave**
   Rationale: IABP inflation will be triggered to occur in the middle of the T wave, which corresponds with ventricular diastole. Balloon inflation displaces blood proximally; there is increased diastolic pressure and coronary perfusion.

2. **C. before the end of the QRS**
   Rationale: Deflation occurs during isometric contraction at the end of diastole leading to a reduction of the impedance against which the left ventricle must eject. Deflation occurs during systole, which coincides with QRS-T interval.

3. **D. increased / decreased / increased**
   Rationale: Increased LV function; it is anticipated that the cardiac output increases 20% or 0.5 to 1 L/min with IABP support.

4. **D. decreased myocardial oxygen demand**
   Rationale: The IABP can decrease myocardial oxygen demand by decreasing afterload.

5. **B. increased coronary perfusion pressure**
   Rationale: Inflation occurs during ventricular diastole. This displaces blood proximally to the coronary arteries and the rest of the body.

6. **D. refractory ventricular dysrhythmias**
   Rationale: The IABP can stabilize patients with medically refractory ventricular arrhythmias. The mechanism of action is unclear and may be due to an improvement in coronary blood flow and decreased afterload. Some suggest that the IABP reduces potentially proarrhythmic adrenergic drive; or by reducing afterload and myocardial stretch the IABP could potentially make the myocardium less arrhythmogenic.

7. **D. aortic insufficiency**
   Rationale: Aortic regurgitation is problematic in the face of counterpulsation due to increased valvular regurgitation from

increased diastolic root pressure. Balloon inflation during diastole will worsen the degree of regurgitation.

8. **A. aortic regurgitation**
Rationale: Early balloon inflation would result in the IABP inflating before the dicrotic notch (which represents closure of the aortic valve) and this would result in aortic regurgitation, decreased stroke volume, premature closure of the aortic valve, and increased left ventricular volume.

9. **A. increased diastolic blood pressure**
Rationale: Early deflation will result in loss of afterload reduction (increased diastolic blood pressure) and an increase in myocardial oxygen demand.

10. **D. balloon rupture**
Rationale: IABP rupture is probably caused by rubbing of an abrasive aortic plaque against the smooth surface of the balloon. Blood or any discoloration in the helium tubing indicates balloon perforation and the presence of arterial blood.

CLINICAL INQUIRY BOX

Question: What are the outcomes of patients who underwent IABP therapy after an acute myocardial infarction?

Reference: Fan, Z.-G., Gao, X.-F., Chen, L.-W., Li, X.-B., Shao, M.-X., Ji, Q., . . . Tian, N.-L. (2016). The outcomes of intra-aortic balloon pump usage in patients with acute myocardial infarction: A comprehensive meta-analysis of 33 clinical trials and 18,889 patients. *Patient Preference and Adherence, 10,* 297–312.

Objective: To determine the outcomes of patients who underwent IABP therapy after an acute myocardial infarction.

Method: Meta-analysis.

Results: A total of 33 clinical trials, which included 18,889 patients, were identified in the meta-analysis. There was a decrease in mortality rate in patients who sustained a myocardial infarction and who underwent IABP therapy. There was no difference in in-hospital and midterm mortality rate between patients who did and did not receive IABP therapy. Patients who developed cardiogenic shock and those on thrombolytic therapy had a decreased mortality rate but with an increased incidence of bleeding and stroke.

Conclusion: Patients receiving IABP therapy following a myocardial infarction had better long-term survival rates, especially those who developed cardiogenic shock as a result of the MI. Negative sequelae included bleeding from thrombolytic therapy and stroke.

References

Bhamidipaty, M., Mees, B., & Wagner, T. (2016). Management of intra-aortic balloon pump rupture and entrapment. *Aorta, 4*(2), 61–63.

Bridgewater, B., & Soon, S. Y. (2014). The intra-aortic balloon pump. *Surgery, 33*(2), 62–63.

Chen, S., Yin, Y., Ling, Z., & Krucoff, M. W. (2014). Short and long term effect of adjunctive intra-aortic balloon pump use for patients undergoing high risk reperfusion therapy: A meta-analysis of 10 international randomised trials. *Heart (British Cardiac Society), 100*(4), 303–310.

De Jong, M. M., Lorusso, R., Awami, F. A., Matteuci, F., Parise, O., Lozekoot, P., . . . Gelsomino, S. (2018). Vascular complications following intra-aortic balloon pump implantation: An updated review. *Perfusion, 33*(2), 96–104.

Deppe, A. C., Weber, C., Liakopoulos, O. J., Zeriouh, M., Slottosch, I., Scherner, M., . . . Wahlers, T. (2017). Preoperative intra-aortic balloon pump use in high-risk patients prior to coronary artery bypass graft surgery decreases the risk for morbidity and mortality—a meta-analysis of 9,212 patients. *Journal of Cardiac Surgery, 32*(3), 177–185.

DeWaha, S., Desch, S., Eitel, I., Fuernau, G., Lurz, P., Sandri, M., . . . Thiele, H. (2014). Intra-aortic balloon counterpulsation—basic principles and clinical evidence. *Vascular Pharmacology, 60*(2), 52–56.

Goldich, G. (2014). Getting in sync with intraaortic balloon pump therapy. *Nursing, 11*, 10–13.

Grieshaber, P., Schneider, T., Oster, L., Orhan, C., Roth, P., Neimann, B., & Boning, A. (2018). Prophylactic intra-aortic balloon counterpulsation before surgical myocardial revascularization in patients with acute myocardial infarction. *Perfusion, 18*(6), 1–11.

Haddad, E. V. (2015). *Intra-aortic balloon counterpulsation.* Retrieved from https://emedicine.medscape.com/article/1847715-overview.

Harper, J. P. (2017). Intraaortic balloon pump management. In D. L. Wiegand (Ed.), *AACN procedure manual for high acuity, progressive and critical care* (7th ed., pp. 431–449). St. Louis, MO: Elsevier.

Hatch, J., & Baklanov, D. (2014). Percutaneous hemodynamic support in PCI. *Current Treatment Options in Cardiovascular Medicine, 16*, 293, 1–13.

Hochman, J. S., & Reyentovich, A. (2014). *Prognosis and treatment of cardiogenic shock complicating acute myocardial infarction.* Retrieved from http://www.uptodate.com/contents/prognosis-and-treatment-of-cardiogenic-shock-complicating-acute-myocardial-infarction.

Ihdayhid, A. R., Chopra, S., & Rankin, J. (2014). Intra-aortic balloon pump: Indications, efficacy, guidelines and future directions. *Current Opinion in Cardiology, 29*, 285–292.

Jones, B. M., Kapadia, S. R., Smedira, N. G., Robich, M., Tuzcu, E. M., Menon, V., . . . Krishnaswamy, A. (2014). Ventricular septal rupture complicating acute myocardial infarction: A contemporary review. *European Heart Journal, 35*, 2060–2068.

Kaneko, S., Isoda, S., Matsuki, Y., Yamazaki, I., & Masuda, M. (2017). Post-infarction ventricular septal defect due to an isolated septal myocardial infarct. *Journal of Cardiac Surgery, 32*, 487–488.

Lomivorotov, V. V., Efremov, S. M., Kirov, M. Y., Fominskiy, E. V., & Karaskov, A. M. (2017). Low-cardiac output syndrome after cardiac surgery. *Journal of Cardiothoracic and Vascular Anesthesia, 31*(2017), 291–308.

Murks, C., & Juricek, C. (2016). Balloon pumps inserted via the subclavian artery. *AACN Advanced Critical Care, 27*(3), 301–315.

Nwaejike, N., Son, A. Y., Milano, C. A., & Daneshmand, M. A. (2017). Is there a role for upper-extremity intra-aortic balloon counterpulsation as a bridge-to-recovery or a bridge-to-transplant in the treatment of end-stage heart failure? *Interactive Cardiovascular and Thoracic Surgery, 25*(4), 654–658.

Parissis, H., Graham, V., Lampridis, S., Lau, M., Hooks, G., & Mhandu, P. C. (2016). IABP: History-evolution-pathophysiology-indications: What we need to know. *Journal of Cardiothoracic Surgery, 2016*, 1–13.

Sari, M., Kahveci, G., Kilicgedik, A., Ayturk, M., & Pala, S. (2018). Acute myocardial infarction complicated with ventricular septal rupture and intracranial hemorrhage. *Echocardiography, 35*, 559–562.

Ternus, B., Jentzer, J., Joyce, D., Stulak, J., & Barsness, G. (2016). Hemodynamic effects of the intra-aortic balloon pump in patients awaiting surgical LVAD placement. *Critical Care Medicine, 44*(2). doi:10.1097/01.ccm.0000508871.84076.47

Townsley, M. (2018). Prophylactic intra-aortic balloon counterpulsation—still searching for answers. *Journal of Cardiothoracic and Vascular Anesthesia.* doi:10.1053/j.jvca.2018.01.051

Van Nunen, L. X., Noc, M., Kapur, N. K., Patel, M. R., Perera, D., & Pijls, N. H. (2016). Usefulness of intra-aortic balloon pump counterpulsation. *The American Journal of Cardiology, 117*(3), 469–476.

Webb, C. A., Weyker, P. D., & Flynn, B. C. (2015). Management of intra-aortic balloon pumps. *Seminars in Cardiothoracic and Vascular Anesthesia, 19*(2), 106–121.

White, J. M., & Ruygrok, P. N. (2015). Intra-aortic balloon counterpulsation in contemporary practice—where are we? *Heart, Lung and Circulation, 24*(4), 335–341.

Xiushui, R. (2014). *Cardiogenic shock.* Retrieved from http://emedicine.medscape.com/article/152191.

Web Resources

Intra-aortic balloon pump: https://www.youtube.com/watch?v=o11fhdVOYWA

Intra-aortic balloon pump information: http://www.cprworks.com/IABP.html

Timing and triggering of the intra-aortic balloon pump: https://www.youtube.com/watch?v=Ff-1YXaUBO0

CHAPTER 11

Mechanical Ventilation After Cardiac Surgery

Mary Jane Bowles, Roberta Kaplow

▶ Introduction

Mechanical ventilation may be essential in the postoperative management of patients undergoing cardiac surgery and cardiopulmonary bypass (CPB). Prior to the 1990s, patients were mechanically ventilated until the morning after surgery before weaning was attempted. In more recent decades, the need for cost containment has resulted in "fast-tracking" patients by implementing early weaning protocols and reversible sedation. By utilizing appropriate anesthetic techniques and postoperative management, the cardiac surgery patient may be extubated within 6 hours without complications, thus leading to better patient outcomes.

The reported benefits of earlier extubation include improved preload, decreased hemodynamic compromise, early discharge from the intensive care unit (ICU), early ambulation, prevention of potential complications of prolonged intubation, and decreased neurologic compromise (in elderly patients). It is undisputed that mechanical ventilation saves lives but is associated with risks to the cardiac surgery patient.

Early extubation protocols have also shown a decrease in morbidity associated with both cardiac and respiratory complications (Crawford et al., 2016; Garcia-Delgado, Navarrete-Sànchez, & Colmenero, 2014). Data from one recent study revealed increased ICU length of stay in patients extubated within 6 hours of surgery. There was no increased length of hospital stay in this patient cohort (Richey et al., 2018).

The majority of patients are extubated within 24 hours following coronary artery bypass grafting (CABG) procedures. However, prolonged mechanical ventilation may occur in up to 20% of cardiac surgery patients (Govender, Bihari, & Dixon, 2015). In open heart surgery, mechanical ventilation is most often defined as at least 24 hours but is often referred to in segments of at least 6 hours, 8 hours, 24 hours, or 72 hours but as long as 2 weeks (Govender et al., 2015).

The Society of Thoracic Surgeons (STS; 2014) was formed to provide the highest quality patient care through education, research, and advocacy in chest surgery. In 2007, the Virginia Cardiac Surgery Quality Initiative (VCSQI), a subgroup of STS, identified the timely extubation of patients and reduction in rates of prolonged ventilation as a priority to improve outcomes. In the VCSQI review, the ability to achieve early extubation included the use of less sedation and shorter acting muscle relaxants. Some institutions utilized bispectral index monitoring as part of the cardiac anesthesia protocol, extubations while still maintained on the intra-aortic balloon pump (IABP), moderate hypothermia intraoperatively with more aggressive rewarming postoperatively, standard protocol orders, and transparency regarding results of extubation times (VCSQI, 2014).

Nurses in the ICU who are caring for patients in the immediate postoperative period following cardiac surgery must have an understanding of the pathophysiology of the lungs, use of mechanical ventilation, weaning protocols, and ability to interpret the clinical significance of diagnostic tests such as arterial blood gases (ABGs) and radiographic findings. They must be able to identify complications of patients on mechanical ventilation and implement measures to prevent morbidities associated with therapy so optimal patient outcomes can be attained.

▶ Predictors of Prolonged Mechanical Ventilation

Several factors have been identified as predictors of the need for prolonged mechanical ventilation following cardiac surgery. Preoperative risk factors include female gender, higher body mass index (BMI), lower ejection fraction, or history of chronic obstructive pulmonary disease (COPD), chronic kidney disease, hypertension, heart failure, recent myocardial infarction, atrial fibrillation, or endocarditis. Intraoperative risk factors include type of surgery, use of CPB, intraoperative time, and transfusion requirements in the operating room (OR). Postoperative risk factors reported include bleeding within the first 24 hours of surgery and postoperative inotrope requirements, admission to the ICU on IABP therapy, and reexploration procedure because of bleeding (Govender et al., 2015; Pulido, 2017; Totonchi, Baazm, Chitsazan, Seifi, & Chitsazan, 2014; Wise et al., 2017).

Anesthesia and Postoperative Complications

General anesthesia is used for pain control, muscle relaxation, and amnesia effect during cardiac surgery. A combination of medications are utilized: inhalation, intravenous, and sometimes epidural agents; these agents all have an effect on the patient related to duration, mechanism of action, and side effects and will impact duration of ventilation and extubation.

Acute respiratory distress syndrome (ARDS) is the leading cause of respiratory failure, but in the cardiac surgery population the impact is greater. No cardiac surgery patient is considered without ARDS risk (Rong, DiFranco, & Gaudino, 2016). Data suggest that patients who undergo cardiac surgery and have prolonged ventilator time postoperatively have lower probability of being discharged from the ICU to a general unit, or have higher in-hospital mortality rates (Kang, 2016). Similarly, postoperative cardiac surgery patients who developed pneumonia also had a higher mortality rate (Ibañez et al., 2014).

Delays Related to Bypass Complications

Several clinical conditions, when present, are likely to result in failure of ventilator weaning. When these conditions are compounded with complications associated with CPB, ventilation time may be prolonged due to a decrease in surfactant production, potential for pulmonary microemboli, and interstitial fluid accumulation in the lungs. Furthermore, red blood cell damage in the pump circuit may potentially occur, decreasing the number of oxygen-carrying capacity cells (Bignami et al., 2016).

Complications of Prolonged Ventilation

Prolonged use of mechanical ventilation is not without risk. In one study, patients who required prolonged ventilation (>72 hours) were more likely to experience infection (Garcia-Delgado et al., 2014). Other complications such as sepsis, multiple organ dysfunction syndrome, and death have been reported in patients who required prolonged mechanical ventilation after cardiac surgery (Fernandez-Zamora et al., 2018).

▶ Pathophysiology of the Lungs

The main function of the respiratory system is to transport air into the lungs so that oxygen can enter the body and carbon dioxide (CO_2) can be eliminated. Air enters the nose or mouth and moves through the trachea into the bronchi and then into each lung. Once air is in the lungs, gas exchange occurs in the approximately 300 million alveoli. Oxygen and carbon dioxide can cross between the lung capillaries and the alveolar spaces, allowing gas exchange to occur. The nasal passages and bronchi warm and moisten the air before it enters the alveoli as a method of preventing damage to delicate alveolar structures.

The mechanism of breathing involves the diaphragm and the intercostal muscles. During normal breathing, inspiration is an active process and expiration is a passive process. Inspiration involves contraction of the diaphragm and the intercostal muscles to allow for the movement of air into the respiratory tract. The diaphragm and intercostal muscles then relax during expiration.

The respiratory center, which is located in the medulla oblongata (the lower part of the brainstem), receives neural, chemical, and hormonal signals that can control the rate and depth of movements of the diaphragm and other respiratory muscles. An increase in carbon dioxide or a decrease in oxygenation, for example, will increase the rate or depth of breathing. Injury, medications, and disease processes can affect the respiratory center's ability to respond to changes in carbon dioxide or oxygen, resulting in respiratory compromise. The use of mechanical ventilation may be needed in these circumstances.

The autonomic nervous system is also involved in breathing. The parasympathetic nervous system may stimulate bronchoconstriction, whereas stimulation of the sympathetic nervous system may cause bronchodilation.

▶ Assessment of Readiness for Weaning

While many postoperative cardiac surgery patients are extubated prior to their admission to the ICU and others remain on mechanical ventilation for only a few hours after surgery, all intubated patients should be evaluated for their readiness for weaning. Data suggest that it may be safe to extubate patients 2 hours following cardiac surgery (Parmer, Clarke, Lau, Porter, & Allsager, 2014).

A number of criteria have been suggested for the ICU nurse to use to determine patient readiness, including the patient's ability to cough adequately, presence of minimal secretions, pulmonary mechanics, and being awake and cooperative. In addition, hemodynamic stability, bleeding control, normothermia, and ability to follow commands must be assessed when deciding if a patient is ready for extubation (Dirks & Waters, 2014; Hefner et al., 2016).

General Physiologic and Hemodynamic Stability

The patient's overall condition should be assessed, because a number of conditions may potentially influence the success of weaning from mechanical ventilation. Presence of excessive bleeding or an electrolyte imbalance may affect the patient's ability to oxygenate or eliminate carbon dioxide (Dirks & Waters, 2014). Similarly, if the patient is not hemodynamically stable—a common finding in the postoperative cardiac surgery patient—success with weaning may be impaired. The ICU nurse should assess vital signs and hemodynamic parameters, and evaluate the patient for presence of dysrhythmias, tachycardia, bradycardia, weak peripheral pulses, and signs of heart failure (e.g., increase in pulmonary artery occlusive pressure or decrease in cardiac output or mixed venous saturation) (Dirks & Waters, 2014).

A number of clinical conditions have been found to influence the ability to wean by affecting either the capacity of or the demand on the respiratory system. In addition to hemodynamic instability and electrolyte imbalances, administration of morphine causes delays in weaning from mechanical ventilation (Parmar et al., 2014). Patient factors that should be optimized prior to extubation include hemodynamic instability, respiratory, metabolic/temperature, resolution of acidosis, amount of bleeding, patient cognition, and neuromuscular factors (Fitch et al., 2014).

A patient's mental status should be adequate enough to allow for maintenance of a patent airway and the ability to cooperate with coughing and deep breathing to prevent postextubation respiratory compromise and complications (Garcia-Delgado et al., 2014).

Mechanical weaning parameters are, in general, insufficient at predicting weaning success because they do not take into account cardiac reserves. Therefore it is necessary for nurses to understand cardiovascular response to mechanical ventilator weaning. In one study, Porhomayon, Papadakos, Nader, and El-Solh (2013) reported serum B-type natriuretic peptide (BNP) and N-terminal pro B-type natriuretic peptide (NT-proBNP) appear to signify patients with heart failure during the weaning process. Ischemic heart disease, valvular heart disease, or systolic or diastolic dysfunction can be part of the cause of cardiac load increase and weaning failure. The extra demand on cardiac load during spontaneous breathing trials may become apparent when transferring patients from positive to spontaneous ventilation. In these situations, diuretic therapy may be considered for excessive preload, and weaning to noninvasive positive pressure ventilation may be beneficial (Porhomayon et al., 2013). However, BNP levels are increased in multiple disorders, such as sepsis unrelated to cardiac disease (e.g., cirrhosis, hyperthyroidism), and further research is needed in the usefulness as an indicator of weaning in cardiac surgery (Mangia, 2014).

Pulmonary Mechanics

Evaluation of certain parameters is suggested to evaluate patient readiness to wean—namely, vital capacity, minute ventilation (or volume), respiratory rate, oxygenation, tidal volume, intact airway protection, and negative inspiratory pressure (or force) (Amitai 2018):

- Vital capacity is the amount of air that can be exhaled forcibly following a full inspiration (Green, 2017).
- Minute ventilation is the volume of gas exchange (inhaled and exhaled) in 1 min. It is measured by multiplying respiratory rate and tidal volume (Green, 2017).
- Respiratory rate is the number of breaths taken by a patient in 1 min.
- Tidal volume refers to the amount of air inhaled by the patient during a normal breath (versus a forced inhalation) (Green, 2017). If tidal volume is too low, it is surmised that the patient will develop atelectasis or pneumonia postextubation.
- Negative inspiratory pressure refers to the amount of negative pressure that the patient generates during a forced inspiration when working against an obstruction to flow (Green, 2017). It is a reflection of the patient's ability to take a deep breath and generate a cough that is strong enough to clear secretions.

The ICU nurse should be mindful that these physiologic weaning parameters are not perfect predictors of a patient's success with extubation. Rather, when assessed in combination with the other criteria discussed in this section, these data will provide some insight into the patient's condition and possible tolerance to breathing without mechanical support.

Assessment of readiness to wean has been studied extensively utilizing the Burns Weaning Assessment Program (BWAP). The BWAP consists of a 26-factor bedside checklist; the BWAP score is derived by simply dividing the number of factors scored as "yes" by 26. Not all BWAP factors are significantly associated with weaning success but are predicative of weaning success (Burns et al., 2012). When studied in a variety of units, including cardiovascular, the BWAP scores of less than 50 were weaned successfully 74% of the time. However, the patients with BWAP scores of 50 or more were weaned successfully 96% of the time. After 3 consecutive days of mechanical ventilation, several conditions complicate and delay weaning (Burns et al., 2012).

Respiratory Physiologic Issues

Infrequently, a postoperative patient may require prolonged ventilatory support for more than several days. Failure to wean has two primary causes: failure of gas exchange at the alveolar level and failure to ventilate adequately.

Atelectasis

One of the most common reasons for deficiency in gas exchange in the postoperative cardiac surgery patient is atelectasis. Atelectasis affects as many as 70% of cardiac surgery patients. It is the most common respiratory complication following cardiac surgery. Etiologic factors identified include preoperative risks such as diabetes, hyperlipidemia, smoking, and preoperative alcohol use. Transfusion with 4 units of packed red blood cells intraoperatively is another identified risk factor for the development of postoperative atelectasis (Saffari et al., 2015). Pain from median sternotomy or thoracotomy incisions inhibits deep breathing efforts, which can result in atelectasis and pneumonia (Silvestry, 2017). Aggressive pulmonary toileting and pain management are needed postextubation to prevent further respiratory compromise. Atelectasis is discussed in more detail in Chapter 13.

Left Ventricular Failure

Persistent left ventricular failure after cardiac surgery causes an increase in hydrostatic pressure, with resultant fluid extravasation into alveoli. Interstitial fluid in the alveoli inhibits oxygen transfer and increases shunting.

Pleural Effusion

Postoperative cardiac surgery patients may also develop a pleural effusion, usually on the left side. Although the specific etiology of this condition is not known, contributing factors are thought to include volume overload, hypoalbuminemia,

inflammation of the pericardium and pleura (postpericardiotomy syndrome), atelectasis, and pneumonia. Development of a pleural effusion may lead to hypoxia, thereby affecting the success of weaning from mechanical ventilation although it is not listed as a strong predictor for length of mechanical ventilation (Govender et al., 2015).

A small pleural effusion is common in the early postoperative course following CABG procedures. It occurs with less frequency in patients who have undergone mitral or aortic valve replacement surgery, and typically occurs more commonly on the left side than on the right side. Effusions may necessitate thoracentesis or occasionally placement of a chest tube. Pleural effusions can present with different symptoms depending on the size of the effusion. Typically, the ICU nurse can expect to percuss dullness or decreased resonance and to auscultate diminished or inaudible breath sounds or a pleural friction rub. Pleural effusions rarely result in an increased mortality rate or increased length of stay (Heffner, 2013). Pleural effusion is discussed in more detail in Chapter 13.

Phrenic Nerve Injury

Another potential cause of weaning failure is phrenic nerve injury. This can result from cold cardioplegia or mechanical stretching during cardiac surgery. It can also result from harvesting procedures for internal thoracic artery grafts (Alassal et al., 2015), dissection of the internal thoracic artery, or use of cold slush (topical hypothermia solution) (Aguirre et al., 2013). The reported incidence of phrenic nerve injury during cardiac surgery is up to 6% (Gavazzi, de Rino, Boveri, Picozza, & Franceschi, 2016).

Phrenic nerve injury may be associated with either unilateral or bilateral paralysis; the former is more common. It is more common to occur on the left side than the right (Aguirre et al., 2013). Patients with unilateral involvement typically do not experience respiratory symptoms and will be successfully extubated. It is noted that patients with COPD may experience shortness of breath and may require reintubation. Patients with bilateral involvement typically have tachypnea, paradoxical abdominal breathing, and hypercarbia during weaning attempts (Aguirre et al., 2013).

Arterial Blood Gas

Another method of evaluating the effectiveness of breathing and determining readiness for weaning from mechanical ventilation following cardiac surgery is by obtaining an ABG. An ABG provides data with which to evaluate the patient's condition and the need for potential intervention; specifically, it includes pH, partial pressure of oxygen (PaO_2), oxygen saturation (SaO_2), partial pressure of carbon dioxide ($PaCO_2$), and bicarbonate (HCO_3) levels. Accurate interpretation will assist in determining the patient's acid–base balance and any required interventions. **TABLE 11.1** lists normal values for an ABG.

Acid–Base Disorders

The pH is a measurement of acidity and alkalinity of the blood. If a patient has an acidic pH, a decrease in myocardial contractility, vascular response to catecholamines, and response to

effects and actions of certain medications may result. An alkalotic pH may result in interference with tissue oxygenation, normal neurologic functioning, and normal muscular functioning.

Respiratory Acidosis. The definition of respiratory acidosis is a pH of less than 7.35 with a $PaCO_2$ greater than 45 mmHg. It is important to treat respiratory acidosis, because its presence increases the minute ventilation required to normalize pH (Rogers & McCutcheon, 2015). **BOX 11.1**

BOX 11.1 Causes of Respiratory Acidosis

Impaired Respiratory Muscle Function Related To:
- Neuromuscular blocking agents
- Phrenic nerve paralysis

Pulmonary Disorders
- Atelectasis
- Acute respiratory distress syndrome
- Pleural effusion
- Pneumonia
- Pneumothorax
- Pulmonary edema
- Pulmonary embolism

Increased Carbon Dioxide Production
- Bronchospasm
- Shivering
- Sepsis

Hypoventilation Secondary To:
- Pain
- Sternal incision
- Residual anesthesia
- Awakening with inadequate analgesia and impaired respiratory mechanics
- Opioid side effects

User Error
- Inappropriate ventilator settings
- Hypoventilation during transfer from the operating room

Data from Bignami et al., 2016; Rogers & McCutcheon, 2015.

TABLE 11.1 Components and Normal Values of Arterial Blood Gas	
ABG Component	**Normal Value**
pH	7.35–7.45
PaO_2	80–100 mmHg
$PaCO_2$	35–45 mmHg
HCO_3	22–26 mEq/L
SaO_2	94%–100%
Base excess	–2 to +2 (A negative base excess indicates a base deficit in the blood.)

HCO_3, bicarbonate; $PaCO_2$, partial pressure of carbon dioxide; PaO_2, partial pressure of oxygen; SaO_2, oxygen saturation.

lists common causes of respiratory acidosis in the postoperative cardiac surgery patient.

Signs and symptoms of respiratory acidosis are respiratory, neurologic, and cardiovascular in nature. Respiratory symptoms may include dyspnea, respiratory distress, and shallow respirations. Headache, restlessness, combativeness, hallucinations, and confusion are neurologic symptoms. If CO_2 levels continue to increase, symptoms can progress to agitation or delirium, somnolence, stuporousness, constricted pupils, drowsiness, seizures, and coma. Cyanosis may be present if the acidosis is accompanied by hypoxemia. Superficial blood vessels may become dilated and papilledema may be noted on retinal examination (Byrd, 2014a). Treatment for respiratory acidosis entails treating the underlying cause of hypoventilation and increasing ventilation.

Respiratory Alkalosis. Respiratory alkalosis is defined as a pH greater than 7.45 with a $PaCO_2$ less than 35 mmHg. Conditions that cause hyperventilation can result in respiratory alkalosis. **BOX 11.2** lists common causes of respiratory alkalosis in the postoperative cardiac surgery patient.

Respiratory alkalosis is associated with both nervous and cardiac system sequelae. Lightheadedness, dizziness, agitation, numbness or tingling of the extremities, laryngospasm, confusion, and blurred vision are common neurologic symptoms. Cardiac symptoms may include chest pain, ischemic changes on electrocardiogram (ECG), peripheral vasoconstriction, dysrhythmias, and palpitations (Rogers & McCutcheon, 2015).

Treatment of respiratory alkalosis focuses on eradicating the underlying cause. The patient must be monitored for respiratory muscle fatigue and acute respiratory failure. If these situations occur, temporary reinstitution of mechanical ventilation may be indicated.

Metabolic Acidosis. Metabolic acidosis is defined as a bicarbonate level less than 22 mEq/L and a pH less than 7.35. **BOX 11.3** lists possible causes of metabolic acidosis in the postoperative cardiac surgery patient.

Metabolic acidosis symptoms arise in relation to the neurologic, cardiovascular, gastrointestinal,

---

> **BOX 11.2** Causes of Respiratory Alkalosis
>
> ### Hypoventilation Secondary To:
> - Anxiety or fear
> - Pain or generalized discomfort
>
> ### Increased Oxygen Demand
> - Fever
> - Sepsis
>
> ### Pulmonary Disorders
> - Pneumonia
> - Pulmonary edema
> - Pneumothorax/hemothorax
> - Aspiration
> - Asthma
> - Emphysema
> - Chronic bronchitis
>
> ### Medication
> - Respiratory stimulants
> - Catecholamines
> - Nicotine
>
> ### User Error
> - Inappropriate ventilator settings
> - Hyperventilation during transfer from operating room

Data from Bignami et al., 2016; Byrd, 2014b.

---

and respiratory systems. Fatigue, dyspnea on exertion, nausea and vomiting, deep respirations, use of accessory muscles, tachycardia, and hypotension are possible (Rogers & McCutcheon, 2015). Kussmaul respirations occur when the body attempts to maintain a normal pH by blowing off CO_2. Laboratory findings may include hyperkalemia, hyperphosphatemia, hyperuricemia, and hypocalcemia (Thomas, 2017a). The ICU nurse should attempt to identify the underlying cause of the metabolic acidosis. Hypoxia of any tissues will produce metabolic acids from anaerobic metabolism even if the PaO_2 is normal. The only way to treat acidosis is to restore tissue perfusion, thereby preventing further hypoxemia and hypoxia from developing. If renal failure is the etiology of the

---

BOX 11.3 Causes of Metabolic Acidosis

Hemodynamics

- Decreased cardiac output
- Inadequate systemic perfusion
- Decreased cardiac function
- Decreased peripheral perfusion
- Hypotension
- Hypovolemia
- Vasoconstriction from hypothermia

Physiologic Conditions (Increasing Acids)

- Sepsis
- Low cardiac output
- Tissue hypoperfusion
- Impaired renal perfusion
- Low filling pressures
- Renal failure
- Regional ischemia
- Diabetic ketoacidosis
- Anaerobic metabolism

Medication

- Metformin (Glucophage®)

Data from Mehta & Alston, 2017; Rogers & McCutcheon, 2015.

BOX 11.4 Causes of Metabolic Alkalosis

Loss of Acids

- Nasogastric suctioning
- Excessive administration of diuretics without adequate potassium and chloride repletion
- Hypochloremia

Hypokalemia

Massive Transfusion (from Citrate)

Data from Rogers & McCutcheon, 2015.

---

metabolic acidosis, the ICU nurse should attempt to attain and maintain normovolemia, administer diuretics based on the patient's hemodynamic profile, and possibly support the patient during dialysis or hemofiltration. Treatment may also entail administration of sodium bicarbonate (depending on the severity of the acidosis or pH level) (Thomas, 2017b).

Metabolic Alkalosis. Metabolic alkalosis is defined as a bicarbonate level greater than 26 mEq/L with a pH greater than 7.45. **BOX 11.4** lists conditions that may cause a metabolic alkalosis in the postoperative cardiac surgery patient.

Metabolic alkalosis symptoms are primarily associated with the neurologic and musculoskeletal systems. Weakness, myalgia, polyuria, and cardiac dysrhythmias may be expected. The patient also may develop hypoventilation, which can manifest with feeling jittery, perioral tingling,

and muscle spasms (Thomas, 2017c). Electrolyte imbalances associated with metabolic alkalosis include hypokalemia, hypocalcemia, hypomagnesemia, and hypophosphatemia (Thomas, 2017d). Treatment of metabolic alkalosis can be difficult. Acetazolamide (Diamox®) is commonly given after cardiac surgery when excess diuretics have been administered. It may take hours to days to resolve the alkalosis. Acetazolamide blocks the action of carbonic anhydrase, thereby promoting renal excretion of sodium, potassium, phosphorus, bicarbonate, and water (Thomas, 2017d). Renal excretion of potassium and phosphorus may be excessive with acetazolamide therapy, however. In severe cases (pH at least 7.55), intravenous administration of hydrochloric acid may be necessary. It may also be considered in patients who cannot receive sodium chloride or potassium chloride because of fluid overload or acute kidney injury. Administration of hydrochloric acid may also be indicated for patients who require rapid correction of this metabolic imbalance (Thomas, 2017d).

Administration of ammonium chloride may be considered in severe cases of metabolic alkalosis. Ammonium chloride converts in the liver to ammonia and hydrochloric acid. Release of hydrochloric acid may help to correct the metabolic alkalosis (Thomas, 2017d).

Supplementation with potassium may be part of the treatment plan for patients with a metabolic alkalosis. This is typically done in patients who have a metabolic alkalosis due to hypokalemia (Thomas, 2017d).

Intrapulmonary Shunt

Intrapulmonary shunt (IPS) is the percentage of cardiac output that does not participate in gas exchange. This blood passes through the lungs but is not exposed to ventilated alveoli, so gas exchange does not take place; as a consequence, the blood leaves the lungs in a desaturated state. IPS can occur as a result of a number of conditions (e.g., collapsed or fluid-filled alveoli) and is a major cause of hypoxemia in the ICU. A frequent cause of IPS following cardiac surgery is atelectasis (Lone, 2016).

A normal shunt is in the range of approximately 2% to 5%. Some patients, however, may have a shunt as high as 40% or 50%, such as with ARDS. Following cardiac surgery, the increased risk of ARDS has been associated with CPB, blood product transfusions, large volume shifts, and prolonged mechanical ventilation. The impact of ARDS affects survival, morbidity, and in-hospital length of stay (Rong et al., 2016). Because the desaturated blood has not been exposed to ventilated alveoli, increasing oxygen delivery will not correct the resultant hypoxia. Instead, correction of the underlying pathology is necessary to resolve this condition.

A-a Gradient

In addition to assessing acid–base balance, another assessment criterion that may be used to determine patient readiness to wean from mechanical ventilation is calculation of the alveolar-arterial (A-a) oxygen gradient, a method of measuring IPS. This calculation determines the difference between the percentage of alveolar oxygen entering the alveoli and the percentage of oxygen diffusing into the arterial blood. The result of this calculation will aid the clinician in assessing for the presence of dysfunction in oxygenation as well as the degree of IPS (Sarkar, Niranjan, & Banyal, 2017). The higher the A-a gradient, the more severe the problem with oxygen

reaching the blood. If the shunt is too extensive, the patient is not ready for weaning from mechanical ventilation.

Hypoventilation during cardiac surgery results in atelectasis, increasing the A-a gradient. As the alveoli reexpand postoperatively, the A-a gradient normalizes (300 mmHg), revealing the patient's readiness for weaning.

The formula for calculating an A-a gradient is complex. Fortunately, Internet sources offer calculator programs to facilitate the process. In one such calculator, the ICU nurse would need to insert the local barometric pressure (P_B, which is preset at 760 mmHg), PaO_2, and $PaCO_2$ data from the ABG, and the patient's fraction of inspired oxygen (FiO_2) level, and then click the "Calculate Aa Gradient" button for the result to appear (McAuley, 1993–2014).

PaO_2/FiO_2 Ratio

A suggested alternative to the A-a gradient that is easy to calculate and considered a reliable indicator of gas exchange is the PaO_2/FiO_2 (P/F) ratio. This ratio is an index of oxygenation that is commonly used by clinicians because of its ease in calculation. To use this ratio, you must have the PaO_2 from the blood gas and the FiO_2 at the time the blood gas was drawn. Normal $PaO_2/FiO_2 = 100$ mmHg/0.21 ≈ 500. The lower the ratio, the worse the disease process. PaO_2/FiO_2 less than 300 is consistent with acute lung injury (ALI); PaO_2/FiO_2 less than 200 is consistent with ARDS (Bignami et al., 2016). Criticisms of the PaO_2/FiO_2 ratio include the fact that it is affected by changes in $PaCO_2$ and mixed venous oxygen saturation (SvO_2), it is reportedly not equally sensitive across the entire range of FiO_2, and it cannot provide information about the functional status of the lungs based on interventions to augment oxygenation (e.g., positive end-expiratory pressure [PEEP], lateral or prone positioning) (Slutsky, 2014).

$PaO_2/(FiO_2 \times$ Mean $P_{aw})$

Another oxygenation index, $PaO_2/(FiO_2 \times$ mean $P_{aw})$, where P_{aw} is mean airway pressure, takes into account the effects of PEEP.

Mild ARDS	200 mmHg less than PaO_2/FiO_2, 300 mmHg or less with positive end-expiratory pressure (PEEP) or continuous positive airway pressure at least 5 cmH$_2$O
Moderate ARDS	100 mmHg $<$ PaO_2/FiO_2, 200 mmHg with PEEP $\geq$5 cmH$_2$O
Severe ARDS	$PaO_2/FiO_2 <$ 100 mmHg with PEEP $\geq$5 cmH$_2$O

Data from Ferguson ND, Fan E, Camporota L, Antonelli M, Anzueto A, Beale R, Brochard L, Brower R, Esteban A, Gattinoni L, et al., The Berlin definition of ARDS: an expanded rationale, justification, and supplementary material. Intensive Care Med 2012;38:1573–1582; Rong, DiFranco & Gaudino, 2016.

▶ Postoperative Mechanical Ventilation

Prolonged mechanical ventilation following cardiac surgery is associated with increased ICU and hospital lengths of stay, resource use, costs, and poorer physiologic outcomes (Bignami et al., 2016; Garcia-Delgado et al., 2014). Results of "fast-track" programs have shown that postoperative intubation can be safely limited in cardiac surgery patients.

If not extubated in the OR, the patient is placed on mechanical ventilation upon arrival to the ICU. The mode of ventilation and settings used will depend on the patient's clinical status. Cardiac surgical patients have multiple risk factors for postoperative respiratory dysfunction. Because patients are at risk for surgery-related complications (e.g., hemodynamic instability, temperature dysregulation, blood loss from the mediastinum) for the first 2 to 6 hours postoperatively, it is suggested that extubation occurs after that period of time. It is further recommended that the extubation process be based on a protocol (Fitch et al., 2014).

Initial Postoperative Ventilator Settings

For patients who remain on mechanical ventilation in the postoperative period, the settings used should be based on a plan intended to optimize gas exchange, decrease work of breathing, and minimize complications associated with positive-pressure ventilation (Garcia-Delgado et al., 2014). **TABLE 11.2** shows the initial ventilator settings. **BOX 11.5** reveals an example of a weaning

TABLE 11.2 Initial Postoperative Ventilator Settings	
Mode	IMV, Assist Control, Pressure Support Ventilation, Airway Pressure Release Ventilation, or Pressure Control
FiO_2	Range = 0.4 to 1.0. Depends on the patient's ABG results and SpO$_2$ measurements. It is modified to the lowest level while maintaining SpO$_2$ levels at least 92% or what is reasonable according to the patient's baseline and past medical history.
Tidal volume	5 to 8 mL/kg ideal body weight. Tidal volume may be increased to decrease carbon dioxide levels, and vice versa. Tidal volume may also be adjusted to maintain pH within appropriate limits for the patient and to achieve a minute ventilation of 100 mL/kg/min. It may also be adjusted to maintain peak inspiratory pressure less than 35 cmH$_2$O.
Rate	8 to 12 breaths/min. Respiratory rate may be increased to decrease carbon dioxide levels and to achieve a minute ventilation of 100 mL/kg/min.
Minute volume	100 to 120 mL/kg/min. Minute volume may be increased by increasing the rate, the tidal volume, or both to decrease carbon dioxide levels.
PEEP	3 to 10 cmH$_2$O. PEEP levels may be increased to improve oxygenation particularly in the immediately postoperative period to recruit alveoli.

Pressure support	5 to 10 cmH$_2$O
I:E ratio	1:2 to 1:3. This can be reduced to 1:4 or 1:5 in the presence of obstructive airway disease to prevent air trapping. If a patient has difficulty with oxygenation, the ratio may be changed to either 1:1 or 2:1 (inverse I:E ratio when patient has ARDS).
Inspiratory flow rate	30 to 60 L/min

ABG, arterial blood gas; ARDS, acute respiratory distress syndrome; FiO$_2$, fraction of inspired oxygen; I:E, inspiratory:expiratory; IMV, intermittent mandatory ventilation; PEEP, positive end-expiratory pressure; SpO$_2$, peripheral capillary oxygen saturation.
Data from Amitai, 2018.

BOX 11.5 Respiratory Therapy (RT) and Registered Nurse (RN)–Driven Cardiac Surgery Weaning Protocol

Patient determined candidate for extubation. Propofol: Titrate to a RASS Scale of 0 to −2 for one hour or hemodynamic stability, then discontinue. Preferably within 45–60 minutes of arrival.

Readiness for Extubation Criteria:

- Patient can lift head off bed.
- Respiratory rate less than 10–30 breaths per minute.
- Minute ventilation 4–8 liters per minute.
- Tidal volume 3–5 mL/kg/ideal body weight.
- FiO$_2$ less than or equal to 50%.
- PEEP less than or equal to 8 cmH$_2$O.

Spontaneous Breathing Trial Successful: Yes or No

Assess Readiness to Wean Criteria:

- Bleeding less than 200 mL/hour 1st hour and decrease each hour
- Temperature 37°C
- PaO$_2$/FiO$_2$ ratio greater than 200 and PEEP weaned to 5 cmH$_2$O
- Hemodynamically stable (CI >2.2 L/min/m^2)

Both respiratory and hemodynamically stable
Extubate to Oxygen Protocol per RT and RN

Post Extubation RT and RN Care

- Cough and deep breathe every hour while awake post extubation × 12 hours, then every 2 hours while awake
- Incentive spirometry every hour while awake post extubation × 12 hours, then every 2 hours while awake
- Maintain sternal precautions
- Patient "dangled" on side of bed
- Utilize foot pedometer ASAP when patient in chair
- Ambulate patient postoperative day 1
- Wean: (Specify) oxygen to maintain SpO$_2$ greater than 91%.
- If patient is short of breath, return patient to previous oxygen level and reattempt to wean in 2 hours.

Breathing Trial Failed

- Return to previous settings, re-evaluate every 30 minutes
- RT to evaluate and initiate per RT Protocol for Intermittent Therapies

Reproduced from Mary Washington Hospital, 2017.

protocol driven by a respiratory therapist and registered nurse.

Patient Monitoring

When the patient is admitted to the ICU, the nurse should auscultate breath sounds to confirm good bilateral air entry and absence of bronchospasm and adventitious sounds. The postoperative cardiac surgery patient will be monitored with pulse oximetry and potentially with waveform capnometry (end-tidal carbon dioxide [$ETCO_2$]) (Amitai, 2018). These noninvasive monitoring devices provide the ICU nurse with continuous estimates of the patient's oxygenation and ventilation status, respectively, and will likely expedite the weaning process. For capnography, an infrared gas analyzer is placed in the exhalation port of the ventilator or closest to the endotracheal tube. The normal $ETCO_2$ is 2 to 6 mmHg less than the $PaCO_2$.

▶ Weaning Criteria

Anesthesia traditionally utilizes short-acting anesthetic agents so that the patient will wake up quickly. The ICU nurse assesses the patient for readiness to wean on an ongoing basis.

Initiating the weaning process commences when the patient is hemodynamically stable, normothermic, and adequately resuscitated; has no clinically significant dysrhythmias; is draining less than 100 mL/hr from the chest tube; is not shivering; and is on minimal vasoactive support. The patient must be awake, oriented, able to cooperate with instructions, and breathe spontaneously.

However, readiness for extubation should be monitored by a dynamic assessment with key considerations emphasizing trends and stability, rather than by rigid numbers (Conti, Mantz, Longrois, & Tonner, 2014). A chest radiograph should be reviewed prior to extubation to ascertain the presence of any indicators that the patient might not tolerate extubation. Lab values (e.g., electrolytes, lactate level) should be within normal ranges. The ABG results should be at or close to the patient's baseline or normalized.

The patient should be normothermic before weaning is attempted, because shivering causes an increase in carbon dioxide production. Shivering following hypothermic CPB causes a two- to threefold increase in oxygen consumption as well as carbon dioxide production and increased release of catecholamines. The latter results in tachycardia, hypertension, increased cardiac output, postoperative pain, intraocular pressure, and intracranial pressure (Golembiewski, 2015).

Conti and colleagues (2014) summarize weaning criteria as follows:

- Underlying cause of acute respiratory failure resolved
- Hemodynamic stability, defined as minimal or no vasoactive/inotropic drugs
- Adequate neurologic status, defined as Glasgow Coma Scale score greater than 8 or, if sedated, target Richmond Agitation-Sedation Scale score in the range −2 to 0 achieved with minimal sedation
- Absence of fever or temperature less than 38°C
- Adequate gas exchange, as indicated by a partial pressure of oxygen: fraction of inspired oxygen ratio greater than 200 with PEEP of 5 cmH$_2$O
- Partial pressure of carbon dioxide adjusted to bring blood pH into normal range

Weaning from Mechanical Ventilation

Optimal management of mechanical ventilation and weaning require dynamic and collaborative decision making among nursing, respiratory therapists, and health care providers to minimize complications and avoid delays in liberation from the ventilator. Recruitment maneuvers (RMs) are a key element of protective ventilation to reexpand collapsed lung tissue. During RMs, high airway pressures are maintained over a short period of time. Documented studies demonstrate a reduction in shunt fraction and better blood oxygenation when RMs were applied after CPB. High pressures will recruit alveoli, and significantly shorten ICU and hospital stay, but caution must be maintained to not overdistend the lungs (Bignami et al., 2016; Neto & Schultz, 2017).

Weaning may be accomplished in several different ways, depending on the mode of ventilation and the patient's condition. The first goal is to wean the patient as tolerated while maintaining SpO_2 of at least 92% to 94% on FiO_2 0.40 and PEEP 5 cmH_2O. If the patient is receiving pressure support, as the patient's respiratory effort increases, mechanical ventilation support levels can be gradually titrated down (Rose, 2015).

Once physiologic parameters have been met, the amount of support the patient receives from the ventilator is gradually decreased or else the patient typically undergoes a spontaneous breathing trial (SBT). Data suggest more successful weaning and extubation with SBTs (Rose, 2015). An alternative to an SBT for weaning is to gradually and incrementally decrease the amount of support from pressure support ventilation or the intermittent mandatory ventilation (IMV) rate. Data are conflicting regarding whether earlier weaning occurs with SBTs versus pressure support ventilation or use of IMV. Regardless of the method used, once the patient has satisfactory ABG results and has demonstrated the ability to breathe independently without signs of distress, extubation can be considered. In addition to assessment of pulmonary mechanics, if the patient is able to maintain a patent airway and manage secretions and the criteria in **BOX 11.6** are met, the patient is considered ready to be extubated.

The ICU nurse plays a pivotal role in assessing tolerance to weaning. Signs and symptoms that would indicate poor tolerance to weaning include a respiratory rate of 35 or greater; SpO_2 less than 90%; heart rate greater than 140; systolic or diastolic blood pressure higher than 180 or 90 mmHg, respectively; and presence of agitation, diaphoresis, or anxiety. Hammash, Moser, Frazier, Lennie, and Hardin-Pierce (2015) found early detection and effective management of cardiac dysrhythmias during weaning are important as the arrhythmias can contribute to unstable hemodynamic status, unsuccessful weaning, and the need for longer duration of

---

BOX 11.6 Readiness for Extubation Criteria

NIP –25 cmH_2O
RR less than 25 bpm
HR less than 140
VE 10 L/min
VC 10 to 15 mL/kg
RSBI f/V_T less than 105

Cardiac status:

- No signs of ischemia
- Not receiving vasopressor therapy or low-dose inotropic agents

Neurologic status:

- Alert
- Able to respond to commands
- Cough and gag reflex
- Able to protect airway and clear secretions
- Able to sustain a head lift for at least 5 sec

bpm, beats/min; f/V_T, ratio of respiratory frequency to tidal volume; NIP, negative inspiratory pressure; RR, respiratory rate; RSBI, Rapid Shallow Breathing Index; VC, vital capacity; VE, minute volume.
Data from Conti, Mantz, Longrois, & Tonner, 2014; Epstein, 2017; Godard et al., 2016.

---

mechanical ventilation. Further, if the patient has an inadequate minute volume, tidal volume, episodes of apnea lasting more than 25 sec, mental status changes, a decrease in SpO_2 to less than 92%, or $ETCO_2$ greater than 55 mmHg, the trial is stopped, the patient is restored to the prior ventilator settings, and an ABG is obtained. It has been recommended that spontaneous breathing trials be attempted hourly until weaning is successful (Rose, 2015).

When ABG results are obtained and are within the appropriate range, collaboration with the health care provider regarding extubation is indicated. If the ABG results are not acceptable, the patient should be placed back on the previous support settings and reassessed in 30 to 60 minutes (Rose, 2015).

Researchers have compared intubation times using automated weaning systems, a knowledge-based system for automated weaning with conventional health care provider–controlled weaning after off-pump coronary artery bypass.

No complications or increase in reintubations occurred with the computer-driven weaning system, and the weaning system reduced the duration of mechanical ventilation (Rose, 2015). Another study evaluated the Siemens Servo 300A ventilator, which has an automode function allowing for automated weaning from mechanical ventilation. Data suggest that the automode along with SBT as part of the protocol decreased ventilation time, time to successful extubation, ICU length of stay, and the number of patients requiring prolonged mechanical ventilation (Rose, 2015).

Noninvasive ventilation (NIV) is the deliverance of positive pressure via a face mask, mouthpiece, or helmet. Non-invasive ventilation can avoid the complications associated with artificial airways such as ventilator-associated events or pharyngolaryngeal dysfunction or injuries. Non-invasive ventilation may be utilized to optimize successful weaning and extubation. It has been used for early extubation to NIV, thereby reducing associated risks and preventing reintubation or rescue therapy that can develop following extubation (Rose, 2015).

Weaning from Prolonged Ventilation

In long-term weaning, the physiologic or rapid, shallow breathing index is a reliable predictive indicator of failure to wean and extubation. The physiologic index is determined by assessing the minute frequency of spontaneous ventilation (f) and dividing this value by the tidal volume (V_T) in liters. When this index is high, it reflects a clinical picture of a patient with rapid, shallow breathing. When f/V_T is less than 105, 78% of patients can be weaned and extubated successfully. When f/V_T is greater than 105, 95% of patients cannot be weaned and extubated successfully (Hefner et al., 2016). Long-term care in the patient on mechanical ventilation should include application of ventilator care bundles.

This includes handwashing, cleansing of the oral cavity with chlorhexidine, low tidal volume of ideal body weight, application of PEEP, monitoring of endotracheal cuff pressures with goal pressure of 20 to 30 cmH$_2$O, and head of the bed at least 30 to 45 degrees (Amitai, 2018; Garcia-Delgado et al., 2014).

▶ Postextubation Care

Prior to extubation with the cuff of the endotracheal tube deflated and then upon extubation, the patient is assessed for a patent airway and absence of laryngeal edema. The ICU nurse should ask the patient to speak a few words. Once extubated, the patient should be placed on a humidified face mask set to deliver an FiO$_2$ 0.40 greater than what was received when on mechanical ventilation. The FiO$_2$ level may be titrated down according to SpO$_2$ values, which should initially be maintained above the range of 97% to 98%. After the initial postextubation period, FiO$_2$ can be titrated to maintain SpO$_2$ at least 95% for the first 2 to 3 days. After that point, a nasal cannula can be used to maintain SpO$_2$ at least 90%. In a recent study, high-flow nasal cannula was compared to NIV. The data suggest no difference between these two modalities in preventing reintubation or postextubation respiratory failure. The researchers cite comfort, availability, and lower costs as advantages to nasal cannula use postextubation (Hernández et al., 2016).

Identified risk factors of extubation failure include older age, severity of illness upon admission to the ICU, prolonged ventilation before attempting extubation, and use of continuous sedation. Reasons for extubation failure include upper airway obstruction, impaired ability to clear secretions, respiratory failure, hypoxemia, hypercarbia, cardiac failure, neurologic impairment, and insecure airway. Renal failure, IABP requirement, longer surgical time, and longer time on bypass have also been implicated (Garcia-Delgado et al., 2014). Hefner and colleagues (2016) found with a standardized early extubation protocol, they reduced the median hours of initial mechanical ventilation to 6.9 hours and the percentage of patients reintubated decreased to 3.5% from 11.8%.

The awakening and breathing coordination bundled with delirium monitoring that is a component of the Awakening and Breathing, Choosing the right sedative, Delirium monitoring, Early mobilization and integrating Family (ABCDEF) bundle has been shown to be an effective strategy for weaning, decrease in ventilator time, and extubation readiness with a reduction in delirium incidence (Society of Critical Care Medicine, n.d.).

Postextubation, the ICU nurse should initially observe for laryngospasm for as long as 1 hour and stridor for as long as 24 hours; both conditions may result in the need for reintubation. Prophylactic administration of dexamethasone has been shown to be effective in decreasing the incidence of postextubation stridor in patients who are at risk for developing laryngeal edema (Bean, 2014).

After cardiac surgery, many patients will have decreased breath sounds secondary to lower lobe atelectasis. For this reason, the ICU nurse must frequently evaluate the patient in terms of work of breathing, respiratory rate, use of accessory muscles, and expiratory phase of breathing. Nursing care must include encouraging early mobility, deep breathing exercises, bronchial hygiene, and frequent auscultation of breath sounds. Chest physiotherapy will promote lung expansion, mobilize secretions, encourage coughing, and prevent the side effect of retained secretions, which might otherwise cause atelectasis and potentially pneumonia (Waugaman, VanNortwick, Dionne, Whitmore, & Bradley, 2015).

One of the sequelae of bypass procedures is activation of the inflammatory response, which can cause marked pulmonary dysfunction (Bignami et al., 2016). A variety of interventions are being studied for their potential to mitigate the deleterious effects of bypass procedures that can cause delays in weaning from mechanical ventilation. These interventions include use of a leukocyte filtration to reduce the effects of CPB, ultrafiltration to reduce fluid overload, intraoperative use of heparin-bonded circuits designed to prevent complement activation and subsequent increase in neutrophil activation, and use of antioxidants and anti-inflammatory drugs with the serine protease inhibitor activity of aprotinin in combination with leukocyte-reduction filters. The last combination has been shown to improve post-bypass lung performance by reducing inflammatory response and its sequelae (Bignami et al., 2016; Rong et al., 2016).

▶ Summary

Caring for patients following cardiac surgery is often challenging. While many patients are admitted to the ICU having already been extubated, others require management with mechanical ventilation for either a short or prolonged period of time. Mechanical ventilation is suggested to be associated with—and may even cause—lung damage and many other complications.

Prolonged use of mechanical ventilation is correlated with an increased mortality rate. The cardiac surgery ICU nurse must continuously assess the post–cardiac surgery patient for tolerance to therapy, prevent complications associated with mechanical ventilation, minimize the effects of the patient's comorbidities and the procedure-associated complications, and assess the patient's readiness for and tolerance of weaning from mechanical ventilation in collaboration with respiratory therapy. Although the majority of patients are quickly weaned from mechanical ventilation and extubated, extubation failure must be minimized or recognized promptly. Identifying patients at risk for prolonged mechanical ventilation following cardiac surgery based on preoperative assessment variables may assist to mitigate complications postoperatively. Using high levels of clinical judgment and caring practices will affect the ICU nurse's ability to optimize outcomes of the postoperative cardiac surgery patient.

⌕ CASE STUDY

A 76-year-old patient, has a history of hyperlipidemia, hypertension, congestive heart failure (with an ejection fraction [EF] of 20%), aortic stenosis, peripheral vascular disease, and COPD. The patient presented with substernal pain and "heaviness" in his chest. Upon admission, the 12-lead ECG revealed ST segment elevation in leads II, III, and aVF, and elevation in V5 and V6 with additional ST segment depression in V3 and V4. The patient reported his chest pain to be 8 of 10; he was treated with sublingual nitroglycerin, which decreased the pain to 6 of 10. Initial electrolytes and complete blood count were within normal limits although troponin I was elevated and hemoglobin A1c (HbA_{1c}) was 7.5%. Cardiac catheterization revealed severe three-vessel coronary artery disease. The patient was scheduled for on-pump CABG and aortic valve replacement. The left internal thoracic artery was used to bypass the left anterior descending (LAD) artery, and the saphenous vein was used to bypass the remaining blockages. The intraoperative course was uneventful, and the patient was admitted to the ICU postoperatively. He remained intubated for 2 days postoperatively.

Critical Thinking Questions

1. What risk factors to prolonged mechanical ventilation did this patient have?
2. Which pulmonary interventions will be necessary to facilitate respiratory functioning in this patient?
3. What are possible pulmonary complications from cardiac surgery?

Answers to Critical Thinking Questions

1. This patient was over the age of 65 years, has a history of peripheral vascular disease and valvular disease (aortic stenosis), and underwent valve surgery.
2. Nursing care must include mobility, bronchial hygiene, and frequent auscultation of breath sounds. Bronchial hygiene will promote lung expansion, mobilize secretions, and prevent retention of secretions that cause atelectasis and potentially pneumonia. This care should include pulmonary toileting of effective coughing and incentive spirometry. Incentive spirometry has only limited effectiveness, however, because many patients are unable to cooperate adequately to use it correctly. Care for this patient should include early mobility beginning with dangling at beside upon extubation and walking on postoperative day 1.
3. Potential pulmonary complications include phrenic nerve injury, atelectasis, pleural effusions, and air leak syndrome.

Self-Assessment Questions

1. A 70-year-old man is transferred to the cardiovascular ICU after CABG. Respirations are being assisted by mechanical ventilation. A spontaneous breathing trial is planned within the hour. Which is an appropriate criterion for extubation in this patient?
   A. Heart rate 160/min
   B. Hemoglobin level 6 g/dL
   C. Inspiratory force -25 cmH_2O
   D. Minute ventilation 15 L/min

2. Which ABG values would be *most likely* interpreted as acute respiratory failure?

	pH	pCO_2	pO_2	HCO_3
A.	7.19	72	52	26
B.	7.26	68	65	42
C.	7.30	55	82	28
D.	7.35	45	69	22

3. The purpose of using high PEEP in the immediate postoperative period after heart surgery is to:
   A. allow for a low ventilatory rate.
   B. promote healing of the alveolar membranes.
   C. increase alveolar recruitment.
   D. decrease pulmonary shunting.

4. An otherwise healthy 75-kg patient was admitted following CABG × 3 with the left internal thoracic artery (LITA). The patient has developed ARDS and is being ventilated on the following settings:

VT	350 mL
Rate	20 bpm
Mode	Assist/Control
FiO_2	0.80
PEEP	5 cmH$_2$O

The ABG reveals:

pH	7.35
pCO_2	55
pO_2	44
HCO_3	25

Which ventilator change would most effectively correct the hypoxemia?
   A. Increasing tidal volume
   B. Increasing I:E ratio
   C. Change to SIMV
   D. Increasing PEEP to 10 cmH$_2$O

5. A metabolic acidosis would be indicated by:
   A. pH greater than 7.35
   B. pCO_2 less than 45
   C. HCO_3 less than 18
   D. pO_2 greater than 80

6. Which best defines hypoventilation in an extubated post-CABG patient?
   A. RR less than 12
   B. pCO_2 greater than 45
   C. pO_2 less than 80
   D. pH greater than 7.35

7. The post-CABG patient with mitral valve replacement had initial postoperative coagulopathy requiring 6 units of packed red blood cells (PRBCs), 2 units of fresh frozen plasma (FFP), and 6 packs of platelets pooled to one unit. The nurse's primary respiratory concern should be:
   A. hypoxemia.
   B. acute lung injury.
   C. respiratory acidosis.
   D. metabolic alkalosis.

8. A patient who is 72 hours postoperative aortic valve replacement suddenly becomes dyspneic and RR increases from 24 to 40/min. An ABG sample was obtained, with the patient receiving 6 L via nasal cannula, and returns as pH 7.50, pCO_2 31, and pO_2 48. Chest x-ray results show a ground glass–like appearance. Auscultation reveals crackles up the nipple line on both right and left sides. The nurse should suspect the patient has developed:
   A. aspiration pneumonia.
   B. pulmonary fibrosis.
   C. pulmonary embolism.
   D. ARDS.

9. A postoperative CABG patient has a temperature of 37.0°C, cardiac index (CI) of 3.0/min/m^2 on 2.5 mcg/kg/min dobutamine, chest drainage of 50 mL/hr, mean arterial pressure (MAP) of 70 mmHg, normal sinus rhythm (NSR), and serum glucose of 180 mg/dL. The patient has been successful during spontaneous breathing/awakening trials (SBT/SAT). The next most anticipated step should be:
   A. wean the dobutamine.
   B. insulin for the elevated blood glucose.
   C. proceed to extubation.
   D. monitor for an additional hour.

10. Which parameter can be used to predict readiness for removing a patient from mechanical ventilator?
   A. PaO_2/FiO_2 less than 200
   B. Minute ventilation 12 L/min
   C. NIP −10 cmH$_2$O
   D. Respiratory rate 20 bpm

Answers to Self-Assessment Questions

1. C. **inspiratory force −25 cmH$_2$O**
   Rationale: Negative inspiratory force is an indicator of respiratory muscle strength. At least −25 cmH$_2$O is a predictor of successful liberation from mechanical ventilation. A heart rate of 160, hemoglobin of 6 g/dL, and minute ventilation of greater than 15 L/min are all indicators that the patient will likely not tolerate liberation from mechanical ventilation.

2.   A. **7.19 / 72 / 52 / 26**
     Rationale: An elevated CO_2 (>50) and pO_2 less than 60 are indicators of acute respiratory failure.

3.   C. **increase alveolar recruitment**
     Rationale: Application of PEEP opens collapsed alveoli, which is common in postoperative cardiac surgery patients.

4.   D. **increasing PEEP to 10 cmH$_2$O**
     Rationale: The patient is hypoxemic and is receiving high concentrations of oxygen at this time. Increasing the PEEP can help improve oxygenation. Changing the mode will not correct the patient's hypoxemia and may increase the patient's level of instability. Increasing the tidal volume is not recommended in patients with ARDS. Increasing the I:E ratio will increase the CO_2 level by increasing inspiratory time.

5.   C. **HCO$_3$ less than 18**
     Rationale: A metabolic acidosis is indicated by a pH less than 7.35 and HCO$_3$ less than 22 mEq/L.

6.   B. **pCO$_2$ greater than 45**
     Rationale: A pCO$_2$ greater than 45 indicates hypoventilation.

7.   B. **acute lung injury**
     Rationale: Transfusion-associated acute lung injury can occur following administration of blood products.

8.   D. **ARDS**
     Rationale: This patient has signs and symptoms and ABG and chest x-ray results consistent with ARDS. Aspiration pneumonia manifests with bilateral opacities on chest film. Pulmonary fibrosis will manifest with opacities. In addition, the patient has no risk factors for pulmonary fibrosis. Patients with a pulmonary embolism will have an enlarged pulmonary artery.

9.   C. **proceed to extubation**
     Rationale: This patient meets criteria for consideration to extubate.

10. D. **respiratory rate 20 bpm**
     Rationale: An RR of 20 is one criterion for considering the patient ready for extubation. The PaO2/FiO2 ratio is too low and is suggestive of ARDS. The minute ventilation is too high, and the negative inspiratory force (NIF) is too low to consider the patient ready for extubation.

CLINICAL INQUIRY BOX

Question: What are the predictors of postoperative prolonged ventilation following cardiac surgery?

Reference: Sharma, V., Rao, V., Manlhiot, C., Boruvka, A., Fremes, S., & Wasowicz, M. (2107). A derived and validated score to predict prolonged mechanical ventilation in patients undergoing cardiac surgery. *The Journal of Thoracic and Cardiovascular Surgery, 153,* 108–115.

Objective: To derive and validate a risk index predicting prolonged mechanical ventilation following cardiac surgery.

Methods: Retrospective analysis of two databases.

Results: Strong predictors of prolonged mechanical ventilation following cardiac surgery included previous cardiac surgery, lower left ventricular ejection fraction (LVEF), shock, surgery for repair of congenital heart disease, and CPB time.

Conclusion: Prolonged mechanical ventilation following cardiac surgery can be predicted by preoperative and intraoperative data.

References

Aguirre, V. J., Sinha, P., Zimmet, A., Lee, G. A., Kwa, L., & Rosenfeldt, F. (2013). Phrenic nerve injury during cardiac surgery: Mechanisms, management and prevention. *Heart, Lung and Circulation, 22*(11), 895–902.

Alassal, M. A., Baker, N. F., Shallan, A. M., Raghunayakula, S. N., Elwakeel, E., Elrakhawy, H., . . . Ibrahim, M. F. (2015). Right phrenic nerve palsy post coronary artery bypass grafting (CABG) without harvesting right internal mammary artery (RIMA): A rare and unexpected complication. *Journal of Clinical and Experimental Cardiology.* Retrieved from https://www.omicsonline.org /open-access/right-phrenic-nerve-palsy-post-coronary -artery-bypass-grafting-cabg-without-harvesting-right -internal-mammary-artery-rima-a-rare-and-unexpected -complication-2155-9880-1000406.pdf.

Amitai, A. (2018). *Ventilator management.* Retrieved from http://emedicine.medscape.com/article/810126-overview.

Bean, J. P. (2014). Post extubation stridor. *International Student Journal of Nurse Anesthesia, 13*(2), 14–16.

Bignami, E., Guarnieri, M., Saglietti, F., Belletti, A., Trumello, C., Giambuzzi, I., . . . Alfieri, O. (2016). Mechanical ventilation during cardiopulmonary bypass: A review. *Journal of Cardiothoracic and Vascular Anesthesia, 30*(6), 1668–1675.

Burns, S. M., Fisher, C., Tribble, S. S., Lewis, R., Merrel, R., Conaway, M., & Beck, T. P. (2012). The relationship of 26 clinical factors to weaning outcome. *American Journal of Critical Care, 12*(21), 52–59.

Byrd, R. P. (2014a). *Respiratory acidosis clinical presentation.* Retrieved from http://emedicine.medscape.com/article /301574-clinical#aw2aab6b3b3.

Byrd, R. P. (2014b). *Respiratory alkalosis clinical presentation.* Retrieved from http://emedicine.medscape.com/article /301680-clinical#a0218.

Conti, G., Mantz, J., Longrois, D., & Tonner, P. (2014). Sedation and weaning from mechanical ventilation: time for "best practice" to catch up with new realities? *Multidisciplinary respiratory medicine, 9*(1), 45. doi:10.1186/2049-6958-9-45

Crawford, T. C., Magruder, J. T., Grimm, J. C., Sciurtino, C., Conte, J.-V., Kim, B. S., . . . Whitman, G. J. (2016). Early extubation: A proposed new metric. *Seminars in Thoracic and Cardiovascular Surgery, 28*(2), 290–299.

Dirks, J., & Waters, J. (2014). Cardiovascular therapeutic management. In L. D. Urden, K. M. Stacy, & M. E. Lough (Eds.), *Critical care nursing: Diagnosis and management* (7th ed., pp. 412–466). St. Louis, MO: Elsevier Mosby.

Epstein, S. K. (2017). Weaning from ventilatory support. *Current Opinion in Critical Care, 15*(1), 36–43.

Fernandez-Zamora, M. D., Gordillo-Brenes, A., Banderas-Bravo, E., Arboleda-Sànchez, J. A., Hinojosa-Pérez, R., Aguilar-Alonso, E., . . . Rivera-Fernàndez, R. (2018). Prolonged mechanical ventilation as a predictor of mortality after cardiac surgery. *Respiratory Care, 63*(5), 550–557.

Fitch, Z. W., Debesa, O., Ohkuma, R., Duquaine, D., Steppan, J., Schneider, E. B., . . . Whitman, G. J. R. (2014). A protocol-driven approach to early extubation after cardiac surgery. *The Journal of Thoracic and Cardiovascular Surgery, 147*(4), 1344–1350.

Garcia-Delgado, M., Navarrete-Sanchez, I., & Colmenero, M. (2014). Preventing and managing perioperative pulmonary complications following cardiac surgery. *Current Opinion in Anesthesiology, 27*, 146–152.

Gavazzi, A., de Rino, F., Boveri, M. C., Picozzi, A., & Franceschi, M. (2016). Prevention of peripheral nervous system complications after major heart surgery. *Neurological Sciences, 37*, 205–209.

Godard, S., Herry, C., Westergaard, P., Scales, N., Brown, S. M., Burns, K., . . . Seely, A. J. C. (2016). Practice variation in spontaneous breathing trial performance and reporting. *Canadian Respiratory Journal, 2016.* doi:10.1155/2016/9848942

Golembiewski, J. (2015). Pharmacological management of perioperative shivering. *Journal of PeriAnesthesia Nursing.* doi:101016/j.jopan.2015:05.002

Govender, M., Bihari, S., & Dixon, D.L. (2015). Risk factors for prolonged mechanical ventilation after cardiopulmonary bypass for open-heart surgery in adults. *Clinical Research in Pulmonology, 3*(1), 1033.

Green, R. J. (2017). Selected topics in physiologic ventilation. In R. J. Green Jr. (Ed.), *Green's respiratory therapy: A practical and essential tutorial on the concepts of respiratory care* (pp. 11–118). Chula Vista, CA: Aventine Press.

Hammash, M. H., Moser, D. K., Frazier, S. K., Lennie, T. A., & Hardin-Pierce, M. (2015). Heart rate variability as a predictor of cardiac dysrhythmias during weaning from mechanical ventilation. *American Journal of Critical Care, 24*(2), 118–127.

Heffner, J. E. (2013). *Pleural effusions following cardiac surgery.* Retrieved from http://www.utdol.com/online /content/topic.do?topicKey=pleurdis/8523&selected Title=1~150&source=search_result.

Hefner, J. L., Tripathi, R. S., Abel, E. E., Farneman, M., Galloway, J. & Moffatt-Bruce, S.D. (2016). Quality improvement intervention to decrease prolonged mechanical ventilation aster coronary artery bypass surgery. *American Journal of Critical Care, 25*(5), 423–430.

Hernàndez, G., Vaquero, C., Colinas, L., Cuena, R., Gonzàlez, P., Canabal, A., . . . Fernandez, R. (2016). Effect of postextubation high-flow nasal cannula vs noninvasive ventilation on reintubation and postextubation respiratory failure in high-risk patients: A randomized clinical trial. *Journal of the American Medical Association, 316*(15), 1565–1574.

Ibañez, J., Riera, M., Amezaga, R., Herrero, J., Colomar, A., Campillo-Artero, C., . . . Bonnin, O. (2014). Long-term mortality after pneumonia in cardiac surgery patients. A propensity-matched analysis. *Journal of Intensive Care*

Medicine, 10. Retrieved from http://jic.sagepub.com/content/early/2014/02/26/0885066614523918.abstract.

Kang, Y. A. (2016). Risk factors and outcomes associated with unplanned ICU readmission after cardiac surgery. *AACN Advanced Critical Care, 27*(1), 29–39.

Lone, N. A. (2016). *Pulmonary atelectasis.* Retrieved from https://emedicine.medscape.com/article/100160-overview.

Mangia, A. (2014). *Brain-type natriuretic peptide (BNP).* Retrieved from https;//emedicine.medscape.com/article/2087425-overview.

Mary Washington Hospital. (2017). Policies and Procedures, Mary Washington Mechanical Ventilation Cardiac Surgery Weaning Protocol.

McAuley, D. (1993–2014). *A-a gradient calculator.* Retrieved from http://www.globalrph.com/aagrad.htm.

Mehta, M., & Alston, P. (2017). Metabolic acidosis after heart surgery and intraoperative red cell salvage. *Cardiothoracic and Vascular Anesthesia, 31*(Suppl 1), S81–S82.

Neto, A. S., & Schultz, M. J. (2017). Optimizing the settings on the ventilator high PEEP for all? *Journal of the American Medical Association, 317*(14), 1413–1414.

Parmer, J., Clarke, J., Lau, G., Porter, R., & Allsager, C. (2014). Delays in extubation following elective adult cardiac surgery. *Critical Care. 18*(Suppl1). Retrieved from http://ccforum.com/content/18/S1/P185.

Porhomayon, J., Papadakos, P., Nader, N. D., & El-Solh, A. A. (2013). Weaning failure: My heart is not up to it. *Chronic Respiratory Disease, 10*(3), 165–174.

Pulido, J. N. (2017). Prediction of prolonged mechanical ventilation after cardiac surgery: An imperfect crystal ball. *The Journal of Thoracic and Cardiovascular Surgery, 153*(1), 116–117.

Richey, M., Mann, A., He, J., Daon, E., Wirtz, K., Dalton, A., . . . Flynn, B. C. (2018). Implementation of an early extubation protocol in cardiac surgery patients decreased ventilator time but not intensive care unit or hospital length of stay. *Journal of Cardiovascular and Vascular Anesthesia, 32*(2), 739–744.

Rogers, K. A., & McCutcheon, K. (2015). Four steps to interpreting arterial blood gases. *Journal of Perioperative Practice, 25*(3), 46–52.

Rong, L. Q., DiFranco, A., & Gaudino, M. (2016). Acute respiratory distress syndrome after cardiac surgery. *Journal of Thoracic Diseases, 8*(10), E1177– E1186.

Saffari, N., Nasiri, E., Mousavinasab, S. N., Ghafari, R., Soleimani, A., & Esmaeili, R. (2015). Frequency rate of atelectasis in patients following coronary artery bypass grafting and its associated factors as at Mazandaran Heart Center in 2013–2014. *Global Journal of Health Science, 7*(7), 97–105.

Sarkar, M., Niranjan, N., & Banyal, P. K. (2017). Mechanisms of hypoxemia. *Lung India, 34*(1), 47–60.

Silvestry, F. E. (2017). *Postoperative complications among patients undergoing cardiac surgery.* Retrieved from https://www.uptodate.com/contents/postoperative-complications-among-patients-undergoing-cardiac-surgery.

Slutsky, A. S. (2014). *Optimizing gas exchange in mechanically ventilated patients with acute respiratory failure.* Retrieved from http://www.medscape.org/viewarticle/443575.

Society of Critical Care Medicine (n.d.). *ABCDEF bundle.* Retrieved from http://www.sccm.org/ICULiberation/ABCDEF-Bundles

Society of Thoracic Surgeons. (2014). *About STS.* Retrieved from http://www.sts.org/about-sts.

Thomas, C. P. (2017a). *Metabolic acidosis workup.* Retrieved from https://emedicine.medscape.com/article/242975-workup.

Thomas, C. P. (2017b). *Metabolic acidosis. Treatment and management.* Retrieved from https://emedicine.medscape.com/article/242975-treatment.

Thomas, C. P. (2017c). *Metabolic alkalosis. Clinical presentation.* Retrieved from https://emedicine.medscape.com/article/243160-clinical.

Thomas, C. P. (2017d). *Metabolic alkalosis. Treatment and management.* Retrieved from https://emedicine.medscape.com/article/243160-treatment.

Totonchi, Z., Baazm, F., Chitsazan, M., Seifi, J., & Chitsazan, M. (2014). Predictors of prolonged mechanical ventilation after open heart surgery. *Journal of Cardiovascular and Thoracic Research, 6*(4), 211–216.

Virginia Cardiac Surgery Quality Initiative. (2014). *The Virginia Cardiac Surgery Quality Initiative.* Retrieved from http://www.vcsqi.org/about_us.php.

Waugaman, S., VanNortwick, C., Dionne, H., Whitmore, E., & Bradley, L. (2015). Early mobilization in cardiac surgery patients decreases complications, length of stay, and readmission. *Critical Care Nurse, 35*(2), E24–E25.

Wise, E. S., Stonko, D. P., Glaser, Z. A., Garcia, K. L., Huang, J. J., Kim, J. S., . . . Eagle, S. J. (2017). Prediction of prolonged ventilation after coronary artery bypass grafting: Data from an artificial neural network. *Heart Surgery Forum, 20*(1), E007–E014.

Web Resources

Patient education guides on mechanical ventilation: http://patients.thoracic.org/information-series/en/resources/mechanical-ventilation.pdf

Respiratory assessment: http://www.youtube.com/watch?v=IepL5u5lAtEMechanical ventilation tutorial: http://www.ccmtutorials.com/rs/mv/

Ventilator case studies: http://www.ventworld.com/education/casestudies.asp

© LeslieLauren/iStock/Getty Images

CHAPTER 12

Pharmacologic Support Following Cardiac Surgery

Carrie L. Griffiths

▸ Introduction

Hemodynamic compromise, dysrhythmias, and coagulopathy following cardiac surgery are common therapeutic challenges. The etiology of these complications may be the patient's underlying cardiac disease, postoperative filling pressures, decreased ventricular compliance, loss of vasomotor tone, increased capillary permeability, increased urinary output, inflammatory response to cardiopulmonary bypass (CPB), poor myocardial protection during aortic cross-clamping, pulmonary edema, cardiac tamponade, or ventricular dysfunction. Even though the surgery has been completed, there may not be an immediate improvement in contractility in some patients (Chung & Carlese, 2017).

In the care of the postoperative cardiac surgery patient, the intensive care unit (ICU) nurse must be aware of the intricate balance between physiologic data and the medications utilized to treat and prevent complications. This chapter discusses several medications used in the immediate

postoperative setting, including their mechanism of action, therapeutic uses, and side effects. In addition, nurse precautions that are utilized in the delivery of care are described. Many of the medications profiled in this chapter have a number of mechanisms of action and indications. Because of the potential for interaction of some of these medications and their sometimes burdensome side effect profiles, the ICU nurse needs a high level of clinical judgment to help optimize the patient's outcome.

▸ Agents Used to Manage Postoperative Hypertension

Hypertension is common following postoperative cardiac surgery and is frequently linked to vasoconstriction and decreased sensitivity of baroreceptors. The vasoconstriction may be linked to induced hypothermia during CPB (Silvestry,

Original contributions from Tim Murphy, Roberta Kaplow, and Sonya R. Hardin

2017). Development of hypertension, vasoconstriction, or both may be due to decreased oxygen levels or inflammatory responses to CPB (Silvestry, 2017). Hypertension leads to increased afterload with resultant metabolic acidosis, increased systemic vascular resistance (SVR), decreased cardiac output (CO), decreased stroke volume (SV), tissue hypoxia of skeletal muscles, and increased myocardial oxygen consumption (Silvestry, 2017). From previous studies of anesthesia and postoperative complications, potential causes of increased afterload include hypothermia, hypovolemia, hypercarbia, inadequate rewarming, volume overload, cardiogenic shock, pain, and anxiety. The latter two causes arise as a result of increased sympathetic nervous system stimulation. Hypertension must be managed after cardiac surgery because extreme vasoconstriction places patients at risk of developing life-threatening hypertension and decreased CO. Controlling hypertension is also important after cardiac surgery to reduce bleeding from surgical sites and enhance CO. Refer to **TABLE 12.1** for a summary of medications used to treat hypertension following cardiac surgery.

TABLE 12.1 Antihypertensive Agents Used in Postoperative Cardiac Surgery Patients and Hemodynamic Effects

Agent	Dose	Mechanism of Action	Hemodynamic Effects
Vasodilators			
Nitroglycerin (Tridil®)	3 to 10 mcg/min; titrated in 5-mcg increments every 3 to 5 min	Venous and arterial vasodilation (dose dependent). Increases coronary blood flow, dilates coronary arteries	Decreases preload and afterload (dose dependent). Decreases PAP, CVP, SVR, PVR, myocardial oxygen consumption
Nitroprusside (Nitropress®, Nipride®)	0.3 to 0.5 mcg/kg/min; titrated in 0.5-mcg/kg/min increments every 10 min up to 10 mcg/kg/min	Smooth muscle relaxant; arterial vasodilation. Generates nitric oxide	Decreases SVR and PVR; increases venous capacitance, decreases coronary vascular resistance
Nicardipine (Cardene®)	Infusion at 5 mg/h; dose may be slowly increased by 2.5 mg/hr to a maximum of 15 mg/hr. May reduce by 3 mg/hr once goal blood pressure is reached	Inhibits calcium ion influx into vascular smooth muscle and myocardium. Acts directly on arterioles. Also been shown to dilate the coronary vasculature	Peripheral vascular and coronary vasodilation and lower blood pressure

Agent	Dose	Mechanism of Action	Hemodynamic Effects
Clevidipine (Cleviprex®)	1 to 2 mg/hr via continuous infusion; dose may be doubled in 90-sec intervals. Once blood pressure begins to approach goal, incremental dosing should be every 5 to 10 min and be less than double the dose. A maximum initial dose is 16 mg/hr. Total 24-hr dosing should not exceed 21 mg/hr	Blocks calcium channels. Smooth muscle relaxant and arterial vasodilator.	Decreases MAP and SVR
Fenoldopam mesylate (Corlopam®)	Initial dose of 0.01 to 0.3 mcg/kg/min. Titration in increments of 0.05 to 0.1 mcg/kg/min every 5 to 15 min, to maximum of 1.6 mcg/kg/min, to achieve desired blood pressure. Should not be used for more than 48 hr	Selective dopamine-1 receptor agonist and moderately binds to alpha$_2$ receptors	Vasodilator; increases renal blood flow; decreases SVR and PVR and enhances cardiac output
Beta Blockers			
Esmolol (Brevibloc®)	Loading dose: 500 to 1,000 mcg/kg IV bolus over 1 min. Maintenance dose: 50 mcg/kg/min titrated in 50-mcg/kg/min increments every 4 min to a maximum dose of 300 mcg/kg/min	Cardioselective beta-adrenergic receptor blocker. Inhibits effects at beta$_1$ receptors. Inhibits beta$_2$ receptors at higher doses	Decreases heart rate, blood pressure, contractility, and cardiac output
Labetalol (Normo-dyne®, Trandate®)	10 to 20 mg IV push over 2 min; additional 10- to 20-mg doses every 10 min up to a maximum of 300 mg in 24 hr may be given. Infusion dosing: Initial rate 2 mg/min to a maximum cumulative dose of 300 mg	Noncardioselective adrenergic blocking agent. Exerts inhibitory effects on beta$_1$, beta$_2$, and alpha$_1$ receptors	
ACE Inhibitors			
Enalaprilat (Vasotec®)	0.625 to 1.25 mg, infused over 5 min every 6 hr; additional doses, up to a maximum of 5 mg every 6 hr, may be administered	Prevents conversion of angiotensin I to angiotensin II (a potent vasoconstrictor) by inhibiting ACE in the pulmonary and systemic vascular endothelium	Vasodilation; decreases SVR

(continues)

TABLE 12.1 Antihypertensive Agents Used in Postoperative Cardiac Surgery Patients and Hemodynamic Effects *(continued)*

Agent	Dose	Mechanism of Action	Hemodynamic Effects
ARBs			
No specific ARB recommendations noted in literature and no commercially available IV ARB agents	Dosage is drug dependent	Blocks production of angiotensin II from sources of angiotensin II other than the liver (i.e., blood vessels, in the adrenals, and within all other tissues)	The adrenal-related blockage results in a decrease in aldosterone levels, thereby leading to increased excretion of sodium and water from kidneys
Calcium Channel Blockers			
Nicardipine (Cardene®)	See page 218 in "Vasodilators"		
Clevidipine (Cleviplex®)	See page 219 in "Vasodilators"		
Selective Dopamine-1 Receptor Agonist			
Fenoldopam Mesylate (Corlopam®)	See page 219 in "Vasodilators"		

ACE, angiotensin-converting enzyme; ARB, angiotensin receptor blocker; CVP, central venous pressure; IV, intravenous; MAP, mean arterial pressure; PAP, pulmonary artery pressure; PVR, pulmonary vascular resistance; SVR, systemic vascular resistance.
Adams, Holland, & Urban, 2017; Lexicomp Online, 2017; Parra, Roman, Anasthasia, & Straka, 2016.

Vasodilators

Vasodilators are the agents of choice to decrease hypertension in the immediate postoperative cardiac surgery patient. Nitroprusside is the agent of choice (Silvestry, 2017). Vasodilators are utilized to control hypertension, reduce afterload by decreasing vasoconstriction, and prevent angina pectoris, myocardial infarction (MI), and heart failure, all of which could occur in the postoperative cardiac surgery patient. These agents may also be used in postoperative cardiac surgery patients who have normal blood pressure (BP) despite poor pump function (Silvestry, 2017). Agents may dilate either the arterial or venous system, or both. The most commonly used vasodilators in this patient population are nitroglycerin (Tridil®), nitroprusside (Nipride®), nicardipine (Cardene®), clevidipine (Cleviprex®), and fenoldopam mesylate (Corlopam®).

Care must be taken to correct hypovolemia in hypertensive patients prior to administering a vasodilator. Abrupt, life-threatening hypotension may develop when vasodilators are used and there is an inadequate volume to fill the vasculature. The ICU nurse should always be prepared to administer a rapid fluid bolus when starting any vasodilator, should hypotension occur. As with all vasoactive agents, use of the smallest dose necessary to accomplish the desired effect is recommended. The risk of side effects escalates with higher infusion rates.

Nitroglycerin

Mechanism of Action. Nitroglycerin (NTG) has many uses in postoperative cardiac surgery patients. It decreases preload and, in higher doses, afterload. Patients with high preload benefit because NTG lowers pulmonary artery pressure (PAP) and central venous pressure (CVP) via its vasodilatory action. Nitroglycerin also decreases SVR and pulmonary vascular resistance (PVR). Whenever myocardial ischemia is suspected postoperatively, NTG may be ordered because of its ability to dilate the coronary arteries and increase coronary blood flow. This agent also decreases pulmonary congestion and myocardial oxygen consumption (Treavor, Katzung, & Kruidering-Hall, 2015).

In addition to treating hypertension, decreasing preload or afterload, and treating myocardial ischemia, NTG is also used in some centers on a short-term basis (12–48 hr) to prevent spasm of internal thoracic arteries in the postoperative period.

Dosage. Infusion rates for NTG may be set as low as 5 to 10 mcg/min. The rate is titrated in 5-mcg increments until a mean arterial pressure (MAP) goal has been attained. Titration to effect can occur as often as every 5 to 10 min owing to the short half-life of NTG. This agent has an immediate onset of action and the drug effects last 30 min (Alexander, 2014).

Side Effects. One potential side effect of NTG is hypoxia—a condition caused by the drug's inhibition of pulmonary arterial vasoconstriction, which in turn increases blood flow through poorly oxygenated lung areas (Lumb & Slinger, 2015). Other side effects that are often reported with NTG administration include lightheadedness, headache, hypotension, reflex tachycardia, dizziness, and flushing of the face and neck. Tachyphylaxis occurs within 6 hours of initiation of therapy (Alexander, 2014). Although rare, methemoglobinemia has been reported as being associated with intravenous (IV) administration of NTG (Ladha et al., 2017).

Nursing Implications. Abrupt discontinuation of NTG can cause coronary vasospasm. For this reason, close monitoring of rhythm, blood pressure, and hemodynamic parameters is warranted when the infusion is stopped. The drug dosage used depends on the desired effect, the patient's blood pressure, and hemodynamics, bearing in mind that increasing coronary blood flow may improve cardiac function. The advantages of NTG are its ease of titration and short half-life.

Nitroprusside

Mechanism of Action. Nitroprusside is a smooth muscle relaxant that is used to control hypertension and reduce afterload (SVR and PVR). A powerful arterial vasodilator, it lowers blood pressure by generating nitric oxide. Nitroprusside also increases venous capacitance and decreases coronary vascular resistance (Treavor et al., 2015).

Dosage. For afterload reduction, initial doses as low as 0.3 to 0.5 mcg/kg/min should be used and slowly titrated (every 10 min) up to 10 mcg/kg/min to maintain the blood pressure within specified goals. Nitroprusside has an immediate onset of action (the peak effect occurs in 2 min), and its effects dissipate rapidly (within 3 min) when the infusion is discontinued (Treavor et al., 2015). It rapidly reduces blood pressure and is converted in the body to cyanide and then to thiocyanate. Its adverse effects can be attributed mainly to excessive hypotension and excessive cyanide accumulation; thiocyanate toxicity may also occur. To avoid cyanide toxicity, its use should be limited to low doses (<2 mcg/kg/min) for less than 72 hours, and use at the maximum dose (10 mcg/kg/min) should not occur for more than 10 min. Thiocyanate toxicity can also occur, especially in patients with renal impairment who receive an infusion for more than 72 hours (Rodgers & Reed, 2017).

Side Effects. Administration of nitroprusside may produce reflex tachycardia, hypotension, and renal dysfunction. Rarely, patients may develop a decreased platelet count or hypothyroidism (thiocyanate impairs iodine transport). Owing to its dilation of the pulmonary arterioles, nitroprusside can decrease arterial oxygen content or worsen any existing ventilation/perfusion mismatch, leading to hypoxia. Methemoglobinemia may also occur, which will decrease the blood's oxygen-carrying capacity. Cerebral vasodilation with resultant increased intracranial pressure may occur, and it should be avoided in patients with suspected stroke or head injury. Nitroprusside may also inhibit platelet function; cause hypothyroidism, bradycardia or tachycardia, and electrocardiogram (ECG) changes; and decrease renal and cerebral blood flow (Hotlinger, Beebe, Kozhimannil, Prielipp, & Belani, 2014).

An excessive amount of cyanide in the plasma (>80 ng/mL) following nitroprusside administration—as a consequence of overdosage or depletion of endogenous thiosulfate (which converts cyanide to thiocyanate)—may result in nonspecific features such as nausea, malaise, headache, vertigo, dizziness, disorientation, confusion, psychosis, weakness, muscle spasm, and shortness of breath or more specific features such as generalized seizures (Udeh, Ting, Arango, & Mick, 2015). Metabolic or lactic acidosis may be the first sign of cyanide toxicity. Cyanide poisoning occurs when the infusion rate of the drug exceeds the excretion rate of cyanide (Udeh et al., 2015). Thiocyanate levels should be monitored daily; excess amounts can be removed with dialysis.

Nursing Implications. Nitroprusside can cause sudden, life-threatening hypotension if its use is not closely monitored. Care should be taken not to flush or initiate new medications in lines that contain nitroprusside, because doing so can result in abrupt hypotension. When nitroprusside is discontinued, the line should be aspirated and then flushed to avoid this possibility.

Like NTG, nitroprusside can cause pulmonary vasodilation with shunting of blood to atelectatic areas of the lung, resulting in hypoxia and a need for higher oxygen delivery. This effect is usually seen immediately and can be dose dependent. If it occurs, another therapy may be chosen. Increasing positive end-expiratory pressure is helpful in resolving atelectasis.

Beta-Adrenergic Antagonists

Depending on the etiology of hypertension, beta-adrenergic antagonists (also called beta blockers) may be effective. The net effects of beta blockers are a decrease in heart rate (HR), BP, and CO. Beta blockers are discussed in detail later in this chapter.

Esmolol (Brevibloc®)

Mechanism of Action. Esmolol is an ultra-short-acting, cardioselective, beta-adrenergic receptor blocker. It inhibits the effects of $beta_1$ receptors. At higher doses, this agent inhibits $beta_2$ receptors located in bronchial musculature and blood vessels (Adams, Holland, & Urban, 2017; Parra, Roman, Anasthasia, & Straka, 2016).

Indications. Esmolol is indicated for intraoperative and postoperative hypertension, management of acute MI, and management of intraoperative and postoperative tachydysrhythmias. It is also used in the management of hypertension in patients with aortic dissection (Parra et al., 2016).

Dosage. For postoperative hypertension, the dose of esmolol is 500 mcg/kg, given as an IV bolus administered over 1 min. This bolus should be followed by a maintenance dose of 50 mcg/kg/min given over 4 min. If additional dosing is required after 5 min, the same loading dose followed by 100 mcg/kg/min may be infused over 4 min. This titration may continue by increasing the maintenance dose in 50-mcg/kg/min increments until the desired therapeutic endpoint or a maintenance dosage of 300 mcg/kg/min is reached. Because esmolol has a short half-life, it is a practical choice for treating patients with a labile blood pressure (Nagelhout, 2014).

Side Effects. Side effects commonly associated with esmolol include bradycardia, chest pain, hypotension, confusion, headache, dizziness, agitation, dyspnea, wheezing, fatigue, constipation, and nausea and vomiting. Serious but less common side effects include seizures, bronchospasm, and pulmonary edema. Anemia may prolong the half-life of esmolol. Esmolol should not be used in patients with acute heart failure, bradycardia, heart block (greater than first degree), or bronchospasm (Butterworth, 2013; Ramos & Varon, 2014).

Nursing Implications. Logically, any patient who requires an agent that causes beta-receptor stimulation should not receive beta blocker therapy. Esmolol is contraindicated in patients with cardiogenic shock, hemodynamic compromise, second- or third-degree atrioventricular (AV) block, first-degree AV block (if the PR interval is 0.24 sec or greater), or severe sinus bradycardia. Caution should be exercised when this agent is administered to patients with heart failure, bronchospastic disease, atrial fibrillation (AF) with associated hypotension, diabetes, renal impairment, or hyperthyroidism (Minczak, 2014). Because esmolol may require large volumes of fluid for its administration, thought should be given as to whether it is the appropriate drug for patients who may not be able to tolerate this excessive fluid intake.

The ICU nurse should monitor heart rate, blood pressure, and for signs of heart failure in patients receiving esmolol. Similarly, patients with diabetes should have their blood glucose monitored on a regular basis because esmolol may mask symptoms of hypoglycemia. Sudden withdrawal of therapy should be avoided because it can cause myocardial ischemia and hyperdynamic circulation (Butterworth, 2013).

Labetalol (Normodyne®, Trandate®)

Mechanism of Action. Labetalol is a nonselective, adrenergic blocking agent that exerts inhibitory effects on beta$_1$, beta$_2$, and alpha$_1$ receptors.

Indications. Labetalol is used on an off-label basis for postoperative hypertension. Data suggest it is effective when used on postoperative vascular surgery patients and in patients with aortic dissection (Upadhye & Schiff, 2012).

Dosage. For postoperative hypertension, patients receive 10 mg IV over 2 min. If additional doses are needed, 10 to 20 mg may be given every 10 min, up to a maximum dose of 300 mg in a 24-hour period (Butterworth, 2013). A continuous infusion starting at 2 mg/min may be used, with the same maximum cumulative 300-mg dose in 24 hours.

Side Effects. When labetalol is given for on-label conditions, serious side effects have included bronchospasm, hyperkalemia, and ventricular dysrhythmias. Commonly experienced side effects include bradycardias, edema, postural hypotension, diaphoresis, increased liver enzymes (less common), dizziness, paresthesias, elevated renal function tests, dyspnea, wheezing, and fatigue (Parra et al., 2016).

Nursing Implications. Like esmolol, labetalol is contraindicated in patients with cardiogenic shock, second- or third-degree AV block, or severe sinus bradycardia. It is also contraindicated in patients with bronchial asthma or chronic obstructive pulmonary disease. Caution should be exercised when labetalol is administered to patients with heart failure, bronchospastic disease, diabetes, heart failure, ischemic heart disease, liver disease, peripheral vascular disease (PVD), or hyperthyroidism. Monitoring by the ICU nurse should include heart rate, blood pressure, and signs of heart failure. Similarly, patients with diabetes should have their serum glucose monitored on a regular basis due to the potential masking of the signs and symptoms of hypoglycemia. Sudden withdrawal of therapy should be avoided (Butterworth, 2013). As with esmolol, any patient who requires an agent that causes beta receptor stimulation should not receive beta blocker therapy.

Angiotensin-Converting Enzyme Inhibitors
Enalaprilat (Vasotec®)

Hemodynamic Effects. Angiotensin-converting enzyme (ACE) inhibitors act on the renin–angiotensin–aldosterone system (RAAS). Specifically, they prevent the conversion of angiotensin I to angiotensin II by inhibiting ACE in the pulmonary and systemic vascular endothelium (Alexander, 2014). Because angiotensin II is a potent vasoconstrictor, inhibition results in vasodilation. Additionally, these agents prevent the production of aldosterone, which blocks the reabsorption of sodium in the kidneys. These agents cause a decrease in SVR and typically have little effect on heart rate. With the dosage described in this section, patients should experience improvements in both blood pressure and CO (Parra et al., 2016).

Indications. Angiotensin-converting enzyme inhibitors may be administered early after cardiac surgery to patients with mild left ventricular (LV) dysfunction, even in the face of moderate renal impairment (Hillis et al., 2011). Enalaprilat is the only ACE inhibitor available in an IV dosage form.

Dosage. The initial dose of enalaprilat is 0.625 to 1.25 mg, infused over 5 min. Additional doses, up to a maximum of 5 mg every 6 hours, may be administered.

Side Effects. The most common side effects with enalaprilat are cough, hyperkalemia, and renal failure. The cough is thought to occur due to the accumulation of bradykinin in the lung and vasculature (Benowitz, 2015). While benign, it should be treated by discontinuation of enalaprilat rather than with antitussive agents. Hyperkalemia occurs when aldosterone is inhibited secondary to the inhibition of angiotensin II. Enalaprilat should be avoided in patients with bilateral renal artery stenosis because a decrease in glomerular filtration rate (GFR) may occur. If acute kidney injury should occur, enalaprilat should be discontinued (Townsend, 2016). Angioedema with potential airway compromise is a rare side effect. The ICU nurse should observe the patient for facial or tongue swelling or reported airway swelling. Neutropenia can be a rare but serious complication. Patients may also rarely report dysgeusia (altered sense of taste) or blurred vision. The ICU nurse should observe for signs of onset of these complications and anticipate possible discontinuation of the medication if they occur.

Nursing Implications. For patients who have a history of renal insufficiency and who are receiving enalaprilat, nurses should monitor serum creatinine levels (Townsend, 2016). Meticulous monitoring of the patient's hemodynamic profile and hourly measurement of urinary output may help avoid the development of renal failure sometimes associated with ACE inhibitors.

Angiotensin Receptor Blockers

Angiotensin receptor blockers (ARBs) influence the RAAS by blocking production of angiotensin II from sources of angiotensin II other than the liver. The blocking of angiotensin receptors occurs on blood vessels, in the adrenals, and within all other tissues. The adrenal-related blockage results in a decrease in aldosterone levels, thereby leading to increased excretion of sodium and water from the kidneys. While there are many drugs in this class, common ARBs include oral losartan (Cozaar®), valsartan (Diovan®), and candesartan (Atacand®). There are no parenteral dosage forms.

ARBs cause less cough than ACE inhibitors, but otherwise have similar side effects. They are utilized predominately for hypertension management and require blood pressure monitoring after their initiation. Both ACE inhibitors and ARBs are contraindicated in patients with bilateral renal artery stenosis.

Calcium Channel Blockers
Nicardipine

Hemodynamic Effects. Nicardipine blocks the flow of calcium on vascular smooth muscle. It acts directly on arterioles to cause peripheral vascular and coronary vasodilation and lower blood pressure. It has little effect on contractility or AV node conduction. Nicardipine has also been shown to dilate the coronary vasculature (Krakoff, 2017). Administration did not affect ventricular preload or afterload or CO despite significant decreases in blood pressure (Aronson et al., 2008).

Indications. Nicardipine is indicated for the treatment of hypertension, including in the postoperative period (Adams et al., 2017; Parra et al., 2016).

Dosage. Therapy is initiated at an infusion rate of 5 mg/hr. The dose may be slowly increased by 2.5 mg/hr to a maximum of 15 mg/hr. Once the blood pressure endpoint is reached, a maintenance infusion may be run at 3 mg/hr (Cannon et al., 2013).

Side Effects. The most common side effects of nicardipine are headache, hypotension, nausea, vomiting, peripheral edema, headache, dizziness, and tachycardia. Serious adverse events that have been reported include angina and myocardial ischemia or infarction. Severe bradycardia has also been reported (Cannon et al., 2013).

Nursing Implications. Because of nicardipine's potential to cause negative inotropic effects, especially in patients with heart failure, portal hypertension, or significant LV dysfunction, caution should be exercised when administering this agent with a beta blocker. Close blood pressure and heart rate monitoring are required during therapy. Nicardipine is contraindicated in patients with advanced aortic stenosis, because this may reduce coronary perfusion resulting in ischemia (Parra et al., 2016). Nicardipine is prepared as a dilute solution; patients requiring large doses for extended periods may receive too much fluid.

Clevidipine (Cleviprex®)

Hemodynamic Effects. Clevidipine is an ultra-short-acting IV calcium channel blocker. It functions as both a smooth muscle relaxant and an arterial vasodilator. This agent causes a decrease in MAP and SVR, but it does not reduce filling pressures (Espinosa et al., 2016).

Indications. Clevidipine is used to treat postoperative hypertension without impairing cardiac function. In one study of postoperative cardiac surgery patients, treatment with this calcium channel blocker was effective in 91.8% of patients (Adams et al., 2017).

Dosage. The initial dose of clevidipine is 1 to 2 mg/hr via continuous infusion. The dose may be doubled in 90-sec intervals. Once the patient's blood pressure begins to approach the goal, less rapid dose titration (every 5–10 min) should occur. A maximum initial dose of 16 mg/hr is recommended, and a therapeutic effect is achieved for most patients at infusion rates of 4 to 6 mg/hr. The total 24-hour dosing should not exceed an average of 21 mg/hr (or 1,000 mL total) because of lipid load restrictions.

Side Effects. Reported side effects of clevidipine include headache, sinus tachycardia, hypotension, nausea, vomiting, and dizziness. Other side effects that have been reported include AF and acute renal failure. Although rare, cardiac arrest, MI, hypotension, and reflex tachycardia have occurred with use of this agent (Adams et al., 2017; Parra et al., 2016).

Nursing Implications. Administration of clevidipine is contraindicated in patients with an allergy to soy or egg products or with alterations in lipid metabolism (e.g., hyperlipidemia) due to its formulation in a lipid vehicle. Because of the phospholipid vehicle, it is recommended that the IV tubing be changed every 4 hours. Clevidipine is also contraindicated in patients with severe aortic stenosis, because it may reduce myocardial oxygen delivery secondary to afterload reduction. Caution should be exercised when administering clevidipine concomitantly with a beta blocker. Heart failure symptoms may be exacerbated due to this agent's negative inotropic effects. Patients may develop hypotension and reflex tachycardia when rapid titration takes place in an effort to increase the dosage.

When a patient is receiving clevidipine, the ICU nurse should continuously monitor heart rate and blood pressure during the infusion and until vital signs become stable. Blood pressure monitoring should continue for a minimum of 8 hours following discontinuation of clevidipine if the patient is not converted to another antihypertensive agent. Patients should also be monitored for exacerbation of heart failure symptoms because of its negative inotropic effects (Hempel & Prescott, 2018).

Selective Dopamine-1 Receptor Agonists

Fenoldopam Mesylate

Hemodynamic Effects. Fenoldopam mesylate is a dopamine-1 receptor agonist. The dopamine-1 (D_1) receptors are located in the coronary, mesenteric, and renal vasculature; when stimulated, they cause vasodilation (Bove et al., 2014). Fenoldopam also moderately binds to alpha$_2$ receptors, which results in lowered SVR and PVR and enhanced CO. This agent has rapid action as a vasodilator and increases renal blood flow (Parra et al., 2016).

Indications. Fenoldopam is indicated for the short-term treatment of severe hypertension, including during the perioperative period (Adams et al., 2017). It is believed to be especially useful in patients with renal insufficiency when administered in the prescribed dose range. Due to stimulation of dopamine-1 receptors in the kidneys, fenoldopam causes an increase in GFR, renal blood flow, and sodium excretion (Bove et al., 2014).

Dosage. The initial dose of fenoldopam is 0.01 to 1.6 mcg/kg/min. Titration can occur in increments of 0.05 to 0.1 mcg/kg/min every 5 to 15 min, to a maximum of 1.6 mcg/kg/min, to achieve the desired blood pressure. The doses must be administered as a continuous infusion; no bolus doses should be given. Fenoldopam should not be used for more than 48 hours. Fenoldopam may be discontinued progressively or rapidly once the desired effect has been achieved (Gillies, Kakar, Parker, Honoré, & Ostermann, 2015).

Side Effects. Possible adverse effects of fenoldopam include hypotension, dose-related tachyarrhythmias, flushing, nausea, vomiting, dizziness, headache, angina, cardiac dysrhythmias, heart failure, MI, hypokalemia (to <3 mEq/L), and serum creatinine elevation (Parra et al., 2016).

Nursing Implications. Caution should be used when fenoldopam is administered to patients who are concomitantly receiving beta blockers or in patients with hypokalemia, hypotension, liver disease, tachycardia, or glaucoma (increased intraocular pressure may result). During administration of this agent, the ICU nurse should monitor blood pressure, heart rate, and serum electrolytes, particularly potassium (Adams et al., 2017).

▶ Agents Used to Manage Postoperative Low Cardiac Output and Hypotension

Some degree of myocardial depression, low CO, and hypotension are common in the immediate postoperative period following cardiac surgery. These conditions can be related to preexisting cardiac disease, inflammation related to CPB, postischemic dysfunction, or reperfusion injury (Kouchoukos, Blackstone, Hanley, & Kirklin, 2013).

Low CO following CPB procedures is primarily due to LV dysfunction. This LV dysfunction may occur secondary to cardioplegic arrest, decreased preload, loss of vasomotor tone, intraoperative blood loss, increased capillary permeability, increased urinary output from hypothermia, dysrhythmias, or intraoperative MI (Kato & Matsui, 2017). Low cardiac output syndrome (LCOS), which may occur in postoperative cardiac surgery patients, is a decrease in CO secondary to a brief episode of myocardial dysfunction.

Contributing factors to postoperative hypotension include hypovolemia, vasodilation (relative hypovolemia), anemia, pneumothorax, hemothorax, cardiac tamponade, electrolyte imbalance, hemorrhage, metabolic alterations, and dysrhythmias.

Effective treatment of low CO and hypotension depends on quickly identifying the causes and initiating the appropriate treatment. Detrimental complications can occur even with brief periods of hypotension, so aggressive and prompt intervention is warranted.

When low CO or hypotension is accompanied by low CVP and pulmonary artery occlusive pressure (PAOP), volume resuscitation is needed to correct hypovolemia. A combination of crystalloids, colloids, and blood products may be used for this purpose. An in-depth discussion of volume resuscitation appears in Chapter 17.

If hypotension persists after volume resuscitation, it may be secondary to significant vasodilation. In this scenario, adrenergic agonists or vasopressors may be required to normalize blood pressure if the patient has normal pump function and remains unresponsive to volume repletion alone. It is best to begin pharmacologic intervention once the patient has adequate filling pressures and acid–base and electrolyte balance has been achieved (Silvestry, 2017).

Many cardiac surgery patients require vasopressor and inotropic support. In these patients, volume repletion, administration of vasodilators, pacing, or any combination of these may not be adequate (Silvestry, 2017). Typically, patients who improve with inotropic support are those with a cardiac index (CI) less than 2 L/min/m^2 who have optimal heart rate, cardiac rhythm, filling pressures, afterload, and absence of tamponade (Khalpey, Schmitto, & Rawn, 2012).

Adrenergic Agonists

Adrenergic agonists are used to normalize blood pressure when all known causative factors are corrected but hypotension persists. Any patient receiving an adrenergic agonist should be continuously assessed for hypovolemia, which may occur even after adequate volume repletion. Adrenergic agonists are often referred to as sympathomimetics, reflecting their ability to activate adrenergic receptors by direct receptor binding, promotion of norepinephrine (NE) release, blockade of NE reuptake, and inhibition of NE inactivation.

Adrenergic agonists are classified as either catecholamines or noncatecholamines. Catecholamines include epinephrine (Adrenaline®), norepinephrine (Levophed®), dopamine (Intropin®), and dobutamine (Dobutrex®). An example of a noncatecholamine is phenylephrine (Neo-Synephrine®).

Adrenergic agonists are notable for their specificity, with the various agents acting on $alpha_1$, $alpha_2$, $beta_1$, $beta_2$, or a combination of these receptors (**TABLE 12.2**). The precise ability of a drug to selectively activate certain receptors to the exclusion of others is dose dependent. Clinical activation of $alpha_1$ receptors results in vasoconstriction. Activation of $alpha_2$ receptors inhibits NE release and often has central effects. When $beta_1$ receptors are activated, patients experience a positive inotropic effect (increased force of

TABLE 12.2 Adrenergic Receptors and Effects When Stimulated

Adrenergic Receptor Type	Effects When Stimulated
β_1	Increased heart rate, blood pressure, contractility (increased inotropic effect), cardiac output, conduction velocity, and automaticity
β_2	Bronchodilation
α_1	Vasoconstriction
α_2	Vasodilation by inhibition of central norepinephrine release
Dopamine$_1$ (D$_1$), postsynaptic	Direct vasodilation
D$_2$, presynaptic	Vasodilation by inhibition of norepinephrine release
Vasopressin (V$_1$) (on vascular smooth muscle)	Increased peripheral vascular resistance and vasoconstriction of capillaries and arterioles

Adams et al., 2017; Maclaren, Mueller, & Dasta, 2017.

contraction) and increased blood pressure, heart rate, CO, and impulse conduction through the AV node. Activation of beta$_2$ receptors can also have positive inotropic (increase in contractility) and chronotropic (increase in heart rate) effects on the heart and cause peripheral vasodilation (especially in skeletal and muscle vasculature). When beta$_2$ receptors in the lung are stimulated, bronchodilation occurs.

Stimulation of dopamine-1 (D$_1$, postsynaptic) receptors, by contrast, causes direct vasodilation. Stimulation of dopamine-2 (D$_2$, presynaptic) receptors causes vasodilation by inhibiting the release of NE (Maclaren, Mueller, & Dasta, 2017).

Use of adrenergic agonists is typically initiated in the operating room (OR) during cardiac surgery, and patients can often be weaned from their agents rapidly after recovery from anesthesia. These drugs are titrated so as to maintain blood pressure within the ordered parameters—typically a MAP of more than 65 mmHg or a systolic blood pressure (SBP) of at least 90 mmHg. Higher pressures may be required to perfuse organs when patients have a history of extreme hypertension, carotid artery disease, PVD, or renal dysfunction (Adams et al., 2017).

All adrenergic agonists cause vasoconstriction such that significant tissue damage can occur if extravasation of these agents into the subcutaneous tissue occurs. Decreased blood flow to tissue as a result of vasoconstriction may lead to tissue death. Immediate treatment with an appropriate agent should be utilized promptly after extravasation of adrenergic agonists is suspected or identified. These agents should be given ideally via a central line to limit the risk of extravasation.

Six adrenergic agonists are typically used after cardiac surgery: phenylephrine, norepinephrine, epinephrine, vasopressin (antidiuretic hormone), dopamine, and dobutamine. These medications are used to elevate blood pressure for patients in hypotensive states.

Phenylephrine

Hemodynamic Effects and Indications. Phenylephrine is a vasoconstrictor that is often used after cardiac surgery to manage mild to moderate hypotension and to increase SVR when hypotension coexists. It causes vasoconstriction by activating alpha$_1$ receptors on vascular smooth muscle; no other adrenergic receptors are stimulated. The vasoconstrictor effects lead to an increase in SVR. Phenylephrine is also valuable in patients with a high CI who are profoundly vasodilated. A decrease in CO is seen with use of this agent, and either an increase or a decrease in heart rate may be seen (Jentzer, Coons, Link, & Schmidhofer, 2015).

Dosage. Phenylephrine should be started at a dose relative to the clinical situation. Effects are often seen immediately. The dose range is 0.05 to 1.5 mcg/kg/min (Levy, Schrader, & Ramsay, 2018). Patients may become refractory after several hours of phenylephrine infusing; a change to norepinephrine may be required.

Side Effects. Because of its vasoconstrictor activity, phenylephrine causes hypoperfusion to tissues and end organs, which can lead to visceral and renal ischemia. It also causes an increase in myocardial oxygen consumption and may exacerbate metabolic acidosis. Other reported side effects include hypertension, MI, tachyarrhythmias, ventricular dysrhythmias, and pulmonary edema. Care should be taken when administering phenylephrine or any other alpha agonist to patients who have undergone revascularization procedures with arterial grafts; spasm may occur (He & Taggart, 2016).

Nursing Implications. The patient should receive adequate volume resuscitation prior to receiving phenylephrine or receiving a significantly increased dose of this agent. Phenylephrine is contraindicated for use in patients with severe hypertension and tachycardia. Caution should be exercised when administering this drug to patients with bronchial asthma, diabetes, or hypertension. Heart rate and blood pressure should be monitored, preferably continuously.

Norepinephrine

Hemodynamic Effects and Indications. Norepinephrine is a powerful vasopressor and adrenergic agonist that stimulates alpha$_1$ and beta$_1$ receptors, causing vasoconstriction, increased inotropic effects, and cardiac stimulation. A small amount of beta$_2$ receptor stimulation occurs as well. Norepinephrine is classified as a vasopressor and an inotrope (Jentzer et al., 2015). It is typically used in profound hypotension when volume repletion is inadequate; it can also be administered concomitantly with fluid resuscitation if the patient's blood pressure and CO are significantly impaired (Jentzer et al., 2015).

Indications. Norepinephrine is indicated when patients have slightly low blood pressure due to low SVR.

Dosage. Norepinephrine is used in the dose range of 2 to 20 mcg/min or 0.01 to 3 mcg/kg/min and titrated so as to reach the desired response, usually a MAP of at least 70 mmHg (Levy et al., 2018). This dose will likely produce decreased peripheral and visceral blood flow, which may lead to the development of a metabolic acidosis.

Side Effects. The most clinically significant side effects experienced by the postoperative cardiac surgery patient receiving norepinephrine are an increase in myocardial workload and oxygen consumption. End-organ damage (e.g., damage to the kidneys and mesentery) may also occur secondary to alpha$_1$ receptor stimulation (Levy et al., 2018). Norepinephrine exacerbates hyperglycemia and metabolic acidosis, with acidosis occurring secondary to an increase in lactate production (Maclaren et al., 2017).

Nursing Implications. High doses and long-term use of norepinephrine cause decreased perfusion to the skin and can lead to tissue necrosis and limb loss. Patients should be assessed regularly for cyanosis, decreased capillary refill time, and diminished peripheral pulses, all of which are signs of decreased perfusion (Le & Patel, 2014). The patient should receive adequate volume resuscitation prior to receiving this therapy or receive a significantly increased dose of norepinephrine.

Epinephrine

Hemodynamic Effects and Indications. Epinephrine stimulates alpha$_1$, beta$_1$, and beta$_2$ receptors. It may be used after cardiac surgery as an inotrope to improve cardiac function and enhance SV, as an adrenergic agonist and vasopressor for refractory hypotension, or as a positive chronotropic agent to increase heart rate in bradycardia (Maclaren et al., 2017). Epinephrine is also useful in the cardiac arrest situation owing to its ability to enhance automaticity (Shah, 2015).

Dosage. Epinephrine's effects on different adrenergic receptors vary with the dosage used. At low doses (<0.02 mcg/kg/min), epinephrine causes stimulation of beta$_2$ receptors with resultant mild peripheral vasodilation and relaxation of the bronchial smooth muscle. At higher doses (0.008–0.06 mcg/kg/min), beta$_1$ stimulation results in an increased blood pressure, CO, and contractility. At doses of 0.5 to 4.0 mcg/kg/min, positive chronotropic effects are noted. At the highest dosage (>2 mcg/kg/min), alpha$_1$ receptor stimulation causes vasoconstriction, which results in an increase in SVR. The blood pressure effects of epinephrine vary in postoperative cardiac surgery patients. In particular, patients who are post-CPB demonstrate inconsistent hemodynamic responses to epinephrine administration. Variable responses in CO, heart rate, and MAP have been reported (Maclaren et al., 2017).

Side Effects. When higher doses of epinephrine are administered, patients may develop atrial or ventricular ectopy and tachyarrhythmias owing to beta$_1$ receptor stimulation. The higher the dose, the more likely that atrial or ventricular ectopy and tachyarrhythmias will be seen (Maclaren et al., 2017).

Epinephrine can raise the serum glucose levels so profoundly that insulin drips should be anticipated. Higher than normal doses of insulin may be required to maintain adequate glycemic control. The hyperglycemia is attributable to increased gluconeogenesis and the stress response to catecholamine administration (Maclaren et al., 2017). Hyperglycemia typically occurs in patients who receive epinephrine within the first 6 to 8 postoperative hours and usually disappears within a few hours after epinephrine is discontinued (Levy et al., 2018).

Patients receiving low doses of epinephrine may also develop metabolic acidosis due to low serum bicarbonate levels (typically between 17 and 21 mEq/L). This metabolic acidosis may occur secondary to the inadequate metabolism and lactate buildup that occurs in response to beta$_1$ stimulation. It is not related to hypoperfusion, as patients' cardiac performance is acceptable when the acidosis develops. Cardiac output and mixed venous saturation levels also remain within acceptable parameters. As with hyperglycemia, metabolic acidosis typically occurs in patients who receive epinephrine within the first 6 to 8 postoperative hours and usually disappears within a few hours of epinephrine's discontinuation (Maclaren et al., 2017).

Nursing Implications. While on epinephrine, the patient must be monitored closely for tachycardia and signs of myocardial ischemia—administration of this agent will increase PVR, SVR, lactate, and myocardial oxygen consumption. Adequate oxygenation should be maintained and the patient monitored for signs of ischemia, given that epinephrine increases myocardial oxygen demand. The ICU nurse should be prepared to quickly wean the patient from insulin if the epinephrine drip is reduced or discontinued. Hyperglycemia usually resolves within 6 hours or fewer after the epinephrine infusion is discontinued.

While increasing blood pressure and CO/CI are goals of therapy, vasodilators may be necessary to control elevated blood pressure when epinephrine must be used at high doses to maintain CO. Similarly, when epinephrine is infused at higher doses, alpha$_1$ stimulation causes an increase in myocardial workload, SVR, and PAOP (Maclaren et al., 2017).

Vasopressin

Cardiopulmonary bypass frequently causes the release of vasopressin (antidiuretic hormone), which may contribute to post-bypass vasoconstriction. Data indicate that vasopressin levels may diminish as hypotension continues. This finding suggests that the body may have a limited supply of vasopressin that is depleted following the initial hypotensive episode (Maclaren et al., 2017).

Hemodynamic Effects and Indications. Vasopressin is used to treat vasodilatory shock following CPB procedures in patients with profound hypotension (MAP <70 mmHg) despite fluid resuscitation, afterload reduction, inotropic therapy, and norepinephrine administration. Postoperative CPB patients who have protracted hypotension can demonstrate poor vascular smooth muscle response to catecholamines. Vasopressin, when administered in high doses, promotes contraction of vascular smooth muscle, which in turn causes vasoconstriction of the capillaries and small arterioles and can increase MAP. It is also believed that some patients have low vasopressin concentrations, such that exogenous administration may improve these patients' clinical status (Yimin, Xiaoyu, Yuping, Weiyan, & Ning, 2013). The postoperative cardiac surgery patients with vasodilatory shock who benefit most from vasopressin are those with a deficiency, often manifested by reduced response to high doses of other vasopressors. Those with a low ejection fraction (EF) who take chronic ACE inhibitors may also benefit (Thoma, 2013). In the VANCS randomized controlled trial, patients who received vasopressin (32%) versus norepinephrine (49%) showed a decrease in mortality (p=0.0014) and a lower occurrence of atrial fibrillation in the vasopressin group (63.8% versus 82.1%, p=0.0004) (Hajjar et al., 2017).

Vasopressin stimulates V$_1$ receptors on vascular smooth muscle, which causes an increase in peripheral vascular resistance and vasoconstriction of capillaries and arterioles. Vasopressin may improve LV function, which would result in an increase in CO and coronary blood flow (Yimin et al., 2013). Vasopressin increases secretion of corticotropin, a hormone produced by the anterior pituitary gland that stimulates the adrenal cortex. The adrenal cortex produces cortisol, a major hormone responsible for blood pressure regulation.

Dosage. The dosage of vasopressin needed to achieve vasoconstrictor effects is 0.01 to 0.1 unit/min by continuous IV infusion (Levy et al., 2018).

Side Effects. Side effects of vasopressin are rare but include end-organ damage from vasoconstriction, leading to hypoperfusion, hyponatremia, and increased SVR. All of these effects occur secondary to the drug's vasoconstrictive effects. Patients may also develop nausea, abdominal cramping, bronchoconstriction, water intoxication with resultant hyponatremia, and decreased myocardial oxygen delivery secondary to constriction of the coronary arteries (Hajjar et al., 2017).

Nursing Implications. Extreme caution should be used in patients with coronary artery disease who are receiving vasopressin because of the potential for extreme vasoconstriction associated with this agent. The ICU nurse should monitor for a number of adverse effects in the postoperative cardiac surgery patient, including decreased CO, chest pain, myocardial ischemia, ventricular dysrhythmias, bronchoconstriction, metabolic acidosis, tremors, gastrointestinal infarction, abdominal cramping, and water intoxication (Hajjar et al., 2017).

Dopamine and Dobutamine

The use of dopamine and dobutamine is required in many postoperative cardiac surgery patients even when careful attention is paid to intraoperative myocardial protection. Prolonged surgery, myocardial edema, advanced age, reperfusion injuries, and poor preoperative cardiac function are all factors that put the patient at higher risk for low CO postoperatively. Both dopamine and dobutamine cause an increase in CO and heart rate (Alexander, 2014).

Before these agents are administered, CO/CI should be high enough to sustain end-organ perfusion and deliver adequate amounts of oxygen to tissues. This criterion should be judged subjectively for each patient based on adequate urine output, normal capillary refill time, appropriate mentation, adequate blood pressure, warm skin temperature, and lack of acidosis. Objectively, CI should be more than 2 L/min/m^2 before use of dopamine and dobutamine is considered; normal CI in the nondiseased heart is in the range of 2.5 to 4.5 L/min/m^2. When preload has been optimized and SV remains low, poor contractility is the likely etiology and inotropes are indicated. Adding inotropes will increase the amount

of contractile force and result in an improved SV and CO/CI.

Dopamine

Hemodynamic Effects and Indications. Like epinephrine, dopamine's effects on different adrenergic receptors vary with dosage. Dopamine stimulates dopaminergic, alpha$_1$, beta$_1$, and beta$_2$ receptors, resulting in either vasoconstriction or positive inotropic and chronotropic effects (Jentzer et al., 2015). Stimulation of beta$_2$ receptors is less than that seen with the other adrenergic agents. Dopamine is used to increase blood pressure, CO, and perfusion through the renal vasculature. At higher doses, this drug has vasopressor properties, as it stimulates the release of endogenous NE. Dopamine also stimulates D$_1$ and D$_2$ receptors when administered in doses less than 8 mcg/kg/min (Jentzer et al., 2015).

Some data suggest that dopamine administration to post–cardiac surgery patients results in an increase in renal oxygenation secondary to vasodilation. No increase in GFR, sodium reabsorption, or renal oxygen consumption were reported (Ricksten, Bragadottir, & Redfors, 2013).

Dosage. Renal vasodilation occurs due to stimulation of dopaminergic receptors in the kidneys at doses of 0.5 to 4.0 mcg/kg/min. At infusion rates of 4 to 10 mcg/kg/min, beta$_1$ stimulation is seen. Positive inotropic and chronotropic effects lead to an increase in heart rate, blood pressure, contractility, and CO. At doses exceeding 10 mcg/kg/min, alpha$_1$ stimulation occurs, along with associated vasoconstriction and increased SVR (Jentzer et al., 2015). Dopamine's effect on renal perfusion in long-term outcomes remains controversial (Silvestry, 2017). This agent should be started at a low dose and doses titrated upward slowly to achieve the desired effect.

Side Effects. Common side effects of dopamine include chest pain, hypertension, palpitations, tachyarrhythmias, headache, anxiety, dyspnea, oliguria, nausea, and vomiting. Serious side effects include ectopic beats (including ventricular dysrhythmias), widening QRS complex, and gangrenous disorder (Levy et al., 2018).

Nursing Implications. Systolic pressures are often elevated with dopamine use, making it a poor choice in patients with pulmonary hypertension. Dopamine is also contraindicated in patients with tachyarrhythmias. As with other inotropes, caution should be exercised when administering this agent to patients with angina, hypovolemia, or ventricular dysrhythmias.

Like epinephrine, dopamine causes vasoconstriction, such that significant tissue damage can result if extravasation into the subcutaneous tissue occurs. Decreased blood flow to tissue from vasoconstriction may lead to tissue sloughing and death. Immediate infiltration with phentolamine (Regitine®) to the ischemic area should be implemented promptly after extravasation of adrenergic agonists is suspected or identified (Le & Patel, 2014).

Dobutamine

Hemodynamic Effects and Indications. Dobutamine is a synthetic catecholamine and positive inotrope that acts primarily as a beta$_1$ agonist. It causes an increase in CO/CI, while lowering SVR at high doses and increasing heart rate. It achieves these effects by increasing contractility and causing peripheral vasodilation (Jentzer et al., 2015). Dobutamine causes minimal amounts of alpha$_1$ receptor stimulation and a small amount of beta$_2$ receptor stimulation. This agent is useful when patients have low CO with high SVR or PVR and cannot tolerate vasodilators to decrease afterload. Dobutamine administration also results in enhanced coronary blood flow and decreased LV preload and afterload—more so than is noted with dopamine. Following cardiac surgery, vasodilation is frequently present with LCOS. Due to its inotropic effects, dobutamine is the drug of choice in this situation (Lomivorotov, Efremov, Kirov, Fominskiy, & Karaskov, 2017).

Patients with high pulmonary pressures, including those who have undergone mitral valve replacement, with or without a history of pulmonary hypertension, and with low heart rates may benefit more from dobutamine than from dopamine. This preference arises because dobutamine administration is associated with a decrease in PAP, LV stroke work index, CI, PAOP, and SVR (Adams et al., 2017).

Dosage. The onset of action of dobutamine is rapid, and it is rapidly cleared (2–3 min) when discontinued, allowing for rapid titration of the drug. The dose is 2 to 20 mcg/kg/min, and doses as high as 40 mcg/kg/min have been reported (Yancy et al., 2013).

Side Effects. While administering dobutamine, the ICU nurse should observe for hypotension, ventricular dysrhythmias, nausea, palpitations, shortness of breath, and myocardial ischemia. Other reported side effects include angina, dyspnea, tachyarrhythmias (increase in heart rate 5–15 beats/min), hypertension (increase in SBP 10–20 mmHg), and headache (Vardeny & Ng, 2016). Of note, dobutamine is less likely to cause dysrhythmias than other positive inotropic agents. As with other catecholamines, mild hypokalemia may develop.

Nursing Implications. Like other agents in this category, dobutamine should not be given to hypovolemic patients. Monitoring of blood pressure, heart rate, PAP, PAOP, CVP, CO, SVR, and urinary output should be performed on an ongoing basis to determine the drug's efficacy and the patient's tolerance of therapy. Evaluation of the patient's ECG and electrolyte status should also be performed on a regular basis.

Phosphodiesterase Inhibitors

Another category of medications that may be used to treat low CO after cardiac surgery comprises the phosphodiesterase (PDE) inhibitors. Two direct phosphodiesterase inhibitors—inamrinone (formerly amrinone, Inocor®) and milrinone (Primacor®)—are especially well-known agents. Inamrinone is no longer commercially available in the United States.

Milrinone

Hemodynamic Effects and Indications. Milrinone is a positive inotrope with vasodilator properties. Its administration will cause a decrease in

SVR and PVR, making it an ideal agent for patients with right ventricular (RV) failure. Milrinone also decreases coronary vascular resistance and, therefore, has a highly favorable effect on myocardial oxygen consumption (Yancy et al., 2013).

Milrinone enhances CO by directly inhibiting phosphodiesterase from metabolizing cyclic adenosine monophosphate (AMP) in myocardial cells. An increase in cyclic AMP causes an increase in the amount of calcium that moves into cells through the ion channels, thereby resulting in a more forceful contraction (i.e., inotropic effect).

Milrinone also produces venous and arterial vasodilation, and decreases SVR, PVR, and LV preload (PAOP), while minimally affecting myocardial oxygen demand and heart rate (Jentzer et al., 2015). All of these actions contribute to an improvement in CO/CI. It also produces vasodilation in vascular smooth muscle by decreasing intracellular calcium concentration. This effect causes relaxation of the vasculature and ventricles, thereby increasing SV and CO/CI and lowering afterload. In addition, milrinone promotes myocardial relaxation and improves coronary and mesenteric blood flow (Bangash, Kong, & Pearse, 2012).

Milrinone is indicated for the management of ventricular failure in the postoperative cardiac surgery patient. Because of its vasodilator properties, it is a valuable option in the management of patients with pulmonary vasoconstriction and RV dysfunction (Adams et al., 2017; Levy et al., 2018).

Dosage. A loading dose of 50 mcg/kg of milrinone may be given over 10 min, but is no longer recommended by heart failure guidelines. It should be administered via continuous infusion at a rate of 0.375 to 0.75 mcg/kg/min (Levy et al., 2018). Milrinone has a rapid onset of action, and a half-life of 2 to 3 hours following titration or discontinuation. The half-life is longer than that for dobutamine, making milrinone more challenging to titrate. As well, the half-life is prolonged in patients with renal insufficiency as the drug can accumulate (Jentzer et al., 2015).

Side Effects. Ventricular tachycardia or supraventricular tachycardia (SVT) may occur when milrinone is given, owing to the drug's proarrhythmic

properties. Hypotension should be anticipated related to the vasodilatory properties of milrinone (Yancy et al., 2013).

Nursing Implications. Patients receiving milrinone may require concomitant administration of an adrenergic agonist to counteract the profound vasodilation that occurs (Jentzer et al., 2015). Aggressive replacement of potassium and magnesium are recommended as well, because the dysrhythmias are more likely to occur when an electrolyte imbalance is present. Patients receiving milrinone should also be observed for hypotension during therapy. Patient improvement may be reflected by increased CO, decreased PAOP, and favorable changes in clinical indices. **TABLE 12.3** and **BOX 12.1** provide a summary of medications used to treat LCOS and hypotension following cardiac surgery.

Other Agents Used to Control Postoperative Hypotension

Methylene Blue (ProvayBlue®)

Hemodynamic Effects and Indications. Methylene blue is an inhibitor of nitric oxide, which is released in large quantities in patients following CPB. Nitric oxide produces profound vasodilation and vasoplegia (hypotension with normal or high CO, low CVP, low PAOP, and low peripheral vascular resistance) (Manghelli, Brown, Tadros, & Munfakh, 2015; Mehaffey et al., 2017). Methylene blue is not U.S. Food and Drug Administration (FDA) approved for the indication, but is frequently used in the treatment of vasodilatory shock or vasoplegia syndrome in the immediate postoperative CPB period (Lexicomp Online, 2017).

Dosage. The dosage of methylene blue is most commonly 1 to 2 mg/kg via bolus followed by a continuous infusion of 0.5 to 1 mg/kg/hr if the patient doesn't respond to the bolus dose (Manghelli et al., 2015).

Side Effects. The two main side effects of methylene blue administration are hypertension and a brief period of artificial low oxygen saturation

TABLE 12.3 Select Agents Used to Manage Postoperative Low Cardiac Output and Hypotension and Hemodynamic Effects

Agent	Dose	Mechanism of Action	Hemodynamic Effects
Adrenergic Agonists			
Epinephrine (Adrenaline®)	0.008 to 0.06 mcg/kg/min by continuous IV infusion	Stimulation of β_1 receptors	Increased contractility and stroke volume, and cardiac stimulation
	0.5 to 4.0 mcg/min by continuous IV infusion		Increased heart rate
	Less than 0.02 mcg/kg/min by continuous IV infusion	Stimulation of β_2 receptors	Vasodilation and relaxation of the bronchial smooth muscle
	Greater than 2 mcg/min by continuous IV infusion	Stimulation of α_1 receptors	Vasoconstriction; increased SVR
Norepinephrine (Levophed®)	2 to 20 mcg/min or 0.01 to 3 mcg/kg/min by continuous IV infusion	Stimulation of α_1 receptors	Vasoconstriction; increased SVR; decreased cardiac output; increase or decrease in heart rate
		Stimulation of β_1 receptors	Increased inotropic effects and cardiac stimulation
Dopamine (Intropin®)	0.5 to 3.0 mcg/kg/min	Stimulation of dopaminergic receptors	Renal vasodilation
	4 to 10 mcg/kg/min by continuous IV infusion	Stimulation of β_1 receptors	Increased heart rate, blood pressure, contractility, and CO
	Greater than 10 mcg/kg/min	Stimulation of α_1 receptors	Vasoconstriction; increased SVR
	Less than 8 mcg/kg/min by continuous IV infusion	Stimulation of D_1 and D_2 receptors	Vasodilation
Dobutamine (Dobutrex®)	2 to 20 mcg/kg/min by continuous IV infusion	Stimulation of β_1 receptors (increased contractility) and peripheral vasodilation	Increased CO/CI, and heart rate; decreased SVR and PAOP (more so than dopamine), PAP, left ventricular stroke work index, enhanced coronary blood flow

Agent	Dose	Mechanism of Action	Hemodynamic Effects
		Minimal amounts of α_1 stimulation	Vasoconstriction
		Small amount of β_2 receptor stimulation	Relaxation of the bronchial smooth muscle
Phenylephrine (Neo-Synephrine®)	100 to 200 mcg/min OR 0.4 to 9.1 mcg/kg/min by continuous IV infusion	Activation of α_1 receptors	Vasoconstriction; increased SVR; decreased CO; increase or decrease in heart rate
Vasopressin (antidiuretic hormone)	0.01 to 0.1 unit/min by continuous IV infusion	Stimulates V_1 receptors	Contraction of vascular smooth muscle, which causes vasoconstriction of the capillaries and small arterioles and can increase mean arterial pressure
PDE Inhibitors			
Inamrinone (Inocor®)	Loading dose: 0.75 mg/kg administered over 2 to 3 min Maintenance dose: 10 to 30 mcg/kg/min by continuous infusion Additional loading doses at 0.75 mg/kg may be administered. Total daily dose should not exceed 10 mg/kg/day	PDE inhibitor; venous and arterial vasodilation; vasodilation in vascular smooth muscle by decreasing intracellular calcium concentration	Increased CO/CI and SV; decreased SVR, PVR, and PAOP; promotes myocardial relaxation and improves coronary skeletal muscle, and mesenteric blood flow
Milrinone (Primacor®)	Maintenance dose: 0.125 to 0.75 mcg/kg/min by continuous infusion	PDE inhibitor; positive inotrope and vasodilator	Increased CO/CI and SV; decreased SVR, PVR, and PAOP; promotes myocardial relaxation and improves coronary skeletal muscle, and mesenteric blood flow
Other Agent			
Methylene blue (Urolene Blue®)	1 to 2 mg/kg administered as a slow IV push	Inhibitor of nitric oxide	Vasodilation

CO/CI, cardiac output/cardiac index; IV, intravenous; PAOP, pulmonary artery occlusive pressure; PAP, pulmonary artery pressure; PDE, phosphodiesterase; PVR, pulmonary vascular resistance; SV, stroke volume; SVR, systemic vascular resistance.

Adams et al., 2017; Alexander, 2014; Jentzer et al., 2015; Levy et al., 2018; Yancy et al., 2013.

BOX 12.1 Vasoactive Agents Used to Manage Postoperative Low Cardiac Output and Hypotension and Hemodynamic Effects

Agent	MAP	PAP	PAOP	CO/CI	SVR	PVR
Epinephrine	+	+/–	+/–	+	+/–	+/–
Norepinephrine	++	++	++	+	++	++
Dopamine	+/–	+/–	+/–	+	+/–	+/–
Dobutamine	+/–	–	–	+	–	–
Phenylephrine	++	~	+	~	++	++
Vasopressin	++	–	~	~	++	–/~
Inamrinone	–	–	–	+	–	–
Milrinone	–	–	–	+	–	–
Methylene blue	+	+	~	~	+	+

CI, cardiac index; CO, cardiac output; MAP, mean arterial pressure; PAOP, pulmonary artery occlusive pressure; PAP, pulmonary artery pressure; PVR, pulmonary vascular resistance; SVR, systemic vascular resistance.

+, increase; –, decrease; ~, no change

Alexander, 2014; Jentzer et al., 2015; Vardeny & Ng, 2016.

on pulse oximetry. Other reported side effects include hypotension, abdominal pain, dizziness, headache, confusion, nausea, vomiting, and diarrhea. Serious adverse events reported include cardiac dysrhythmias, malignant hyperthermia, and methemoglobinemia (Manghelli et al., 2015).

Nursing Implications. Following administration of methylene blue, the ICU nurse should observe for hypertension, urine discoloration, and transiently low oxygen saturation on pulse oximetry. The (false) decreased oxygenation saturation on pulse oximetry is short lived, lasting less than 10 min and results from interference with light absorption (Chan, Chan, & Chan, 2013). If the patient's oxygen saturation is in question during this time, evaluation with an arterial blood gas should be performed (Ladha et al., 2017). The ICU nurse should anticipate immediate increases in SVR and MAP and the need to significantly lower the infusion rate of norepinephrine. The ICU nurse should also monitor methemoglobin levels, complete blood count results, and blood pressure during administration of methylene blue. Caution should be exercised when this agent is administered to patients with renal impairment or glucose-6-phosphate dehydrogenase (G6PD) deficiency (Hassan, Al-Riyami,

Al-Huneini, Al-Farsi, & Al-Khabori, 2014; Manghelli et al., 2015).

Dexamethasone (Decadron®)

Despite supportive data, and possibly because the data are inconsistent (Murphy, Whitlock, Gutsche, & Augoustides, 2013), the routine use of steroids remains controversial in cardiac surgery patients. Their mechanism of action and the pathophysiologic changes that occur during cardiac surgery, which can result in adrenal insufficiency, have been cited as justifications for their administration in this scenario.

Any postoperative cardiac surgery patient exhibiting protracted vasodilatory shock should be suspected of having adrenal insufficiency. In cardiac surgery patients with physiologic stress, a low or normal cortisol level can be assumed to be associated with adrenal insufficiency (Krüger & Ludman, 2014). Cortisol plays a vital role in regulating blood pressure by increasing the sensitivity of the vasculature to endogenous epinephrine and norepinephrine. In the absence of normal cortisol levels, widespread vasodilation occurs secondary to the effects of proinflammatory mediators.

Mechanism of Action. Steroids decrease inflammation by suppressing neutrophil migration, decreasing production of proinflammatory mediators, and reversing the increase in capillary permeability. In patients with adrenal insufficiency, their mineralocorticoid effects can promote sodium and water retention (Nieman, 2017).

Indications. Corticosteroids are used in cardiac surgery cases involving persistent postoperative hemodynamic instability associated with a CPB-induced inflammatory response. They are additionally used in patients with known preoperative adrenal insufficiency (e.g., those on preoperative chronic steroid therapy).

Hydrocortisone (Solu-Cortef®)

Indications. Hydrocortisone is used in cases involving postoperative hemodynamic instability associated with a CPB-induced inflammatory response.

Dosage. The dosage of hydrocortisone is based on the indication. For acute adrenal insufficiency, the recommended dose is an initial 100-mg IV bolus, then 200 to 300 mg/day. Common doses include 100 mg every 8 hours or 50 mg every 6 hours. Alternatively, the total daily dose may be administered as a continuous infusion. Doses should be gradually tapered down over 3 to 7 days depending on patient response (Nieman, 2016). In patients receiving chronic preoperative steroids, patients should be tapered to their preoperative regimen.

Side Effects. Side effects that are reported as being related to administration of hydrocortisone include insomnia, hyperglycemia, and delirium. Potentially serious adverse events include, but are not limited to, hypertension, edema, headache, seizure, mood swings, bruising, hypokalemia, Cushing's syndrome, sodium and water retention, abdominal distention, stress ulcer, and immunosuppression (Nieman, 2017).

Nursing Implications. Withdrawal and discontinuation of hydrocortisone should be done slowly, with gradual tapering of the dose (Nieman, 2016). Patients receiving chronic preoperative steroids should be tapered to their preoperative regimen.

▶ Agents Used to Prevent or Control Postoperative Dysrhythmias

As discussed in Chapter 15, postoperative dysrhythmias are common in cardiac surgery patients. Several potential etiologic factors have been identified, including preexisting cardiac conditions (e.g., pericarditis), structural heart disease; infarction, ischemia, or enlargement; respiratory complications (e.g., acute respiratory distress syndrome [ARDS]); electrolyte imbalance (e.g., hypokalemia, hyperkalemia, hypomagnesemia); surgical trauma (intraoperative injury to the atrium, inadequate cardioprotection during CPB); hypothermia; hyperadrenergic state; acid–base imbalance; anxiety; and pain (Peretto, Durante, Limite, & Cianflone, 2014). Prior to intervening with pharmacotherapy, any underlying causes should be treated. Atrial and ventricular dysrhythmias, including bradyarrhythmias and tachyarrhythmias, may be experienced by cardiac surgery patients.

The most common antiarrhythmic medications used in the immediate postoperative phase are categorized as Class I, II, III, or IV agents. Class I agents are sodium channel blockers and include quinidine (Quinaglute®), procainamide (Pronestyl®), disopyramide (Norpace®), lidocaine (Xylocaine®), propafenone (Rythmol®), and flecainide (Tambocor®). Class II agents are beta blockers and include metoprolol (Lopressor®, Toprol®) and carvedilol (Coreg®). Class III agents delay repolarization and include amiodarone (Cordarone®) and ibutilide (Corvert®). Class IV agents include the calcium channel blockers diltiazem (Cardizem®) and verapamil (Calan®) (**BOX 12.2**). The agents used most often for postoperative cardiac surgery patients are discussed here and are summarized in **TABLE 12.4**.

Agents Used to Manage Atrial Dysrhythmias

As noted in Chapter 15, AF is a common dysrhythmia that may occur in 20% to 50% of postoperative

BOX 12.2 Categories of Antiarrhythmic Therapy

Category	Mechanism of Action
Class I	Sodium channel blockers
Class II	Beta blockers
Class III	Delays repolarization; prolongs action potential by affecting potassium channels
Class IV	Calcium channel blockers

cardiac surgery patients. Given that most patients remain in the ICU for 24 hours or less, AF may not appear until after the patient leaves the ICU. However, this complication can have major consequences for both the patient and the health care system (Gillinov et al., 2016; Peretto et al., 2014).

A wide array of medications are used to treat atrial dysrhythmias after cardiac surgery. The particular medication selected will depend on the drug's mechanism of action, the suspected cause of the dysrhythmia, and the drug's side effect profile.

TABLE 12.4 Agents Used to Manage Postoperative Dysrhythmias

Dysrhythmia	Agent	Dose	Mechanism of Action
Atrial fibrillation	Metoprolol	**PO**: Initial dose of 25 to 50 mg, followed by additional doses of 25 mg until heart rate is less than 100 beats/min **IV**: 5 to 15 mg (usually 5 mg) over 2.5 min; additional doses may be given at 7.5-min intervals	Class II, cardioselective beta blocker
	Carvedilol	**PO**: 6.25 mg BID or 3.125 mg BID in patients with heart failure. Titrated to a maximum dose of 25 mg PO BID	Class II, nonselective beta blocker, alpha blocker
	Amiodarone	**IV**: 150 mg given over 10 min, followed by a 24-hr infusion given at a rate of 1 mg/min for the first 6 hr and at a rate of 0.5 mg/min for the next 18 hr, if required Total loading dose: 5 to 10 g	Class III but possesses properties in all four categories of agents Blocks potassium channels, which prolongs the duration of the action potential and decreases membrane excitability Slows heart rate by depressing SA node Increases refractoriness of AV node Decreases impulse conduction by indirectly blocking sodium channels, and blocking beta-adrenergic receptors Increases atrial and ventricular refractoriness Inhibits alpha-adrenergic receptors

Dysrhythmia	Agent	Dose	Mechanism of Action
	Ibutilide	**IV**: For patients who weigh 60 kg or greater: 1 mg over 10 min For patients who weigh less than 60 kg: 0.01 mg/kg over 10 min A second dose of equal strength may be administered over 10 min if conversion does not take place with initial dose	Class III antiarrhythmic
	Diltiazem	**IV**: Initial bolus: 0.25 mg/kg over 5 to 10 min Subsequent bolus: 0.35 mg/kg over 5 to 10 min after 15 min if needed Maintenance infusion: 5 to 15 mg/hr	Class IV Blocks calcium ion influx during depolarization of cardiac and vascular smooth muscle Decreases vascular resistance and causes relaxation of the vascular smooth muscle, resulting in a decrease in blood pressure Negative inotropic effect
	Digoxin	**IV or PO**: Total loading dose: 0.5 to 1 mg, given as ½ total dose initially, then ¼ total dose given at intervals of 6 to 8 hr in 2 follow-up doses **PO maintenance dose**: 0.125 to 0.375 mg daily **IV maintenance dose**: 0.125 to 0.25 mg daily	May control ventricular rate Slows conduction at the AV node and increases refractory period Positive inotrope
	Adenosine	**IV Initial dose**: 6-mg rapid IV push followed by 20 mL normal saline **Subsequent IV doses**: 12-mg IV push followed by 20 mL normal saline	Transient depression of LV function. Slows SA node impulse formation. Slows conduction through the AV node. Can interrupt reentry pathways through the AV node. Coronary vasodilation.
Ventricular dysrhythmias	Amiodarone	**VF, pulseless VT initial bolus**: 300-mg IV push A maximum of 2.2 g may be given in 24 hr **Continuous infusion**: 1 mg/min for the first 6 hr and at a rate of 0.5 mg/min for the next 18 hr, if required Total loading dose: 10 g	See description in AF.

(continues)

TABLE 12.4 Agents Used to Manage Postoperative Dysrhythmias			*(continued)*
Dysrhythmia	**Agent**	**Dose**	**Mechanism of Action**
	Lidocaine	**VF, pulseless VT initial bolus**: 1 to 1.5 mg/kg **Subsequent bolus doses**: 0.5 to 0.75 mg/kg every 5 to 10 min **Continuous infusion**: 1 to 4 mg/min Maximum dose is 3 mg/kg in 24 hr	Class I antiarrhythmic agent.
	Sotalol	**PO**: 80 to 160 mg every 12 hr; if necessary, may increase dose to 240 to 320 mg/day ***IV initial**: 75 mg over 5 hr daily or BID **IV maintenance**: 75 to 300 mg over 5 hr daily or BID; may increase by 75 mg/day every 3 days * Start IV therapy only if baseline QT interval is less than 450 msec.	Classes II and III; non-cardioselective beta blocker

AF, atrial fibrillation; AV, atrioventricular; BID, two times per day; CPB, cardiopulmonary bypass; IV, intravenous; PO, by mouth; LV, left ventricular; VF, ventricular fibrillation; VT, ventricular tachycardia.
Alexander, 2014; Sanoski & Bauman, 2017.

Prior to initiating treatment of AF, three criteria are considered. First, determination is made as to whether the patient is hemodynamically stable or unstable with the presence of AF. The ICU nurse can identify the presence of hemodynamic compromise by assessing for hypotension, altered mental status, presence of chest pain, shortness of breath, poor peripheral perfusion, decreased urinary output, signs of impaired CO, or increased preload (Khalpey et al., 2012).

Next, precipitating factors should be identified. These conditions may include patient-related risk factors such as age, comorbidities, structural heart disease, ischemia, increased sympathetic tone, electrolyte or acid–base imbalance, pulmonary disorders, and surgery-related risk factors such as perioperative drugs and hemodynamic stress (Peretto et al., 2014).

Lastly, the goal of therapy needs to be decided. Therapy can be aimed at restoring normal sinus rhythm (rhythm control) or at controlling the rate

of AF (rate control). Direct current cardioversion can also be used alone or in combination with medications. The ultimate goal is hemodynamic stability (Gillinov et al., 2016; Peretto et al., 2014). Unfortunately, the evidence remains inconclusive on whether rate control versus rhythm control is better in these patients (Gillinov et al., 2016). Agents that may be used to control rate include beta blockers or calcium channel blockers. Refer to Chapter 15 for details on each of the agents used to control postoperative cardiac surgery dysrhythmias.

Agents to Treat Electrolyte Imbalances

Correcting electrolyte imbalances is paramount in preventing and correcting all dysrhythmias. The goal of treatment is to lower the heart rate, thereby reducing the workload on the heart and promoting conversion back to sinus rhythm as soon as possible. As described in Chapter 17, numerous factors related to cardiac surgery put the patient at risk for developing postoperative acid–base and electrolyte disturbances. These factors include anesthesia, induced hypothermia, physiologic effects of CPB techniques, shock resulting in acute kidney injury, cardioplegia, rapid fluid and electrolyte shifts across fluid compartments following CPB, stress associated with surgery, intraoperative volume repletion, hemodilution, and the rewarming process that follows hypothermia (Khalpey et al., 2012). An in-depth discussion of the management of the common electrolyte imbalances experienced by postoperative cardiac surgery patients appears in Chapter 17.

▶ Other Agents That May Be Required in Postoperative Cardiac Surgery Patients

Naloxone (Narcan®)

Mechanism of Action

Naloxone is an opioid antagonist that effectively blocks the effects of opioids that have been administered. It has the greatest affinity for the mu receptor but competes for the mu, kappa, and sigma opiate receptor sites in the central nervous system (Butterworth, Mackey, & Wasnick, 2013).

Indications

Naloxone may be used in patients with hypoventilation following opioid analgesic administration.

Dosage

For reversal of opioid-induced respiratory depression, the dose is 0.4 to 2 mg IV. It may be repeated every 2 to 3 min as needed until the desired effect is achieved (Butterworth et al., 2013).

Side Effects

Side effects associated with naloxone are rare, but include cardiac dysrhythmias, tachycardia, hypertension, hypotension, ventricular fibrillation (VF), pulmonary edema, and hepatotoxicity (Butterworth et al., 2013). Additionally, in patients with opioid dependence, it can precipitate acute withdrawal symptoms.

Nursing Implications

Care should be taken to closely monitor for continued hypoventilation, because naloxone's duration is much shorter than many opioids. The dose should be titrated to patient effect. The ICU nurse should monitor blood pressure, heart rate, and respiratory rate following administration of naloxone. In addition, a decline in opioid medication effects, including worsening pain and possible withdrawal symptoms, should be anticipated.

▶ Prophylactic Antibiotics

Patients who undergo CPB are at an increased risk of postoperative infection if they do not receive prophylactic antibiotic therapy. Administration of prophylactic antibiotics preoperatively and continuing for up to 24 hours postoperatively significantly decreases postoperative infection rates (Bratzler et al., 2013). These infections have high mortality rates (e.g., mediastinitis is as high as 47%) (Paruk, Sime, Lipman, & Roberts, 2017).

Cardiopulmonary bypass causes a number of physiologic consequences that suggest that stopping antibiotics may not be advisable. Specifically, CPB compromises humeral immunologic defenses, decreases phagocytosis, and activates white blood cells. Further, the length of the procedure, prolonged perfusion times, amount of time on mechanical ventilation, use of intra-aortic counterpulsation devices, and redo surgery are among the risk factors of surgical site infections (Cove, Spelman, & MacLaren, 2012).

Antibiotic selection is area and facility specific, typically based on the institutional antibiograms that are reported. However, first generation cephalosporins, such as cefazolin, are generally recommended both preoperatively and for up to 24 hours postoperatively provided the population does not have a high incidence of methicillin-resistant *Staphylococcus aureus* (Bratzler et al., 2013).

▶ Agents Used to Control Postoperative Bleeding

As discussed further in Chapter 13, the incidence of excessive postoperative bleeding (defined as loss of more than 500 mL of blood in the first postoperative hour) following cardiac surgery can lead to increased morbidity and mortality; the actual incidence is procedure dependent (Ranucci, Baryshnikova, Pistuddi, Menicanti, & Frigiola, 2017). Postoperative bleeding may be surgical in origin or multifactorial, related to the effects of preoperative medications (anticoagulants and antiplatelet agents), coagulation system dysfunction from exposure to CPB circuitry, or attributable to inadequate heparin reversal at the end of CPB (Ranucci et al., 2017). Depending on the etiology of the bleeding, pharmacologic intervention may be warranted.

Protamine Sulfate

Mechanism of Action

Protamine sulfate acts a reversal agent for heparin that when combined with heparin forms an inactive salt. It can also partially reverse the activity of low-molecular-weight heparin, such as enoxaparin (Lovenox®) or dalteparin (Fragmin®) (Welsh et al., 2014).

Indications

In the intraoperative period, protamine sulfate is routinely given to reverse the effects of heparin administered during CPB. Postoperatively, protamine sulfate is indicated for patients with a postoperative coagulopathy due to inadequate heparin reversal (Welsh et al., 2014).

Dosage

There are conflicting opinions about how to dose protamine. One way is based on the amount of heparin that needs to be reversed. In this case, the dosage is 1 to 1.5 mg protamine sulfate for every 100 units of heparin that needs to be reversed, up to a maximum dose of 50 mg. This dose should be administered no faster than 5 mg/min. The other method is based on heparin levels; it has been suggested that this method results in less postoperative bleeding (Welsh et al., 2014). Heparin is neutralized within 5 min of administration and the effect lasts for 2 hours (Levy et al., 2018).

Side Effects

Side effects of protamine sulfate administration include hypotension, bronchospasm, pulmonary artery hypertension (from pulmonary vasoconstriction secondary to a nonimmunologic reaction), bradycardia, flushing, decreased myocardial contractility, cardiac arrest from VF, urticaria, angioedema, platelet dysfunction, and non-cardiogenic pulmonary edema (Levy et al., 2018).

A protamine reaction may manifest in any of several ways. If this medication is administered too quickly, a histamine reaction can occur. Hypotension develops as a result of histamine release, with resultant decreases in SVR and PVR. These effects can be reversed with administration of an alpha receptor agonist.

A Type I reaction is either an anaphylactic or anaphylactoid reaction with associated hypotension, tachycardia, bronchospasm, flushing, and pulmonary edema. This reaction is often related to immunoglobulin E (IgE), causing release of histamine, leukotrienes, and kinins. The release of these substances results in capillary leak, hypotension, and pulmonary edema. Type I reactions may occur within the first 10 to 20 min (or more) following administration of protamine.

Protamine can also cause catastrophic pulmonary vasoconstriction, with associated increases in PAP, hypotension (secondary to peripheral vasodilation), left atrial depression, RV dilation, and myocardial depression. This kind of reaction is hypothesized to result from activation of various mediators of the inflammatory response. Complement activation leads to leukocyte aggregation, which causes pulmonary edema; the arachidonic acid pathway stimulates production of thromboxane, which causes constriction of pulmonary vasculature. The latter effect subsides in approximately 10 min (Bakchoul, Jouni, & Warkentin, 2016).

Nursing Implications

Patients with allergies to fish have a high risk of the anaphylactoid type of protamine reaction, because protamine sulfate is made of a protein found in fish sperm. In addition, caution should be used when administering protamine to men who are infertile or who have undergone a vasectomy, because antiprotamine antibodies may be present in these individuals (Bakchoul et al., 2013). There is also a 30- to 50-fold increased risk of protamine reaction in patients who take NPH insulin (Shokri, Ali, & El Sayed, 2016).

While a protamine reaction is more likely to occur in the OR, administration of protamine also may take place in the ICU if the patient experiences inadequate heparin reversal. If a protamine reaction occurs, in addition to administration of an alpha receptor agonist to increase SVR, management strategies that may be implemented include administration of the following therapies: 500 mg IV calcium chloride to increase SVR and promote contractility, an inotropic agent (e.g., low-dose epinephrine, dobutamine, inamrinone, milrinone) to decrease PVR, a vasodilator (e.g., nitroglycerin, nitric oxide) to decrease preload and PVR, aminophylline to manage wheezing, and heparin to reverse a protamine reaction.

Desmopressin (DDAVP®)
Mechanism of Action

For patients with CPB-induced platelet dysfunction, desmopressin stimulates the release of von Willebrand factor, which increases levels of endogenous factor VIII, factor XII, prostacyclin, and tissue plasminogen activator, thereby decreasing bleeding time and activated partial thromboplastin time (Mirmansoori et al., 2016).

Indications

Desmopressin may be used in patients with platelet dysfunction and bleeding secondary to CPB, and for prophylaxis of bleeding in patients with uremia (Mirmansoori et al., 2016).

Dosage

In cardiac surgery patients, a dose of 0.3 mcg/kg IV over 30 min is used. It is typically administered as a single dose, but dose may be repeated one additional time (Wademan & Galvin, 2014). Use should be limited to two doses total because of the lack of effect after two doses secondary to depletion of endogenous von Willebrand factor.

Side Effects

Desmopressin may cause hyponatremia, headache, or dizziness. While rare, thrombosis, including MI and cerebrovascular thrombosis, can occur (Levy et al., 2018).

Nursing Implications

The ICU nurse should observe for improvement in bleeding, including chest tube output, hemoglobin/hematocrit, and platelet counts. Urine output and serum sodium levels should also be monitored (Adams et al., 2017).

Recombinant Activated Factor VII (NovoSeven® RT)
Mechanism of Action

Recombinant activated factor VII activates the extrinsic pathway of the coagulation system. This action stimulates the generation of thrombin and leads to a subsequently rapid correction of the patient's prothrombin time. Factor VII also expedites platelet activation and ultimate fibrin clot formation (Hoffman, 2017).

Indications

As described further in Chapter 13, recombinant activated factor VII may prove helpful in achieving hemostasis in cardiac surgery patients with intractable bleeding. Factor VII is sometimes used following cardiac surgery in patients with coagulopathies who have already received standard therapies with blood and product replacement (Hoffman, 2017). It should be used with extreme caution, because it carries a thrombotic risk that could be detrimental to patients immediately following bypass grafting. In fact, although there are mixed results, some data suggest that because of an increased risk of stroke, factor VIIa is not recommended for routine use in cardiac surgery patients (Alfirevic, Duncan, You, Lober, & Soltesz, 2014).

Dosage

A wide range of activated factor VIIa doses have been used in the cardiac surgery population, with doses ranging from 20 to 90 mcg/kg, and 50 mcg/kg being a common dose (Alfirevic et al., 2014). The smallest effective dose should be used due to thrombotic risk (Hoffman, 2017).

Side Effects

Serious adverse effects that have been reported with recombinant activated factor VII use include SVT and thrombotic events—including MI, arterial thromboembolism, bleeding, coagulopathies, venous thromboembolism, cerebral artery occlusion, cerebral ischemia, acute renal failure, and pulmonary embolism (Hoffman, 2017).

Nursing Implications

The ICU nurse must carefully observe for and anticipate thromboembolic complications when the patient receives recombinant activated factor VII. Monitoring of coagulation profile results (i.e., prothrombin time, activated partial thromboplastin time, platelets, and international normalized ratio) and assessing for decreased postoperative bleeding are steps that should be taken to determine the efficacy of this treatment. Caution should be exercised when administering recombinant activated factor VII to patients with advanced atherosclerotic disease, coagulopathies, or septicemia because of the increased risk of thrombotic events associated with use of this medication.

Epsilon-Aminocaproic Acid (Amicar®)

Mechanism of Action

Epsilon-aminocaproic acid is an antifibrinolytic agent. It works by preventing plasminogen from binding to fibrin, thereby stopping the activation of plasmin and preventing clot breakdown (Network for the Advancement of Patient Blood Management, Haemostasis and Thrombosis, n.d.).

Indications

Aminocaproic acid is indicated for patients with postoperative bleeding that occurs secondary to fibrinolysis. It may be used to treat excessive bleeding following CPB, to decrease chest tube output, minimize blood transfusion requirements, and for fibrinolysis prophylaxis (Koster, Faraoni, & Levy, 2015; Ortmann, Besser, & Klein, 2013).

Dosage

For prevention of bleeding, the dose of aminocaproic acid is 75 to 150 mg/kg over 20 to 30 min followed by 10 to 15 mg/kg/hr intraoperatively (Lexicomp Online, 2017). For postoperative bleeding, additional bolus doses of 100 mg/kg IV can be given.

Side Effects

Side effects of aminocaproic acid include thrombocytopenia, agranulocytosis, leukopenia, coagulation disorders, dysrhythmias, pulmonary embolism, decreased vision, seizures, delirium, dizziness, headache, malaise, hallucinations, intracranial hypertension, muscle weakness, elevated creatine phosphokinase, stroke, and abdominal pain (Ortmann et al., 2013). Reported serious adverse events include bradyarrhythmias, hypotension, renal failure, and rhabdomyolysis (Levy et al., 2018).

Nursing Implications

Administration of aminocaproic acid is contraindicated in patients with disseminated intravascular coagulopathy. This medication should be used with caution in patients with cardiac, hepatic, or renal insufficiency. A definitive diagnosis of primary fibrinolysis must be made before administering aminocaproic acid.

Aminocaproic acid should not be administered rapidly. The ICU nurse should monitor the patient's complete blood count and coagulation profile prior to and after therapy. Evaluation for bradycardia, hypotension, dyspnea, and renal function tests should be conducted as well. The ICU nurse should observe the patient for signs and symptoms of thrombosis, including pulmonary embolism or stroke and arrange for appropriate testing as needed.

Other Coagulation Factors

In addition to fresh frozen plasma, factor eight inhibitor bypassing activity (FEIBA) and prothrombin complex concentrate (PCC) (Bebulin®, Profilnine®, Kcentra®) formulations have been used in off-label capacity in patients following cardiac surgery who have excessive bleeding. Prothrombin Complex Concentrate (PCC) (Human), as the name connotes, is a concentrate of coagulation factors derived from humans. Depending on the manufacturer, the product contains either three factors (II, IX, and X) or four factors (II, VII, IX, and X). It may also contain proteins C and S, which are natural coagulation inhibitors. Most preparations contain a small amount of heparin (Seller & Peng, 2013). Further studies are needed on the use of these agents for cardiac surgery patients.

Mechanisms of Action

FEIBA is a procoagulant (Maeda et al., 2013). Prothrombin complex concentrate increases plasma levels of factor IX and other factors in the concentrate to temporarily correct a coagulation defect caused by deficiency in these clotting factors (Rao et al., 2014).

Indications

FEIBA is used for hemophilia A (those with factor VIII deficiency). It has been used off label in patients following cardiac surgery with cardiopulmonary bypass who have life-threatening coagulopathies or excessive bleeding (Rao et al., 2014; Song et al., 2014). FEIBA is contraindicated in patients who underwent cardiac surgery under CPB and those procedures involving extracorporeal membrane oxygenation because of the high risk of thrombotic events, including a clotted hemothorax and distal extremity ischemia in one patient each (Balsam, Timek, & Pelletier, 2008).

Prothrombin complex concentrate is approved for use in patients with hemophilia B (those with factor IX deficiency) to prevent or control bleeding episodes. One formulation, Kcentra® PCC, is indicated for adult patients with a need for reversal of acute major bleeding related to acquired factor deficiency induced by vitamin K antagonist (e.g., warfarin [Coumadin®]) therapy (Cada, Levien, & Baker, 2013). Prothrombin complex concentrate is also used off label to control excessive bleeding after CPB (Arnékian et al., 2012).

Dosage

FEIBA is dosed based on body weight and is administered IV either with a syringe or with an infusion. Prothrombin complex concentrate is administered by IV infusion. The dose is based on different criteria, per product. For example, Kcentra® dosage is individualized based on the patient's current predose International Normalized Ratio (INR) and body weight (CSL Behring, 2017). Other product dosage is based on the number of factor IX international units (IU) required and body weight. Dosage may also be based on the amount of postoperative bleeding (i.e., whether major bleeding exists or not). A 1% increase in factor IX (0.01 IU)/IU administered/kg can be expected.

Side Effects

FEIBA side effects include thrombotic events and myocardial infarction. In one study, there were three deaths—two from multiple organ failure and one from respiratory failure (Balsam et al., 2008). The most common side effects reported for PCC include disseminated intravascular coagulation, myocardial infarction, and thrombosis. The most serious adverse reactions of Kcentra® were venous thromboembolic events (VTEs) (e.g., ischemic stroke, pulmonary embolism, deep vein thrombosis). There is a boxed warning on Kcentra® literature addressing VTEs. Common side effects of this agent include headache, nausea/vomiting, hypotension, dizziness, uricaria, fever, chills, and anemia (Cada et al., 2013).

Nursing Implications

Because many of the PPC formulations contain heparin, their use is contraindicated in patients with heparin-induced thrombocytopenia. Other contraindications are product specific. The nurse should refer to the package insert or other facility-specific reference to obtain contraindications. Patient education should include the risk of bloodborne pathogens and Creutzfeldt-Jakob disease since this product is derived from humans; no cases have been reported to date. The nurse should also monitor for a hypersensitivity reaction (HSR), as this complication is a possibility. If HSR occurs, the infusion should be stopped and facility-specific protocol for HSR should be followed. Monitoring for intravascular clotting (e.g., disseminated intravascular coagulation) is essential. Upon suspicion of a thrombotic event, the infusion should be stopped and the patient should be evaluated.

▶ Summary

Patients who undergo cardiac surgery may develop several alterations in their hemodynamic profile and their cardiac rate and rhythm in the immediate postoperative period. Alterations in preload, afterload, and CO may be treated with a variety of agents, each of which has its own side effect profile. An understanding of the pharmacologic agents used in the immediate postoperative period is essential. Part of the role of the ICU nurse is to stay current with data regarding pharmacologic agents used in the management of postoperative cardiac surgery patients. Implementation of recommendations published in updates and U.S. boxed warnings issued by the FDA is essential to help ensure patient safety. (**TABLE 12.5**). The ICU nurse must be vigilant in managing the complexities associated with administration of these agents and in using sound clinical judgment to help ensure optimal patient outcomes.

TABLE 12.5 U.S. Boxed Warnings Issued by the FDA

Agent	Black Box Warning
Nitroprusside (Nipride®)	Medication must be diluted. Frequent blood pressure monitoring required due to hypotension. Cyanide toxicity can occur; therefore, monitoring of acid–base balance and venous oxygen concentration is needed.
Norepinephrine (Levophed®), dopamine (Intropin®)	Infiltration requires the use of phentolamine mesylate (Regitine®) as soon as possible to treat extravasation.
Phenylephrine (Neo-Synephrine®)	The complete contents of the package insert should be reviewed prior to prescribing.

http://www.fda.gov.

🔍 CASE STUDY

A 67-year-old patient, has a history of class III angina. She has sustained a non–ST elevation myocardial infarction (NSTEMI). Three-vessel disease is noted on angiography. A left ventricular ejection fraction (LVEF) of 48% is reported. The patient underwent on-pump coronary artery bypass grafting (CABG), which included use of the left internal thoracic artery for the left anterior descending coronary artery and the saphenous vein graft to the posterior descending artery. The patient required vasopressor support to be weaned from CPB; total CPB time was 105 min. The patient received protamine to reverse the effect of heparin. At closure of the procedure, the patient remained hypotensive and tachycardic and remained on vasopressor support with norepinephrine at 0.35 mcg/kg/min. Upon admission postoperatively to the cardiovascular ICU, the patient remains intubated and on mechanical ventilation. Data are BP 70/30 (43), HR 115, CI 2.7 L/min/m², PAOP 8 mmHg, CVP 3 mmHg, and SVR 720 dyne/sec/cm⁻⁵.

Critical Thinking Questions

1. What is the etiology of this patient's hypotension?
2. Is her clinical picture consistent with vasodilatory (vasoplegic) shock?
3. What treatment can be added to the norepinephrine infusion?

Answers to Critical Thinking Questions

1. This patient likely has vasodilatory (vasoplegic) shock. This condition is a common complication following CPB, as CPB causes an inflammatory response; the associated mediators cause vasodilation. It is characterized by CO within normal range or elevated, low MAP, end-organ ischemia (e.g., oliguria), and elevated serum lactate levels.
2. The patient's clinical condition is consistent with vasodilatory (vasoplegic) shock. This type of shock is usually manifested with a MAP less than 50 mmHg, CVP less than 5 mmHg, PAOP less than 10 mmHg, CI at least 2.5 L/min/m², and low SVR.
3. In addition to norepinephrine, since the patient appears to be refractory to this infusion alone, methylene blue may be added. Steroids may be added as an anti-inflammatory agent. Phenylephrine may also be added to increase MAP.

Self-Assessment Questions

1. Which arterial blood gas (ABG) result should the nurse anticipate as a result of hypertension?

	pH	pCO_2	pO_2	HCO_3	SaO_2
A.	7.30	50	76	27	94%
B.	7.32	32	70	19	92%
C.	7.52	29	82	22	95%
D.	7.49	49	89	28	97%

2. Which change in hemodynamic parameters should the nurse anticipate when caring for a patient receiving nitroglycerin for post–cardiac surgery hypertension?
   A. CVP 12 to 14 mmHg
   B. MVO_2 35 to 48 mL/min
   C. SVR 1,400 to 11 dyne/sec/cm⁻⁵
   D. DO_2 900 to 760 mL/min

3. For which should the nurse teach the patient, who is being discharged with an angiotensin receptor blocker after cardiopulmonary bypass surgery, to observe?
   A. Decreased sodium levels
   B. Bounding peripheral pulses
   C. Fluid retention
   D. Cold intolerance

4. Which hemodynamic effect should the nurse anticipate when administering clevidipine to a patient following cardiac surgery?
   A. CVP 14 to 11 mmHg
   B. SVR 100 to 1,250 dyne/sec/cm⁻⁵
   C. PAOP 12 to 14 mmHg
   D. MAP 95 to 75 mmHg

5. A nurse should question an order to administer phenylephrine to a patient with:
   A. BP 190/100.
   B. RR 32.
   C. SVR 1450 dyne/sec/cm^{-5}.
   D. HR 156.

6. A patient receiving a low-dose epinephrine infusion should be monitored for:
   A. serum glucose 286 mg/dL.
   B. serum sodium 130 mEq/L.
   C. serum lactate 1.2 mmol/L.
   D. serum HCO_3 26 mEq/L.

7. Which should the nurse anticipate when administering milrinone to a patient with ventricular failure following cardiac surgery?
   A. SVR 900 to 1,100 dyne/sec/cm^{-5}
   B. HR 90 to 136
   C. PAOP 16 to 12 mmHg
   D. MVO_2 35 to 20 mL/min

8. The nurse should observe for which after administering methylene blue to a patient following cardiopulmonary bypass surgery?
   A. $PaCO_2$ 50 mmHg
   B. T 35.1°C (95.2°F)
   C. SpO_2 81%
   D. HR 56

9. A patient with a cardiopulmonary bypass–induced inflammatory response is to receive hydrocortisone for hemodynamic instability. For which should the nurse observe?
   A. Fluid retention
   B. Serum glucose 56 mg/dL
   C. Serum sodium 130 mEq/L
   D. Serum potassium 5.8 mEq/L

10. A patient is to receive naloxone for opioid-induced respiratory depression. For which should the nurse observe?
    A. Sinus bradycardia
    B. First-degree AV block
    C. Atrial flutter
    D. Ventricular fibrillation

Answers to Self-Assessment Questions

1. B. **7.32 / 32 / 70 / 19 / 92%**
   Rationale: Hypertension leads to increased afterload with a resultant metabolic acidosis.

2. C. **SVR 1,400 to 11 dyne/sec/cm^{-5}**
   Rationale: Nitroglycerin decreases preload and afterload. Decreases in PAP, CVP, SVR, PVR, and myocardial oxygen consumption (normal = 30–35 mL/min).

3. A. **decreased sodium levels**
   Rationale: Administration of an angiotensin receptor blocker can result in increased sodium and water excretion from the kidneys.

4. D. **MAP 95 to 75 mmHg**
   Rationale: Clevidipine causes a decrease in MAP and SVR but does not reduce filling pressures.

5. D. **HR 156**
   Rationale: Phenylephrine is contraindicated for use in patients with severe hypertension and tachycardia.

6. A. **serum glucose 286 mg/dL**
   Rationale: Patients on a low-dose epinephrine infusion may develop a metabolic acidosis, low serum bicarbonate levels, hyperglycemia, and lactate buildup.

7. C. **PAOP 16 to 12 mmHg**
   Rationale: Milrinone produces venous and arterial vasodilation and decreases SVR, PVR, and PAOP, while minimally affecting myocardial oxygen demand and heart rate. It increases SV and CI/CO by producing vasodilation in vascular smooth muscle and by decreasing intracellular calcium concentration.

8. C. **SpO_2 81%**
   Rationale: The two main side effects of methylene blue are hypertension and a brief period of artificially low oxygen saturation on pulse oximetry. Other side effects include hypotension, abdominal

pain, dizziness, headache, confusion, nausea, vomiting, and diarrhea. Serious adverse events include cardiac dysrhythmias, malignant hyperthermia, and methemoglobinemia.

9. A. **fluid retention**
Rationale: Side effects of hydrocortisone include insomnia, hyperglycemia, and delirium. Potentially serious adverse events include hypertension, edema, headache, seizure, mood swings, bruising, hypokalemia, sodium and water retention, abdominal distention, Cushing's syndrome, stress ulcer development, and immunosuppression.

10. D. **ventricular fibrillation**
Rationale: Side effects associated with naloxone are rare but include cardiac dysrhythmias, tachycardia with hypertension, hypotension, ventricular fibrillation, pulmonary edema, and hepatotoxicity.

CLINICAL INQUIRY BOX

Question: What is the rate of secondary prevention use of cardiovascular drugs in a cohort of patients who underwent CABG surgery from admission until 1 year postoperatively?

Reference: Barry, A. R., Koshman, S. L., Norris, C. M., Ross, D. B., & Pearson, G. J. (2014). Evaluation of preventive cardiovascular pharmacotherapy after coronary artery bypass graft surgery. *Pharmacotherapy, 34*(5), 464–472.

Objectives: To determine the rate of secondary prevention use of cardiovascular drugs in a cohort of patients who underwent CABG surgery from admission until 1 year postoperatively.

Method: Retrospective analysis.

Results: The percentage of patients discharged on aspirin, beta blockers, statins, and angiotensin-converting enzyme inhibitors (ACEIs) or angiotensin II receptor blockers (ARBs) was 35%. Patient use at discharge was 96%, 94%, 95%, and 42%, respectively. At 1 year postoperatively, adherence rates were 95%, 84%, 84%, and 65%, respectively.

Conclusion: The utilization rate for the four classes of cardiovascular medications was 35% at discharge and 48% at 1 year postoperatively. Adherence rates were high for aspirin, beta blockers, and statins at both time points. Adherence rates for ACEIs or ARBs were lower but showed an increase from discharge to the 1-year mark.

References

Adams, M., Holland, N., & Urban, C. (2017). Drugs for hypertension. In M. Adams, N. Holland, & C. Urban (Eds.), *Pharmacology for nurses. A pathophysiologic approach* (5th ed., pp. 375–394). Boston, MA: Pearson.

Alexander, E. (2014). Pharmacology. In S. Burns (Ed.), *AACN essentials of progressive care nursing* (3rd ed., pp. 151–180). New York, NY: McGraw-Hill.

Alfirevic, A., Duncan, A., You, J., Lober, C., & Soltesz, E. (2014). Recombinant factor VII is associated with worse survival in complex cardiac surgical patients. *Annals of Thoracic Surgery, 98*(2), 618–624.

Arnékian, V., Camous, J., Fattal, S., Rézaiguia-Delclaux, S., Nottin, R., & Stéphan, F. (2012). Use of prothrombin complex concentrate for excessive bleeding after cardiac surgery. *Interactive Cardiovascular and Thoracic Surgery, 15*(3), 382–389.

Aronson, S., Kyke, C. M., Stierer, K. A., Levy, J. H., Cheung, A. T., Lumb, P. D., . . . Newman, M. F. (2008). The ECLIPSE trials: Comparative studies of clevidipine to nitroglycerin, sodium nitroprusside, and nicardipine for acute hypertension treatment in cardiac surgery patients. *Anesthesia and Analgesia, 107*(4), 1110–1121.

Bangash, M. W., Kong, M. L., & Pearse, R. M. (2012). Use of inotropes and vasopressor agents in critically ill patients. *British Journal of Pharmacology, 165*(7), 2015–2033.

Bakchoul, T., Jouni, R., & Warkentin, T. E. (2016). Protamine (heparin)-induced thrombocytopenia: A review of the serological and clinical features associated with anti-protamine/heparin antibodies. *Journal of Thrombosis and Haemostasis, 14*, 1685–1695.

Bakchoul, T., Zöllner, H., Amiral, J., Panzar, S., Selleng, S., Kohlmann, T., . . . Greinacher, A. (2013). Anti-protamine-heparin antibodies: Incidence, clinical reference and pathogenesis. *Blood, 121*(15). Retrieved from http://www.bloodjournal.org/content/121/15/2821?550-checked=true.

Balsam, L. B., Timek, T. A., & Pelletier, M. P. (2008). Factor eight inhibitor bypassing activity (FEIBA) for refractory bleeding in cardiac surgery: Review of clinical outcomes. *Journal of Cardiac Surgery, 23*(6), 614–621.

Benowitz, N. L. (2015). Antihypertensive agents. In B. G. Katzung & A. J. Trevor (Eds.), *Basic & clinical pharmacology* (13th ed.). Retrieved from http://accesspharmacy.mhm edical.com/content.aspx?bookid=1193&sectionid=69104839.

Bove, T., Zangrillo, A., Guarracino, F., Alavaro, G., Persi, B., Maglioni, E., . . . Landoni, G. (2014). Effect of fenoldopam on use of renal replacement therapy among patients with acute kidney injury after cardiac surgery: A randomized clinical trial. *Journal of the American Medical Association, 312*(21), 2244–2253.

Bratzler, D. W., Dellinger, E. P., Olsen, K. M., Peri, T. M., Auwaerter, P. G., Bolon, M. K., . . . Weinstein, R. A. (2013). Clinical practice guidelines for antimicrobial prophylaxis in surgery. *American Journal of Health-System Pharmacy, 70*, 195–283.

Butterworth, J. F. (2013). Cardiovascular drugs. In J. F. Butterworth, F. A. Hansley, D. E. Martin Jr., & G. P. Gravlee (Eds.), *A practical approach to cardiac anesthesia* (5th ed., pp. 23–88). Philadelphia, PA: Lippincott Williams & Wilkins.

Butterworth, J. F., Mackey, D. C., & Wasnick, J. D. (2013). Adjuncts to anesthesia. In J. F. Butterworth, D. C. Mackey, & J. D. Wasnick (Eds.), *Morgan & Mikhail's clinical anesthesiology* (5th ed., pp. 277–294). Philadelphia, PA: Lippincott Williams & Wilkins.

Cada, D. J., Levien, T. L., & Baker, B. E. (2013). Prothrombin complex concentrate. *Hospital Pharmacy, 48*(11), 951–957.

Cannon, C. M., Levy, P., Baumann, B. M., Borczuk, P., Chandra, A., Cline, D. M., . . . Peacock, W. F. (2013). Intravenous nicardipine and labetalol use in hypertensive patients with signs or symptoms suggestive of end-organ damage in the emergency department: A subgroup analysis of the CLUE trial. *British Medical Journal, 3*(3), ii.

Chan, E. D., Chan, M. M., & Chan, M. M. (2013). Pulse oximetry: Understanding its basic principles facilitates appreciation of its limitations. *Respiratory Medicine, 107*(6), 789–799.

Chung, M., & Carlese, A. (2017). Postcardiothoracic surgery care. In J. M. Oropello, S. M. Pastores, & V. Kvetan (Eds.), *Critical care*. Retrieved from http://accessmedicine.mhmedical.com/content.aspx?bookid=1944&sectionid=143519793.

Cove, M. E., Spelman, D. W., & MacLaren, G. (2012). Infectious complications of cardiac surgery: A clinical review. *Journal of Cardiovascular and Vascular Anesthesia, 26*(6), 1094–1100.

CSL Behring. (2017). *Kcentra® package insert*. Retrieved from http://labeling.cslbehring.com/PI/US/Kcentra/EN/Kcentra-Prescribing-Information.pdf.

Espinosa, A., Ripollés–Melchor, J., CasansFrancés, R., Abad-Gurumeta, A., Bergese, S. D., ZuletaAlarcon, A., . . .

Valvo-Vecino, J. M. (2016). Perioperative use of clevidipine: A systematic review and meta-analysis. *PLoS ONE, 11*(3), e0150625.

Gillies, M. A., Kakar, V., Parker, R. J., Honoré, P. M., & Ostermann, M. (2015). Fenoldopam to prevent acute kidney injury after major surgery—a systematic review and meta-analysis. *Critical Care, 19*. Retrieved from https://www.ncbi.nlm.nih.gov/pmc/articles/PMC4699343/.

Gillinov, A. M., Bagiella, E., Moskowitz, A. J., Raiten, J. M., Groh, M. A., Bowdish, M. E., . . . Mack, M. J. (2016). Rate control versus rhythm control for atrial fibrillation after cardiac surgery. *The New England Journal of Medicine, 374*, 1911–1921.

Hajjar, L. A., Vincent, J. L., Galas, F. R. B. G., Rhodes, A., Landoni, G., Osawa, E. A., . . . Filho, R. K. (2017). Vasopressin versus norepinephrine in patients with vasoplegic shock after cardiac surgery: The VANCS randomized controlled trial. *Anesthesiology, 126*, 85–93.

Hassan, K. S., Al-Riyami, A. Z., Al-Huneini, M., Al-Farsi, K., & Al-Khabori, M. (2014). Methemoglobinemia in an elderly patient with glucose-6-phosphate dehydrogenase deficiency: A case report. *Oman Medical Journal, 29*(2), 135–137.

He, G. W., & Taggart, D. P. (2016). Spasm in arterial grafts in coronary artery bypass grafting surgery. *Annals of Thoracic Surgery, 101,* 1222–1229.

Hempel, C., & Prescott, G. (2018). Cardiovascular drugs. In T. L. Demler & J. Rhoads (Eds.), *Pharmacotherapeutics for advanced nursing practice* (pp. 311–368). Burlington, MA: Jones and Bartlett Learning.

Hillis, D. L., Smith, P. K., Anderson, J. L., Bittl, J. A., Bridges, C. R., Byrne, J. G., . . . Winniford, M. D. (2011). ACCF/AHA guideline for coronary artery bypass graft surgery: A report of the American College of Cardiology Foundation/American Heart Association Task Force on practice guidelines. *Journal of the American College of Cardiology, 58*(24), 2584–2614.

Hoffman, M. (2017). *Recombinant factor VIIa: Clinical uses, dosing, and adverse events*. Retrieved from https://www.uptodate.com/contents/recombinant-factor-viia-clinical-uses-dosing-and-adverse-effects.

Hotlinger, D. G., Beebe, D. S., Kozhimannil, T., Prielipp, R. C., & Belani, K. G. (2014). Sodium nitroprusside in 2014: A clinical concepts review. *Journal of Anaesthesiology Clinical Pharmacology, 30*(4), 462–471.

Jentzer, J. C., Coons, J. C., Link, C. B., & Schmidhofer, M. (2015). Pharmacotherapy update on the use of vasopressors and inotropes in the intensive care unit. *Journal of Cardiovascular Pharmacology and Therapeutics, 20*(3), 249–260.

Kato, H., & Matsui, Y. (2017). Perioperative care of low cardiac output syndrome. *Kyobu Geka, 70*(8), 565–570.

Khalpey, Z. I., Schmitto, J. D., & Rawn, J. D. (2012). Postoperative care of cardiac surgery patients. In L. H. Cohn (Ed.), *Cardiac surgery in the adult* (4th ed.). Retrieved from http://accesssurgery.mhmedical.com/content.aspx?bookid=476&Sectionid=39679028.

Koster, A., Faraoni, D., & Levy, J. H. (2015). Antifibrinolytic therapy for cardiac surgery: An update. *Anesthesiology, 123*, 214–221.

Kouchoukos, N. T., Blackstone, E. H., Hanley, F. L., & Kirklin, J. K. (2013). Postoperative care. In N. T. Kouchoukos, E. H. Blackstone, F. L. Hanley, & J. K. Kirklin (Eds.), *Kirklin/Barratt-Boyes cardiac surgery* (4th ed., pp. 133–162). Philadelphia, PA: Elsevier.

Krakoff, L. R. (2017). Diagnosis and treatment of hypertension. In V. Fuster, R. A. Harrington, J. Narula, & Z. J. Eapen (Eds.), *Hurst's the heart* (14th ed.). Retrieved from http://accessmedicine.mhmedical.com/content.aspx?bookid=2046&sectionid=155632214.

Krüger, W., & Ludman, A. J. (2014). Shock. In W. Krüger & A. J. Ludman (Eds.), *Core knowledge in critical care medicine* (pp. 159–272). London, UK: Springer.

Ladha, S., Aggarway, S., Kiran, U., Choudhary, A., Kapoor, P. M., & Choudhary, U. K. (2017). Diagnostic dilemma: Low oxygen saturation during cardiac surgery. *Annals of Cardiac Anaesthesia, 20*(2), 262–264.

Le, A., & Patel, S. (2014). Extravasation of noncytotoxic drugs: A review of the literature. *Annals of Pharmacotherapy, 48*(7), 870–886.

Levy, J. H., Schrader, J. N., & Ramsay, J. G. (2018). Cardiac surgery pharmacology. In L. H. Cohn & D. H. Adams (Eds.), *Cardiac surgery in the adult patient* (5th ed., pp. 71–98). New York, NY: McGraw-Hill.

Lexicomp Online. (2017). Retrieved from https://online.lexi.com/lco/action/home.

Lomivorotov, V. V., Efremov, S. M., Kirov, M. Y., Fominskiy, E. V., & Karaskov, A. M. (2017). Low-cardiac-output syndrome after cardiac surgery. *Journal of Cardiothoracic and Vascular Anesthesia, 31*(1), 291–308.

Lumb, A. B., & Slinger, P. (2015). Hypoxic pulmonary vasoconstriction: Physiology and anesthetic implications. *Anesthesiology, 122*, 932–946.

Maclaren, R., Mueller, S. W., & Dasta, J. F. (2017). Use of vasopressors and inotropes in the pharmacotherapy of shock. In J. T. DiPiro, R. L. Talbert, G. C. Yee, G. R. Matzke, B. G. Wells, & L. Posey (Eds.), *Pharmacotherapy: A pathophysiologic approach* (10th ed.). Retrieved from http://accesspharmacy.mhmedical.com/content.aspx?bookid=1861&sectionid=146057724.

Maeda, K., Asija, R., Hollander, S., Williams, G., Yeh, J., Rosenthal, D., . . . Reinhartz, O. (2013). Low dose factor eight inhibitor bypassing activity (FEIBA) for incessant bleeding in pediatric patients on mechanical circulatory support (MCS). *The Journal of Heart and Lung Transplantation, 32*(4), S290.

Manghelli, J., Brown, L., Tadros, H. B., & Munfakh, N. A. (2015). A reminder of methylene blue's effectiveness in treating vasoplegic syndrome after on-pump cardiac surgery. *Texas Heart Institute Journal, 42*(5), 491–494.

Mehaffey, J. H., Johnston, L. E., Hawkins, R. B., Charles, E. J., Yarboro, L. Kern, J. A., . . . Ghantal, R. K. (2017). Methylene blue for vasoplegic syndrome after cardiac operation: Early administration improves survival. *Annals of Thoracic Surgery, 104*(1), 36–41.

Minczak, B. M. (2014). Cardiac procedures. In J. R. Roberts & J. R. Hedges (Eds.), *Clinical procedures in emergency medicine* (6th ed., pp. 213–227). Philadelphia, PA: Elsevier Saunders.

Mirmansoori, A., Farzi, F., Sedighinejad, A., Imantalab, V., Mohammadzadeh, A., Roushan Z. A., . . . Dehghan, A. (2016). The effect of desmopressin on the amount of bleeding in patients undergoing coronary artery bypass graft surgery with a cardiopulmonary bypass pump after taking anti-platelet medicine. *Anesthesia and Pain Medicine, 6*(5), e39226. doi:10.5812/aapm.39226

Murphy, G. S., Whitlock, R. P., Gutsche, J. T., & Augoustides, J. G. T. (2013). Steroids for adult cardiac surgery with cardiopulmonary bypass: Update on dose and key randomized trials. *Journal of Cardiothoracic and Vascular Anesthesia, 27*(5), 1053–1059.

Nagelhout, J. J. (2014). Autonomic and cardiac pharmacology. In J. J. Nagelhout & K. L. Plaus (Eds.), *Nurse anesthesia* (5th ed., pp. 158–211). St. Louis, MO: Elsevier Saunders.

Network for the Advancement of Patient Blood Management, Haemostasis and Thrombosis. (n.d.). *Antifibrinolytics in open-heart surgery*. Retrieved from http://www.nataonline.com/np/419/antifibrinolytics-cardiac-surgery.

Nieman, L. K. (2016). Treatment of adrenal insufficiency in adults. Retrieved from https://www.uptodate.com/contents/treatment-of-adrenal-insufficiency-in-adults?source=see_link&sectionName=ADRENAL%20CRISIS&anchor=H2#H2.

Nieman, L. K. (2017). Pharmacologic use of glucocorticoids. Retrieved from https://www.uptodate.com/contents/pharmacologic-use-of-glucocorticoids?source=search_result&search=corticosteroids&selectedTitle=2~150.

Ortmann, E., Besser, M. W., & Klein, A. A. (2013). Antifibrinolytic agents in current anesthesia practice. *British Journal of Anaesthesia, 111*(4), 549–563.

Parra, D., Roman, Y. M., Anasthasia, E., & Straka, R. J. (2016). Hypertension. In M. A. Chisholm-Burns, T. L. Schwinghammer, B. G. Wells, & J. T. DiPiro (Eds.), Pharmacotherapy. Principles and practice (4th ed., pp. 45–64). New York, NY: McGraw-Hill.

Paruk, F., Sime, F. B., Lipman, J., & Roberts, J. (2017). Dosing antibiotic prophylaxis during cardiopulmonary bypass—a higher level of complexity? A structured review. *International Journal of Antimicrobial Agents, 49*, 395–402.

Peretto, G., Durante, A., Limite, L. R., & Cianflone, D. (2014). Postoperative arrhythmias after cardiac surgery: Incidence, risk factors, and therapeutic management. *Cardiology Research and Practice, 2014*, 1–15.

Ramos, A. P., & Varon, J. (2014). Current and newer agents for hypertensive emergencies. *Current Hypertension Reports, 16*, 450.

Ranucci, M., Baryshnikova, E., Pistuddi, V., Menicanti, L., & Frigiola, M. (2017). The effectiveness of 10 years of interventions to control postoperative bleeding in adult cardiac surgery. *Interactive Cardiovascular and Thoracic Surgery, 24*, 196–202.

Rao, V. K., Lobato, R. L., Bartlett, B., Klanjac, M., Mora-Mangano, C. T., Soran, P. D., . . . Van der Starre, P. J. (2014). Factor VIII inhibitor bypass activity and recombinant activated factor VII in cardiac surgery. *Journal of Cardiothoracic and Vascular Anesthesia, 28*(5), 1221–1226.

Ricksten, S., Bragadottir, G., & Redfors, B. (2013). Renal oxygenation in clinical acute kidney injury. *Critical Care, 17*, 221.

Rodgers, J. E., & Reed, B. N. (2017). Acute decompensated heart failure. In J. T. DiPiro, R. L. Talbert, G. C. Yee, G. R. Matzke, B. G. Wells, & L. Posey (Eds.), *Pharmacotherapy: A pathophysiologic approach* (10th ed.). Retrieved from http://accesspharmacy.mhmedical.com/content .aspx?bookid=1861&sectionid=146056502.

Sanoski, C. A., & Bauman, J. L. (2017). The arrhythmias. In J. T. DiPiro, R. L. Talbert, G. C. Yee, G. R. Matzke, B. G. Wells, & L. Posey (Eds.), *Pharmacotherapy: A pathophysiologic approach* (10th ed.). Retrieved from http://accesspharmacy.mhmedical.com/content .aspx?bookid=1861&sectionid=146057036#1145802698.

Seller, A., & Peng, Y. G. (2013). Drug innovation update: Prothrombin complex concentrate use during cardiac surgery. *SCA Bulletin, 12*(7). Retrieved from http://www .scahq.org/sca3/newsletters/2013dec/drug-innovation -update.html.

Shah, S. N. (2015). Asystole medication. Retrieved from http:// emedicine.medscape.com/article/757257-medication#3.

Shokri, H., Ali, I., & El Sayed H. M. (2016). Protamine adverse reactions in NPH insulin treated diabetics undergoing coronary artery bypass grafting. *The Egyptian Journal of Cardiothoracic Anesthesia, 10*, 25–30.

Silvestry, F. E. (2017). *Postoperative complications among patients undergoing cardiac surgery*. Retrieved from http://www.uptodate.com/contents/postoperative -complications-among-patients-undergoing-cardiac -surgery.

Song, H. K., Tibayan, F. A., Kahl, E. A., Sera, V. A., Slater, M. S., Deloughery, T. G., . . . Scanlan, M. M. (2014). Safety and efficacy of prothrombin complex concentrates for the treatment of coagulopathy after cardiac surgery. *The Journal of Thoracic and Cardiovascular Surgery, 147*(3), 1036–1040.

Thoma, A. (2013). Pathophysiology and management of angiotensin-converting enzyme inhibitor-associated refractory hypotension during the perioperative period. *American Association of Nurse Anesthetists Journal, 81*(2), 133–140.

Townsend, R. R. (2016). Major side effects of angiotensin- converting enzyme inhibitors and angiotensin II receptor blockers. Retrieved from http://www.uptodate.com /contents/major-side-effects-of-angiotensin-converting -enzyme-inhibitors-and-angiotensin-ii-receptor-blockers.

Treavor, A. J., Katzung, B. G., & Kruidering-Hall, M. (2015). Drugs used in hypertension. In A. J. Trevor, B. G. Katzung, & M. Kruidering-Hall (Eds.), *Katzung & Trevor's pharmacology: Examination & board review* (11th ed.). Retrieved from http://accesspharmacy.mhmedical.com/ Content.aspx?bookid=1568&sectionid=95701518.

Udeh, C. I., Ting, M., Arango, M., & Mick, S. (2015). Delayed presentation of nitroprusside-induced cyanide toxicity. *Annals of Thoracic Surgery, 99*, 1432–1434.

Upadhye, S., & Schiff, K. (2012). Acute aortic dissection in the emergency department: Diagnostic challenges and evidence-based management. *Emergency Medical Clinics of North America, 30*(2), 307–327.

Vardeny, O, & Ng, T. M. H. (2016). Heart failure. In M. A. Chisholm-Burns, Schwinghammer, T. L., Wells, B. G., Malone, P. M., J. M. Kolesar, & J. T. DiPiro (Eds). *Pharmacology Principles & Practice* (4th ed., pp. 65–90). New York, NY: McGraw-Hill.

Wademan, B. H., & Galvin, S. D. (2014). Desmopressin for reducing postoperative blood loss and transfusion re- quirements following cardiac surgery in adults. *Interactive Cardiovascular and Thoracic Surgery, 18*(3), 360–370.

Welsh, K. J., Nedelcu, E., Bai, Y., Whaed, A., Klein, K., Tint, H., . . . Nguyen, A. N. D. (2014). How do we manage cardiopulmonary bypass coagulopathy? *Transfusion, 54*(9), 2158–2166.

Yancy, C. W., Jessup, M., Bozkurt, B., Butler, J., Casey Jr., D. E., Drazner, M. A., . . . American College of Cardiology Foundation/American Heart Association Task Force on Practice Guidelines. (2013). ACCF/AHA guideline for the management of heart failure: A report of the American College of Cardiology Foundation/American Heart Association Task Force on practice guidelines. *Circulation, 128*(16), e240–e327.

Yimin, H., Xiaoyu, L., Yuping, H., Weiyan, L., & Ning, L. (2013). The effect of vasopressin on the hemodynamics in CABG patients. *Journal of Cardiothoracic Surgery, 16*(8), 49.

Web Resources

Adverse event reporting system (case reports): http://www. fda.gov/cder/aers/extract.htm U.S. Food and Drug Administration: http://www.fda.gov/

Clinical drug trials (lists studies by drug intervention): http:// www.clinicaltrials.gov Safety-related drug labeling changes: http://www.fda.gov/medwatch/safety.htm

FDA Safety News (recalls and safety alerts and preventing medical errors): http://www.accessdata.fda.gov/scripts /cdrh/cfdocs/psn/index.cfm

Herbal drug and supplement information: http://www.nlm .nih.gov/medlineplus/druginformation.html

Scientific Review of Alternative Medicine: http://www.sram .org/

CHAPTER 13

Postoperative Complications of Cardiac Surgery and Nursing Interventions

Barbara Leeper, Roberta Kaplow

▶ Introduction

Coronary artery bypass grafting (CABG) and valve replacement procedures are among the most frequently performed surgical procedures, with more than 2 million operations being performed worldwide. Patients who are candidates for cardiac surgery often present with a number of comorbidities. Some of these comorbidities are directly related to the need for surgery, whereas others are attributable to advanced age and other noncardiac conditions. An extensive presurgical evaluation should always be performed, as discussed in Chapter 4. From these data and a thorough assessment of the patient's condition, management of the patient's complex problems may take place before, during, and following cardiac surgery.

Despite the trend toward cardiac surgery being performed on older persons and those with more complex health issues, the 30-day mortality associated with cardiac surgical procedures continues to decline. The overall mortality rate is now reported to be 1% to 5.6% (Allyn et al., 2017; Mariscalco et al., 2017; Pieri et al., 2016; Silvestry, 2017). An important focus for the patient undergoing cardiac surgery is an assessment of cardiac risk. Calculation of risk potential affords patients and their families insight into the risk of complications and possible mortality of the surgical procedure. It also heightens the health care team's awareness of the high-risk patient for whom more aggressive therapy may be warranted and alerts caregivers to the potential for postoperative complications. This chapter describes the most common postoperative complications associated with cardiac surgery and the intensive care unit (ICU) nursing management of these complications.

Once a patient has been deemed an acceptable candidate for cardiac surgery, a comprehensive

Original contributions from Tamara S. Goda

preoperative evaluation must occur. The patient's history and presence of noncardiac comorbidities must be fully assessed to determine what, if any, perioperative complications should be factored into the patient's recovery. Additionally, numerous cardiac surgery risk models are available that can provide a patient with specific risk assessment, allowing for calculation and prediction of perioperative morbidity and mortality. Examples include but are not limited to the Society of Thoracic Surgery (STS) database and the EuroSCORE II. Many cardiac surgery centers will input patient-specific data into one of these systems for the purpose of identifying the risk of morbidity and mortality preoperatively. Some cardiac surgery centers will have a "high risk" meeting preoperatively to present those patients that are deemed to be very high risk for adverse outcomes following the surgical procedure. This meeting may consist of surgeons reviewing films and discussing appropriateness of the surgery. Others may have a multidisciplinary team approach, including not only surgeons, anesthesiologists, perfusionists, cardiologists, nurses (operating room, ICU, telemetry), advanced practice providers, physical therapists, social workers, among others. Once the patient is presented, discussion ensues for each level of care about what needs to be in place to ensure the patient has the best possible outcome. **BOX 13.1** lists the most common risk factors that have been shown to have predictive value when determining postoperative complications and higher rates of mortality.

Complications of cardiac surgery have negative and variable effects on patient outcomes. Postoperative complications may occur secondary to patient comorbidities, the complexity of the surgical procedure, the use of cardiopulmonary bypass (CPB), or any combination of these. However, advances in surgical techniques and technology, improved understanding of CPB, and the creation of highly specialized critical care teams have positively influenced both postoperative management and outcomes. Perhaps the greatest advances have been related to the evolution of minimally invasive surgical procedures, allowing operations to be offered to older persons and those patients with multiple comorbidities who might previously not have been considered

---

BOX 13.1 Risk Factors for Postoperative Complications

Older age (>65 years)
Female gender
BSA
Emergent need for procedure (versus urgent need)
Hearing impairment
Recent smoking
Resternotomy or previous cardiac surgery
Preexisting preoperative comorbidities: COPD, diabetes, peripheral vascular disease, heart failure, chronic kidney disease or other preexisting kidney disease, peripheral vascular disease, left main coronary artery disease, malnutrition
CABG/valve surgery
Low ejection fraction/cardiac output
Pulmonary dysfunction
Preoperative presence of intra-aortic balloon pump
Preoperative vasoactive drug support
Cardiogenic shock
Anemia
Duration of anesthesia
Duration of surgery
Duration of CPB
Duration of aortic cross-clamping
Intraoperative phrenic nerve damage
Lactate level greater than 2.5 mmol/L
Inotropic support following CPB
Postoperative fluid balance
Need for RBC transfusion
Need for FFP transfusion
Postoperative CVA
Postoperative new onset atrial fibrillation
Postoperative development of acute kidney injury
Incomplete revascularization

BSA, body surface area; CABG, coronary artery bypass grafting; COPD, chronic obstructive pulmonary disease; CPB, cardiopulmonary bypass; CVA, cerebrovascular accident; FFP, fresh frozen plasma; RBC, red blood cell. Data from Ji et al., 2013; Lomivorotov, Efremov, Kirov, Fominskiy, & Karaskov, 2017; Norkienė, Ringaitienė, Kuzminskaitė, & Šipylaitė, 2013; Pieri et al., 2016; Wang & Bellomo, 2017.

---

surgical candidates. Additionally, postoperative care rendered in the ICU in terms of early extubation protocols, decreased utilization of blood products, and strict glycemic control has been directly correlated with lower morbidity and mortality rates (Ji et al., 2013).

Despite these improvements, a few complications continue to be associated with a mortality rate of 50% or greater. The deleterious side effects of CPB, circulatory arrest, hypothermia, and aortic cross-clamping can cause a number of physiologic abnormalities in major organs in the perioperative period. Most notably, the loss of pulsatile blood flow while on CPB results in decreased perfusion pressure. Therefore, many organ systems—the brain, gut, and kidneys—can suffer damage when the surgical procedure and CPB time are protracted. Knowledge and early identification of potential postoperative complications are essential to successful patient management and outcomes following cardiac surgery.

▶ Systemic Inflammatory Response to Cardiac Surgery

The body's complement system is composed of more than 30 proteins; activation of this system and the resulting inflammatory response can have serious effects on the cardiac surgery patient (Stoppelkamp et al., 2015). The etiology is felt to be related to exposure of blood with the extracorporeal circuit (Pagowska-Klimek et al., 2016). Inflammation is the body's response to the disruption within the tissues and involves a series of controlled humoral and cellular reactions. Complement activation during cardiac surgery can be triggered by a number of mechanisms: tissue trauma during the procedure and the resulting release of plasmin; intravenous administration of protamine following CPB; and, most recently, cardiac dysrhythmias have been directly correlated with high levels of C-reactive protein markers following CABG (Zakkar, Ascione, James, Angelini, & Suleiman, 2015). Additionally, a very specific activator of the response can be seen as a result of CPB when a patient's blood comes into contact with the foreign surface of the CPB circuit.

The systemic inflammatory response is characterized by the release of proinflammatory factors such as interleukins 6 and 8 (IL-6 and IL-8) and tumor necrosis factor, and it has been directly linked to several postoperative complications. This inflammatory response has been directly correlated to myocardial ischemia and reperfusion injury, pulmonary dysfunction, acute respiratory distress syndrome (ARDS), and severe systemic peripheral vasodilation, often requiring vasopressor support (Zakkar et al., 2015).

Current recommendations for treatment call for supportive care until the inflammatory response resolves. Much research is being conducted on specific complement pathway inhibitors. Investigational studies are being conducted to both identify a genetic component to complement response and specific pathway inhibitors to improve outcomes. Likewise, the use of statins (e.g., atorvastatin [Lipitor®] or simvastatin [Zocor®]) has been shown to play a role in the reduction of oxidative stress and C-reactive protein and may diminish the associated inflammatory response (Rezaei, 2016). Additionally, advances in CPB technology have resulted in the routine use of heparin-coated circuits, thereby making them more biocompatible, reducing the complement and platelet activation and local immune response (Evora et al., 2016).

▶ Cardiac Complications

Adequate cardiac function is the most important factor associated with recovery from cardiac surgery. Perioperatively, patients with poor cardiac function and low cardiac output (CO) have a higher mortality risk. Hence, the ICU nurse plays a vital role in identifying and treating a low CO state and preventing subsequent complications.

Hemodynamic compromise in the cardiac surgery patient is challenging to manage, because the status of such patients tends to be labile in the immediate postoperative period. The etiology of hemodynamic compromise is multifactorial. It may be caused by the patient's underlying cardiac function, volume status, dysrhythmias, decreased ventricular compliance, loss of vasomotor tone, increased capillary permeability, postoperative bleeding, poor myocardial protection during aortic cross-clamping, or a systemic inflammatory response to CPB. Data suggest that a release of inflammatory mediators occurs in patients who undergo cardiac surgery, further contributing to these individuals' postoperative hemodynamic instability. Secretion of prostaglandins and other proinflammatory mediators (cytokines) stimulates release of nitric oxide, leading to profound vasodilation (Rodrigues, Evora, & Evora, 2014). Nitric oxide causes resistance to vasopressors by preventing vessels of some patients from vasoconstricting.

Perhaps the factor that influences cardiac performance most in the immediate postoperative period is the underlying preoperative cardiac pathology. Even though surgery has been performed, the patient will not experience an immediate improvement in contractility; inadequate inotropy is not uncommon after cardiac surgery (Silvestry, 2017). When decreased ventricular function is present, compensatory mechanisms such as sympathetic nervous system (SNS) stimulation and endogenous catecholamine production cause an increase in heart rate, contractility, and vasoconstriction. In turn, both preload and afterload increase (Guarracino, Baldassarri, & Pinsky, 2013). Initially, these compensatory factors will improve CO and blood pressure, albeit usually at the cost of increasing myocardial oxygen consumption, which can exacerbate myocardial ischemia. The compensatory mechanisms are temporary, however; when they are exhausted, poor tissue perfusion will ensue. Initial signs of poor tissue perfusion include tachycardia, diminished peripheral pulses, delayed capillary refill time, increased serum lactate, dyspnea, confusion, agitation, decreased urinary output, hypotension, and (possibly) metabolic acidosis (Lumley & Hirst, 2016).

The primary objective of postoperative management of the cardiac surgery patient is attainment of an adequate CO. Optimal hemodynamic parameters in a postoperative cardiac surgery patient include a cardiac index (CI) of 2.2 to 4.4 L/min/m^2, pulmonary artery occlusive pressure (PAOP) 10 to 15 mmHg, central venous pressure (CVP) 5 to 15 mmHg, mean arterial pressure (MAP) 60 to 90 mmHg, systolic blood pressure in the 90 to 140 mmHg range, and systemic vascular

resistance in the 1,400 to 2,800 dynes/sec/cm^{-5} range (Silvestry, 2017). The patient should also have warm, well-perfused extremities and urine output at least 0.5 mL/kg/hr. Patients with a history of hypertension or renal insufficiency may require a higher MAP. Patients with a history of ventricular dysfunction, mitral valve repair surgery, active bleeding, or weak aortic suture lines may need to be maintained with a lower MAP (Stephens & Whitman, 2015a).

Low Cardiac Output Syndrome

To help ensure oxygen delivery, CO (the amount of blood ejected by the heart each minute) must be adequate. A related parameter to CO is cardiac index, the amount of blood ejected by the heart each minute in relation to a patient's body surface area (BSA). Adequate tissue perfusion is dependent on satisfactory CO. Cardiac output and index are functions of stroke volume (SV), the amount of blood ejected by the heart with each beat, and heart rate. Stroke volume depends on myocardial contractility, preload (the amount of volume returning to the right or left side of the heart), and afterload (the amount of work the heart has to do to eject blood (Mohrman & Heller, 2014).

Low cardiac output syndrome (LCOS) is most likely the result of left ventricular dysfunction and decreased SV, which may be due to decreased preload, increased afterload, or decreased contractility (Aranki & Cutlip, 2018; Silvestry, 2017).

Low cardiac output syndrome is often seen after cardiac surgery and is associated with increased morbidity and mortality. Low cardiac output states are seen most commonly in patients with advanced age, left ventricular dysfunction, acute myocardial ischemia, combined CABG/valve procedures, extended cross-clamping and CPB times, mitral valve procedures, and chronic kidney disease (Kouchoukos, Blackstone, Hanley, & Kirklin, 2013). Low cardiac output syndrome can be defined as CI less than 2 L/min/m^2, SBP less than 90 mmHg, pulmonary artery diastolic (PAD) pressure greater than 20 mmHg, systemic vascular resistance (SVR) exceeding 1,500 dynes/sec/cm^{-5}, elevated serum lactate, mental status changes, cold and clammy skin, the need for administration of an inotropic infusion for more than 30 minutes, intra-aortic balloon pump (IABP) therapy, or any combination of these. Postoperative cardiac surgery patients may develop LCOS transiently within the first 6 to 8 hours due to myocardial ischemia and reperfusion injury following cardioplegic arrest (Lomivorotov, Efremov, Kirov, Fominskiy, & Karaskov, 2017).

The ICU nurse must monitor for signs and symptoms of impaired CO. Assessment of the patient with LCOS reveals decreased MAP, tachycardia, cool extremities and decreased or weak peripheral pulses, oliguria or anuria, and distended neck veins.

Hemodynamic monitoring reveals mixed venous oxygen saturation (SvO_2) levels lower than normal in the setting of LCOS. Venous oxygen saturation is the percentage of hemoglobin saturated with oxygen in the pulmonary artery after blood has circulated systemically and oxygen has been extracted based on cellular need. Normal SvO_2 values are in the range of 70% to 75%. If the SvO_2 is less than 70%, it indicates that cells are sensing hypoperfusion or an increased metabolic rate and are extracting more oxygen from hemoglobin. Venous oxygen saturation monitoring provides data on the balance between oxygen supply and demand. Lab data that will help support a diagnosis of low CO include a metabolic acidosis or increasing base deficit on arterial blood gas and an elevated serum lactate level (Kouchoukos et al., 2013).

Management of the patient with low CO depends on the underlying cause, hemodynamic profile, and patient assessment findings. Use of fluids, vasopressors, and inotropic agents will vary based on whether the patient has low preload or whether the SVR is elevated or low (Silvestry, 2017). If inotropic support is required, the chosen drug's efficacy must be carefully monitored, because inotropic agents increase myocardial workload and metabolic rate. Low-dose epinephrine or dobutamine (Dobutrex®) may be administered if contractility (ejection fraction [EF]) is below the expected values for the patient. These agents may have decreased efficacy in patients with chronic systolic dysfunction due to down regulation of beta receptors. Use of a phosphodiesterase inhibitor (e.g., milrinone [Primacor®])

may be a more effective means to augment contractility in this group of patients. Phosphodiesterase inhibitors augment myocardial contractility and coronary blood flow, and decrease SVR. These will result in increased CO and decreased preload and afterload of the left ventricle with minimal increase in myocardial oxygen demand. If vasodilation is the cause of the LCOS, administration of a vasoconstrictor (e.g., phenylephrine [Neosynephrine®]), norepinephrine [Levophed®], or vasopressin (antidiuretic hormone, [ADH]) is warranted (Silvestry, 2017).

If afterload is elevated, administration of nitroprusside (Nipride®), dobutamine, or IABP therapy may be indicated (Silvestry, 2017). Regardless of the cause of low CO, the primary goal of management focuses on decreasing metabolic demand. Interventions such as preventing hyperthermia, administering sedation and analgesia, decreasing work of breathing with mechanical ventilation, and preventing or treating tachycardia, dysrhythmias, and electrolyte and acid–base imbalances may need to be considered.

Preload Issues

Preload refers to the amount of volume returning to the right or left heart at the end of filling (diastole). It may be assessed by CVP and PAOP, which are the filling pressures of the right and left heart, respectively. Pulmonary artery occlusive pressure is a reflection of left ventricular end-diastolic pressure (LVEDP), from which estimates of left ventricular end-diastolic volume can be made (Silvestry, 2017). In recent years studies have demonstrated limited usefulness of CVP and PAOP accurately reflecting the preload status. Additionally, there is a trend to move away from the use of pulmonary artery catheters to less invasive or noninvasive devices. These newer devices offer continuous CO/CI and SVR measurements along with dynamic variables, including stroke volume variation, pulse pressure variation, and systolic pressure variation. These have been shown to be a more accurate indicator of the patient's need for volume (Soliman, Samir, el Naggar, & El Dehely, 2015; Stephens & Whitman, 2015a). The majority of patients are admitted to the ICU from the operating room (OR) with alterations in preload despite having a positive fluid balance. The volume, however, is not in the intravascular space; instead, much of the fluid is located in the interstitium or other third space (e.g., pleural cavity).

Adequate preload is essential to maintain a satisfactory CO and tissue perfusion. Decreased preload in the immediate postoperative cardiac surgery patient can result from several factors, including excessive fluid output from diuresis or hypothermia, vasodilation during rewarming, inadequate intraoperative fluid resuscitation, intraoperative or postoperative bleeding, loss of vasomotor tone, infusion of vasodilator agents, decreased LV compliance, or capillary leak leading to third spacing of fluid. Further, after cardiac surgery, compliance of the left ventricle is typically decreased, which causes diastolic dysfunction. A higher LVEDP will be required during this time to maintain preload (Silvestry, 2017).

The type and amount of fluid resuscitation required will be based on the patient's history, cardiac function, amount and type of fluid lost, and hematocrit level. If the patient experiences excessive postoperative bleeding, transfusion of blood and blood products should be initiated while the source of the blood loss is being determined. The hemoglobin requirement should be determined by the patient's cardiac and hemodynamic status, age, and other clinical issues pertinent to the situation (Najafi & Faraoni, 2015). Coagulation factors such as fresh frozen plasma and cryoprecipitate may also need to be given to correct coagulopathies usually caused by CPB.

If bleeding is not present, bolus administration of isotonic crystalloids (e.g., 0.9% normal saline, lactated Ringer's solution) or colloid (e.g., 5% albumin) may be used to optimize preload, usually to a PAOP of 18 to 20 mmHg. Administration of inotropic agents is not recommended for patients with decreased preload; intravascular volume repletion is required (Silvestry, 2017). Patients with a history of ventricular hypertrophy or diastolic dysfunction usually require a higher preload (Klabunde, 2013). Volume requirements may decrease after the patient has been removed from positive pressure ventilation, as this change is often associated with an increase in venous return

owing to the decrease in intrathoracic pressure (Cherpanath, Lagrand, Schultz, & Groeneveld, 2013). Vasodilation is reported as the major contributor to a decrease in preload in the initial postoperative period, therefore volume repletion is typically required (Silvestry, 2017).

A therapeutic endpoint for volume resuscitation may be the MAP. The goal of a MAP in the range of 60 to 90 mmHg is suggested. Tachycardia is not believed to be an appropriate indicator of adequacy of preload, given the many preoperative and intraoperative factors that can affect the correlation between heart rate and hypovolemia. Ongoing monitoring of the patient's hemodynamic profile must take place concomitantly with volume repletion. Care must be taken not to overstretch the ventricle with excessive volume, because an impaired CO may ensue (Beebe & Myers, 2011).

Cardiac Dysrhythmias

Dysrhythmias are a common complication following cardiac surgery. Additionally, they are a major source of morbidity and mortality, exposing patients to both extra days in the hospital and high-risk medications. As discussed in Chapter 15, atrial dysrhythmias are the most commonly encountered rhythm abnormalities in the postoperative CABG patient. The overall incidence of atrial dysrhythmias is reported at 15% to 40% following CABG procedures, 37% to 50% following valve surgery, and up to 60% in patients who underwent valve procedures with CABG (Lee, 2016). Many factors have been implicated in the development of postoperative dysrhythmias (**BOX 13.2**). Postoperative dysrhythmias are discussed in detail in Chapter 15.

Dysrhythmias can compromise CO when they interfere with diastolic filling. If a disturbance in heart rhythm is present, prompt identification and close assessment of the patient are essential. Assessment of the patient with cardiac dysrhythmias following cardiac surgery requires evaluation of the rhythm, presence of atrial kick and its effects on systemic perfusion, as well as evaluation of precipitating factors. Treatment is based on whether the goal of therapy is to control the

BOX 13.2 Common Causes of Dysrhythmias Following Cardiac Surgery

Patient-Related Factors

Age
Female gender
Caucasian
Preexisting heart disease
History of atrial fibrillation
Mitral stenosis
Cardiomegaly
Previous cardiac surgery
Severe right coronary artery stenosis
Unstable angina
Hypertension
Extracardiac morbidities—obesity or BMI less than 25 kg/m^2, COPD, elevated hemoglobin A1c, stroke

Surgery-Related Factors

Tissue trauma and inflammation
Hemodynamic stress
Poor intraoperative myocardial protection/ ischemic injury
Prolonged CPB time
Long aortic cross-clamp time
Pulmonary complications—hypoxia/hypercapnia, ET tube misplacement, and pneumothorax
Electrolyte disturbances (hypokalemia, hypomagnesemia)
Need for inotropes
Need for IABP therapy
Medications
Fever, pain, and anxiety
Hypothermia

COPD, chronic obstructive pulmonary disease; CPB, cardiopulmonary bypass; ET, endotracheal tube; IABP, intra-aortic balloon pump.
Data from Aranki, Cutlip, & Aroesty, 2016; Lee, 2016; Peretto, Durante, Limite, & Cianflone, 2014.

rate or to convert the rhythm. Postoperative dysrhythmias are discussed in detail in Chapter 15; the pharmacologic management of dysrhythmias is discussed in Chapters 12 and 15.

Diastolic Dysfunction

Diastolic dysfunction is characterized by reduced ventricular compliance and can be exacerbated by myocardial ischemia or edema from reperfusion injury. Diastolic dysfunction commonly occurs following aortic valve replacement and is largely due to the LV hypertrophy that results from standing aortic stenosis. A second very common cause of postoperative diastolic dysfunction is poor intraoperative myocardial protection. The hemodynamic picture is one of elevated PAOP and low CO, EF greater than in preoperative setting, and small left ventricle (Ferreira, Northington, Huang, Aranki, & Muehlschlegel, 2015; Stephens & Whitman, 2015a). If the left ventricle becomes stiff during filling (diastole), it may not be able to fill completely. As a result, fluid may back up to the lungs, and heart failure may ensue.

Treatment of diastolic dysfunction includes volume administration to maximize preload and administration of vasodilators. Patients with diastolic dysfunction from decreased LV compliance will require a higher PAOP to maintain adequate preload than do patients with a reduced preload from the other etiologies listed earlier. Because the ventricle has decreased compliance in this case, the PAOP may be elevated despite the need for additional preload (Stephens & Whitman, 2015a). Infusion of an inotropic agent should be administered at low doses if the patient's EF is low to normal. A combination of dobutamine and norepinephrine may be effective. Monitoring for tachycardia is essential when using these agents, because an increased heart rate will decrease ventricular filling time, which can result in decreased SV and CO. Milrinone (discussed later in this chapter) causes vasodilation and may improve EF. If a vasodilator is used, it is important not to exceed baseline levels of dilation. Administration of a vasoconstrictor may be required in diastolic dysfunction after cardiac surgery if the patient is vasodilated from the inflammatory response common after these procedures. In this case, the goal is to normalize vascular resistance, but not elevate it (Stephens & Whitman, 2015a).

Right Ventricular Failure

Although most low output states following cardiac surgery are attributable to LV failure, low CO can also be the result of right ventricular (RV) failure.

Right ventricular failure after cardiac surgery is a significant cause of postoperative morbidity and mortality. The incidence is low (Estrada, Franco, Moreno, Gambasica, & Nunez, 2016). Etiology of RV dysfunction may include a sudden change in preload or afterload, myocardial ischemia or stunning, infarction from right coronary artery disease, pulmonary hypertension of any cause, coronary malperfusion, CPB, left ventricular failure, or any combination of these (Stephens & Whitman, 2015b). Inadequate function of the right ventricle leads to decreased filling of the left ventricle, reduced LV output, and poor systemic perfusion. The right ventricle then becomes distended, which increases RV preload, with RV failure being the ultimate outcome. Right ventricular failure can also occur following a heart transplant (Lomivorotov et al., 2017). The diagnosis of RV failure is based on the presence of elevated CVP and low PAOP and CO (Kouchoukos et al., 2013). Often, a transesophageal echocardiogram will be performed to visualize the dilated RV and confirm RV failure. A pulmonary artery catheter can also provide RV function data (Stephens & Whitman, 2015b).

Management of RV failure includes optimizing preload, ensuring atrioventricular (AV) conduction, reducing RV afterload (pulmonary vascular resistance [PVR]), improving RV contractility, and maintaining systemic blood pressure (Stephens & Whitman, 2015b). Nitric oxide or prostacyclin, both pulmonary vasodilators, can be administered to decrease RV afterload, which will improve RV function. Mitigation of hypoxemia, acidosis, and hypercarbia will also reduce potentiation of RV failure. Maintaining a partial pressure of oxygen (PaO_2) greater than 90 mmHg and pH greater than 7.45 will also improve RV function. If the right ventricle is extremely dilated and is leading to decreased LV preload, diuretics and ultrafiltration may be indicated to remove excess volume. If these interventions are not effective, use of dobutamine or milrinone may be indicated to decrease pulmonary vascular resistance and CO. Monitoring for hypotension is essential when administering either of these agents as they are both peripheral vasodilators and adequate blood pressure is needed to

maintain RV perfusion. Concomitant administration of norepinephrine or vasopressin, both vasoconstrictors, may be needed. In some cases, a right ventricular assist device may be required (Stephens & Whitman, 2015b).

Decreased Myocardial Contractility

Contractility is the shortening of myocardial fibers during systole (ventricular emptying) and the force produced by the myocardium to eject blood. It is evaluated with EF by echocardiography (Silvestry, 2017).

Cardiac contractility may be impaired postoperatively due to cross-clamping of the aorta without adequate myocardial protection, valve lesions that are not corrected, myocardial hibernation, ischemia, decreased coronary blood flow, cardiac tamponade, myocardial infarction (MI), or coronary graft vasospasm or thrombosis (Silvestry, 2017). Other implicating factors include hypoxia, acidosis, electrolyte imbalance, narcotics, anesthesia, transient ischemic/reperfusion injury, impaired preoperative function (EF <35%), inadequate intraoperative myocardial protection, duration and extent of postoperative hypothermia, CPB time (especially if >120 min), tamponade, valve function, or myocardial ischemia or infarction (Kouchoukos et al., 2013; Silvestry, 2017).

Left ventricular function/contractility may be reduced following cardiac surgery. It reaches its lowest point 24 hours after surgery and gradually returns to baseline within a week (Cool, Thomas, Nolan, & Parr, 2014). Decreased contractility may require inotropic support along with vasoactive medications to support cardiac function. Both inotropic and vasodilator support with medications such as dobutamine, milrinone, and low-dose epinephrine, used alone or in combination, may prove effective in improving cardiac contractility. No data support the use of inotropes to improve patient outcomes following cardiac surgery, nor do any data support use of one inotrope over another (Cool et al., 2014). Epinephrine, however, is associated with the development of temporary but significant hyperglycemia, metabolic acidosis, and increased serum lactate when used in the initial 6 to 8 postoperative hours. These effects usually resolve in

12 hours (Rosas, Giocoechea-Turcott, Ortiz, Salazar, & Palma, 2012). It also initially elevates serum lactate levels (Silvestry, 2017).

In addition to titrating medications based on the patient's hemodynamic profile, the ICU nurse must monitor for signs and symptoms of inadequate perfusion related to the impaired contractility. Evaluation of CI, hypotension, mottling, end-organ dysfunction (e.g., inadequate urinary output), and presence of a metabolic acidosis is vital. Urinary output may be increased in the initial postoperative period, however, so it is considered a less reliable indicator of poor perfusion.

Myocardial Stunning and Hibernation

Cardiovascular research has led to the identification of two important phenomena: myocardial stunning and myocardial hibernation.

Myocardial stunning is a period of impaired contractility following temporary ischemia, in which the dysfunction persists despite return of blood flow. Myocardial stunning may occur after CPB, and postoperative cardiac dysfunction (i.e., decreased ventricular function) is often attributed to its effects (Kouchoukos et al., 2013).

Hibernating myocardium is a condition of impaired LV function when the patient is at rest; it reflects a chronic reduction in blood flow. Heart function can be partially or totally normalized by improving blood flow or decreasing oxygen demand (Shavelle, 2014). Myocardial hibernation is considered a compensatory or protective mechanism to safeguard the capacity and integrity of the myocardium during times of decreased blood flow (Shavelle, 2014).

Increased Systemic Vascular Resistance (Afterload)

As with preload, right- and left-sided afterload can be evaluated to help determine cardiac performance. Right-sided afterload is reflected by PVR; left-sided afterload is reflected by SVR. Most of the discussion in this section refers to left-sided afterload.

Afterload is determined by intraventricular systolic pressure and the thickness of the ventricular wall. The latter factor is minimally affected with cardiac surgery. Systolic blood pressure will have the greatest effect on afterload and, therefore, SV and myocardial oxygen demand. By decreasing afterload, CO will improve (Silvestry, 2017).

Increased SVR is also often a compensatory result of the sympathetic nervous system (SNS) response to low CO. Increased SVR may be poorly tolerated in a patient with already poor myocardial function.

Hypertension is a well-known complication of patients who undergo cardiac surgery and is often associated with vasoconstriction related to hypothermia during CPB. Development of hypertension, vasoconstriction, or both may be related to decreased oxygen levels in the muscle with concomitant metabolic acidosis or inflammatory responses to CPB. Other potential causes of increased afterload include hypothermia, hypovolemia, hypercarbia, inadequate rewarming, volume overload, cardiogenic shock, pain, and anxiety. The latter two etiologies result from increased SNS stimulation. If vasoconstriction is extreme, the patient is at risk of developing life-threatening hypertension and decreased CO (Silvestry, 2017).

Treatment of increased afterload may entail administration of vasodilator therapy with medications such as sodium nitroprusside, nitroglycerin (Tridil®), or milrinone. Sodium nitroprusside is the treatment of choice (Silvestry, 2017). Given that vasodilators cause a decrease in preload, concomitant administration of fluids may be required to maintain adequate intravascular volume during their use. As the potential for abrupt hypotension exists when nitroprusside is administered, frequent blood pressure monitoring is essential, especially during rewarming (Silvestry, 2017). In severe cases of LV failure, IABP counterpulsation may be used to reduce afterload. Intra-aortic balloon pump therapy is discussed in detail in Chapter 10.

Decreased Systemic Vascular Resistance

While an increase in afterload is common following cardiac surgery, some patients develop a decreased SVR postoperatively. This condition, which is also referred to as vasodilatory shock, is associated with a CO that is either normal or increased (Silvestry, 2017). The incidence of vasodilatory shock is reported to range from 5% to 8% following CPB. The incidence is reported at 42% in patients who are undergoing placement of a ventricular assist device for end-stage heart failure and 27% in patients with a left ventricular ejection fraction (LVEF) less than 35%. Risk factors of vasodilatory shock include a decreased EF, extended time of aortic cross-clamping, and use of angiotensin-converting enzyme (ACE) inhibitors preoperatively (Silvestry, 2017). Vasodilatory shock also may be caused by an inflammatory response to CPB. Management entails administration of a vasoconstrictor agent such as phenylephrine or norepinephrine. If patients do not respond to this therapy, vasopressin administration may be attempted. Finally, methylene blue administration may be considered, because this agent inhibits nitric oxide production (Silvestry, 2017).

Mechanical Issues

A number of mechanical issues can contribute to the development of hemodynamic compromise in the postoperative cardiac surgery patient. These complications include cardiac tamponade, coronary artery or radial artery graft spasm or occlusion, acute graft closure, hematoma, prosthetic valve regurgitation, pneumothorax, and hemothorax. Treatment of mechanical complications typically involves surgery (Silvestry, 2017).

Cardiac Tamponade

During cardiac surgery, the pericardial sac is excised to gain access to the epicardial surface of the heart. At the end of the procedure, the pericardial sac remains open, leaving a communication between the heart and the mediastinum. Excessive bleeding in the perioperative period may lead to the potential accumulation of blood and fluid in the mediastinal space. This may lead to compression of the atria, restriction of venous return to the heart, and reduced ventricular filling, resulting in a decrease or cessation of preload, causing a

precipitous fall in CO (Floerchinger et al., 2013). Cardiac tamponade is most often the result of persistent mediastinal bleeding that is not adequately being evacuated by chest tubes.

Cardiac tamponade is one of several potential complications that may result in ventricular dysfunction (Silvestry, 2017). Diagnosis may be difficult because hypotension, tachycardia, and elevated filling pressures are common scenarios in most immediate postoperative cardiac surgery patients. In addition, some of the other characteristic symptoms of cardiac tamponade (e.g., muffled heart sounds, pulsus paradoxus, and neck vein distention) are not helpful in the cardiac surgery patient. While the patient may experience equalization of intracardiac pressures (CVP equal with PAOP or PAD), other signs and symptoms will likely suggest the presence of cardiac tamponade prior to this manifestation (Yarlagadda, 2017). Heightened awareness for tamponade should be present when the patient develops the signs and symptoms listed in **BOX 13.3**.

Pericardial effusions occur in as many as 85% of patients following a CABG procedure. The effusion usually becomes apparent on postoperative day 2, but may occur on postoperative day 10 (Aranki et al., 2016).

Continuous hypotension that does not respond to fluid administration and the use of inotropic support with the presence of signs and symptoms listed in Box 13.3 requires prompt intervention with a bedside echocardiogram to differentiate between ventricular dysfunction and cardiac tamponade (Yarlagadda, 2017). The patient may need to return to the OR for clot evacuation, bleeding site repair, or both. When an echocardiogram is not feasible or there is impending cardiac arrest, emergency mediastinal exploration is warranted for accurate diagnosis (Čanádyová, Zmeko, & Mikráček, 2012). **BOX 13.4** lists the steps undertaken in an emergency resternotomy.

Coronary Vasospasm

A frequently unrecognized cause of sudden cardiovascular collapse in the early postoperative period is coronary artery/graft vasospasm. This

BOX 13.3 Signs and Symptoms of Cardiac Tamponade

Sudden decrease or cessation of significant mediastinal bleeding
Persistent low cardiac output state with hypotension
Narrowing pulse pressure
Pulsus paradoxus
Diminished heart sounds
Kussmaul sign (elevated jugular venous pressure and distention during inspiration)
Palpitations
Cold, clammy skin
Weak pulse (due to hypotension)
Inappropriately fluctuating MAP/ Systolic Pressure Variation (>15 mmHg)
Increased central venous pressure or equalization of intracardiac pressures: RA = PAOP = LA pressures
An increasing requirement for inotropic or vasopressor medications
Chest radiograph findings of an enlarged cardiac silhouette or widened mediastinum
ECG changes, including decreased voltage QRS complex, a compensatory tachycardia, dysrhythmias, or pulseless electrical activity
Sudden oliguria
Altered mental status, drowsiness
Dizziness
Dyspnea, tachypnea
Diaphoresis
Cyanosis or pallor
Anxiety, restlessness, or both

ECG, electrocardiogram; MAP, mean arterial pressure; RA, right atrial; PAOP, pulmonary artery occlusive pressure; LA, left atrial.
Data from Kaplow, & Iyere, 2017; Schiavone, 2013; Yarlagadda, 2016.

BOX 13.4 Emergency Resternotomy Procedures

1. Alert the surgeon and operating team.
2. Obtain an emergency open chest tray.
3. Obtain an electrocautery device, and apply the ground pads to the patient's skin to prevent a Bovie burn.
4. Set up sterile suction.
5. Obtain personal protective equipment, sterile gowns, antiseptic solution, and drapes.
6. Remove the dressing.
7. Cleanse skin with chlorhexidine solution.
8. Place sterile towels and drapes on the patient's skin.
9. Assist the surgeon by supplying scalpel and wire cutters.
10. Open the incision down to the sternum with the scalpel.
11. Cut the sternal wires with the wire cutters.
12. Place the sternal retractor to expose the heart, carefully locating the existing coronary artery bypass grafts.
13. Assist with controlling bleeding and suctioning, if needed.
14. Assist in irrigation of mediastinum with warm saline or antibiotics.
15. Assist in closing the sternum.
16. Apply a dressing to the incision, securing the epicardial pacer wires and chest tube sites.
17. Assess the patient's cardiovascular and hemodynamic status every 15 minutes until stable.
18. Monitor coagulation and hematology laboratory studies as needed.
19. Monitor chest tube drainage.

complication usually presents itself as acute hypotension, ST segment elevation in multiple leads, and low CO. All types of coronary grafts are implicated in the development of coronary vasospasm—saphenous vein grafts, arterial conduits, and normal cardiac vessels alike (He, 2013). In addition, vasoconstriction of an arterial conduit may occur; patients who received a radial artery graft are routinely given a prophylactic "cocktail," which includes a vasodilator, such as nitroglycerin, and a calcium channel blocker. Other regimens are reported as well (He, 2013). Vasospasm usually resolves on its own; however, treatment is aimed primarily at supportive care to maintain hemodynamic instability.

Myocardial Ischemia and Infarction

Myocardial ischemia, whether transient or leading to MI, may occur after cardiac surgery. Causative factors leading to perioperative myocardial ischemia include poor myocardial protection during CBP (e.g., insufficient cardioplegia, incomplete revascularization, coronary vasospasm, or coronary artery or intracoronary embolism). Other risk factors that have been identified include age over 70 years, female gender, acute kidney injury, diabetes, peripheral artery disease, emergency or redo surgery, LVEF less than 35%, cardiogenic shock, or preoperative MI (Al-Attar, 2011). Myocardial infarction may also occur in the early postoperative period related to acute closure of a bypass graft. Patients may be started on aspirin, clopidogrel, or both within the initial few postoperative hours to reduce prevalence of MI. The incidence of postoperative MI is 4% to 5% for patients who have undergone CABG specifically. It is typically due to poor perfusion of the more proximal coronary arteries after bypass grafting. The incidence of MI following other cardiac surgical procedures is unknown (Silvestry, 2017).

The diagnosis of perioperative MI can be determined by electrocardiogram (ECG) changes (e.g., the presence of Q waves or ST elevation), evidence of new wall motion abnormalities, and the presence of elevated cardiac markers (troponin I or creatine kinase [CK-MB]). Significant ST elevation on a postoperative ECG may indicate acute graft closure; other suspect ECG findings include new bundle branch block, ventricular dysrhythmias, or complete heart block (Silvestry, 2017).

Continuous ST segment monitoring is helpful for identification of new or acute ST segment changes indicating myocardial ischemia/injury (Sandau, 2017). Troponin I is a myocardial protein that is a very sensitive and specific marker for myocardial damage. However, troponin elevation is common in the immediate postoperative period following cardiac surgery. The troponin elevation varies among surgical procedures. In fact, troponin concentrations may be present upon admission to the ICU. Higher levels are reported following CABG alone or associated with procedures of the ascending aorta and with valve replacement. Inflammation has been implicated as a possible reason for troponin release even in the absence of myocardial injury. Lower troponin levels are reported following off-pump

CABG and non-CABG procedures (Silvestry, 2017). This makes diagnosis of postoperative MI more difficult (Aranki & Cutlip, 2018; Harskamp et al., 2014). Use of the Joint European Society of Cardiology/American College of Cardiology Foundation/American Heart Association/World Health Federation Task Force definition of MI has been recommended. That is, a CABG-related MI be diagnosed based on biomarkers that are elevated more than five times the 99th percentile of the upper limit of normal and either new pathologic Q waves or new left bundle branch block for the first 72 hours after surgery (Aranki & Cutlip, 2018).

Patients with suspected MI or persistent ischemia follow the same course as uncomplicated postoperative patients, with beta blockade and intravenous nitroglycerin being administered to them if the blood pressure permits (Zafari, 2014). Serial troponin levels should be obtained and monitored as well as 12-lead ECG for the presence of acute changes indicating ischemia/injury (i.e., T-wave inversion, ST segment elevation). Interventional cardiology should be notified to determine if a percutaneous coronary intervention (PCI) is warranted. Intra-aortic balloon pump therapy may be used to diminish inotrope use, infarct size, and myocardial oxygen demand depending upon the patient's hemodynamic status (Parissis, Soo, & Al-Alao, 2012).

Cardiac Arrest

Cardiac arrest is the most serious complication of any cardiac surgery procedure, with the incidence of occurrence estimated to be 0.7% to 5.2% (Pulido, 2014). It can occur unexpectedly at any time from the OR until discharge. It must be managed immediately and in accordance with either the American Heart Association Advanced Cardiac Life Support (ACLS) standards or the Cardiac Advanced Life Support (CALS) standards. Because of the need for and emergent and highly organized approach to resuscitation following cardiac arrest in the cardiac surgery population, hospitals in Europe and the Society of Thoracic Surgery have adopted cardiac surgery–specific protocols designed to assist staff with

> **BOX 13.5** Internal Defibrillation Procedure
>
> 1. Follow the procedure for chest reentry.
> 2. Follow the procedures for advanced cardiac life support (ACLS).
> 3. Prepare the defibrillator for internal defibrillation by gathering sterile internal defibrillation paddles.
> 4. Assist with positioning the internal paddles on the heart.
>   a. One paddle is placed over the right atrium or right ventricle.
>   b. The other paddle is placed over the apex of the heart.
> 5. Charge the defibrillator paddles (5–20 joules).
> 6. Verify providers are clear of the patient and all equipment before defibrillation.
> 7. Assess the patient's cardiac rhythm for conversion and presence of pulse.
> 8. If needed, repeat the defibrillation, following ACLS guidelines.
> 9. Assist with transport to the operating room or closure at the bedside.
> 10. Monitor the patient's neurologic, cardiac, and pulmonary status until stable.

resuscitation efforts (Society of Thoracic Surgeons Task Force on Resuscitation After Cardiac Surgery, 2017). Following the CALS protocol, cardiac surgery patients who were defibrillated immediately (within 60 sec) had survival rates of 54% to 79% (Ley, 2015). The CALS guidelines have yet to be endorsed by the American Heart Association. Potential causes for unexpected cardiac arrest in an otherwise hemodynamically stable patient include mechanical issues such as bleeding/cardiac tamponade and acute graft closure; ventricular arrhythmias are another common scenario. Cardiac arrest may also occur from postoperative shock (Stephens & Whitman, 2015b). Overall mortality rates for cardiac arrest following cardiac surgery is reported at 50% to 83% (LaPar et al., 2014).

As resuscitation efforts are started, evaluation for potential causes—including those unique to cardiac surgery patients—should begin. Checking the position of the endotracheal tube, signs of hypovolemia, patient temperature, chest tube drainage, proper ventilator functioning, results from chest radiograph (for widened mediastinum, tension pneumothorax, or tamponade), arterial blood gas, and electrolytes may help identify the underlying cause of cardiac arrest. Noting the infusion rates of vasoactive agents may provide additional clues. Treating and reversing the cause is the priority here, occurring simultaneously with an established protocol for high-quality cardiopulmonary resuscitation, epinephrine, early defibrillation, and emergency chest reentry. **BOX 13.5** lists the steps for internal defibrillation.

▶ Pulmonary Complications

Pulmonary dysfunction following cardiac surgery is a major cause of death (Silvestry, 2017). Pneumonia is the most common complication seen following surgery of the mitral valve (5.5% of patients). Other common causes of pulmonary dysfunction following cardiac surgery include pleural effusions, atelectasis, decreased thoracic compliance, difficulty weaning, dysfunction of the diaphragm, and pulmonary edema (Stephens & Whitman, 2015b; Silvestry, 2017). While pulmonary complications are common following cardiac surgery, only 5% to 8% of patients require mechanical ventilation for more than 3 days (Stephens & Whitman, 2015b).

Virtually all patients undergoing cardiac surgical procedures will have some degree of postoperative respiratory dysfunction. Cardiac surgery patients are at risk for developing postoperative pulmonary complications due to a number of factors. Preoperative factors include age over 65 years, female gender, recent smoking, chronic obstructive pulmonary disease (COPD), congestive heart failure, diabetes, hypercarbia, and use of vasoactive drug support. Intraoperative risk factors include phrenic nerve injury, aortic cross-clamping, use of IABP, and duration of CPB time. Postoperative risk factors that have been identified include presence of bacteremia, endocarditis, gastrointestinal hemorrhage, acute kidney injury, sternal infection, stroke, new-onset AF, anemia, and reoperation for postoperative bleeding (Ji et al., 2013). Protocols have been developed and are widely utilized that allow for rapid weaning and successful extubation for the majority of cardiac surgery patients (Kiessling et al., 2013).

Preoperative identification of patients with pulmonary risk factors should facilitate provision of proper perioperative intervention. Early identification and intervention to maximize lung function prior to surgery can prevent the incidence of most postoperative pulmonary dysfunction.

Developing an understanding of the postoperative changes in pulmonary function, routine pulmonary management, and contributory factors of pulmonary dysfunction allows for the early identification and management of such problems.

Postoperative Effects on Pulmonary Function

Respiratory complications are noted to be among the top contributors of postoperative morbidity for the cardiac surgery patient. This is especially true of patients who develop ARDS, which is associated with a morality rate as high as 80% (Stephens & Whitman, 2015b). The development of pulmonary dysfunction after cardiac surgery is associated with inconsistencies in gas exchange, ventilation/perfusion mismatch, decreased functional residual capacity, and pulmonary shunting. Patients will often manifest signs of respiratory dysfunction, including shortness of breath, tachypnea, and decreased oxygen saturation. Dysfunction may be related to the use of general anesthesia and neuromuscular blocking agents, a decreased vital capacity from a median sternotomy, and thoracic manipulation. Atelectasis, increased capillary leak, and inflammation for CPB may also contribute to pulmonary dysfunction, as will administration of blood products and crystalloids during surgery (Badenes, Lozano, & Belda,

2015). **TABLE 13-1** lists other factors contributing to higher risk of pulmonary dysfunction.

Atelectasis

Atelectasis occurs in most patients who undergo general anesthesia. Collapse of the individual alveoli, particularly in the dependent parts of the lungs leading to atelectasis, is prevalent in cardiac surgery patients. The absence of traditional ventilation while on CPB as well as deliberate intraoperative lung collapse contribute to this problem, with the incidence of atelectasis reported to be as high as 85% (Badenes et al., 2015). The development of atelectasis is thought to be due to intraoperative displacement of the diaphragm from a sternotomy, lack of lung activity while the patient is on CPB, and from high oxygen concentration during surgery. In patients undergoing CPB, atelectasis is related to increased extravascular lung water, which changes surfactant activity, causes activation of the inflammatory process, and results in coagulation. This results in decreased gas exchange, changes in ventilation to perfusion ratio, decreased functional residual capacity, increased shunt, and hypoxemia. Decreased oxygenation and lung compliance result, continue into the postoperative period, and can have a substantial impact on patient recovery. Areas of atelectasis can lead to an increased risk of postoperative respiratory infection. Pneumonia is a common hospital-acquired infection in postoperative cardiac surgery patients and is a leading cause of morbidity and mortality in these patients (Ibañez et al., 2016).

Techniques or devices that encourage patients to inspire deeply are beneficial. The aim of therapy is to produce a large and sustained increase in the transpulmonary pressure, thereby distending the lung and reexpanding the collapsed alveoli. Several alveolar recruitment methods while intubated include increased levels of positive end-expiratory pressure (PEEP) for short periods of time (sustained inflation) (Santos, Silva, Pelosi, & Rocco, 2015). Once extubated, methods such as noninvasive ventilation, nebulization, deep-breathing exercises, incentive spirometry, and chest physiotherapy have been shown to be helpful in reexpansion of the collapsed lung units (Madappa, 2014).

TABLE 13.1 Factors Contributing to Development of Pulmonary Dysfunction After Cardiac Surgery

Contributing Factors	Effects on Pulmonary System
General anesthesia Paralytics Narcotics Supine positioning	Decreased central respiratory drive leading to decreased use of respiratory muscles Upward shift of diaphragm Chest wall relaxation Changes in compliance of chest wall
Cardiopulmonary bypass	Pulmonary edema from fluid overload and hemodilution Interstitial pulmonary edema from a systemic inflammatory response, which produces capillary leak Complement activation, release of cytokines, and neutrophil activation, which cause increased endothelial permeability Insufficient alveolar distention to activate production of surfactant, which may lead to alveolar collapse, retention of secretions, and atelectasis
Cooling for myocardial protection	Phrenic nerve injury
Median sternotomy incision and chest tubes	Chest wall splinting, which reduces the patient's ability to take deep breaths
Use of ITA for coronary artery bypass conduit	Use of ITA requires pleural dissection, which causes a potential decrease in chest wall compliance
Blood transfusion	Can cause TRALI
Sternal or thoracotomy incisional pain Obesity Age Diaphragmatic injury Smoking history History of COPD, heart failure	Decreased respiratory muscle use

COPD, chronic obstructive pulmonary disease; ITA, internal thoracic artery; TRALI, transfusion-related acute lung injury.
Data from Badenes, Lozano, & Belda, 2015; Ji et al., 2017; Roekaert & Heijmar, 2012.

Vigorous pulmonary toileting along with early ambulation are generally effective therapies for the postoperative cardiac surgery patient who is recovering from atelectasis.

Pleural Effusion

Postoperative pleural effusions, or fluid collections in the pleural space, occur in about 41% of cardiac surgery patients, occurring more frequently in those who undergo takedown of the internal thoracic artery (ITA) (Bejar et al., 2016). Causes of pleural effusions in postoperative cardiac surgery patients include heart failure, postpericardiotomy syndrome, pneumonia, pulmonary embolism, chylothorax, hemothorax, and erosion of a central venous catheter through central venous structures, or they can be related to the surgical procedure (Heffner, 2017). Chest tubes left in place at the end of the cardiac surgery procedure are often strategically placed to avoid postoperative pleural effusions. Pleural effusions are easily diagnosed on a chest radiograph.

Patients with small pleural effusions (less than two intercostal spaces [ICSs] on a chest radiograph) are usually asymptomatic. A small percentage of patients with an ITA (7%) and saphenous vein (2%) CABG procedures have pleural effusions that can be seen in more than two ICSs. Pleural effusions are typically left sided. Small pleural effusions will likely resolve on their own, with the body reabsorbing the fluid collection (Heffner, 2017). Diuretics can also be used when pleural effusions are bilateral and appear to be related to congestive heart failure. Moderate to large effusions may occupy more than 25% of the lung and may cause activity-limiting dyspnea and require intervention. In this situation, a thoracentesis or chest tube insertion is indicated (Boka, 2017).

Phrenic Nerve Injury

There has been a decline in phrenic nerve injury with diaphragmatic dysfunction as a result of improved techniques used in cardiac surgical procedures. The incidence is related to the cardiac surgical procedure (Kodric et al., 2013). Historically, the primary etiology of this morbid complication was cold injury to the phrenic nerve caused from the use of ice in the pericardial region as a method of myocardial protection. Phrenic nerve injury is also thought to be related to the pleurotomy required for ITA harvesting; this results in more chest wall trauma, pain, and decreased ability to cough and deep breathe (Kamanger, 2013). Ice is no longer used routinely in the pericardium; however, phrenic nerve injury may also occur with the takedown of the ITA. Dissection of the ITA may also decrease blood supply to the intercostal muscles, which may result in injury to the phrenic nerve (Kamanger, 2013).

Signs and symptoms depend on whether the paralysis is unilateral or bilateral. Unilateral phrenic nerve injuries rarely produce significant respiratory symptoms, and patients can usually be extubated without difficulty. Some patients may be asymptomatic at rest but develop dyspnea on

exertion and activity intolerance. If the patient has a history of lung disease, dyspnea at rest may be present; orthopnea may occur. In contrast, bilateral phrenic nerve injury, although rare, results in paradoxical breathing, tachypnea, shallow respirations, dyspnea, and carbon dioxide retention when attempts are made at extubation. Symptoms may increase when the patient is in a supine position. Other symptoms may include anxiety, insomnia, morning headache, extreme sleepiness during the day, and poor sleep. Gastrointestinal symptoms such as dyspepsia, regurgitation, nausea, and epigastric pain may occur. Arterial blood gas analysis will reveal hypoxia and progressive hypercarbia. The hypoxia is related to atelectasis and ventilation/perfusion mismatching. Chest radiograph may reveal an elevated hemidiaphragm at end expiration with spontaneous ventilation, small lung volumes, and atelectasis; these will not be apparent while the patient is mechanically ventilated owing to the effects of the positive pressure ventilation. Treatment may involve plication of the diaphragm, which attempts to stabilize the diaphragmatic muscle and prevents paradoxical motion with breathing. Phrenic pacing, diaphragmatic pacing, or noninvasive ventilation at night may be required. A tracheostomy with positive pressure ventilation may be required if less invasive methods are not successful. Inspiratory muscle strength and endurance training may be successful. Nerve reconstruction techniques may be attempted on some patients. Many patients improve with chest physiotherapy and prevention and treatment of pneumonia (Kamanger, 2013). Phrenic nerve injury is discussed in more detail in Chapter 11.

Pneumothorax

A pneumothorax (PTX) is air in the pleural space. If a pleural space is opened at the time of surgery (e.g., during the takedown of an ITA), a chest tube must be placed to drain both air and fluid to avoid complications (Mohammed, 2015). A small PTX can also occur because of direct injury to the lung during surgery, central venous cannulation, or barotrauma during positive pressure ventilation. This is usually noted in the immediate postoperative period and detected on the initial postoperative chest radiograph (Stark, 2013). The incidence of PTX may increase in patients with preexisting bullous lung disease or in those requiring high levels of PEEP. A PTX that is small will usually reabsorb on its own and can be monitored with serial chest radiographs. A chest tube must be inserted for any large PTX, because it could potentially enlarge with the use of positive pressure ventilation (Mohammed, 2015).

It is not uncommon for a tension PTX to develop following cardiac surgery. The most common causes are regional block, airway instrumentation, and central line placement. Patients with COPD are at greater risk. Although rare, it can also occur intraoperatively. Signs may be masked during general anesthesia. When the patient is admitted to the ICU, peak airway pressures are elevated; more pressure is required to deliver the same tidal volume. Expiratory volumes are decreased and are due to air leaking into the pleural space. An increase in end-expiratory pressure will be noted even in patients not receiving PEEP (Jain, Arora, Juneja, Mehta, & Trehan, 2014). In this situation, the patient acutely decompensates. Although breath sounds may be diminished, it may be difficult to assess given ventilator sounds and various alarms in the unit. Other signs and symptoms of tension PTX can include distended neck veins, hypotension, and tracheal deviation away from the collapsed lung. If the patient is hemodynamically unstable and a tension PTX is suspected, decompression with a 16-gauge needle at the second intercostal space, midclavicular line, is indicated. A rush of air and an improvement in hemodynamics confirm the diagnosis (Jain et al., 2014). A chest radiograph should be obtained to assess the involved structures and the severity of the tension PTX. Treatment also includes immediate placement of a chest tube, usually at the fifth intercostal space, anterior axillary line, for the residual PTX (Daley, 2014).

Prolonged Mechanical Ventilation

A small number of patients will require prolonged mechanical ventilation after cardiac surgery. Prolonged mechanical ventilation beyond 48 hours occurs in about 5% to 10% of patients and is usually the result of cardiac or hemodynamic dysfunction, surgical reexploration, neurologic complications, or acute renal failure (Totonchi, Baazm, Chitsazan, Seifi, & Chitsazan, 2014). These patients typically do not have gas exchange or oxygenation issues but require an airway support because of critical illness. Prolonged mechanical ventilation is discussed in detail in Chapter 11.

Acute Respiratory Distress Syndrome

Acute respiratory distress syndrome is characterized by inflammation of the lung parenchyma and increased microvascular permeability, which causes leakage of fluid into the alveolar space, hypoxemia, increased work of breathing, and pulmonary infiltrates on a chest radiograph. Acute respiratory distress syndrome usually becomes evident within the first 24 to 48 hours following cardiac surgery and can be a direct result of the acute inflammatory reaction and systemic response seen with CPB. The reported incidence of patients developing ARDS after cardiac surgery is up to 20%; mortality rates are as high as 80% (Stephens & Whitman, 2015b). Up to 17% of patients who undergo aortic valve procedures develop ARDS. Previous cardiac surgery, use of CPB, large volume shifts, mechanical ventilation, direct surgical insult, shock, and excessive administration of blood products are important predictive factors for this complication (Rong, Di Franco, & Ginadino, 2016). Transfusion-related acute lung injury (TRALI) presents a similar clinical picture to that of ARDS, resulting in diffuse pulmonary edema due to increased alveolar permeability. Transfusion-related acute lung injury is thought to be an immune-mediated response between donor plasma antibodies and the recipient leukocyte antigens; criteria defining TRALI include hypoxemia with increased oxygen requirements, along with the development of pulmonary infiltrates within 6 hours of transfusion (Zah-Bogović, Mesarić, Hrabač, & Majerić-Kogler, 2014).

The risk of ARDS can be decreased with lung protective strategies such as use of low tidal volume (6 mL/kg ideal body weight) (Stephens & Whitman, 2015a). Treatment of ARDS and TRALI is mainly supportive, with maintenance of adequate oxygenation being the primary goal. The use of smaller tidal volumes (6 mL/kg) and PEEP has been associated with improved outcomes. In some cases the use of extracorporeal mechanical circulatory oxygenation (ECMO) may be needed to maintain tissue perfusion and oxygenation. Use of judicious fluid administration, minimizing administration of blood products, nutrition, and early mobility may improve outcomes as well (Stephens, Shah, & Whitman, 2013).

Oxygen concentration should be titrated to achieve a PaO_2 of at least 70 mmHg. Patients with actual or potential RV failure may require a PaO_2 of 85 to 100 mmHg to decrease RV preload. Positive end-expiratory pressure should be added to promote oxygenation. Normal partial pressure of carbon dioxide ($PaCO_2$) levels should be maintained with a normal pH (7.35–7.45) because elevated $PaCO_2$ levels can increase RV afterload. Carbon dioxide and lactate levels increase as the patient warms from surgery; this can lead to a respiratory and metabolic acidosis. To correct this, the respiratory rate should be increased to increase minute volume (rather than increasing tidal volume) (Stephens & Whitman, 2015a). Patients should be assessed on an ongoing basis for readiness for weaning from mechanical ventilation. The head of the bed should be elevated at 30 degrees to prevent risk of aspiration, unless contraindicated. Arterial blood gas results should be monitored.

Pneumonia

Postoperative pneumonia is the most common infection following cardiac surgery. It usually occurs within 5 days of surgery but may develop within the first 24 to 48 hours. The reported incidence of postoperative pneumonia is 1% to 5% (Silvestry, 2017). As discussed in Chapter 11, patients with persistent left ventricular (LV) failure are also at risk for the development of pneumonia. Additionally, patients with perioperative renal failure and those who receive excessive blood product administration are also at a higher risk because of the additional fluid volume burden

on the pulmonary system. Other identified independent predictors of postoperative pneumonia include COPD, postoperative AF, diabetes, smoking, older age, longer ICU length of stay (LOS), hypertension, preoperative corticosteroid use, and length of CPB time. Patients with incisional pain from either a sternotomy or thoracotomy are also at risk for developing pneumonia if the pain interferes with effective coughing and deep breathing (Silvestry, 2017).

Signs and symptoms may include fever, elevated white blood cell count, increased pulmonary secretions, and pulmonary infiltrates on chest radiograph. Hypoxemia may develop with associated increased oxygen requirements (Allou et al., 2015).

Aggressive use of incentive spirometry, chest physiotherapy, and early mobilization are all strategies to avoid postoperative pneumonia in the cardiac surgery population. Finally, one key to the avoidance of postoperative pneumonia is to follow evidence-based guidelines for the prevention and management of ventilator-associated events (VAEs). Basic strategies for avoidance of VAEs are oral hygiene using chlorhexidine solution, keeping patients semirecumbent, avoiding gastric overdistention, early nutrition, and daily sedation interruption for early weaning and extubation from the ventilator.

▸ Hematologic Complications

Bleeding

Bleeding and clotting are common postoperative scenarios in the cardiac surgery patient population. Approximately 30% of patients undergoing CABG require a blood transfusion (Aranki, Aroesty, & Suri, 2017). Severe bleeding (i.e., bleeding requiring transfusion of more than 10 units of packed red blood cells) is reported to occur in up to 5% of patients. It is typically related to incomplete hemostasis, heparin used during CPB, decreased circulating clotting factors, hypothermia, dilutional decrease in platelets, coagulopathies, or platelet dysfunction (Silvestry,

2017). Predictors of the need for transfusion are female gender, older age, lower body weight, lower hemoglobin preoperatively, preoperative use of antiplatelet or antithrombotic agents, reoperation, emergency or complex procedures, and coagulation abnormalities (Aranki et al., 2017). Postoperative bleeding typically subsides within the first few hours; however, 1% to 3% of patients will require mediastinal reexploration (Colson et al., 2016). Typically, bleeding following cardiac surgery can be classified into two categories: surgical versus nonsurgical (coagulopathy). The etiology of postoperative bleeding may be surgical incision sites, platelet inhibition from exposure to preoperative antiplatelet drugs, platelet dysfunction from exposure to the CPB circuit, the effects of heparin, or a combination of these. Excessive bleeding is defined as loss of more than 500 mL of blood in the first postoperative hour. Bleeding is a significant contributor to postoperative morbidity and mortality, therefore prompt assessment and treatment in the ICU are critical. Administration of blood products may be enough to correct bleeding caused from coagulopathies. However, bleeding that persists despite correction of coagulation factors will require a return to the OR for early mediastinal reexploration (Silvestry, 2017). Usual sources of surgical bleeding include, but are not limited to, coronary anastomoses sites, saphenous vein branches, ITA takedown sites or the ITAs themselves, cannulation sites, or sternal wire sites.

Bleeding following cardiac surgery typically leads to administration of blood products (Silvestry, 2017). Packed red blood cells are often used to maintain adequate hemodynamic parameters and to correct hemoglobin to ensure adequate tissue oxygen delivery. Additionally, fresh frozen plasma, platelets, and cryoprecipitate are often required to correct other postoperative coagulopathies. It has been projected that cardiac surgery operations account for 15% of the nation's blood supply annually, with approximately 30% of all patients who undergo CABG requiring a blood transfusion (Silvestry, 2017).

There are various risk factors that predispose patients to postoperative bleeding following cardiac surgery. These are summarized in **BOX 13.6**.

BOX 13.6 Risk Factors for Postoperative Bleeding Following Cardiac Surgery

Patient-Related Risk Factors
Advanced age
Females or those with small BSA
Advanced cardiac disease, LV dysfunction, shock, or any combination of these
Preoperative anemia
Known coagulopathies (e.g., von Willebrand's disease, hemophilia)
Other extracardiac comorbidities—renal or hepatic disease, thrombocytopenia

Preoperative Medications
High-dose aspirin
Antiplatelet drugs such as clopidogrel (Plavix®), prasugrel (Effient®), and ticagrelor (Brilinta®)
Low-molecular-weight heparin or fondaparinux within 24 hours of procedure
Incomplete reversal of INR off warfarin
Emergency surgery while on glycoprotein IIb/IIIa inhibitors eptifibatide (Integrilin®) or abciximab (ReoPro®)

Surgical Procedure–Related Risk Factors
Complex procedures—combined CABG/valve and others with long CPB time, circulatory arrest
Emergent procedures
Reoperations
Use of bilateral ITAs
Heparin rebound or incomplete reversal of heparin with protamine

BSA, body surface area; CABG, coronary artery bypass grafting; CPB, cardiopulmonary bypass; INR, international normalized ratio; ITAs, internal thoracic arteries; LV, left ventricular
Data from Aranki, Aroesty, & Suri, 2017; Silvestry, 2017

Quantitative assessment of postoperative bleeding is critical to document the extent of hemorrhage and the associated patient response while rectifying the situation. General guidelines for excessive mediastinal bleeding are characterized by continuous chest tube output of greater than 200 mL/hr for 2 hours. Ensuring the chest tubes remain patent and documenting the color and consistency of chest tube output are important. Additionally, accurate and frequent documentation (every 15–30 min) of blood loss is key to keeping up with volume replacement when excessive bleeding occurs. Assessment of hemodynamics using a pulmonary artery catheter is important to provide information about filling pressures and CO. Maintenance of adequate hemodynamics is crucial. This is generally accomplished through administration of crystalloid and colloid solutions along with administration of packed red blood cells to keep hemoglobin 8 g/dL or above (hematocrit ≥24%) (Aranki et al., 2017). There are variable definitions of excessive bleeding following cardiac surgery. These include 200 mL/hr or 1,500 mL/8 hr (Stephens & Whitman, 2015a). Of note, surgical reexploration is associated with a twofold increase in early mortality after 90 days (Fröyd & Jeppsson, 2016). Researchers of a recent study report a mortality rate of 8% versus 12% in patients who required reexploration for bleeding following cardiac surgery (Ruel et al., 2017).

In addition to hemodynamics, coagulation studies should be monitored. Prothrombin time (PT)/activated partial thromboplastin time (aPTT), international normalized ratio (INR), fibrinogen level, platelet function testing, or thromboelastogram (TEG) should be obtained and trended so that platelets, cryoprecipitate, and fresh frozen plasma can be administered to correct abnormalities in platelets, fibrinogen, and coagulation factors, respectively (Stephens & Whitman, 2015a). Additionally, medications that improve platelet function (e.g., desmopressin [DDAVP®]) or prevent fibrinolysis (e.g., epsilon-aminocaproic acid [Amicar®]) may also help in improving postoperative coagulopathy (Silvestry, 2017). Protamine sulfate is also administered to reverse the heparin given during CPB. Therefore, activated clotting times and TEG may be utilized to assess for heparin rebound or incomplete reversal as a factor in postoperative bleeding. There are several potential side effects related to protamine sulfate infusion—bradycardia and hypotension being most common.

A frequently used medication that may help in patients with severe and uncontrollable bleeding is factor VIIa. Recombinant activated factor VIIa provides a sudden surge of thrombin-expediting platelet activation and fibrin clot formation and produces a rapid improvement in the INR (Habib, Mousa, & Al-Halees, 2016), although evidence suggests that recombinant factor VIIa may be helpful in achieving hemostasis at the site of vessel injury, thereby reducing transfusion requirements. Activated platelets are present throughout the body following CPB; therefore, systemic thrombosis may occur. Current recommendations exist for dosing factor VIIa for use in cardiac surgery patients (60 mcg/kg), because it is expensive. There are specific dosing guidelines that are critical to avoid complications. Factor VIIa was discussed in more detail in Chapter 12.

Thrombosis

Patients who have undergone CABG procedures are also at risk for developing clots. This is believed to be related to increased platelet activity. Aspirin may not be effective in mitigating clot formation (Silvestry, 2017).

Heparin-Induced Thrombocytopenia (HIT)

Thrombocytopenia is common following cardiac surgery. It may occur in over 94% of postoperative patients (Hamid, Akhtar, Naqvi, & Ahsan, 2017). In one study, 31.5% of patients developed a platelet count at least 33% lower than baseline (Chandra et al., 2013). In another study, platelet counts decreased by 50% (Hamid et al., 2017). In a third study, HIT was present in 0.3% of cardiac surgery patients; secondary thrombocytopenia was present in 8.7% of patients. Patients with HIT had a mortality rate of 11.1% (vs. 4.5% of patients with thrombocytopenia and 4% of patients with secondary thrombocytopenia) (Seigerman, Cavallaro, Hagaki, Chung, & Chikwe, 2014). This condition has numerous etiologies in cardiac surgery patients. Predictors of HIT include female gender, congestive heart failure, cardiac insufficiency, atrial fibrillation, hepatic disease, and chronic kidney injury. HIT is associated with increased risk of death, stroke, amputation, acute kidney injury, respiratory failure, and need for a tracheostomy (Seigerman et al., 2014). Factors such as effects of the CPB circuitry (e.g., mechanical destruction of platelets), hemodilution, platelet dysfunction, depletion of platelets, intravascular devices, use of IABP therapy, and effects of medications (e.g., antibiotics, antiarrhythmics) are common causes of thrombocytopenia in this population. A multitude of medications used in the cardiac surgery setting can also cause thrombocytopenia. One medication of significance is heparin, which is used to counteract exposure of the blood to surfaces of the CPB machines (Cheung & Stafford-Smith, 2017).

Heparin-induced thrombocytopenia is a prothrombotic disorder of coagulation caused by platelet-activating, heparin-dependent antibodies. The platelet activation effect leads to excessive thrombin generation, evolving into a hypercoagulable state eliciting both venous and arterial thrombosis. Patients undergoing cardiac surgery are at a higher risk for HIT secondary to the large systemic dose and long exposure to unfractionated heparin required for both preoperative and intraoperative systemic anticoagulation (Cheung & Stafford-Smith, 2017). Heparin-induced thrombocytopenia develops in approximately 1% of all inpatients receiving heparin. However, major thrombotic complications can be avoided when HIT is suspected by using alternative direct thrombin inhibitors for anticoagulation (e.g., bivalirudin [Angiomax®] and argatroban). The diagnosis of HIT should be considered when the platelet count falls to less than 150,000 mm^3 or by greater than 50% of the baseline count between 3 and 14 days of exposure. Laboratory testing with platelet factor-4/heparin enzyme-linked immunosorbent assay (ELISA) antibody and serotonin release assay are necessary to identify whether the patient has acquired the antibodies (Eke, 2014). When HIT is suspected, all heparin products must be discontinued, including use of heparin-coated vascular access catheters and heparin flushes for intravenous (IV) lines. Nonheparin anticoagulants (direct thrombin inhibitors), such as argatroban, should be administered even when confirmatory lab results are not yet available to prevent new thrombosis. Argatroban has been approved by the U.S. Food

and Drug Administration for the prevention and treatment of HIT (Eke, 2014).

Correlation of laboratory data with clinical symptoms is important for an accurate diagnosis. Careful and thorough assessment for areas of new thrombosis should occur by monitoring skin temperature, color, sensation, and peripheral pulses. In addition, ongoing recognition of signs and symptoms of stroke, MI, pulmonary embolism, and renal impairment are important, because they signal a much more serious complication of HIT. Postoperative care should include use of measures to prevent venous thrombotic events, including early mobility (ambulation if possible), isometric exercises, sequential compression devices, graduated compression stockings, or combinations of these interventions (Aranki et al., 2017).

▶ Renal Complications

Cardiac surgery–associated acute kidney injury (CSA-AKI) is a common and serious complication of the use CPB and is among the top two causes of AKI in the ICU (Mao et al., 2013). The incidence of postoperative renal complications is reported as high as over 92% (do Nascimento, Aguiar, da Silva, da Paixão Duarte, & da Silva Magro, 2015) and mortality rates for those developing CSA-AKI requiring dialysis can be upwards of 55% (Mao et al., 2013; Silvestry, 2017). Other data suggest an incidence of renal complications at 24% or 30% based on an increase in serum creatinine by 25% or 50% (Aranki et al., 2017; Silvesty, 2017). The associated mortality rate following cardiac surgery is 1% to 5%, depending on the type of cardiac surgical procedure, preoperative performance status, and comorbidities. Up to 1% to 5% of patients require dialysis (Silvestry, 2017).

Preoperative risk factors for development of AKI include hemodynamic instability, advanced atherosclerotic vascular disease, decreased creatinine clearance, long cardiopulmonary bypass time, use of contrast agents before surgery hypertension, hyperlipidemia, liver dysfunction, stroke, smoking, anemia, and decreased creatinine clearance (glomerular filtration rate <60 mL/min) (O'Neal, Shaw, & Billings, 2016; Silvestry, 2017).

Long duration of CPB is thought to put the patient at risk for AKI. It is believed to be related to renal artery vasoconstriction, hypothermia, loss of pulsatile blood flow while on CPB, and atheroembolic disease (Silvestry, 2017). Other intraoperative risk factors include complex surgery, the need to be placed back on CPB, decrease in hematocrit while on CPB, aortic cross-clamp time, hypoperfusion, hypovolemia, venous congestion, emboli, and exposure to inotropes (O'Neal et al., 2016). There are also several intraoperative measures that should be employed to avoid renal complications and preserve renal blood flow during cardiac surgical procedures. Development of CSA-AKI is associated with a variety of factors. The most critical factor is maintenance of adequate mean perfusion pressures to ensure renal perfusion while on CPB. For that reason, keeping the CPB run as short as possible, off-pump coronary artery surgery, or minimally invasive procedures are good options for preservation of renal function. Additional intraoperative measures include optimizing hemodynamics (avoiding hypotension and hypovolemia). Avoidance of nephrotoxic agents (e.g., aminoglycosides, angiotensin-converting enzyme inhibitors, and contrast media) in the immediate postoperative period is also suggested (Silvestry, 2017).

Postoperative risk factors for the development of CSA-AKI include exposure to vasopressors, inotropes, or diuretics; blood transfusion; anemia; hypovolemia; venous congestion; and cardiogenic shock (O'Neal et al., 2016). Postoperatively, aggressive intervention and early recognition of CSA-AKI may prevent serious and permanent renal damage. The ICU nurse plays a key role in the optimization of hemodynamics. This can often be challenging in the early postoperative phase when rewarming occurs and fluid shifts may cause extreme blood pressure lability. Additionally, prompt identification of reduced urine output, worsening tissue edema, and discontinuation of any potential nephrotoxic drugs are key to renal function preservation. In nonoliguric renal failure, treatment should be directed toward restriction of fluids, administration of diuretics, and close electrolyte monitoring and replacement. Further, there are no supportive data for the use of aggressive dialysis, although some unease exists that renal function may be augmented with these techniques. Dialysis should be considered with signs and symptoms of uremia, fluid overload, and electrolyte abnormalities (vs. blood urea nitrogen and creatinine levels) (Silvestry, 2017).

Fortunately, only a small percentage (1%–5%) of patients with CSA-AKI require initiation of renal replacement therapy (RRT) (Silvestry, 2017). Optimal timing to initiate RRT following cardiac surgery remains uncertain. The most common forms of RRT used following cardiac surgery include intermittent hemodialysis and continuous venovenous hemofiltration. Regardless of the type of RRT utilized, placement of special vascular access catheters is required. Additionally, patient care is centered on managing the fluid and electrolyte shifts caused by this treatment. The ICU nurse plays a key role in the monitoring and treatment of metabolic acidosis, hyper-/hypokalemia, hypomagnesemia, hypocalcemia, and hyperglycemia. The care of these patients can be quite challenging; therefore, prompt treatment of the underlying cause is critical. Mortality data are variable in patients who developed AKI who were and who were not started on RRT following cardiac surgery (Gaudry, Hejage, & Dreyfuss, 2017; Zou, Hong, & Xu, 2017).

Maintenance of glycemic control (blood sugar <180 mg/dL) for the first 48 hours has been linked to improved outcomes, including reduction of ventilator time as well as ICU and hospital LOS. Infection rates are also lower, including deep sternal wound infections. This may be accomplished with an insulin infusion for 12 to 24 hours with ultimate transition to subcutaneous insulin administration (Stephens & Whitman, 2015b). Likewise, early nutritional intervention and support during critical illness have been shown to improve patient recovery by reducing the risk of development of other additional serious postoperative complications (Abunnaja, Cuviello, & Sanchez, 2012).

▶ Gastrointestinal Complications

Gastrointestinal (GI) complications occur in less than 1% to 4.1% of all patients undergoing cardiac surgical procedures (Schwartz, Lindsey, Khabiri, & Stawicki, 2013). The mortality rate averages up to 63% (Aithoussa et al., 2017). The pathophysiology of the most serious GI complications is related to perioperative low CO, which produces vasoconstriction, hypoxia, and hypoperfusion resulting in intestinal ischemia. Other GI complications include paralytic ileus, GI hemorrhage secondary to gastritis or perforated peptic ulcer disease, acute pancreatitis, acute cholecystitis, and acute hepatic failure (Dong et al., 2012).

Predictive factors for the development of GI complications include advanced age, chronic kidney disease, history of peptic ulcer disease, low LVEF (<40%), reoperations or prolonged CPB time, postoperative need for use of an IABP, prolonged mechanical ventilation, postoperative LCOS, advanced age, postoperative sepsis, postoperative stroke, sternal wound infection, diabetes mellitus, renal failure, peripheral vascular disease, valvular surgery, combined CPB/valvular surgery, prolonged mechanical ventilation, and atrial fibrillation (AF) (Schwartz et al., 2013).

Most GI complications are difficult to diagnose because of their atypical symptoms, and the presence of incisional pain often makes it difficult to accurately describe their symptoms. All of these factors may delay diagnosis or treatment leading to serious and often fatal sequelae of respiratory failure, renal failure, sepsis, and shock.

The hypoperfusion associated with GI complications stems from low CO. Therefore, as with most complications of cardiac surgery, prevention, early recognition, and intervention are key, and maintenance of adequate perfusion pressure while on CPB is critical. Additionally, the presence of atheromatous disease of the aorta and perioperative paroxysmal atrial fibrillation also places the patient at high risk for development of serious embolic/ischemic GI complications.

Postoperatively, all patients return to the ICU with a nasogastric tube in place, which typically remains in place until after extubation. Administration of antacid medications (e.g., famotidine [Pepcid®] or ranitidine [Zantac®]) is standard for all patients admitted to the ICU; proton pump inhibitors (e.g., pantoprazole [Protonix®] or esomeprazole [Nexium®]) are often added for those patients with a history of peptic ulcer disease to prevent serious complications. Postoperatively, diet is advanced as tolerated, but the ICU nurse should monitor the patient for presence and changes in bowel sounds, abdominal pain or distention, nausea, and vomiting. Initial treatment of suspected GI complications is conservative—nothing administered orally (NPO) and supportive care with intravenous fluids and medications. If GI complications are suspected, diagnostic lab tests—complete blood count, comprehensive metabolic panel, liver function tests, amylase and lipase, and lactic acid levels—should be performed. An abdominal radiograph, computed tomography (CT) scan, or both may be obtained. Once a diagnosis has been made, early surgical intervention via a laparotomy is warranted and may be lifesaving in those patients who are attempting to compensate for ischemic bowel or a major GI-induced sepsis or bleed (Dong et al., 2012).

▶ Neurologic Complications

Cardiac surgery patients may develop any of a wide range of neurologic complications. The reported incidence is 2% to 6% in this patient population (Silvestry, 2017). Neurologic complications resulting in central nervous system injury may be divided into two types. Type I is a focal injury such as stroke or encephalopathy. Type II is a neurocognitive insult—memory deficit, a notable decline in intellectual function, memory deficit, and seizure (Silvestry, 2017).

The primary neurologic problems following CABG procedures include stroke, cognitive dysfunction, and peripheral neuropathy

(Aranki et al., 2017). The incidence of stroke following CABG procedures is approximately 4%. Following complex valvular procedures, or aortic surgery, the incidence increases to approximately 10%. Patients may also develop encephalopathy following cardiac surgery; the incidence is reported up to 32%. The etiology of this complication is unknown (Stephens & Whitman, 2015b).

The etiology of neurologic complications following cardiac surgery usually is related to an atheroembolism of aortic debris, a clot from a thrombus from the left atrium or ventricle, cerebral hypoperfusion, air embolism, or a microembolism of white cells, platelets, or fibrin (Silvestry, 2017; Stephens & Whitman, 2015b).

Preoperative risk factors for neurologic complications include prior stroke or transient ischemic attack, increased age, female gender, diabetes, renal failure, LCOS, peripheral artery disease, hypertension, recent MI or unstable angina, and moderate or severe LV dysfunction (McGarvey, Cheung, & Stecker, 2017). Neurologic complications following cardiac surgery are discussed in detail in Chapter 16.

▶ Infectious Complications

The incidence of infectious complications following cardiac surgery depends on the definition for infection that is used—mediastinitis versus superficial surgical site infection. In one study, 4.1% of patients with a median sternotomy developed infectious complications (Lemaignen et al., 2015). In another study, 64% developed a surgical wound infection. There was an associated mortality rate of 17% with this latter group of patients (Dubert et al., 2015).

The most common infections following cardiac surgery are respiratory, surgical site, and those related to devices such as urinary catheters. Several prophylactic measures are taken to minimize a patient's risk for a perioperative infection. Antibiotics administered just prior to skin incision reduce the incidence of mediastinitis. Similarly, the use of preoperative intranasal mupirocin and chlorhexidine oral rinses have been shown to reduce staphylococcal and other nosocomial respiratory infections (Helem, Bootsma, & Bonten, 2015; Lazar, Salm, Engelman, Orgill, & Gordon, 2016).

Surgical site infections (SSIs) following cardiac surgery can present in varying forms of severity, affecting both the graft harvest sites and the sternal incision. SSIs can be classified as either superficial (i.e., limited to the skin or subcutaneous tissue) or deep (i.e., involving the sternal bone, substernal space, or mediastinum [mediastinitis]) (Lemaignen et al., 2015). Fortunately, deep sternal wound infections (DSWIs) occur in less than 2% of patients, as they are potentially lethal—carrying a 50% mortality rate when present (Cologni, Barbero, & Rinaldi, 2015). Identified risk factors for this complication include increased body mass index (BMI), preoperative diabetes or hyperglycemia, COPD, use of an IABP, older age, peripheral vascular disease, female gender, tobacco use, recent treatment with antibiotics, heart failure, and emergent or urgent surgery (Cologni et al., 2015; Lazar et al., 2016; Lemaignen et al., 2015). Additional surgical factors that may lead to DSWI include the use of bilateral ITA grafts, prolonged surgery (>300 min) or CPB time, excessive mediastinal bleeding or reexploration, and hyperglycemia in the ICU (Kubota et al., 2013; Meszaros et al., 2016).

Diligence related to glycemic control—maintenance of glucose levels less than 180 mg/dL for the first 2 postoperative days—has been shown to improve surgical mortality and is therefore one of the core measures of quality following cardiac surgical procedures. The ICU nurse should monitor the patient for purulent discharge from the wound, fever, increased pain or tenderness of the chest wall, or an unstable sternum. In addition to adhering to facility-specific wound care policies, administration of prophylactic antibiotic therapy for 48 hours and tight glycemic control help to minimize the likelihood of serious infections. Wound care is discussed in detail in Chapter 18.

Prevention of Hospital-Acquired Pressure Injury

Cardiac surgery patients have been identified as a group most at risk for developing a hospital-acquired pressure injury (HAPI) with a reported incidence of 29.5% (Rao, Preston, Straus, Stamm, & Zalman, 2016). This high risk is attributed to underlying patient comorbidities and the surgical procedure itself. The formation of pressure injuries during surgery has been reported to be 12% to 66% with an average of 49% (Brindle & Wegelin, 2012). Risk factors for disruption in skin integrity include hypothermia, anesthetic agents, cardiopulmonary bypass time, hemodynamic changes, use of vasopressor agents, position, and length of the surgical procedure. Patients undergoing cardiac surgery have an increased intensity of these risks related to the use of heart-lung bypass for cooling and rewarming, use of underlying water-filled pads to assist with temperature regulation, and delayed return to normothermia in the immediate postoperative period (Brindle & Wegelin, 2012). It is not uncommon for a dark purplish butterfly-shaped area to appear across the buttocks/sacral-coccygeal area within 48 hours of the surgical procedure. This is often called a "butterfly" and classified as a deep tissue injury (DTI), which can evolve into a stage III or IV or unstageable pressure injury. There is thinking that a suspected DTI may represent hypoxic reperfusion versus pressure. Unfortunately, the National Pressure Ulcer Advisory Panel has not adopted this thinking. Costs associated with healing an HAPI can range from $500 to $70,000 per individual. Hospital acquired pressure injuries also increase the length of stay by as much as 11 days and may add $30,000 in additional costs (Rao et al., 2016). Targeted prevention measures must be implemented across the continuum of care beginning with preoperative assessment for risk, intraoperative interventions for prevention, and postoperative interventions in the ICU.

Preoperative assessment should include the patient's nutritional status, including serum albumin, mobility, BMI, comorbid conditions (e.g., diabetes, end-stage renal failure, peripheral vascular disease), and general health status. Initial preventative measures begin when the patient arrives in the preoperative holding area. Studies have shown the use of foam dressings on bony prominences, including heels and sacral-coccygeal area, is associated with a reduction of pressure injury (Santamaria, Gerdtz, Liu, et al., 2015; Santamaria, Gerdtz, Sage, et al., 2015). Application of a foam dressing to both heels and sacrum in the preoperative holding area offers the opportunity to reduce the incidence of pressure injuries during the operative procedure. Another consideration for the OR is the operating table overlay. Use of a dry, viscoelastic polymer overlay on the OR table has been shown to reduce pressure injuries (Huang & Chen, 2013). There are additional support surfaces that can be used under specific areas of the body, such as a small static-air mattress placed under the buttocks. A gel-filled positioner placed under the head has been shown to prevent pressure injuries to the scalp when compared to the typical hard foam donut head rest.

In the ICU, the use of foam dressings on bony prominences (e.g., heels, sacrum, elbows) should continue until the patient is out of bed and mobile. Use of an appropriate ICU low air loss bed is important, particularly if it prevents moisture injuries. A static-air mattress is also available to place under the patient if a low air loss bed is not available. Today, overlays containing thousands of sensors are available to be placed on the bed for pressure mapping. The overlay is connected to a small screen that reflects areas of the body with too much pressure indicating impaired capillary blood flow below the skin surface.

Turning remains an important preventative intervention, although sometimes difficult with hemodynamic instability or if the patient has an open chest. Nevertheless, it is important for the nurse to relieve pressure on bony prominences as much as possible. Tilting the patient from side to side as little as 10 degrees using wedges will relieve pressure (Brindle et al., 2013).

▶ Summary

The initial 24-hour period following cardiac surgery is a challenging and tenuous time. Patients have high levels of vulnerability and instability in the initial postoperative period. While there is some degree of predictability in terms of the postoperative trajectory, the trends toward increasing age and number of preoperative comorbidities in these patients have increased the level of complexity associated with this population.

The role of ICU nurses cannot be overemphasized in terms of their influence in reducing the likelihood of critical events associated with postoperative complications. High levels of clinical judgment, adherence to evidence-based practice guidelines, and caring practices are essential competencies. Prevention and prompt recognition of postoperative complications are pivotal to help ensure optimal patient outcomes.

✎ CASE STUDY

G. A., a 71-year-old female, presented to the emergency department with reports of shortness of breath and fatigue. A stat ECG was obtained revealing an anterior lateral ST segment elevation MI. She was taken immediately to the cardiac catheterization laboratory for a percutaneous coronary intervention. The procedure revealed diffuse coronary artery disease and she was referred for coronary artery bypass procedure.

Her cardiac catheterization revealed the following:

EF: 35% severe apical akinesis, 1+ mitral regurgitation
Left main: distal 80%
Left anterior descending (LAD): proximal 90%
Left circumflex coronary artery (LCx): mid 80%
First oblique marginal artery (OM1): 80%
Right coronary artery (RCA): mid 80%, dominant vessel
Right atrium (RA): 8
Right ventricle (RV): 57/14
Pulmonary artery (PA): 35/15 (19)
PAOP: 5
CO: 3.7 L/min
CI: 2.4 L/min/m^2

She was found to have hypertension (185/90 mmHg) and an elevated troponin I 8.0 ng/L. She also has noninsulin-dependent diabetes and bilateral carotid stenosis. Following the cardiac catheterization, she was started on a nicardipine (Cardene®) infusion to lower her blood pressure.

Two days later, she underwent an on-pump CABG ×4 via median sternotomy (left internal mammary artery to the LAD; saphenous vein graft [SVG] to distal RCA; SVG to the first obtuse marginal; and another SVG to another obtuse marginal branch). There was some difficulty transitioning her off cardiopulmonary bypass. She required inotropic/vasopressor support. Total OR time was 5 hours. Postoperative EF was 30%.

She arrived in the ICU sedated, intubated, on a ventilator with propofol (Diprivan®) infusion and pulmonary artery catheter in place. She has two mediastinal chest tubes and two pleural chest tubes on the left. Handoff communication between the anesthesiologist and the receiving nurse included the goals of care for the immediate postoperative period. These included following the rapid extubation protocol and weaning oxygen, maintaining an SaO$_2$ greater than 93%; and continuing inotropic/vasopressor support, which included milrinone at 0.375 mcg/kg/min and epinephrine at 0.03 mcg/kg/min to achieve a CI greater than 2.2 L/min/m^2, and norepinephrine at 0.02 mcg/kg/min to maintain a MAP at 70 mmHg. Additionally, she was on the cardiac surgery insulin drip protocol to be titrated based on hourly blood glucose measurements (fingerstick) between 120 and 180 mg/dL.

Her hemodynamic measurements were:

BP: 84/62
MAP: 68 mmHg
RA (CVP): 15 mmHg
PA: 40/8 mmHg

PAOP: 10 mmHg
CO: 3.7 L/min
CI: 2.0 L/min/m^2

Her arterial blood gas results on arrival were:

pH: 7.42
PaCO$_2$: 41
PaO$_2$: 98
HCO$_3$: 25

Critical Thinking Questions

1. What immediate postoperative assessments should the nurse make?
2. What are the overall effects of milrinone?
3. Based on her myocardial infarction and her bypass procedure, which ECG leads should you select for continuous ST segment monitoring?

Answers to Critical Thinking Questions

1. Overall assessment should include cardiac, pulmonary, and neurologic status and strength of peripheral pulses.
2. Milrinone is a positive inotrope with some vasodilator properties.
3. Leads III and V3 are ideal for ST segment monitoring.

Self-Assessment Questions

1. Which patient is at greatest risk for developing complications following cardiac surgery? A patient:
   A. with an LVEF of 15%.
   B. with a history of atrial fibrillation diagnosed 1 year ago.
   C. who quit smoking 5 years ago.
   D. with a hemoglobin (Hgb) of 12.8 g/dL.

2. Which patient has the highest mortality risk following cardiac surgery? A patient:
   A. with a creatinine clearance of 80 mL/min.
   B. 73 years of age.
   C. with a cardiac output of 2.8 L/min.
   D. with serum glucose of 180 mg/dL.

3. Which indicates sympathetic nervous system stimulation when decreased ventricular function is present immediately following cardiac surgery?
   A. CVP 13 to 10 mmHg
   B. SVR 1,400 to 1,100 dynes/sec/cm^{-5}
   C. CO 5.3 to 4.2 L/min
   D. MVO$_2$ 35 to 50 mL/min

4. Presence of which hemodynamic parameter indicates further optimization is required following cardiac surgery? A patient with:
   A. CVP 16 mmHg.
   B. CI 2.3 L/min/m^2.
   C. SBP 90 mmHg.
   D. PAOP 15 mmHg.

5. Which patient is at greatest risk for developing low cardiac output syndrome following cardiac surgery? A patient:
   A. who underwent mitral valve replacement.
   B. with an Hgb of 9.8 g/dL.
   C. with acute tubular necrosis.
   D. who underwent a CABG procedure.

6. Which hemodynamic parameter should the nurse anticipate seeing in a patient with low cardiac output syndrome?
   A. CI 2 L/min/m^2
   B. PAP 42/22 mmHg
   C. SVR 1,450 dynes/sec/cm^{-5}
   D. HR 110 bpm

7. Which patient is at greatest risk for developing dysrhythmias following cardiac surgery? A patient with:
   A. temp 37.7°C (99.9°F).
   B. PaCO$_2$ 50 mmHg.

C. K 4.5 mEq/L.

D. BMI 19.2 kg/m^2.

8. Which set of hemodynamic parameters should suggest the presence of right ventricular failure to the nurse who is caring for a postoperative cardiac surgery patient?

	CVP (mmHg)	PAOP (mmHg)	CI (L/min/m^2)
A.	18	16	5.1
B.	8	8	2.1
C.	17	8	2.0
D.	6	18	4.8

9. A postoperative cardiac surgery patient from 6 hours ago is experiencing decreased left ventricular function. A low-dose epinephrine infusion is in progress. For which should the nurse observe?

A. Serum potassium 3.8 mEq/L

B. pH 7.30, PaCO$_2$ 50 mmHg, HCO$_3$ 26 mEq/L

C. Serum lactate 1.1 mmol/L

D. Serum glucose 246 mg/dL

10. Which patient is at greatest risk for developing postoperative hypertension following cardiac surgery? A patient with:

	pH	PaCO$_2$	HCO$_3$
A.	7.30	33	18
B.	7.28	51	20
C.	7.48	49	28
D.	7.50	30	21

Answers to Self-Assessment Questions

1. A. **with an LVEF of 15%**
Rationale: Patients at risk for postoperative complications include those with recent smoking, new-onset atrial fibrillation, low LVEF, and anemia.

2. C. **with a cardiac output of 2.8 L/min**
Rationale: Perioperatively, patients with poor cardiac function and low cardiac output have a higher mortality rate.

3. D. **MVO$_2$ 35 to 50 mL/min**
Rationale: When decreased ventricular function is present, compensatory mechanisms such as sympathetic nervous system stimulation and endogenous catecholamine production cause an increase in heart rate, contractility, and vasoconstriction. In turn, preload and afterload increase. These compensatory factors will improve cardiac output and blood pressure, albeit at the cost of increasing myocardial oxygen consumption.

4. A. **CVP 16 mmHg**
Rationale: Optimal hemodynamic parameters in a postoperative cardiac surgery patient include cardiac index 2.2 to 4.4 L/min/m^2, PAOP 10 to 15 mmHg, CVP less than 15 mmHg, SBP 90 to 110 mmHg, and SVR 1,400 to 2,800 dynes/sec/cm^{-5}.

5. A. **who underwent mitral valve replacement**
Rationale: Low CO states are most commonly seen in patients with advanced age, left ventricular dysfunction, acute myocardial ischemia, combined CABG/valve procedures, extended cross-clamping and cardiopulmonary bypass times, mitral valve procedures, and chronic kidney disease.

6. B. **PAP 42/22 mmHg**
Rationale: Low cardiac output syndrome can be defined as a CI less than 2 L/min/m^2, elevated left-sided filling pressure (PAD) greater than 20 mmHg, and SVR greater than 1,500 dynes/sec/cm^{-5}.

7. B. **PaCO$_2$ 50 mmHg**
Rationale: Patients with hypothermia, electrolyte disturbances, hypercapnia, hypoxia, and obesity are at risk for developing postoperative cardiac surgery dysrhythmias.

8. C. **17 / 8 / 2.0**
Rationale: The diagnosis of right ventricular failure is based on presence of an elevated CVP and low PAOP and CO/CI.

9. D. **serum glucose 246 mg/dL**
Rationale: Epinephrine is associated with development of temporary, but significant hyperglycemia, metabolic acidosis, and increased serum lactate when used in the initial 6 to 8 postoperative hours.

10. A. **7.30 / 33 / 18**
Rationale: Development of hypertension may be related to decreased oxygen levels in the muscles with concomitant metabolic acidosis or inflammatory response to CPB.

CLINICAL INQUIRY BOX

Question: What is the incidence of acute kidney injury following cardiac surgery?

Reference: do Nascimento, M. S., Aguiar, T. C., da Silva, A. V. E., da Paixão Duarte, T. T., & da Silva Magro, M. C. (2015). Acute kidney injury in the postoperative period of cardiac surgery. *Acta Paulista de Enfermagem, 28(4)*. Retrieved from http://www.scielo.br/scielo.php?pid=S0103-21002015000400013&script=sci_arttext&tlng=en.

Objectives: To determine the incidence of acute kidney injury after cardiac surgery.

Method: Prospective cohort study.

Results: Based on the Kidney Disease: Improving Global Outcomes (KDIGO) classification, 92.2% of patients had renal dysfunction. The incidence varied based on the criterion from KDIGO.

Conclusion: A highest percentage of patients who underwent cardiopulmonary bypass, valve replacement, or both developed postoperative acute kidney injury.

References

Abunnaja, A., Cuviello, A., & Sanchez, J. A. (2012). Enteral and parenteral nutrition in the perioperative period: State of the art. *Nutrients, 5,* 608–623.

Aithoussa, M., Atmani, N., Moutakiallah, Y., Abdou, A., Nya, F., Bamous, F., . . . Drissi, M. (2017). Gastro-intestinal complications after heart surgery. *Archives of Digestive Disorders.* Retrieved from http://www.alliedacademies.org/articles/gastrointestinal-complications-after-open-heart-surgery-7790.html.

Al-Attar, N. (2011). *Postoperative myocardial infarction.* Retrieved from http://www.escardio.org/communities/councils/ccp/e-journal/volume10/Pages/Postoperative-myocardial-infarction-Nawwar-Al-Attar.aspx#.VKlfKSeodKo.

Allou, N., Allyn, J., Snauwaert, A., Welsch, C., Lucef, J. C., Kortbaoui, R., . . . Montravers, P. (2015). Postoperative pneumonia following cardiac surgery in non-ventilated patients versus mechanically ventilated patients: Is there any difference? *Critical Care, 19*(6). doi:10.1186/s13054-015-0845-5. Retrieved from https://www.ncbi.nlm.nih.gov/pmc/articles/PMC4372228/.

Allyn, J., Allou, N., Augustin, P., Philip, I., Martinet, O., Belghiti, M., . . . Ferdynus, C. (2017). A comparison of a machine learning model with EuroSCORE II in predicting mortality after elective cardiac surgery: A decision curve analysis. *PLoS ONE, 12*(1), e0169772.

Aranki, S., Aroesty, J. M., & Suri, R. M. (2017). *Early noncardiac complications of coronary artery bypass graft surgery.* Retrieved from https://www.uptodate.com/contents/early-noncardiac-complications-of-coronary-artery-bypass-graft-surgery.

Aranki, S., & Cutlip, D. (2018). *Early cardiac complications of coronary artery bypass graft surgery.* Retrieved from https://www.uptodate.com/contents/early-cardiac-complications-of-coronary-artery-bypass-graft-surgery.

Badenes, R., Lozano, A., & Belda, F. J. (2015). Postoperative pulmonary dysfunction and mechanical ventilation in cardiac surgery. *Critical Care Research and Practice,* *2015.* Retrieved from https://www.hindawi.com/journas/ccrp/2015/420513.

Beebe, R., & Myers, J. (2011). Heart failure. In R. Beebe & J. Myers (Eds.), *Professional paramedic: Medical emergencies, maternal health, and pediatrics* (pp. 66–97). Clifton Park, NY: Delmar.

Bejar, D., Trilei, M., Abouda, M., Yengu, T., Meiki, B., Rejeb, H., . . . Charti, R. (2016). Pleural effusions after cardiac surgery: Etiology and outcomes. *European Respiratory Journal, 48*(Suppl 60). Retrieved from http://erj.ersjournals.com/content/48/suppl_60/PA2528.

Boka, K. (2017). *Pleural effusion treatment & management.* Retrieved from https://emedicine.medscape.com/article/299959-treatment.

Brindle, C. T., Malhotra, R., O'Rourke, S., Currie, L., Falls, P., Adams, C., . . . Creehan, S. (2013). Turning and repositioning the critically ill patient with hemodynamic instability: A literature review and consensus recommendations. *Journal of Wound, Ostomy and Continence Nursing, 40*(3), 254–267.

Brindle, C. T., & Wegelin, J. A. (2012). Prophylactic dressing application to reduce pressure ulcer formation in cardiac surgery patients. *Journal of Wound, Ostomy and Continence Nursing, 39*(2), 133–142.

Čanádyová, J., Zmeko, D., & Mikráček, A. (2012). Re-exploration for bleeding or tamponade after cardiac operation. *Interactive Cardiovascular Thoracic Surgery, 14*(6), 704–707.

Chandra, A. B., Mittal, N., Sanbidi, S., Belur, A., Pathak, S., Pathak, H., . . . Xu, Y. (2013). Low incidence of clinically significant heparin-induced thrombocytopenia after cardiopulmonary bypass surgery. *Journal of Blood Disorders & Transfusion, 5,* 180. doi:10.4172/2155-9864.1000180

Cherpanath, T. G., Lagrand, W. K., Schultz, M. J., & Groeneveld, A. B. (2013). Cardiopulmonary interactions during mechanical ventilation in critically ill patients. *Netherlands Heart Journal, 21,* 166–172.

Cheung, A. T., & Stafford-Smith, M. (2017). *Management of cardiopulmonary bypass in adults*. Retrieved from https://www.uptodate.com/contents/management-of-cardiopulmonary-bypass-in-adults.

Cologni, P., Barbero, C., & Rinaldi, M. (2015). Deep sternal wound infection after cardiac surgery: Evidences and controversies. *World Journal of Critical Care Medicine, 4*(4), 265–273.

Colson, P. H., Gaudard, P., Fellahi, J.-L., Berlet, H., Faucanie, M., Amour, J., . . . ARCOTHOVA Group. (2016). Active bleeding after cardiac surgery: A prospective observational multicenter study. *PLoS ONE, 11*(9), e0162396. doi:10.137/journal.pmc.0162396

Cool, S.-C., Thomas, M., Nolan, J., & Parr, M. (2014). Cardiac surgery—postoperative care. In S.-C. Cool, M. Thomas, J. Nolan, & M. Parr (Eds.), *Key clinical topics in critical care* (pp. 90–95). London: J. P. Medical Ltd.

Daley, B. J. (2014). *Pneumothorax treatment and management*. Retrieved from http://emedicine.medscape.com/article/424547-treatment.

do Nascimento, M. S., Aguiar, T. C., da Silva, A. V. E., da Paixão Duarte, T. T., & da Silva Magro, M. C. (2015). Acute kidney injury in the postoperative period of cardiac surgery. *Acta Paulista de Enfermagem, 28*(4). Retrieved from http://www.scielo.br/scielo.php?pid=S0103-21002015000400013&script=sci_arttext&tlng=en.

Dong, G., Liu, C., Xu, B., Jing, H., Li, D., & Wu, H. (2012). Postoperative abdominal complications after cardio-pulmonary bypass. *Journal of Cardiothoracic Surgery, 7*(108), 1–5.

Dubert, M., Pourbaix, A., Alkhoder, S., Mabileau, G., Lescure, F.-X., Ghodhbane, W., . . . Lucet, J.-C. (2015). Sternal wound infection after cardiac surgery: Management and outcome. *PLoS ONE*. Retrieved from http://journals.plos.org/plosone/article?id=10.1371/journal.pone.0139122.

Eke, S. (2014). *Heparin-induced thrombocytopenia*. Retrieved from http://emedicine.medscape.com/article/1357846-overview.

Estrada, V. H., Franco, D. O., Moreno, A. A., Gambasica, J. A., & Nunez, C. C. (2016). Postoperative right ventricular failure in cardiac surgery. *Cardiology Research, 7*(6), 185–195.

Evora, P. R., Bottura, C., Arcêncio, L., Albuquerque, A. A., Évora, P. M., & Rodrigues, A. J. (2016). Key points for curbing cardiopulmonary bypass inflammation. *Acta Cirurgica Brasileira, 31*(Suppl 1), 45–52.

Ferreira, R. G., Northington, B. A., Huang, C.-C., Aranki, S. F., & Muehlschlegel, J. D. (2015). Sex differences in the prevalence of diastolic dysfunction in cardiac surgical patients. *Journal of Cardiac Surgery, 30*(3), 238–245.

Floerchinger, B., Camboni, D., Schopka, S., Kolat, P., Hilker, M., . . . Schmid, C. (2013). Delayed cardiac tamponade after open heart surgery—Is supplemental CT imaging reasonable? *Journal of Cardiothoracic Surgery, 8*, 158.

Fröyd, V., & Jeppsson, A. (2016). Reexploration for bleeding and its association with mortality after cardiac surgery. *Annals of Thoracic Surgery, 102*(1), 109–117.

Gaudry, S., Hejage, D., & Dreyfuss, D. (2017). Renal replacement therapy after cardiac surgery: Do not ask "when", ask "why." *Critical Care, 21*. Retrieved from https://ccforum.biomedcentral.com/articles/10.1186/s13054-017-1818-7doi: 10.1186/s13054-017-1818-7.

Guarracino, F., Baldassarri, R., & Pinsky, M. R. (2013). Ventriculo-arterial decoupling in acutely altered hemodynamic status. In J.-L. Vincent (Ed.), *2013 annual update in intensive care and emergency medicine* (pp. 225–236). New York, NY: Springer Publishers.

Habib, A. M., Mousa, A. Y., & Al-Halees, Z. (2016). Recombinant activated factor VII for uncontrolled bleeding postcardiac surgery. *Journal of the Saudi Heart Association, 28*(4), 222–231.

Hamid, M., Akhtar, M., Naqvi, H. I., & Ahsan, K. (2017). Incidence and pattern of thrombocytopenia in cardiac surgery patients. *Journal of the Pakistan Medical Association, 67*(7), 1019–1023.

Harskamp, R. E., Abdelsalam, M., Lopes, R. D., Boga, G., Hirji, S., Krishnan, M., . . . Bachinsky, W. B. (2014). Cardiac troponin release following hybrid coronary revascularization versus off-pump coronary artery bypass surgery. *Interactive Cardiovascular and Thoracic Surgery, 12*(6), 1008–1012.

He, G.-W. (2013). Arterial grafts: Clinical classification and pharmacological management. *Annals of Cardiothoracic Surgery, 2*(4), 507–518.

Heffner, J. E. (2017). *Pleural effusions following cardiac surgery*. Retrieved from http://www.uptodate.com/contents/pleural-effusions-following-cardiac-surgery.

Helem, D. J., Bootsma, M. C., & Bonten, M. J. (2015). Prevention of surgical site infections: Decontamination with mupirocin based on preoperative screening for staphylococcus aureus carriers or universal decontamination. *Clinical Infectious Diseases, 62*(15), 631–636.

Huang, H.-V., & Chen, H.-L. (2013). Pressure-redistribution surfaces for prevention of surgery-related pressure ulcers: A meta-analysis. *Ostomy Wound Management, 59*(4), 36–48.

Ibañez, J., Riera, M., Amezaga, R., Herrero, J., Colomar, A., Campillo-Artero, C., . . . Bonnin, O. (2016). Long-term mortality after pneumonia in cardiac surgery patients: A propensity-matched analysis. *Journal of Intensive Care Medicine, 31*(1), 34–40.

Jain, A., Arora, D., Juneja, R., Mehta, Y., & Trehan, N. (2014). Life-threatening tension pneumothorax during cardiac surgery: A case report. *Heart, Lung, & Vessels, 6*(3), 204–207.

Ji, Q., Mei, Y., Wang, X., Feng, J., Cai, J., & Ding, W. (2013). Risk factors for pulmonary complications following cardiac surgery with cardiopulmonary bypass. *International Journal of Medical Sciences, 10*(11), 1578–1583.

Kamanger, N. (2013). *Diaphragmatic paralysis*. Retrieved from http://www.emedicine.medscape.com/article/298200-followup.

Kaplow, R., & Iyere, K. (2017). When cardiac tamponade puts the pressure on. *Nursing, 47*(2), 24–30.

Kiessling, A. H., Huneke, P., Reyher, C., Bingold, T., Zierer, A., & Moritz, A. (2013). Risk factor analysis for fast track protocol failure. *Journal of Cardiothoracic Surgery, 8*, 47. Retrieved from http://www.cardiothoracicsurgery.org/content/8/1/47.

Klabunde, R. E. (2013). *Ventricular and atrial hypertrophy and dilation*. Retrieved from http://www.cvphysiology.com /Heart%20Failure/HF009.htm.

Kodric, M., Trevisan, R., Torregiani, C., Cifaldi, R., Longo, C., Cantarutti, F., . . . Confalonieri, M. (2013). Inspiratory muscle training for diaphragm dysfunction after cardiac surgery. *The Journal of Thoracic and Cardiovascular Surgery, 145*(3), 819–823.

Kouchoukos, N. T., Blackstone, E. H., Hanley, F. L., & Kirklin, J. K. (2013). Postoperative care. In N. T. Kouchoukos, E. H. Blackstone, F. L. Hanley, & J. K. Kirklin (Eds.), *Kirklin/ Barratt-Boyes cardiac surgery* (4th ed., pp. 189–250). Philadelphia, PA: Elsevier.

Kubota, H., Miyata, H., Motomura, N., Ono, M., Takamoto, S., Harii, K., . . . Kyo, S. (2013). Deep sternal wound infections after cardiac surgery. *Journal of Cardiothoracic Surgery, 8*, 132. Retrieved from http://www.cardiothoracicsurgery .org/content/8/1/132.

LaPar, D. J., Ghanta, R. K., Kern, J. A., Crosby, I. K., Rich, J. B., Speir, A. M., . . . Ailawadi, G. (2014). Hospital variation in morality from cardiac arrest after cardiac surgery: An opportunity for improvement. *Annals of Thoracic Surgery, 98*(2), 534–540.

Lazar, H. L., Vander Salm, T., Engelman, R., Orgill, D., & Gordon, S. (2016). Prevention and management of sternal wound infections. *The Journal of Thoracic and Cardiovascular Surgery, 152*(4), 962–972.

Lee, R. (2016). *Atrial fibrillation and flutter after cardiac surgery*. Retrieved from https://www.uptodate.com/contents/atrial -fibrillation-and-flutter-after-cardiac-surgery.

Lemaignen, A., Birgand, G., Ghodhbane, W., Alkhoder, S., Lolom, I., Belorgey, S., . . . Lucet, J. C. (2015). Sternal wound infection after cardiac surgery: Incidence and risk factors according to clinical presentation. *Clinical Microbiology and Infection, 21*(7), e11–e18.

Ley, S. J. (2015). Standards for resuscitation after cardiac surgery. *Critical Care Nurse, 35*(2), 30–38.

Lomivorotov, V. V., Efremov, S. M., Kirov, M. Y., Fominskiy, Z. V., & Karaskov, A. M. (2017). Low-cardiac output syndrome after cardiac surgery. *Journal of Cardiothoracic and Vascular Anesthesia, 31*, 291–303.

Lumley, J. S., & Hirst, N. A. (2016). Distinctive clinical syndromes. In J. S. Lumley, A. K. D'Cruz, J. J. Hoballan, & C. E. H. Scott-Conner (Eds.), *Hamilton Bailey's demonstrations of physical signs in clinical surgery* (19th ed., pp. 23–51). Boca Raton, FL: CRC Press Taylor & Francis Group.

Madappa, T. (2014). *Atelectasis treatment and management*. Retrieved from http://emedicine.medscape.com/article /296468-treatment.

Mao, H., Katz, N., Ariyanon, W., Blanca-Mantos, L., Adýbelli, Z., Giuliani, A., . . . Ronco, C. (2013). Cardiac surgery-associated acute kidney injury. *Cardiorenal Medicine, 3*, 178–199.

Mariscalco, G., Woznick, M. J., Dawson, A. G., Serraino, G. F., Porter, R., Nath, M., . . . Murphy, G. (2017). Body-mass index and mortality among adults undergoing cardiac surgery: A nationwide study with a systematic review and meta-analysis. *Circulation, 135*(9), 850–863.

McGarvey, M. L., Cheung, A. T., & Stecker, M. M. (2017). *Neurologic complications of cardiac surgery*. Retrieved from https://www.uptodate.com/contents/neurologic -complications-of-cardiac-surgery.

Meszaros, K., Fuehrer U., Grogg, S., Sodeck, G., Czerny, M., Marschall, J., . . . Carrel, T. (2016). Risk factors for sternal wound infection after open heart operations vary according to type of operation. *Annals of Thoracic Surgery, 101*(4), 1418–1425.

Mohammed, H. M. (2015). Chest tube care in critically ill patient: A comprehensive review. *The Egyptian Journal of Chest Diseases and Tuberculosis, 64*(4), 849–855.

Mohrman, D. E., & Heller, L. J. (2014). Overview of the cardiovascular system. In D. E. Mohrman & L. J. Heller (Eds.), *Cardiovascular physiology* (pp. 1–18). New York, NY: McGraw-Hill.

Najafi, M., & Faraoni, D. (2015). Hemoglobin optimization and transfusion strategies in patients undergoing cardiac surgery. *World Journal of Cardiology, 7*(7), 377–382.

Norkienė, I., Ringaitienė, D., Kuzminskaitė, V., & Šipylaitė, J. (2013). Incidence and risk factors of early delirium after cardiac surgery. *BioMed Research International.* doi:10.1155/2013/323491

O'Neal, J. B., Shaw, A. D., & Billings, F. T. (2016). Acute kidney injury following cardiac surgery: Current understanding and future directions. *Critical Care, 20.* Retrieved from https://ccforum.biomedcentral.com/articles/10.1186 /s13054-016-1352-z.

Pagowska-Klimek, I., Swierzko, A. S., Michalski, M., Glowacka, E., Szala-Pozdziej, A., Sokolowska, A., . . . Cedzyriski, M. (2016). Activation of the lectin pathway of complement by cardiopulmonary bypass contributes to the development of systemic inflammatory response syndrome after paediatric cardiac surgery. *Clinical and Experimental Immunology, 184*(2), 257–263.

Parissis, H., Soo, A., & Al-Alao, B. (2012). Intra-aortic balloon pump (IABP): From the old trends and studies to the current "extended" indications of its use. *Journal of Cardiothoracic Surgery, 7*, 128. doi:10.1186/1749-8090-6-147

Peretto, G., Durante, A., Limite, L., & Cianflone, D. (2014). Postoperative arrhythmias after cardiac surgery: Incidence, risk factors and therapeutic management. *Cardiology Research and Practice, 2014*, 615987. doi:10.1155/2014 /615987

Pieri, M., Belletti, A., Monaco, F., Pisano, A., Musu, M., Dalessandro, V., . . . Landoni, G. (2016). Outcome of cardiac surgery in patients with low preoperative ejection fraction. *BMC Anesthesiology, 16*(1). doi:10.1186/s12871 -016-0271-5

Pulido, J. N. (2014). Unique aspects of resuscitation practices in postoperative cardiac surgical care: A call to action. *The Journal of Thoracic and Cardiovascular Surgery, 148*(4), 1156–1157.

Rao, A. D., Preston, A. M., Straus, R., Stamm, R., & Zalman, D. C. (2016). Risk factors associated with pressure ulcer formation in critically ill cardiac surgery patients: A systematic review. *Journal of Wound, Ostomy Continence Nursing, 43*(3), 242–247.

Rezaei, Y. (2016). Anti-inflammatory role of statins in preventing postperfusion atrial fibrillation. *American Journal of Cardiology, 117*(2). Retrieved from http://www.ajconline.org/article/50002-9149(15)02216-X/pdf.

Rodrigues, A. J., Evora, P. M., & Evora, P. R. (2014). *Use of inhaled nitric oxide in cardiac surgery: What is going on?* Retrieved from http://www.intechopen.com/books/cardiac-surgery-a-commitment-to-science-technology-and-creativity/use-of-inhaled-nitric-oxide-in-cardiac-surgery-what-is-going-on-.

Roekaert, S., & Heijmar, J. (2012). Postoperative considerations in cardiac surgery. In C. Narin (Ed.), *Perioperative considerations in cardiac surgery.* Retrieved from http://www.intechopen.com/books/howtoreference/perioperative-considerations-in-cardiac-surgery/-early-postoperative-care-after-cardiac-surgery.

Rong, L. Q., Di Franco, A., & Ginadino, M. (2016). Acute respiratory distress syndrome after cardiac surgery. *Journal of Thoracic Disease, 8*(10), E1177–E1186.

Rosas, M. M., Giocoechea-Turcott, E. W., Ortiz, P. L., Salazar, A., & Palma, B. A. (2012). Glycemic control in cardiac surgery. In C. Narin (Ed.), *Perioperative considerations in cardiac surgery* (pp. 247–264). Retrieved from http://www.intechopen.com/books/perioperative-considerations-in-cardiac-surgery/glycemic-control-in-cardiac-surgery.

Ruel, M., Chan, V., Boodhwani, M., McDonald, B., Ni, X., Gill G., . . . Mesana, T. (2017). How detrimental is reexploration for bleeding after cardiac surgery. *Cardiovascular Surgery, 154*(3), 927–935.

Sandau, K. E. (2017). Update to practice standards for electrocardiographic monitoring in hospital settings: A scientific statement from the American Heart Association. *Circulation, 136.* doi:10.1161/CIR.0000000000000527

Santamaria, N., Gerdtz, M., Liu, W., Rakis, S., Sage, S., Ng, A. W., . . . Liew, D. (2015). Clinical effectiveness of a silicone foam dressing for the prevention of heel pressure ulcers in critically ill patients: Border II trial. *Journal of Wound Care, 24*(8), 340–345.

Santamaria, N., Gerdtz, M., Sage, S., McCann, J., Freeman, A., Vassiliou, T., . . . Knott, J. (2015). A randomized controlled trial of the effectiveness of soft silicone multilayers foam dressings in the prevention of sacral and heel pressure ulcers in trauma and critically ill patients: The border trial. *International Wound Journal, 12*(3), 302–308.

Santos, R. S., Silva, P. L., Pelosi, P., & Rocco, P. M. (2015). Recruitment maneuvers in acute respiratory distress syndrome: The safe way is the best way. *World Journal of Critical Care Medicine, 4*(4), 278–286.

Schiavone, W. A. (2013). Cardiac tamponade: 12 pearls. *Cleveland Clinic Journal of Medicine, 80*(2), 109–116.

Schwartz, J., Lindsey, D. E., Khabiri, H., & Stawicki, S. P. (2013). Gastrointestinal complications in cardiothoracic surgery: A synopsis. In M. J. Firstenberg (Ed.), *Principles and practice of cardiothoracic surgery* (pp. 355–371). doi:10.5772/54348

Seigerman, M., Cavallaro, P., Hagaki, S., Chung, I., & Chikwe, J. (2014). Incidence and outcomes of heparin-induced thrombocytopenia in patients undergoing cardiac surgery in North America: An analysis of the nationwide inpatient sample. *Journal of Cardiothoracic and Vascular Anesthesia, 28*(1), 98–102.

Shavelle, D. M. (2014). *Clinical syndromes of stunned or hibernating myocardium.* Retrieved from http://www.uptodate.com/contents/clinical-syndromes-of-stunned-or-hibernating-myocardium.

Silvestry, F. (2017). *Postoperative complications among patients undergoing cardiac surgery.* Retrieved from http://www.uptodate.com/contents/postoperative-complications-among-patients-undergoing-cardiac-surgery.

Society of Thoracic Surgeons Task Force on Resuscitation After Cardiac Surgery. (2017). The Society of Thoracic Surgeons expert consensus for the resuscitation of patients who arrest after cardiac surgery. *Annals of Thoracic Surgery, 103*(3), 1005–1020.

Soliman, R. A., Samir, S., el Naggar, A., & El Dehely, K. (2015). Stroke volume variation compared with pulse pressure variation and cardiac index for prediction for fluid responsiveness in mechanically ventilated patients. *Egyptian Journal of Critical Care Medicine, 3*(1), 9–16.

Stark, P. (2013). *Imaging of pneumothorax.* Retrieved from http://www.uptodate.com/contents/imaging-of-pneumothorax.

Stephens, R. S., Shah, A. S., & Whitman, G. J. (2013). Lung injury and acute respiratory distress syndrome after cardiac surgery. *Annals of Thoracic Surgery, 95*(3), 1122–1129.

Stephens, R. S., & Whitman, G. (2015a). Postoperative critical care of the adult cardiac surgery patient: Part I: Routine postoperative care. *Critical Care Medicine, 43*(7), 1477–1497.

Stephens, R. S., & Whitman, G. (2015b). Postoperative critical care of the adult cardiac surgery patient: Part II: Procedure-specific considerations, management of complications, and quality improvement. *Critical Care Medicine, 43*(9), 1995–2014.

Stoppelkamp, S., Veseli, K., Stang, K., Schlensak, C., Wendel, H. P., & Walker, T. (2015). Identification of predictive early biomarkers for sterile SIRS after cardiovascular surgery. *PLoS ONE, 10*(8), e0135527.

Totonchi, Z., Baazm, F., Chitsazan, M., Seifi, S., & Chitsazan, M. (2014). Predictors of prolonged mechanical ventilation after open heart surgery. *Journal of Cardiovascular and Thoracic Research, 6*(4), 211–216.

Wang, Y., & Bellomo, R. (2017). Cardiac surgery-associated acute kidney injury: Risk factors, pathophysiology, and treatment. *Nature Reviews Nephrology, 13*(11), 697–711.

Yarlagadda, C. (2017). *Cardiac tamponade: Clinical presentation.* Retrieved from http://emedicine.medscape.com/article/152083-clinical.

Zafari, A. M. (2014). *Myocardial infarction treatment and management.* Retrieved from http://emedicine.medscape.com/article/155919-treatment.

Zah-Bogović, T., Mesarić, J., Hrabač, P., & Majerić-Kogler, V. (2014). Possible transfusion-related acute lung injury (TRALI) in cardiac surgery patients. *Croatian Medical Journal, 55*(2), 138–145.

Zakkar, M., Ascione, R., James, A. F., Angelini, G. D., &
Suleiman, M. S. (2015). Inflammation, oxidative stress
and postoperative atrial fibrillation in cardiac surgery.
Pharmacology & Therapeutics, 154, 13–20.

Zou, H., Hong, Q., & Xu, G. (2017). Early versus late initial
of renal replacement therapy impacts mortality in
patients with acute kidney injury post cardiac surgery:
A meta-analysis. *Critical Care, 21.* doi:10.1186/s13054
-017-1707-0

Web Resources

Heparin-induced thrombocytopenia: https://www.youtube
.com/watch?v=SWT5nZjnk_w

Median sternotomy: http://www.youtube.com/watch?v
=r7RsB0BA4EI

Sepsis development and progression: http://www.youtube
.com/watch?v=HoxoeP-l5Uw

CHAPTER 14

Pain Management

Noreen O. Peyatt

▶ Introduction

Cardiac surgery is one of the most common surgical procedures performed worldwide (Miozzo, Stein, Bozzetto, & Plentz, 2016); and one of the most common inquiries patients have prior to surgery is how much pain they will experience postoperatively (Chou et al., 2016). According to patients, pain following intrathoracic, abdominal, and gastric surgeries rank among the most severe, and last anywhere between 2 and 8 days (Gan, 2017). Patients undergoing cardiac surgery also reveal that postoperative pain relief is a significant concern; and pain management is one of the most clinically challenging problems for nurses caring for these patients. Pain following cardiac surgery may be associated with the sternotomy, trauma caused by thoracic cage retractors, graft sites, chest tubes, mechanical ventilation, endotracheal tube suctioning, dressing changes, and even the use of air mattresses (Guimarães-Pereira, Farinha, Azevedo, Abelha, & Catro-Lopes, 2016). Unrelieved postoperative pain is associated with increased length of stay (LOS) and decreased patient satisfaction (Gan, 2017). Health care providers acknowledge that unrelieved postoperative pain can have deleterious effects on cardiac surgery outcomes. In the changing world of health care, decreasing LOS, improving patient outcomes, and increasing patient satisfaction are imperative.

Inadequate pain relief may contribute to numerous complications in the postoperative period. The stress of unrelieved pain on the cardiovascular system results in activation of the sympathetic nervous system (SNS). This SNS activation produces a variety of unwanted effects. Postoperatively, these unwanted effects include hypercoagulation, tachycardia, hypertension, and increased myocardial workload and oxygen demand (Gan, 2017). Additionally, patients may suffer from atelectasis, pneumonia, inability to move bronchial secretions, muscle weakness, hyperglycemia, confusion, and an overwhelming stress response (Kerneis et al., 2015). Aggressive pain control is essential in preventing these complications and improving outcomes. Cardiac morbidity is the primary cause of death following anesthesia and surgery (Pignaton et al., 2016).

Despite these potentially devastating complications, recent reviews report only modest success in effectively managing postoperative pain. A historic look at the undertreatment of pain reveals a landmark study in 1973 by Marks and Sachar in which the authors described that greater than 70% of hospitalized patients experienced moderate to severe pain (Gan, 2017). More than 40 years later, patients continue to describe inadequate pain control, and recent studies report pain is underestimated, undermedicated, and underrelieved (Mukiri, 2015). In a frequently cited study, a random sample of patients described the postoperative pain experience. Incredibly, approximately 80% of the patients surveyed indicated they experienced unrelieved postoperative pain (Gan, 2017). Despite significant advances in care, an estimated 50% to 70% of patients still experience moderate to severe postoperative pain (Gan, 2017). Adding insult to injury, the incidence of chronic pain following cardiac surgery ranges from 21% to 55% (Choiniére et al., 2014).

In a study of almost 200 patients who underwent CABG surgery, authors compared pain intensity in patients whose surgeon used the internal thoracic artery (ITA) to those who had the saphenous vein used (Kamalipour, Vafaei, Kazemi, & Khademi, 2014). Nearly 90% of patients in the ITA group experienced pain that lasted greater than 3 months compared to approximately 75% in the non-ITA group. Additional research supports that chronic chest pain following sternotomy affects as many as 56% of patients. Pain management has become the focus of many multidisciplinary cardiovascular surgery teams after the recognition that poor patient satisfaction is often related to inadequate pain relief. Many providers seek to decrease stress, pain, and anxiety through a systematic pain management approach. These efforts have resulted in the possibility of having excellent clinical outcomes, improved patient satisfaction, and high levels of technical expertise (Mukiri, 2015). And this demonstrates that adequate pain relief is possible especially as clinicians explore the use of multimodal analgesia.

Although significant numbers of research studies support the presence of unmanaged postsurgical pain despite advances in pain management, little to no progress has been made in reducing the incidence of postoperative cardiac surgery pain (Choinière et al., 2014). One possible contributor to inadequate pain management is the lack of regular reassessments following administration of analgesics. Ongoing assessment and reassessment of pain helps to improve pain management and overall patient outcomes (Meissner et al., 2015).

Also, other data support that while there is a high incidence of patients reporting moderate to severe levels of pain following cardiac surgery, those individuals receive only a small percentage of their prescribed or allotted analgesic dosage. Some patients receive less than half of the analgesic prescribed for them, despite sufficient ordering and availability of analgesics by providers (Gan, 2017).

Presence of pain following cardiac surgery has implications for optimal recovery. In addition to surgical pain, patients report incidental pain associated with repositioning, coughing and deep breathing, using the incentive spirometry, moving or turning in bed, and getting up (Gan, 2017; Meissner et al., 2015).

Pain management requires effective and efficient assessment, treatment, and evaluation by all members of the health care team, with nurses playing a fundamental role. Nurses are essential advocates for patients who are experiencing pain. Nurses help ensure that patients receive the best possible pain and symptom management. To be an effective patient advocate, nurses must be able to recognize pain; be available, be ready to act, be empathetic rather than judgmental, and be willing to educate not only the patient but also the health care team (Czarnecki, Turner, & American Society for Pain Management Nursing, 2018).

▶ What Is Pain?

According to the International Association for the Study of Pain (IASP; 2017), "pain is an unpleasant sensory and emotional experience associated with actual or potential tissue damage, or described in terms of such damage" (para. 1). The subcommittee on Taxonomy of IASP first defined pain in 1979. This definition continues to be used in the literature and practice (IASP, 2017). Pain is subjective and uniquely experienced by the individual patient (Czarnecki et al., 2018). Multiple factors, including previous pain experience, culture, mood, and coping skills, influence an individual's pain experience (Czarnecki et al., 2018). "The patient's experience of pain is seen as involving far more than a localized sensation; it encompasses what this sensation means to him" (McCaffery, 1972, p. 7).

Pain is subjective (Czarnecki et al., 2018). The patient's self-report of pain is the most reliable indicator of its presence. Pain is described as "whatever the person says it is and exists whenever he says it does" (McCaffery, 1972, p. 8). However, the inability to communicate does not preclude the fact the patient may still be experiencing pain. The use of the word "says" does not mean the patient must verbalize the existence of pain. All patient behaviors—whether voluntary or involuntary, verbal or nonverbal—may indicate the presence of pain (Chou et al., 2016). Measures must be taken to appropriately assess and treat patients who may be unable to verbally report pain (Chiang, Chia, Lin, & Chen, 2016).

▶ Pain Pathways and Processes

A specialized system, called the nociceptive system, mediates the sensory experience of acute pain. The term *nociception* describes the process by which information about an unpleasant or painful stimulus transmits from the periphery to the brain. Nociception is the total neural activity that occurs prior to the cognitive processes, which enables individuals to identify or experience a sensation as pain. Nociception is necessary for an individual to experience pain. Four unique processes comprise the process of nociception: transduction, transmission, perception, and modulation (Czarnecki et al., 2018). The nociceptive process begins with the initial tissue injury, whether real or perceived.

Transduction, the first step in the nociceptive process, is the conversion of noxious stimuli into electrical energy or nerve impulses. Transduction occurs at nociceptors, or nerve endings that are activated by powerful stimuli. Noxious stimuli such as pressure, temperature extremes, mechanical insults such as a surgical incision, or irritant chemicals trigger the release of numerous chemicals. Chemical release includes bradykinin, histamine, and prostaglandins, which activate or sensitize the nociceptors.

Some analgesic therapies work by preventing or modifying transduction. Local anesthetics and antiepileptic drugs block peripheral sodium channels and thus inhibit the production of action potentials. Nonsteroidal anti-inflammatory drugs (NSAIDs) inhibit the production of prostaglandins that would otherwise sensitize nociceptors (Czarnecki et al., 2018).

Transmission is the actual conduction of painful impulses from the nociceptors in the periphery to the spinal cord and brain via two types of primary afferent neurons: myelinated A-delta fibers and unmyelinated C fibers. The A-delta fibers rapidly produce acute, sharp pain, while the C fibers conduct the impulse more slowly, thereby producing diffuse, dull, aching pain. From the nociceptor, the action potential travels to the dorsal root ganglia and then to the dorsal horn of the spinal cord. The location where nerve fibers enter the spinal cord helps to explain the pattern of pain sensed in cutaneous tissues. The primary afferent neurons release excitatory neurotransmitters such as glutamate in the spinal cord. These transmitters activate spinal neurons that send axons across the spinal cord and up ascending pain pathways via the spinothalamic tracts to the thalamus. Fibers synapse in the thalamus and make connections with other parts of the brain, including the limbic system. Some medications exert their analgesic effects by regulating the release of neurotransmitters. Opioids work at the level of the spinal cord and bind to presynaptic receptors, decreasing calcium conduction and thus the release of neurotransmitters in the dorsal horn (Czarnecki et al., 2018).

Perception is the process by which a conscious individual recognizes the sensation of pain. Perception occurs as the brain processes the information. The spinal cord sends the information carried by the free nerve ending to the thalamus, and the information is then sent to the cortical areas of the brain where pain perception occurs. Sensory information about the pain combines with emotional, cognitive, and sociocultural determinants to create the pain experience. Many interventions can affect the perception of pain. For example, cognitive strategies such as distraction, relaxation, hypnosis, and imagery are effective pain-reducing therapies that operate at this level of the pain pathway and are useful pain management techniques (Czarnecki et al., 2018).

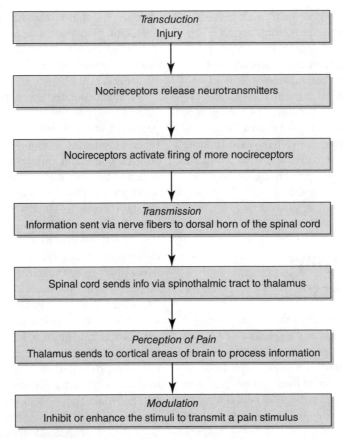

FIGURE 14.1 Pathophysiology of pain.

Modulation, the final step, occurs when stimuli are either enhanced or inhibited by the hypothalamus, pons, and somatosensory cortex so as to process and transmit a pain sensation (Czarnecki et al., 2018). Modulation involves both the peripheral and central nervous systems and many different neurochemicals. Endogenous opioids in the peripheral and central nervous systems, and the central inhibitory neurotransmitters norepinephrine and serotonin, are significant components in modulating pain impulses (Czarnecki et al., 2018). An example of modulation is the use of antidepressants for the management of pain. Some antidepressants block reuptake of the neurotransmitters, norepinephrine, and serotonin, making them available in the fight against pain (Czarnecki et al., 2018). **FIGURE 14.1** depicts the pain physiology process.

Smoking serves as a nicotine-delivery vehicle and produces changes in physiology. Exposure to systemic nicotine has consistent antinociceptive effects. Chronic exposure of nicotine causes the endogenous opioid system to change in ways that may affect processing of nociceptive stimuli. Smoking can produce changes in central nervous system function that persist long after subjects stop smoking. Smokers have been found to complain of greater pain intensity and an increased number of painful sites overall as well as chronic pain. Nicotine withdrawal is thought to enhance the perception of pain. Smoking also causes changes in the neuroendocrine system that could modulate pain perception. Smoking is thought to impair oxygen delivery to tissues by increasing sympathetic outflow and carboxyhemoglobin levels. Hence, smoking may accelerate degenerative processes that interfere with wound healing. Evidence supports that an increase in postoperative analgesic requirements should be anticipated in cigarette smokers (Chiang et al., 2016).

▶ Types of Pain

There are two major classifications of pain: nociceptive and neuropathic. Understanding the type of pain experienced by the patient is key to providing the most effective treatment. Nociceptive pain occurs with direct stimulation of pain receptors. Examples of this type of pain include tissue injury or inflammation. Nociceptive pain can be further classified as either somatic or visceral. Somatic pain refers to the stimulation of pain in the cutaneous and deep layers of skin. Patients are able to localize this pain, which often comprises acute pain due to surgery. Somatic pain often responds best to NSAIDs or acetaminophen. Visceral pain refers to pain resulting from infiltration or compression of the abdominal or thoracic viscera. Patients often have difficulty localizing visceral pain, because the pain is referred to another part of the body. Opioids often work well in the treatment of visceral pain (Chou et al., 2016; Czarnecki et al., 2018).

Postoperative cardiac surgery patients are likely to experience pain from a variety of sources. Incisions from sternotomy, thoracotomy and graft sites, required invasive procedures, tissue retraction and dissection, turning, and presence and removal of chest tubes are some of the identified etiologies (Ziyaeifard, Azarfarin, & Golzari, 2014). Data have shown that patients who underwent painful procedures (e.g., chest tube removal) and were not premedicated for pain subsequently reported moderate to high levels of pain (Gan, 2017).

Neuropathic pain is primarily caused by a dysfunction in the nervous system that can occur either centrally or peripherally. Neuropathic pain is often the consequence of an injury to the nervous system that results in sustained abnormal sensory processing. Patients often describe this pain as burning, fire, stinging, and electric. Examples of neuropathic pain include diabetic neuropathy and phantom pain (Pogatzki-Zahn, Segelcke, & Schug, 2017).

Pain is further categorized as acute or chronic. Acute pain typically has a sudden onset and serves as a warning signal to the body. Acute pain usually results from an insult or injury, and as the insult or injury resolves, so should the pain. Acute pain may last for a moment or it can be more severe and last weeks to months. Experts agree that, by definition, acute pain duration is less than 6 months (Czarnecki et al., 2018). On the other hand, chronic pain, also referred to as persistent pain, persists beyond the time of tissue healing. On average, chronic pain lasts greater than 6 months and is sometimes difficult to manage. Chronic pain often affects function, social and family interactions, and therefore quality of life. Acute and chronic pain can be visualized as a continuum instead of two distinct categories (Dueñas, Ojeda, Salazar, Mico, & Failde, 2016). For patients who undergo cardiac surgery, health care providers' focus remains on acute, nociceptive pain.

Unfortunately, patients who undergo cardiac surgery have a significant risk for developing chronic pain (Gan, 2017). The incidence of chronic pain following cardiac surgery ranges from 21% to 55% (Bouzia et al., 2017). Over time, the patient's pain characteristics may progress from acute, nociceptive pain to chronic, neuropathic pain in origin. This pain is often the result of nerve damage associated with sternal incisions and retractions. Recent studies show that postoperative cardiac pain may be reduced if patients receive pregabalin (Lyrica®) for 2 weeks prior to surgery (American Society of Anesthesiologists [ASA], 2013). Approximately 30% to 44% of patients who undergo thoracotomy exhibit chronic pain 6 months to 1 year after surgery has been reported (Mesbah, Yeung, & Gao, 2015). The risk of developing chronic pain seems to be reduced if postoperative pain is adequately managed (Chou et al., 2016). This places a greater emphasis on the need to control pain during the acute postoperative period.

In another study of cardiac surgery patients, 29% of patients experienced persistent pain from any site (lasting at least 2 months postoperatively), and 25% reported persistent sternotomy pain. Other sites of pain included the shoulder, back, and neck. Pain intensity in these patients was mild, with 7% of the study participants reporting that the pain interfered with activities of daily living (ADLs). There was no significant difference in the incidence in those patients who received postoperative high thoracic epidural anesthesia and opioids (Ziyaeifard et al., 2014).

These findings were corroborated in another study of cardiac surgery patients. Patients who reported moderate to severe postoperative pain were the same patients who reported chronic poststernotomy pain more frequently (Kleiman, Sanders, Nemergut, & Huffmyer, 2017).

Research indicates that individuals who experience uncontrolled acute pain for long periods of time have a greater probability of developing chronic pain (Dueñas et al., 2016). One hypothesis for this phenomenon suggests that a neurophysiologic link results in glial activation following nerve or tissue injury. The signaling molecules involved in glial activation are adenosine triphosphate (ATP); fractalkine (CX3CL1); monocyte chemotactic protein-1 (CCL1); the proinflammatory cytokines interleukin 1-beta (IL-1β), interleukin 6 (IL-6), tumor necrosis factor alpha (TNF-α), and substance P (SP); and glutamate (Czarnecki et al., 2018). This supports the belief that individuals require early cessation of pain to prevent progression to a state of chronic pain. Clearly, early recognition and treatment of acute pain is of prime importance.

▸ Pain Assessment

Pain assessment is the cornerstone of good pain management. Precise and methodical assessment of pain is necessary to determine the most efficacious treatment regimen for patients presenting with pain. The national pain management standards, as delineated by The Joint Commission, require the prompt management of pain once identified (Chou et al., 2016). According to The Joint Commission (2018), health care providers can "improve pain assessment by concentrating more on how pain is affecting patients' physical function." The expectation is for health care providers to perform an initial pain assessment and perform regular reassessments based on the need of the patient. For Joint Commission–accredited organizations, this is mandatory. Having national standards also implies the risk of legal liability if pain is poorly managed. Consumers have the right to have their pain adequately assessed and managed, and there are instances of legal action for poor pain management (Chou et al., 2016).

Typically, during screening, the provider inquires about the patient's present pain state and history of pain. Pain history should always include the use of analgesics, dosing, and efficacy. The progression to a more detailed assessment is determined following the initial screening. Assessment of pain focuses on several key components, including the location, intensity, quality, and duration of the pain; effective pain relief techniques; and the patient's perception of an acceptable pain level or comfort goal (Mukiri, 2015). Pain assessment is a continuous cycle of assessment, intervention, and reassessment. To successfully manage pain, the nurse must first ask about the pain, accept the subjective report of pain, intervene to relieve the pain in accordance with the patients' comfort goal, reassess pain following any intervention, and advocate for changes in the pain management regime as needed (Meissner et al., 2015).

A variety of pain assessment tools exist to aid in the assessment of pain. Self-report of pain is the gold standard for verbal patients. Nurses regularly use pain intensity scales, in clinical practice, to elicit a patient's self-report. Use of pain rating scales facilitates the identification of pain intensity over time and helps to evaluate the effectiveness of pain relieving interventions (Kizza, Muliira, Kohi, & Nabirye, 2016). Pasero and McCaffery (2005) evaluated numerous pain intensity rating scales for use in cognitively intact adolescent and adult patients. The numeric rating scale (NRS) and FACES® pain rating scale are two of the most frequently used tools in daily clinical practice.

Use of the NRS typically involves a horizontal line with a 0 to 5 scale or 0 to 10 scale. The health care provider anchors the scale by explaining that zero is no pain and the opposite end of the scale is the worst imaginable pain. This scale is well established with good validity and reliability. Although health care providers often present the scale verbally without providing a visual copy for the patient, research shows that the use of the written copy results in better patient understanding (Czarnecki et al., 2018). A survey of health care professionals indicated that 70% prefer the use of the 0 to 10 scale for clinical practice (Pasero & McCaffery, 2005). In a recent literature review comparing studies of the NRS, verbal rating scales, and visual analog scales (VASs), the authors report that the NRS showed better overall compliance and was easy to use (Booker & Haedtke, 2016). The 0 to 10 NRS is available in many languages.

Developed originally for use in children, the FACES pain scale is appropriate for use with some adults. The FACES scale is gender, age, and culture neutral. This scale is also translated into several languages. According to Herr and Garand (2001), the FACES pain scale is preferred among African American and Asian adults. The FACES scale contains brief words below the faces to better describe pain. The anchor for zero is still no pain with the opposite end of the scale indicating "hurts worst" (Czarnecki et al., 2018).

Pain Assessment in Patients Who Are Unable to Communicate

Assessment of pain for patients who are unable to communicate can be challenging for nurses. The identification of pain in nonverbal patients can be tedious. It requires obtaining data from various sources to make a clinical judgment that validates a diagnosis of pain (Booker & Haedtke, 2016). Health care providers must not assume that non-communicative patients are not in pain (Czarnecki et al., 2018). A good rule of thumb is to assume pain is present in nonverbal hospitalized patients and then perform a thorough pain assessment to determine if intervention is required (Czarnecki et al., 2018).

Utilization of a behavioral observation pain assessment tool may be necessary based on the patient's condition. Behavioral assessment tools measure behaviors labeled as indicative of pain.

The Checklist of Nonverbal Pain Indicators, the Behavioral Pain Scale, and the Critical-Care Pain Observation Tool (CPOT) are valid and reliable tools that measure the presence or absence of pain (Severgnini et al., 2016). Observable behaviors include facial expressions, body movements, ease of breathing, vocalization, and/or muscle tension. Each observed behavior is scored, and the patient receives a total score that correlates with the presence or absence of pain (Booker & Haedtke, 2016). This score helps guide the health care provider in the management of pain.

The American Society for Pain Management Nursing recommends use of a hierarchical approach for pain assessment. First, all attempts must be made to obtain a patient self-report of pain, the gold standard of pain assessment. Explanation as to the inability of obtaining a self-report should be documented, and further assessment should ensue. A search for the potential cause of pain is conducted, with the provider assuming that pain is present. Behavioral observation is the best approach to assessment when the patient is unable to self-report. Pain behaviors, however, are not always indicative of pain intensity. Health care providers may consider pain reports provided by family members or significant others, because they can often identify subtle changes in the patient's status (Booker & Haedtke, 2016). However, research indicates that discrepancies often exist between a patient's self-report and reports given by other observers. Others often underestimate pain or mistake nonpain behaviors as indicative of pain. Therefore, one must consider all aspects of an assessment and perhaps perform an analgesic trial, monitoring the patient's response to the medication (Czarnecki et al., 2018).

Preoperative Baseline Assessment

Optimal postoperative pain management begins with the preoperative pain assessment. To optimally manage postoperative pain, nurses should obtain a thorough preoperative health history that encompasses topics related to the patient's current and past experiences with pain. Many factors can affect a patient's response and perception of pain (e.g., smoking history, fatigue, sleep deprivation, fear, anxiety, depression, anger, misinformation, altered mental status, educational level, cultural background, ethnic background, pain experience) (Dueñas et al., 2016). Past experiences should alert the nurse to factors that may directly affect the patient's response to the current treatment, including medications that have been effective in the past, acceptable pain levels, concerns about pain, and educational needs. Health care providers must understand that for patients with a history of chronic pain or opioid dependence, postoperative pain management may be more difficult (Chou et al., 2016). Discussions focusing on the patient's expectations help the nurse and patient to mutually develop a plan of care related to pain that includes desirable, predictable outcomes (Mukiri, 2015).

The pain assessment process includes multiple components: initial assessment, treatment, reassessment, and evaluation. Optimal goals include adequate pain management, manageable side effects, and assurance of safety (Chou et al., 2016). Dimensions of the assessment should include the pain's location, description, intensity, duration, alleviating and aggravating factors, associative factors, and impact on ADLs. To identify the location and obtain a description of the pain, the nurse should ask patients to describe the pain in their own words and to point to the location of pain (Czarnecki et al., 2018). Identifying the best pain assessment tool for the patient preoperatively can help the patient provide the most reliable information regarding pain intensity in the postoperative period (Garimella & Cellini, 2013). This may contribute to more effective pain management and, subsequently, increased patient satisfaction.

Determining the duration of pain includes asking questions concerning the timing of when the pain starts, how long it lasts, and which factors alleviate it. Health care providers should also inquire about factors that aggravate the pain. Additionally, determining if any associated factors exist can assist the nurse in developing a more comprehensive treatment plan. For example, do nausea and vomiting accompany the pain? Treatment may need to include measures that control these associated factors. Determining how the pain affects the individual's ADLs provides supplemental information about how the pain interferes with normal functioning. The nurse can develop treatment strategies to target specific challenges the patient faces related to daily life events (Czarnecki et al., 2018).

Although a considerable amount of research on pain over the past several decades exists, only a small percentage of the studies focus on patients undergoing cardiac surgery. In such investigations, the focus was on pain intensity, but other important pain factors were not addressed. In a prospective study exploring the incidence and intensity of pain 1 year after cardiac surgery, results of one study indicated that patients reported more pain than expected. Almost 50% reported severe pain at rest, more than 75% complained of severe pain with coughing, and 62% complained of pain during movement (Huang & Sakata, 2016). The general consensus is that no one technique for managing pain is superior. It is believed that a multimodal approach following cardiac surgery is the most efficacious approach.

The baseline assessment also provides the opportunity to discuss postoperative pain management techniques such as patient-controlled analgesia (PCA), epidural analgesia, and nerve blocks. The nurse has the opportunity to provide education and help frame expectations for the postoperative period. Patients may have numerous questions and anxiety about postoperative pain. The nurse is in a unique position to assist in decreasing anxiety and fear that surround pain, and thus increase the success of postoperative pain management (Glowacki, 2015).

Reassessment of Pain

Following the initial pain assessment and the subsequent pain treatment, regular reassessment of the patient helps determine if the interventions provided are effective or need modification. Reassessment of pain entails comparing pain behaviors and vocalizations exhibited after the intervention to the pain observed during the initial assessment (Meissner et al., 2015). To determine efficacy of interventions, nurses must make it a priority to reassess for pain after any treatment. Reassessments must be comprehensive, timely, and include the presence of adverse side effects. In addition, the reassessment should include whether the patient's comfort goal is met (Glowacki, 2015).

Organizations can assist with ensuring assessment and reassessment compliance by implementing documentation systems that support the nurse to complete the task. Electronic documentation systems that promote ease of obtaining pain assessments before and after interventions will help guide the nurse in completing this crucial component of the care plan and help improve patient outcomes. Electronic documentation systems help promote uniformity, allow data collection and analysis, and promote real-time documentation. Additionally, the ability to easily visualize trends is helpful to all health care providers and can assist in making necessary changes to an analgesic regimen (Chou et al., 2016).

Little research exists in the areas of reevaluation of pain and the measurement tools used to determine patient comfort. One study, however, found a significant lack of pain reassessment by nurses. The authors proposed that knowledge, time, and workload may be factors that limit effective reassessment of pain. Interestingly, these researchers found that nurses had a tendency to be more focused on surgical pain and did not consider other complaints of pain a priority, which resulted in delayed treatment. Nurses must be educated regarding the potential gap in pain control measures due to periods of increased and uncontrolled pain that result directly from lack of timely reevaluation (Glowacki, 2015).

▶ Phases of Pain

The patient experiences pain through three phases: anticipation, presence, and aftermath. The nurse's responsibility is to intervene and assist the patient with each pain phase (Glowacki, 2015). During the anticipation phase, interventions should focus on patient education and the reduction of anxiety. Research supports that anxiety increases intensity of pain scores

(Czarnecki et al., 2018). Anxiety can often be relieved with the knowledge that pain may occur and the development of a realistic plan to manage it when it does. Preoperative discussion of comfort goals and realistic techniques to achieve the goals are essential to successful postoperative reduction of pain and anxiety (Glowacki, 2015).

The presence of pain is the phase where interventions can directly affect the patient's level of comfort and pain intensity. Physiologically, the management of pain revolves around altering the source and perception of pain, and blocking the transmission of pain impulses within the nervous system. Different pharmacologic and nonpharmacologic agents perform differently in relation to the pathology of pain. One strategy is to block or limit the effect of local mediators at the site of injury and decrease inflammation. Nonsteroidal anti-inflammatory drugs are able to block specific mediator production such as prostaglandin, thereby decreasing the inflammatory response. Other medications such as clonidine (Catapres®) block the release of epinephrine from the nerve fibers. A second strategy involves limiting transmission to the secondary neurons in the dorsal horn. The action potential can be blocked or inhibited by local anesthetics and some anticonvulsants such as phenytoin (Dilantin®). Opioids also are used to inhibit both synapses at the dorsal horn. Additionally, nonpharmacologic interventions such as massage and the application of heat or cold may inhibit transmission of pain-related messages (Miozzo et al., 2016). The final strategy in pain management is to enhance the inhibition of the pain sensation. Opioids are the agents of choice in such a case, because they will affect both the primary and secondary neurons. Tricyclic antidepressants can have the same effect by interfering with serotonin uptake and primary neuron transmission (Czarnecki et al., 2018).

▶ Preemptive Analgesia

Preemptive analgesia is the administration of analgesics prior to insult or injury. The goal is to prevent the sensitization to pain, especially prior to surgical intervention (Vadivelu et al., 2014). Data suggest that the administration of preoperative analgesics may indeed help to decrease the sensitization to postoperative pain. This decreased sensitization of nociceptors indicates that preemptive analgesic use has the possibility of greater efficacy than the same treatment administered postoperatively (Jain, 2013). Researchers theorized that the administration of preemptive analgesia would decrease postoperative pain and also prevent the development of chronic pain. Current literature reinforces the premise that the use of preemptive analgesia, which incorporates multimodal antinociceptive interventions, is more effective in decreasing postoperative pain and reducing analgesic consumption in the postoperative period. To be most effective, this regime must be started preoperatively and given for an increased duration, including the postoperative period (Vadivelu et al., 2014).

Data indicate that the benefit of preemptive analgesia might be realized for as long as 1 year after surgery. Effective administration of preemptive analgesia involves the use of various medications and routes of administration. Use of preemptive analgesia includes opiates, local anesthetics, NSAIDs, acetaminophen, antidepressants, and gamma-aminobutyric acid; analgesic therapies target the expected postoperative pain. Depending on the surgical procedure, administration of preemptive analgesia may be oral, intravenous (IV), or epidural or in the form of a nerve block (Gan, 2017).

One study demonstrated that patients who received a single dose of oral gabapentin prior to cardiac surgery required significantly less morphine postoperatively. In addition to decreased morphine consumption, patients reported considerably lower postoperative pain scores and nausea (Jain, 2013). Another study on preemptive use of gabapentin (Neurontin®) prior to coronary artery bypass graft (CABG) surgery describes similar results. Patients who received a single dose of gabapentin preoperatively had substantially lower pain scores and required less tramadol in the postoperative period; however, no significant difference existed in pain scores at 1 and 3 months (Bouzia et al., 2017). Some studies clearly demonstrate the benefit of preemptive analgesia.

▶ Management of Pain

In 1784, surgeon James Monroe first described the advantage of postoperative opium use:

> Opium . . . is highly expedient to abate the smarting of the wound after the operation is over, and to induce sleep; but the stronger dose we dare venture to give has little or no effect in mitigating the suffering of the patient during the operation. (Sattari, Baghdadchi, Kyeyri, Khakzadi, & Mashayekh, 2013, p. 373)

For centuries, health care providers have strived to provide acceptable postoperative pain management. Adequate pain management is essential for the well-being of all patients and is a fundamental human right (Meissner et al., 2015). The consequences of inadequate pain management include physiologic, psychological, social, and economic ramifications. Physiologically, unrelieved pain results in many adverse effects, including increased heart rate, systemic vascular resistance, and increased circulating catecholamines. These effects place patients at greater risk for myocardial ischemia, stroke, and bleeding. Additionally, chronic pain decreases mobility, alters sleep patterns, causes immune dysfunction, and creates dependence on medication and codependence on family members. In terms of psychological effects, studies show that patients with chronic pain are four times more likely to suffer from depression and anxiety. Social and economic factors include the inability or decreased ability to work. This change in work status directly affects the individual's socioeconomic status, impacts unemployment and disability, and increases dependence on government benefits (Sattari et al., 2013).

Opioids, nonopioids, and other analgesics used as adjuvant therapies are the mainstays in pain management (Chou et al., 2016). Treatment modalities may differ, depending on whether the goal is treating acute versus chronic pain, or nociceptive versus neuropathic pain. Health care providers must be cognizant that patients respond uniquely to medications; patients may metabolize medications rapidly, moderately, or slowly. How a patient metabolizes the medication should influence dosing regimens, because genetics play an important role in how patients respond to medications (Chou et al., 2016).

Traditionally, pain management strategies have applied the World Health Organization's (WHO) cancer pain treatment ladder in attempts to manage postoperative pain. This ladder suggests that the first step in treating mild pain should include the use of nonopioids with or without adjuvant medications. Step two entails the addition of opioids to the adjuvants for mild to moderate pain. Step three involves continued opioid use for moderate to severe pain. Postoperative pain reaches its highest level initially after the surgery, but then rapidly improves (Chou et al., 2016).

One study explored the effectiveness of the WHO analgesic ladder following cardiac surgery (Sattari et al., 2013). Under this guideline, most patients received acetaminophen around-the-clock; 89% of patients received an NSAID, and all patients received intermittent morphine. The morphine was converted from the IV route of administration to an oral preparation on the second postoperative day. The amount of morphine administered decreased significantly by the second postoperative day. Effective pain relief was reported in 95% of the patients in this study.

Evidence-based guidelines must direct efforts to manage postoperative pain related to site-specific surgeries. **TABLE 14.1** summarizes

TABLE 14.1 Summary of Site-Specific Pain Treatment Recommendations

	Thoracotomy	**Coronary Artery Bypass Grafting**
Preferred treatment	**Pharmacologic** Epidural ■ Opioids Regional local anesthetics	**Pharmacologic** Intravenous ■ Opioids ■ NSAIDs
	Nonpharmacologic Application of cold TENS Cognitive (patient dependent)	**Nonpharmacologic** None identified
Common usage	**Pharmacologic** PO, IM, IV opioids, and NSAIDs IV PCA opioids Intrathecal opioids Intrathecal local anesthetics	**Pharmacologic** PO, IM opioids, and NSAIDs IV PCA opioids Intrathecal opioids
	Nonpharmacologic Cognitive (patient dependent)	**Nonpharmacologic** None identified
Comments	If there is a risk of or actual bleeding, avoid NSAIDs.	If there is a risk of or actual bleeding, avoid NSAIDs.
		If there is renal hypoperfusion, avoid all NSAIDs.
		Rarely Used Epidural Regional local anesthetics

IM, intramuscular; IV, intravenous; NSAID, nonsteroidal anti-inflammatory drug; PCA, patient-controlled analgesia; PO, per os (by mouth); TENS, transcutaneous electrical nerve stimulation.
Data from Rosenquist & Rosenberg (2003).

recommendations for pain management in conjunction with cardiothoracic surgery.

The use of IV opioids is the preferred method of managing pain in the immediate postoperative period for patients who undergo CABG surgery. These medications can be delivered via nurse- or patient-controlled methods. The use of PCA devices allows for the administration of small, frequent doses of opioids by the patient. One advantage is the ability to obtain and maintain a steady state. Another advantage is the psychologic benefit related to the self-administration of analgesia. In a study by Sattari and colleagues (2013), postoperative cardiac surgery patients received IV morphine and an NSAID either orally or rectally. Although these patients reported moderate pain, they also reported satisfaction with pain management. Additionally, other studies demonstrate the effective use of morphine for various postoperative cardiac surgery patients (Pogatzki-Zahn et al., 2017).

Multimodal Analgesia

The use of multimodal analgesic therapy is fundamental to exceptional pain management and is strongly endorsed by experts in the field of pain management. Data from studies demonstrate significantly lower pain scores and minimal reports of nausea and vomiting for patients who received multimodal analgesia during the postoperative period (Rafiq et al., 2014). The theory of multimodal analgesia is to maximize the efficacy of individual agents to create a synergistic analgesic effect. In turn, the synergy should decrease the dose of medications, thereby decreasing associated side effects and increasing analgesia (Rafiq et al., 2014). Proponents of multimodal analgesia stress the importance of procedure-specific approaches. An example is the use of continuous epidural analgesia that combines an opiate and a local anesthetic. Dosing requirements in the epidural space are significantly lower than IV or oral routes of administration. In turn, patients often experience decreased side effects with improved analgesia. Despite evidence showing the benefits of multimodal analgesia, the technique continues to be underused (Tinsbloom, Muckler, Stoeckel, Whitehurst, & Morgan, 2017).

Epidural and local anesthetics are the preferred methods for managing pain in patients who are undergoing a thoracotomy. Agreement exists that epidural use in these patients provides an excellent method for pain control during the acute pain phase (Ziyaeifard et al., 2014). Other reported benefits of epidural analgesia include early extubation and enhanced pulmonary function (Chou et al., 2016). Some conflicting data exist regarding enhanced pulmonary function with epidural pain management following thoracotomy. Some data suggest that while pain management may be effective and may lead to earlier extubation, pulmonary function may not be enhanced with epidural pain management (Ziyaeifard et al., 2014).

Data are inconsistent regarding the benefits of thoracic epidural anesthesia. In one study involving cardiac surgery patients, participants received either (1) thoracic epidural analgesia in combination with general anesthesia, followed by postoperative patient-controlled thoracic epidural analgesia, or (2) general anesthesia, followed by PCA with IV morphine. No differences between these two groups were observed in terms of pain relief, pulmonary function, ambulation, level of sedation, LOS, or quality of recovery. The study authors concluded, however, that thoracic epidural anesthesia decreases stress response and pain scores (Ziyaeifard et al., 2014). The major concern when using epidural analgesia is the potential for development of an epidural hematoma. When this strategy is used, the intensive care unit (ICU) nurse must monitor for and report lower extremity motor weakness (Chou et al., 2016). The use of thoracic epidurals is not without risk. Risks include failure of the catheter to provide the desired analgesia, hematoma, and motor block; nursing tasks for care and monitoring increase with epidural analgesia.

The use of intrathecal morphine has been reported to be effective in the management of postoperative cardiac surgery pain. In one study, patients undergoing on-pump bypass who received intrathecal morphine prior to induction of general anesthesia were extubated earlier and had a shorter ICU length of stay than a comparison group of patients who did not receive the intrathecal injection prior to induction (Ziyaeifard et al., 2014).

An additional method of pain management for CABG patients is the use of intravenous NSAIDs (Howard, Warhurst, & Sheehan, 2016). The use of NSAIDs in conjunction with opioids in other surgical procedures is well established. These agents are opioid sparing and provide excellent pain relief (Howard et al., 2016). In a retrospective study evaluating the safety of continuous ketorolac (Toradol®) infusions in postoperative CABG patients, the authors conclude there is no association between continuous ketorolac and increased risk of myocardial infarction (MI), or bleeding (Howard et al., 2016). A large single-center retrospective study assessed the ketorolac boxed warning related to use with postoperative cardiac surgery patients. Ketorolac was dosed according to recommended guidelines of 15 to 30 mg every 6 hours as needed. Intermittent dosing with ketorolac was not associated with an increase in the composite outcome of perioperative stroke, transient ischemic attack, MI, renal insufficiency, gastrointestinal (GI) bleeding, or death.

Despite the potential advantages of postoperative NSAID use, its use has been limited in cardiac surgery patients due to the potential for troublesome side effects. The actual occurrence of side effects tends to depend on whether the medication inhibits cyclooxygenase 1 or 2 (COX-1 or COX-2), or both. Serious side effects, including sternal wound infections, MI, infarction, stroke, and pulmonary embolus, have been reported with the use of COX-2 inhibitors; as a consequence, these medications are not recommended for patients deemed to have an increased cardiac risk (Fairweather et al., 2015).

Another promising addition to the multimodal therapy tool kit is the use of acetaminophen. The effective use of oral acetaminophen as an analgesic and antipyretic is well documented; however, the approval of IV acetaminophen by the U.S. Food and Drug Administration adds a new dimension to managing pain. Acetaminophen has an advantage over other analgesic agents because, in appropriate doses, it is safe and well tolerated. As a nonopiate, acetaminophen use does not result in respiratory depression, sedation, constipation, ileus, or pruritus, nor does it have the potential renal or hematologic complications associated with NSAID administration. Moreover, the risk of addiction or diversion is nonexistent (O'Neal, 2013).

Intravenous acetaminophen is an effective and opioid-sparing analgesic. Controversy exists related to cost and therefore, in many instances, its use is limited. Studies in patients undergoing CABG demonstrate that the use of 1 g acetaminophen intravenously every 6 hours may decrease overall morphine consumption (O'Neal, 2013). In a recent single-center, double-blind study in approximately 150 patients following median sternotomy, patients were randomized to receive 1 g IV acetaminophen every 6 hours for 24 hours or comparable placebo. Results demonstrated exceptional pain management in the IV acetaminophen group as evidenced by lower pain intensity scores (Mamoun et al., 2016).

Research supports the use of IV acetaminophen as an adjunct in the postoperative period, despite limited prescribing by some organizations due to cost concerns (Mamoun et al., 2016). Although cost is always a concern, the current research demonstrates improved outcomes and shorter LOS. Cautious use of acetaminophen is warranted in patients with liver dysfunction, a history of alcohol abuse, severe malnourishment, and also in elderly patients. In addition, nurses must be cognizant of other acetaminophen-containing medications (O'Neal, 2013).

▶ Pain Sequelae

Inadequate postoperative pain management may lead to numerous complications and poor patient outcomes. Unrelieved acute pain can have hemodynamic, metabolic, and hemostatic consequences. Patients in pain are less likely to ambulate, delaying early mobilization and increasing the risk for thromboembolic complications. Patients who experience pain, especially following cardiac surgery, may not perform respiratory exercises, such as coughing, deep breathing, or incentive spirometry, leading to an increased risk of pneumonia. Increases in autonomic activity may lead to slowing of the GI system and resultant postoperative ileus; urinary retention may also be a problem. When pain is unrelieved, patients may become anxious, irritable, and agitated, and experience altered sleep cycles (Czarnecki et al., 2018).

▶ Nonpharmacologic Pain Management

Use of nonpharmacologic interventions to augment pain control ranges from relaxation techniques to the application of heat or cold to the use of transcutaneous electrical nerve stimulation (TENS). The success of relaxation techniques typically is patient dependent, although results appear to be better if patients learn the techniques preoperatively (Czarnecki et al., 2018). Unfortunately, little research exists related to the use of nonpharmacologic techniques following cardiac surgery. The research does, however, support the benefit of various nonpharmacologic methods in improving pain management overall.

The use of music to augment pain management appears in the literature and shows some promise. In a review of studies from 1995 through 2007, it was found that 42 studies were conducted to assess the efficacy of music as a means of pain control. Roughly half the studies showed that pain reduction might be achieved through the use of music. A study of postoperative cardiac surgery patients combined analgesics with the use of sedative music for 30 minutes per day over a 3-day period. Results showed a reduction in anxiety and pain as compared to patients receiving the usual course of treatment (Liu & Petrini, 2015). Another study explored the effects of music chosen by patients on their self-reported pain intensity and physiologic pain indicators following open heart surgery. The patients in the music group had significantly lower pain scores and increased oxygen saturation. The researchers concluded that the addition of music is a harmless, effective, and easy technique to help diminish the potentially detrimental effects of pain following open heart surgery (Özer, Karaman Özlű, Arslan, & Gűnes, 2013). Machado, Souza, Poveda, and Costa (2017) conducted a systematic review of nonpharmacologic techniques aimed at improving sleep for patients who underwent cardiac surgery.

The review revealed significant improvement in sleep quality for patients who used interventions such as earplugs, white noise, progressive muscle relaxation, and music.

Transcutaneous electrical nerve stimulation is often used as a complementary therapy in patients with acute and chronic pain (Czarnecki et al., 2018). The supposition is that the effectiveness of TENS is based on the gate control theory of pain, in which the modulation of pain results from the activation of descending inhibitory pathways. In a study of 100 patients who underwent CABG surgery, half received routine postoperative care and half received routine care along with the application of TENS. Pain intensity, using the visual analog scale, and pulmonary function were assessed every 6 hours for 72 hours postoperatively. Results of the study demonstrated statistically significant improvement in pulmonary function, overall opioid consumption, and lower pain scores for the TENS group (Jahangirifard, Razavi, Ahmadi, & Forozeshfard, 2017). However, use of TENS in patients with an implanted cardioverter defibrillator may result in an inappropriate shock and must be used with extreme caution and under the guidance of a health care provider (Badger, Taylor, & Swain, 2017).

The addition and implementation of massage therapy in postoperative cardiac surgery patients helps promote comfort, decrease anxiety, and reduce pain. A meta-analysis of randomized clinical trials compared the traditional pain management of postoperative cardiac surgery patients with massage and reported that massage therapy may assist in decreasing pain and anxiety (Miozzo et al., 2016). A systematic review identified nearly 300 studies reporting efficacy of massage following cardiac surgery. Massage improves mood following cardiac surgery and is a complementary nursing intervention that is simple and inexpensive (Miozzo et al., 2016).

▶ Special Considerations

Pain is a unique, subjective, individualized experience. Nevertheless, some elements that affect the response to pain management techniques may apply across certain groups of people. Recognition of these special considerations may assist the nurse with managing an individual's pain. The special considerations for pain management discussed here are gender differences, cultural influences, and older age.

Gender

Researchers in the study of pain management understand that there are clear differences between the way men and women experience pain; and they recognize the importance of acknowledging these differences. Women tend to have a lower pain threshold for pain than men. Evidence clearly suggests that the perception of pain is different for men and women, and that women have a higher incidence of undertreatment for pain (Olson, 2016). In a study of more than 4,000 postoperative patients, researchers measured pain scores and the total amount of morphine administered to obtain pain relief. Slightly fewer than 50% of the patients were female; however, the female patients required significantly more morphine overall and reported higher pain scores. The difference in morphine requirements was slightly more than 10% between men and women (Olson, 2016). Several studies utilizing video vignettes discovered that nurses were more likely to undertreat pain in women than in men and health care providers were more likely to provide optimal pain treatment regimens for men than women (Pasero & McCaffery, 2005). Gender bias in the treatment of pain is concerning. Research demonstrates that, very often, women experiencing chest pain are much less likely than men to receive invasive and noninvasive diagnostic procedures. Additionally, women are far less likely to receive interventional cardiac procedures when presenting with complaints of chest pain (Olson, 2016). One study revealed that women were more likely to receive sedating medications while prescriptions for men more likely included analgesics. The study also found that women used approximately 40% less opioid medications than men following surgery (Olson, 2016).

Psychological factors also play a part in the role of gender differences. Psychosocial factors shape an individual's expectations, emotions, and social learning (Olson, 2016). Societal norms in how children of both genders are raised, for example, play a part in their pain experience (Edwards, Dworkin, Sullivan, Turk, & Wasan, 2016). Stereotypical norms accept that women may show more emotion around pain while men are less verbal and more stoic.

When studying pain differences reflective of gender, researchers measure gender personality traits in relation to pain. For example, persons identified as possessing more feminine characteristics (women) report experiencing more pain than men. Additionally, reports point to the fact that men—that is, those persons with more masculine traits—report a higher tolerance of pain (Edwards et al., 2016). Gender-related differences exist among pain beliefs, expectations, and behaviors. Gender role expectations can account for the fact that males predominately underreport pain and women are more apt to verbalize pain. Additionally, males demonstrate greater pain endurance, whereas women report a lower threshold and tolerance, resulting in their greater willingness to report pain (Olson, 2016). Similarly, studies suggest that women were more likely to experience severe pain and on a more frequent basis. Some differences in the reports of pain between males and females may be related to the issue of willingness to make a self-report. Males and females have different behaviors regarding the expression of and response to pain (Storesund et al., 2016).

These data on gender differences are corroborated through studies in other patients who have undergone cardiac surgery. Compared to males, females more frequently report less improvement in pain scores or higher pain intensity (Olson, 2016), report lower health-related quality of life after cardiac surgery (Edwards et al., 2016), and experience a more difficult recovery (Bjornnes Rustøen, Lie, Watt-Watson, & Leegaard 2016). Pereira and Pogatzki-Zahn (2015) reviewed nearly 60 studies assessing postoperative gender differences related to pain. Following thoracic, cardiovascular, and neurosurgical procedures, women demonstrated higher postoperative pain scores.

Differences between males and females in the response to analgesia are well documented.

Some studies show greater morphine potency but slower onset of pain relief in females. Additionally, researchers reported that NSAIDs have refractory effects in women when doses exceed 800 mg. Pharmacokinetics may play a role in these differences, although studies to date have not shown significance in clinical practice. One explanation may be that the differences are related to the specific drugs rather than the whole categories of drugs (Giles & Walker, 2000).

The need to explore numerous variables and their influence on gender-related pain responses should be considered for future prospective research studies (Pereira & Pogatzki-Zahn, 2015). These variables include comorbidities, culture, disability, medications, coping, and physical variables. To appropriately respond to an individual's pain experience, nurses need to be sensitive to various societal norms and communication patterns related to gender, and recognize the potential differences in reports of pain and their own potential biases. Health care providers must be mindful of the potential gender differences that exist between males and females; and appreciate the influence psychology and society have on the tolerance, perception, and expression of pain (Olson, 2016).

Race, Ethnicity, and Culture

Distinguishing differences among the definitions of race, ethnicity, and culture has proved difficult in the literature, with many of the terms being used interchangeably. The literature debates whether the term *race* is a biologic or social concept. Typically, race is predominantly used to collect data regarding health disparities. There is no globally accepted definition of race; however, the National Institutes of Health has adopted the use of five racial categories to collect its data (National Institute of Allergy and Infectious Diseases, 2015).

By comparison, *ethnicity* refers to a group of people who share ancestry, social background, culture, and traditions that are sustained over a period of time and provide a sense of identity for group members. Typically, self-identification is the best approach to assigning individuals to a particular ethnic group (Czarnecki et al., 2018).

The term *culture* seems to be derived from behavioral and attitudinal norms in relation to belief systems. Culture is viewed as a factor influencing health care practices and illness beliefs. Regarding pain experience, then, culture affects all areas related to pain, including expression, reporting, and management (Czarnecki et al., 2018).

Given that there are differences in the way these terms are used and studied, findings in this arena must be reviewed carefully. Questions often arise as to whether race, ethnicity, and culture affect how different groups biologically experience pain or how the factors influence the perception of pain. Additionally, culture can influence how the caregiver assesses and treats the pain of persons from different ethnic backgrounds.

A study from Brigham and Women's Hospital found significant racial disparities in the management of pain. Minority patients were almost 30% less likely to receive analgesic medication for abdominal pain than white patients (Pain Doctor, 2016). A 2016 study conducted at the University of Virginia confirmed the overwhelming undertreatment of pain among African Americans in the United States (Pain Doctor, 2016). Some of the disparities exist due to misconceptions and lack of knowledge among medical students and residents. In general, research shows significant differences in terms of the amount of opiate analgesics administered to patients who were white as compared to those who were Hispanic or black. In these cases, patients who were white received higher amounts of opiates than patients of other races. A systematic review of studies investigating the influence of race on analgesic administration further demonstrates disparities in pain management related to ethnicity and race in the United States (Pain Doctor, 2016). The lesson for nurses is that care must be taken to acknowledge potential differences related to race, ethnicity, and culture in how pain is experienced, including the awareness that people are individuals with unique needs.

The Elderly Population

The optimal treatment of pain is a complex endeavor but may be even more complicated in the elderly population. This difference may be explained by elderly patients' tendency to underreport pain, difficulty communicating, and caregiver biases regarding the use of pain medication in the older patient (Czarnecki et al., 2018).

Although older patients may not experience changes in the perception of pain, some physiologic changes do occur with aging that must be considered when utilizing pain medications. In particular, physiologic changes related to renal and liver function may affect the way the older patient metabolizes and eliminates pain medication, resulting in a longer duration of action and the risk for oversedation (Petrini, Matthiesen, & Arendt-Nielsen, 2015). For this reason, care must be taken when prescribing, administering, and monitoring the effects of pain medications in the elderly population (Czarnecki et al., 2018).

Assessment is crucial for managing pain in the older patient. The pain scale chosen is important to the individual functioning of the older patient, and the same scale should be used consistently when assessing a particular patient to ensure reliability of the results (Czarnecki et al., 2018). Trying different scales to determine the best fit for individual patients is a good strategy. Often, older patients have more success using simple word scales, such as "none," "mild," "moderate," and "severe," than with a numeric scale or a VAS. Often, if the older patient has cognitive impairment, rating pain may be difficult. The FACES scale, which seems to be easily used, often produces unreliable results with the elderly. The faces are often seen by these individuals as representing moods like sadness instead of pain, which results in understated pain intensity (Nolan, 2018).

Additional challenges in using pain scales in the elderly population relate to vision and hearing loss, which are more prevalent in older individuals. It is critical that the nurse assess for these deficits and utilize assistive devices as appropriate (Pasero & McCaffery, 2005).

For the patient with vision impairment, the use of a verbal reporting scale might be best; in contrast, patients who are hearing impaired may prefer to use a printed scale that they can point or gesture toward. Depending on the severity of cognitive impairment, the use of "yes" or "no" questions with a behavioral observation scale may be the best option. Studies have found that the use of proxy reports, relying on the assessment of a family member or on nursing judgment of the pain often leads to underestimation of the actual pain experienced (Pasero & McCaffery, 2005).

The older patient's view of pain and pain management may also be a barrier to the effective assessment and treatment of pain. Many older patients may fear addiction to painkillers and therefore underreport their pain. Preparing patients for pain management following surgery provides nurses with a unique opportunity to educate patients and their families about pain, tolerance, dependence, addiction, the patient's disease process, and various pain control techniques (Nolan, 2018). Clearly exploring fears related to addiction and educating about the differences between psychological addiction and physiological dependence may assist in decreasing fear and anxiety.

Treatment strategies for the older patient can include medication regimens in which the patient does not have to request treatment. Options to consider may include nerve blocks, epidural analgesia, and around-the-clock dosing of pain medications; ongoing, vigilant nursing assessment will be crucial to the success of these regimens. Opioids are the most widely utilized therapy with surgical patients, though their dosing needs to be considered carefully. Typically, if communication deficits are present, nurses may be fearful of postoperative delirium and withhold opioids. Nevertheless, even though these medications may potentially contribute to postoperative delirium, recent studies suggest that patients with higher pain scores and uncontrolled pain are more likely to develop delirium (Nolan, 2018). Further complicating matters is the fact that research shows unrelieved acute pain may result in an altered mental status. Pasero and McCaffery (2005) advocate to "assume pain is present" in older patients exhibiting increased agitation.

The level of postoperative pain following cardiac surgery in relation to age has been investigated; results have been inconsistent. Comprehensive patient education regarding the importance of managing pain, attentive nursing assessment, and systematic evaluation of analgesic effectiveness can promote the best possible pain management.

▶ **Summary**

Frequent patient assessment is the key to outstanding management of pain (Glowacki, 2015). Without systematic assessment and reassessment, it becomes impossible to adequately and expertly treat pain. Exceptional pain assessment and management following cardiac surgery are essential to ensuring improved patient outcomes. Knowledge that assessment techniques may need adjustment when providing care to nonverbal and elderly patients may allow for more optimal pain control. Acknowledging the differences in pain perception related to gender and culture allows the nurse to recognize trends and avoid biases when dealing with different groups of people. Recognizing the unique and subjective nature of the pain experience will assist in maximizing positive outcomes for pain management. This multifaceted process involves the timely assessment of pain, appropriate interventions, reassessment, and ongoing evaluation of the pain management regimen.

The use of multimodal analgesia techniques provides superior dynamic pain relief and helps diminish analgesic side effects during the postoperative period (Chou et al., 2016; Vadivelu et al., 2014). The addition of nonpharmacologic techniques aimed at augmenting pain management provides nurses with a relatively simple addition to the arsenal of available modalities. Health care providers must focus on pain management that is acceptable to the patient and remember that inadequate postoperative pain management may contribute to the development of chronic pain syndromes (ASA, 2013). In today's ever-changing health care environment, diminishing complications, decreasing length of stay, and increasing patient satisfaction are imperative to the success of organizations. Good pain management can assist in meeting these goals.

⌕ *CASE STUDY*

F. E., a 66-year-old patient with a history of coronary artery disease, myocardial infarction with multivessel stents, hyperlipidemia, hypertension, and diabetes, underwent an off-pump CABG procedure with median sternotomy and saphenous vein harvesting. Upon completion of surgery, the patient was transferred to the cardiovascular intensive care unit. Upon admission, data are as follows: Vital signs were BP 130/82, HR 112, RR 18, temperature 36°C, CVP 3 mmHg, SpO_2 97%. Chest tube has 150 mL bloody drainage. Ventilator settings: SIMV 12, Vt 420 mL, PEEP 5, Rate 12, Pressure Support 5. The patient is intubated and reversed from anesthesia. An infusion of propofol (Diprivan®) is initiated at 3 mg/kg/hr. The patient grimaces when suctioned, turned, and upon the initiation of early mobility.

Critical Thinking Questions

1. What tool should the nurse use to assess F. E.'s pain at this time?
2. What is/are the etiologic factor(s) of this patient's pain?
3. What treatment modalities should the nurse anticipate using and why?

Answers to Critical Thinking Questions

1. The patient should be assessed for pain using the Critical Care Pain Observation Tool (CPOT), because at this time the patient is unable to self-report pain levels. Physiologic parameters are not ideal to use in this patient, because vital signs are influenced by the cardiac surgery procedure performed and by the associated postoperative inflammatory process.
2. This patient has nociceptive pain. Sources of this patient's pain may include the midsternotomy incision, saphenous vein harvesting, turning and positioning, early mobility, presence of the chest tube, lying on the operating room table during surgery, or any combination of these factors.
3. An opioid is indicated for this postoperative pain. NSAIDs are not ideal at this time as they can interfere with platelet function, impair wound healing, and cause additional postoperative bleeding. IV acetaminophen may be administered if the patient's liver function tests are within range. This latter intervention may decrease the amount of postoperative opioids that may be required.

Self-Assessment Questions

1. Which statement is true regarding pain following cardiac surgery?
   A. The pain decreases over the first postoperative day.
   B. Mild to moderate levels of pain can be expected.
   C. With advances in intraoperative anesthesia care, less than half of cardiac surgery patients experience postoperative pain.
   D. Patients receive less than half of the analgesics prescribed.

2. Which type of pain is of primary concern immediately following cardiac surgery?
   A. Acute, visceral
   B. Chronic, somatic
   C. Chronic, neuropathic
   D. Acute, nociceptive

3. Your cardiac surgery patient is experiencing persistent sternotomy pain but is reluctant to take pain medication. Which is the nurse's best response?
   A. "If you don't let us help you with your pain, you will develop chronic pain."
   B. "Proinflammatory cytokines are mostly causing you to have pain."
   C. "What about taking pain medications is of concern to you?"
   D. "We can wait until your pain level is higher, if you prefer."

4. Which should the nurse use as the initial step to perform a pain assessment of a cardiac surgery patient?
   A. Search for and identify sources of pain.
   B. Ask the patient to quantify the pain level.
   C. Observe the patient for physiologic signs of pain.
   D. Ask family members about the patient's level of pain.

5. Which is a consequence of unrelieved pain?
   A. Decreased circulating catecholamines
   B. Increased systemic vascular resistance
   C. Decreased amounts of interleukins
   D. Increased production of anti-inflammatory mediators

6. Which is a physiologic strategy to decrease pain levels?
   A. Increase prostaglandin levels
   B. Increase release of epinephrine from nerve fibers
   C. Decrease serotonin uptake
   D. Decrease inhibition of primary and secondary neurons

7. Which is the first step in the World Health Organization pain management ladder that can be used for cardiac surgery patients?
   A. Nonopioid
   B. Adjuvant agent
   C. Opioid
   D. Nonpharmacologic intervention

8. Which is the preferred method to manage pain of patients who undergo coronary artery bypass grafting surgery in the immediate postoperative period?
   A. Morphine
   B. Phenytoin (Dilantin®)
   C. Ibuprofen (Motrin®)
   D. Amitriptyline (Elavil®)

9. Your patient is receiving celecoxib (Celebrex®) following cardiac surgery. For which complication is the patient at increased risk?
   A. Sternal wound infection
   B. Hypoglycemia
   C. Pulmonary edema
   D. Hypokalemia

10. Your patient has undergone a thoracotomy. Which should the nurse anticipate using as the preferred method of pain management?
    A. PCA with an opioid
    B. Epidural with local anesthetic
    C. Oral or IV NSAID
    D. Application of heat

Answers to Self-Assessment Questions

1. D. **Patients receive less than half of the analgesics prescribed.**
   Rationale: Data reveal that this statement is correct, even in 2018. Pain decreases over the initial 48 to 72 hours. Severe pain can be expected. Nociceptive, bone, and cutaneous pain can be expected following cardiac surgery

if not managed well. More than half of patients who undergo cardiac surgery experience pain.

2. D. **acute, nociceptive**

Rationale: Acute, nociceptive pain occurs immediately following cardiac surgery. Nociceptive pain originates at the nerve cells and is transmitted to the brain. The patient should not experience visceral (organ) pain. It is too early for the patient to experience chronic pain, which is defined as pain that lasts more than 6 months after the injury has healed. The patient should also not experience neuropathic pain immediately following cardiac surgery unless there was a preexisting condition unrelated to the cardiac surgical procedure.

3. C. **"What about taking pain medications is of concern to you?"**

Rationale: The nurse should explore why the patient does not want to take pain medication. The preference may be based on myths (e.g., fear of addiction), which can be dispelled with education. Option A is a true statement but is not the ideal way to communicate with a patient. Proinflammatory cytokines are involved with peripheral pain. Pain medication will not be as effective if one waits until the pain level is more severe; preemptive analgesia is more effective.

4. B. **Ask the patient to quantify the pain level.**

Rationale: A pain assessment should occur first. The patient's self-report of pain is the most valid and reliable indicator of pain. Searching for causes is not the first step. Physiologic signs of pain are not always the most valid and reliable indicators; other factors can impact physiologic responses (e.g., a patient's hemodynamic parameters). The family should not be asked first; data suggest that family members often underreport patient pain.

5. B. **increased systemic vascular resistance**

Rationale: An increase in systemic vascular resistance is due to the physiologic mechanisms associated with pain. It results in an increase in blood pressure. Levels of circulating catecholamines and interleukins increase as a result of unrelieved pain. There is an associated decrease in production of anti-inflammatory mediators associated with increased pain.

6. C. **decrease serotonin uptake**

Rationale: Selective serotonin reuptake inhibitors are used for pain management; they affect the descending pain pathways. Increased prostaglandin levels cause more pain.

7. A. **nonopioid**

Rationale: It is recommended to start with the least invasive/strong level of pain medication and build up to stronger medications, as indicated. Adjuvant agents, opioids, and nonpharmacologic interventions are not first interventions for the cardiac surgery patient in the immediate postoperative period.

8. A. **morphine**

Rationale: Morphine is indicated for acute, severe pain in the immediate postoperative period following cardiac surgery. Phenytoin is an antiseizure medication and is not used to treat immediate postoperative pain. Ibuprofen is not indicated as a first intervention for severe pain. In addition, it carries the risk of postoperative bleeding. Amitriptyline is indicated for persistent or chronic pain.

9. A. **sternal wound infection**

Rationale: Nonsteroidal anti-inflammatory drugs put the patient at risk for sternal wound infections. COX-2 inhibition is a primary mediator of inflammation. Wound healing is significantly altered with celecoxib. The other three options are not associated with celecoxib administration.

10. B. **epidural with local anesthetic**

Rationale: Epidural administration will get medication to the site causing the pain. Used concomitantly with a local anesthetic will result in good spread once the epidural catheter is inserted. If the patient is experiencing cutaneous pain, an epidural is the most effective treatment strategy. An IV or oral NSAID will not be effective in managing this patient's pain and can increase bleeding risk. Heat will cause vasodilation, which can result in increased pain levels.

CLINICAL INQUIRY BOX

Question: What is the incidence of persistent postoperative pain (lasting >3 months) after excluding other pain sources?

Reference: Guimarães-Pereira, L., Farinha, F., Azevedo, L., Abelha, F., & Castro-Lopes, J. (2016). Persistent postoperative pain after cardiac surgery. Incidence, characterization, associated factors and its impact on quality of life. *European Journal of Pain, 20*(9), 1433–1442.

Objective: To determine the incidence of persistent postoperative pain (lasting >3 months) after excluding other pain sources

Method: Observational, prospective design

Results: Of patients, 43% experienced persistent postoperative pain at 3 months. Of those, 84% were not under any treatment for their pain. Neuropathic pain was present in 50% of patients. Younger age, female gender, high body mass index, CABG procedure, history of osteoarthritis or previous sternotomy, and moderate to severe postoperative pain were predictors of persistent postoperative pain.

Conclusion: Persistent postoperative pain results in a decrease in quality of life. Neuropathic pain was part of the equation in half of the patients experiencing persistent postoperative pain.

References

American Society of Anesthesiologists (ASA). (2013). Persistent pain following cardiac surgery can be predicted, reduced. *ScienceDaily*. Retrieved from http://www.sciencedaily.com/releases/2013/10/131013163318.htm.

Badger, J., Taylor, P., & Swain, I. (2017). The safety of electrical stimulation in patients with pacemakers and implantable cardioverter defibrillators: A systematic review. *Journal of Rehabilitation and Assistive Technologies Engineering, 4*, 1–9.

Bjornnes, A. K., Rustøen, T., Lie, I., Watt-Watson, J., & Leegaard, M. (2016). Pain characteristics and analgesic intake before and following cardiac surgery. *European Journal of Cardiovascular Nursing, 15*(1), 47–54.

Booker, S. Q., & Haedtke, C. (2016). Assessing pain in nonverbal older adults. *Nursing, 46*(5), 66–69.

Bouzia, A., Tassoudis, V., Karanikolas, M., Vretzakis, G., Petsiti, A., Tsilimingas, N., . . . Arnaoutoglou, E. (2017). Pregabalin effect on acute and chronic pain after cardiac surgery. *Anesthesiology Research and Practice, 2017*, Article ID 2753962.

Chiang, H. L., Chia, Y. Y., Lin, H. S., & Chen, C. H. (2016). The implications of tobacco smoking on acute postoperative pain: A prospective observational study. *Pain Research and Management, 216*, Article ID 9432493.

Choinière, M., Watt-Watson, J., Victor, J. C., Baskett, R. J. F., Bussiéres, J. S., Carrier, M., . . . Taillefer, M. C. (2014). Prevalence of and risk factors for persistent postoperative nonanginal pain after cardiac surgery: A 2-year prospective multicentre study. *Canadian Medical Association Journal, 186*(7), E213–E223.

Chou, R., Gordon, D. B., de Leon-Casasola, O. A., Rosenberg, J. M., Bickler, S., Brennan, T., . . . Wu, C. L. (2016). Management of post-operative pain: A clinical practice guideline from the

American Pain Society, the American Society of Regional Anesthesia and Pain Medicine, and the American Society of Anesthesiologists' Committee on Regional Anesthesia, Executive Committee, and Administrative Council. *American Pain Society, 17*(2), 131–157.

Czarnecki, M. L., Turner, H. N., & American Society for Pain Management Nursing. (2018). *Core curriculum for pain management nursing* (3rd ed.). St. Louis, MO: Elsevier.

Dueñas, M., Ojeda, B., Salazar, A., Mico, J. A., & Failde, I. (2016). A review of chronic pain impact on patients, their social environment and the health care system. *Journal of Pain Research, 9*, 457– 467.

Edwards, R. R., Dworkin, R. H., Sullivan, M. D., Turk, D. C., & Wasan, A. D. (2016). The role of psychosocial processes in the development and maintenance of chronic pain. *The Journal of Pain, 17*(9), T70–T92.

Fairweather, M., Heit, Y. I., Buie, J., Rosenberg, L. M., Briggs, A., Orgill, D. P., . . . Bertagnolli, M. M. (2015). Celecoxib inhibits early cutaneous wound healing. *Journal of Surgical Research, 194*(2), 717–724.

Gan, T. J. (2017). Poorly controlled postoperative pain: Prevalence, consequences, and prevention. *Journal of Pain Research, 10*, 2287–2298.

Garimella, V., & Cellini, C. (2013). Postoperative pain control. *Clinics in Colon and Rectal Surgery, 26*(3), 191–196.

Giles, B. E., & Walker, J. S. (2000). Sex differences in pain and analgesia. *Pain Reviews, 7*, 181–193.

Glowacki, D. (2015). Effective pain management and improvement in patients' outcomes and satisfaction. *Critical Care Nurse, 35*(3), 33–41.

Guimarães-Pereira, L., Farinha, F., Azevedo, L., Abelha, F., & Castro-Lopes, J. (2016). Persistent postoperative pain after cardiac surgery: Incidence, characterization, associated factors and its impact on quality of life. *European Journal of Pain, 20*(9), 1433–1442.

Herr, K. A., & Garand, L. (2001). Assessment and measurement of pain in older adults. *Clinics in Geriatric Medicine, 17*(3), 457.

Howard, M. L., Warhurst, R. D., & Sheehan, C. (2016). Safety of continuous infusion of ketorolac in postoperative coronary artery bypass graft surgery patients. *Pharmacy, 4*(22), 2–8.

Huang, A. P. S., & Sakata, R. K. (2016). Pain after sternotomy. *Brasileira de Anestesiologia, 66*(4), 395–401.

International Association for the Study of Pain. (2017). *IASP terminology*. Retrieved from https://www.iasp-pain.org /Education/Content.aspx?ItemNumber=1698.

Jahangirifard, A., Razavi, M., Ahmadi, Z. H., & Forozeshfard, M. (2017). Effect of TENS on postoperative pain and pulmonary function in patients undergoing coronary artery bypass surgery. *Pain Management Nursing.* doi: 10.1016/j.pmn.2017.10.018

Jain, P. (2013). Oral pregabalin holds promise to reduce pain after cardiac surgery. *Annals of Cardiac Anaesthesia, 16*(3), 186–187.

Joint Commission. (2018). *Facts about Joint Commission accreditation standards for health care organizations: Pain assessment and management.* Retrieved from https://www .jointcommission.org/facts_about_joint_commission _accreditation_standards_for_health_care_organizations _pain_assessment_and_management/.

Kamalipour, H., Vafaei, A., Kazemi, A. P., & Khademi, S. (2014). Comparing the prevalence of chronic pain after sternotomy in patients undergoing coronary artery bypass grafting using the internal mammary artery and other open heart surgeries. *Anesthesiology and Pain Medicine, 4*(3), e17969.

Kerneis, C. K., Lafarge, A. L., Larnier, L. L., Scalbert, F., Brusset, A. B., Estagnasie, P. E., . . . Squara, P. S. (2015). Bowel and related complications after cardiac surgery. *Critical Care, 19.* doi:10.1186/cc14455

Kizza, I. B., Muliira, J. K., Kohi, T. W., & Nabirye, R. C. (2016). Nurses' knowledge of the principles of acute pain assessment critically ill adult patients who are able to self-report. *International Journal of Africa Nursing Sciences, 4,* 20–27.

Kleiman, A. M., Sanders, D. T., Nemergut, E. C., & Huffmyer, J. L, (2017). Chronic post-sternotomy pain: Incidence, risk factors, treatment, prevention and the anesthesiologists role. *Regional Anesthesia & Pain Medicine, 42*(6), 698–708.

Liu, Y., & Petrini, M. A. (2015). Effects of music therapy on pain, anxiety and vital signs in patients after thoracic surgery. *Complementary Therapies in Medicine, 23,* 714–718.

Machado, F., Souza, R. C., Poveda, V. B., & Costa, A. L. (2017). Non-pharmacological interventions to promote the sleep of patients after cardiac surgery: A systematic review. *Revista Latino-Americana De Enfermagem, 25,* e2926.

Mamoun, N. F., Lin, P., Zimmerman, N. M., Mascha, E. J., Mick, S. L., Insler, S. R., . . . Duncan, A. E. (2016).

Intravenous acetaminophen analgesia after cardiac surgery: A randomized, blinded, controlled superiority trial. *The Journal of Thoracic and Cardiovascular Surgery, 152*(3), 881–889.

McCaffery, M. (1972). *Nursing management of the patient with pain* (p. 8). Philadelphia, PA: Lippincott.

Meissner, W., Coluzzi, F., Fletcher, D., Huygen, F., Morlion, B., Neugebauer, E., . . . Pergolizzi, J. (2015). Improving the pain management of post-operative acute pain: Priorities for change. *Current Medical Research & Opinion, 31*(11), 2131–2143.

Mesbah, A., Yeung, J., & Gao, F. (2016). Pain after thoracotomy. *British Journal of Anesthesia, 16*(1), 1–7.

Miozzo, A. P., Stein, C., Bozzetto, C. B., & Plentz, R. D. M. (2016). Massage therapy reduces pain and anxiety after cardiac surgery: A systematic review and meta-analysis of randomized clinical trials. *Clinical Trials and Regulatory Science in Cardiology, 23*(24), 1–8.

Mukiri, S. R. K. (2015). Clinical study on post-operative analgesia and pain management for patients undergoing elective surgeries. *International Journal of Surgery, 2*(4), 475–479.

National Institute of Allergy and Infectious Diseases. (2015). *NIH clarifies racial and ethnic categories and definitions.* Retrieved from https://www.niaid.nih.gov/grants-contracts /nih-clarifies-racial-ethnic-categories-definitions.

Nolan, M. R. (2018). *Removing barriers to pain relief in older adults.* Retrieved from https://www.medscape.com/viewarticle /875972.

Olson, K. A. (2016). Gender and the pain experience. *Practical Pain Management, 16*(2), 1–3.

O'Neal, J. B. (2013). The utility of intravenous acetaminophen in the perioperative period. *Frontiers in Public Health, 1,* 25. doi: 10.3389/fpubh.2013.00025.

Özer, N., Karaman Özlü, Z., Arslan, S., & Güneş, N. (2013). Effect of music on postoperative pain and physiologic parameters of patients after open heart surgery. *Pain Management Nursing, 14*(1), 20–28.

Pain Doctor. (2016). *Race and the shocking inequalities in pain management.* Retrieved from https://paindoctor.com/race -inequalities-pain-management/.

Pasero, C., & McCaffery, M. (2005). No self-report means no pain-intensity rating: Assessing pain in patients who cannot provide a report. *American Journal of Nursing, 105*(10), 50–53.

Pereira, M. P., & Pogatzki-Zahn, E. (2015). Gender aspects in postoperative pain. *Current Opinion in Anesthesiology, 28*(5), 546–558.

Petrini, L., Matthiesen, S. T., & Arendt-Nielsen, L. (2015). The effect of age and gender on pressure pain thresholds and suprathreshold stimuli. *Perception, 44,* 587–596.

Pignaton, W., Braz, J. R., Kusano, P., Módolo, M., de Carvalho, L. R., Braz, M., . . . Braz, L. G. (2016). Perioperative and anesthesia-related mortality: An 8-year observational survey from a tertiary teaching hospital. *Medicine, 95*(2), e2208.

Pogatzki-Zahn, E. M., Segelcke, D., & Schug, S. A. (2017). Postoperative pain—from mechanisms to treatment. *Pain Reports, 2*(2), e588.

Pogatzki-Zahn, E. M., Zahn, P. K., & Brennan, T. J. (2007). Postoperative pain: Clinical implications of basic research. *Best Practice & Research Clinical Anaesthesiology, 21*(1), 3–13.

Rafiq, S., Steinbrüchel, D. A., Wanscher, M. J., Andersen, L. W., Navne, A., Lilleoer, N. B., . . . Olsen, P. S. (2014). Multimodal analgesia versus traditional opiate based analgesia after cardiac surgery, a randomized controlled trial. *Journal of Cardiothoracic Surgery, 9*, 52. doi:10.1186/1749-8090-9-52.

Rosenquist, R. W., & Rosenberg, J. (2003). Postoperative pain guidelines. *Regional Anesthesia and Pain Medicine, 28*(4), 279–288.

Sattari, M., Baghdadchi, M. E., Kyeyri, M., Khakzadi, H., & Mashayekh, S. O. (2013). Study of patient pain management after heart surgery. *Advanced Pharmaceutical Bulletin, 3*(2), 373–377.

Severgnini, P., Pelosi, P., Contino, E., Serafinelli, E., Novario, R., & Chiaranda, M. (2016). Accuracy of the critical care pain observation tool and behavioral scale to assess pain in critically ill conscious and unconscious patients: Prospective observational study. *Journal of Intensive Care, 4*(68), 2–8.

Storesund, A., Krukhaug, Y., Olsen, M. V., Rygh, L. J., Nilsen, R. N., & Norekvál, T. M. (2016). Females report higher postoperative pain scores than males after ankle surgery. *Scandinavian Journal of Pain, 12*, 85–93.

Tinsbloom, B., Muckler, V. C., Stoeckel, W. T., Whitehurst, R. L., & Morgan, B. (2017). Evaluating the implementation of preemptive, multimodal analgesia protocol in a plastic surgery office. *Plastic Surgery Nursing, 37*(4), 137–143.

Vadivelu, N., Mitra, S., Schermer, E., Kodumudi, V., Kay, A. D., & Urman, R. D. (2014). Preventive analgesia for postoperative pain control: A broader concept. *Local Regional Anesthesia, 7*, 17–22.

Viscusi, E. R. (2012). *IV acetaminophen improves pain management and reduces opioid requirements in surgical patients: A review of the clinical data and case-based presentations.* Retrieved from http://www.anesthesiologynews.com/download/SR122_WM.pdf.

Watt-Watson, J., Stevens, B., Katz, J., Costello, J., Reid, G., J., & David, T. (2004). Impact of preoperative education on pain outcomes after coronary artery bypass graft surgery. *Pain, 109*(1/2), 73–85.

Ziyaeifard, M., Azarfarin, R., & Golzari, S. E. (2014). A review of current analgesic techniques in cardiac surgery. Is epidural worth it? *Journal of Cardiovascular and Thoracic Research, 6*(3), 133–140.

Web Resources

American Academy of Pain Management: http://www.aapainmanage.org/

American Pain Society: http://www.ampainsoc.org/

American Society for Pain Management Nursing: http://www.aspmn.org/

Daily Pain Diary: https://www.caremark.com/Imagebank/Health_Diaries/DailyPainDiary.pdf

Inside look at chronic pain: http://www.or-live.com/distributors/nlm-flash/chp_1867/rnh.cfm?id=704

International Association for the Study of Pain: https://members.iasp-pain.org/

National Pain Foundation: http://www.nationalpainfoundation.org/default.asp

Pain Management Nursing: http://www.painmanagementnursing.org/

Transcutaneous Electrical Nerve Stimulation (TENS): https://www.intelihealth.com/article/learn-about-transcutaneous-electrical-nerve-stimulation-tens

CHAPTER 15

Postoperative Dysrhythmias

Roberta Kaplow

▶ Introduction

Dysrhythmias following cardiac surgery are known complications and account for high mortality rates, increased hospital length of stay (LOS), and costs. The length of time dysrhythmias last, ventricular response rate, patient's baseline cardiac function, and presence of comorbidities will impact the clinical significance of the dysrhythmias. Atrial fibrillation (AF) and atrial flutter often occur by postoperative day 3. Atrioventricular nodal reentrant tachycardia and ventricular dysrhythmias may also occur (Lee, 2016). Management includes identifying and treating the underlying cause(s) as well as pharmacologic and nonpharmacologic interventions. If the dysrhythmia is self-limiting, treatment may not be necessary, depending on the patient's hemodynamic response. However, treatment may be necessary if systemic infections or persistent pericardial effusion encompass the clinical situation (Peretto, Durante, Limite, & Cianflone, 2014).

Patients may have dysrhythmias prior to surgery or develop them intraoperatively or postoperatively. The origins of dysrhythmias include the atrium, atrioventricular (AV) node, or ventricle. This chapter discusses the most commonly encountered postoperative dysrhythmias, including their incidence, etiology, and suggested management.

▶ Incidence

The incidence of AF is reported at 15% to 40% following coronary artery bypass grafting (CABG), 37% to 50% in patients who undergo valve surgery, and up to 60% of patients who undergo valve replacement and CABG surgery. There is an increased incidence of postoperative dysrhythmias (PODs) associated with age (Lee, 2016). Dysrhythmias may compromise cardiac output (CO) by as much as 15% to 25% (Silvestry, 2018) when they interfere with diastolic filling. It is essential that the nurse working in the intensive care unit (ICU) with postoperative cardiac surgery patients be proficient in identifying and possibly eradicating potential causes and promptly recognizing potentially life-threatening dysrhythmias. Assessment of the patient requires evaluation of cardiac rhythm, its effects on systemic perfusion, and etiologic factors.

▶ Etiology

Several potential etiologic factors related to postoperative cardiac surgery dysrhythmias have been identified. The trauma associated with cardiac surgery itself places the patient at risk for the development of PODs. In addition, advanced age has been implicated in their development (Lee, 2016). This is felt to be related to changes in structure and electrophysiology associated with aging (Peretto et al., 2014). Examples include enlargement of the atrium or cardiomyopathy. Others at risk include chronic obstructive pulmonary disease (COPD), increased hemoglobin A_{1c} (HbA_{1c}), low-intensity physical activity 1 year prior to surgery, Caucasian race, obesity, withdrawal or no use of beta blockers or angiotensin-converting enzyme (ACE) inhibitors preoperatively, mitral valve disease (especially mitral stenosis), low-dose dopamine (Intropin®), severe stenosis of the right coronary artery, increase in P-wave duration, hypokalemia, or hypomagnesemia.

Perioperative risk factors for postoperative dysrhythmias include presence of pericarditis, injury to the atrium, acute atrial enlargement from increased pressure or volume, inadequate cardioprotection during cardiopulmonary bypass (CPB), ischemia of the atrium, long aortic cross-clamp or CPB time, use of postoperative inotropic agents, inflammation, hypokalemia, hypomagnesemia, or oxidative stress (Lee, 2016).

Dysrhythmias in postoperative cardiac surgery patients may result from fluid overload–induced acute atrial enlargement, respiratory complications, electrolyte disturbances (e.g., hypokalemia, hyperkalemia, hypomagnesemia), surgical trauma (inadequate cardioprotection during bypass procedures), hypothermia, hyperadrenergic state, acid–base imbalance, anxiety, or pain. Presence of hypoxia, hypercarbia, excess catecholamines, and use of instrumentation in the operating room may also precipitate the development of PODs. Further, CPB, the amount of cross-clamp time, type of cardioplegia used, and CABG procedures put the patient at risk for the development of PODs (Peretto et al., 2014).

Postoperative dysrhythmias are anticipated following cardiac transplant procedures as well.

They are thought to be due to ischemia of the donor heart, extensive suture lines, rejection, augmented atherosclerosis, and procedure-associated denervation. The incidence is reported at 4% to 24% of heart transplant patients (Eisen & Kusmirek, 2017; Peretto et al., 2014).

▶ Atrial Dysrhythmias

Atrial dysrhythmias are the most commonly encountered rhythm abnormalities in the postoperative CABG patient. The overall incidence of atrial dysrhythmias is reported to be as high as 40%. A higher incidence is reported in patients who undergo valve surgery than CABG (37%–50%) and 60% in patients who undergo valve replacement and CABG (Lee, 2016). Atrial dysrhythmias that may develop in the postoperative cardiac surgery patient may include sïnus tachycardia, premature atrial contractions (PACs) (>60% incidence), supraventricular tachycardia (up to 76%), atrial fibrillation (AF) (10%–24%), atrial flutter, and relative bradycardia (up to 50%).

Sinus tachycardia is a common dysrhythmia following surgery in general, with cardiac surgery being no exception. It can be attributed to the normal stress response. As a general guideline, treatment of sinus tachycardia should focus on ameliorating its underlying cause. Etiology of sinus tachycardia may include pain, fever, anxiety, anemia, medications (e.g., catecholamines), hypermetabolic state (e.g., sepsis), or an increase in adrenergic tone (e.g., in a patient taking a beta blocker preoperatively). The presence of sinus tachycardia is not likely to cause adverse effects if the patient has normal left ventricular (LV) function, and treatment is usually not indicated (Peretto et al., 2014).

Premature atrial contractions may also develop in the postoperative cardiac surgery patient. These abnormal beats are usually not clinically significant and rarely require treatment. However, PACs can predispose patients to postoperative atrial fibrillation (POAF) (Hashemzadeh, Dehdilani, & Dehdilani, 2013). Sixty percent of postoperative cardiac surgery patients were found to have had PACs prior to the onset of POAF. These patients showed either a pattern of sustained uniform PAC activity or spontaneous bursts of high PAC activity interspaced with relatively quiet periods of PAC activity prior to AF (Hashimoto, Yamauchi, & Inoue, 2014). If characteristic PAC patterns predict POAF, pharmacologic interventions with agents used to treat POAF could be initiated when the characteristic PAC pattern is first detected. During the highest POAF risk period (postoperative days 1–5), nurses should maintain a high level of vigilance for potential intervention.

Supraventricular dysrhythmias occur frequently following cardiac surgery and can result in increased hospital LOS, costs of care, and stroke risk. Decreased cardiac output can result from the loss of atrial kick. Risk factors include advanced age, obstructive sleep apnea (OSA), history of heart failure or dysrhythmias, bicaval cannulation, long CPB time, hypothermia, electrolyte disturbances, distention of the atrium, or administration of drugs that can cause dysrhythmias. If preventative measures are not initiated, the incidence of supraventricular dysrhythmias is 30% to 40%. The majority of cases are AF or atrial flutter, which occur more frequently in patients who undergo valve procedures versus CABG. Supraventricular dysrhythmias typically occur on postoperative day 2 or 3. Initiation of prophylactic measures may decrease the incidence of AF by approximately 50%. Prophylaxis may include use of beta blockers (contraindicated in bradycardia), amiodarone (Cordarone®) (contraindicated in bradycardia, conduction disturbances, and chronic interstitial lung disease), sotalol (Betapace®), magnesium (least effective pharmacologic strategy), or biatrial pacing (less effective than beta blockers; equipment costs should be factored in; and requires epicardial pacing wires) (Stephens & Whitman, 2015).

Postoperative Atrial Fibrillation

Atrial fibrillation is the most common dysrhythmia that may occur in the postoperative cardiac surgery patient. It occurs in 15% to 40% of patients who undergo CABG, 37% to 50% of patients following valve surgery, and up to 60% of patients who undergo CABG with valve replacement. The incidence of AF increases with age (Lee, 2016).

Postoperative atrial fibrillation is often self-limiting, with the majority of patients with new-onset POAF converting back to normal sinus rhythm (NSR) within 6 to 8 weeks postoperatively (Peretto et al., 2014). The peak onset of occurrence of POAF is 2 to 4 days following surgery (Lee, 2016; Peretto et al., 2014).

Data suggest that up to 30% of patients who develop POAF did not have a history of this dysrhythmia. Up to 30% of patients transition back to NSR within 12 hours, and 80% convert back within 24 hours (Peretto et al., 2014). Incidence data are variable and depend on the type of procedure performed. Patients who undergo off-pump coronary artery bypass grafting (OPCABG) have less risk of developing POAF. This is felt to be related to the development of less inflammation as compared with on-pump procedures (Peretto et al., 2014).

The pathophysiology of AF involves the rapid release of multiple impulses from the atrium to the AV node; however, the AV node can respond to only a few of these impulses. In AF, the patient's heart does not contract with maximum efficiency. The rapid quivering of the atria may result in hemodynamic compromise from decreased atrial filling and the atrial kick that can normally contribute as much as 25% of CO (Silvestry, 2018). Loss of atrial kick can result in increased pulmonary pressure. This is seen more often in patients with decreased diastolic function. In patients with normal LV function, however, AF is generally well tolerated (Peretto et al., 2014). Because the blood lingers in the atria with AF, small clots may develop, which places the patient at risk for stroke.

Risk Factors for POAF

Many studies have attempted to determine the etiology of AF in the postoperative cardiac surgery patient. The cause of POAF is multifactorial. A patient's demographic data and medical history provide insight into the probability of PODs.

Risk factors may be categorized into preoperative, intraoperative, and postoperative risks. The primary predictor of POAF is age (Lee, 2016). As the body ages, structural and size changes of the atria predispose the individual to develop atrial dysrhythmias. Preoperative risks may also include atrial fibrosis; history of rheumatic heart disease; valve disease; right coronary artery stenosis; increased LV diastolic pressure; hypertension; acute coronary syndrome; heart disease (e.g., LV hypertrophy); enlargement of the left atrium; dilation of the right atrium and right ventricle; history of heart failure, which results in atrial stretch from volume overload; COPD; elevated HbA_{1c}; pulmonary hypertension; tachycardia; hypokalemia; hypomagnesemia; hypothyroidism; preoperative beta blocker withdrawal; preoperative use of digoxin or milrinone (Primacor®); obesity; previous cardiac surgery; Caucasian race; absence of beta blockers or ACE inhibitors; and higher brain natriuretic peptide (Lee, 2016; Peretto et al., 2014). The presence of a pericardial effusion, pericarditis, acute enlargement of the atria, and ischemia have been frequently implicated in the development of POAF (Peretto et al., 2014). Surprisingly, some earlier data suggest that current smokers were less likely to develop dysrhythmias following CABG. This phenomenon is thought to be related to the "hyperadrenergic stimulation" from nicotine in current smokers. This was found not to be true of patients who smoked in the past (Al-Sarraf et al., 2010).

Intraoperative risks that have been identified include sympathetic stimulation from catecholamines, fluid losses, anemia, pain, or administration of adrenergic agents. Sympathetic stimulation leads to an increase in heart rate and contractility from $beta_1$ receptor stimulation. Sympathetic stimulation also leads to an increase in excitability and automaticity (the heart's inherent ability to initiate a beat). Patients with POAF have higher levels of norepinephrine as compared to patients who do not develop POAF. There is also an associated shortened atrial refractoriness associated with sympathetic stimulation. This can put the patient at risk to develop a POD (Peretto et al., 2014).

Inflammation associated with cardiac surgery has been suggested as a mechanism contributing to development of POAF. Inflammation leads to the release of proinflammatory mediators. This is manifested with elevated white blood cell, monocyte, and neutrophil counts (Zakker, Ascione,

James, Angelini, & Suleiman, 2015). A systemic inflammatory response may develop from CPB.

Oxidative stress is another suggested etiologic factor for POAF related to cardiac surgery. A consequence of CPB is ischemia. During reperfusion, there is an increased production of reactive oxygen species (from pro-oxidants [versus antioxidants]). This can result in myocardial stunning, tissue damage, and cell death. The degree of oxidative stress depends on the extent of ischemia and left ventricular ejection fraction (LVEF) (Zakker et al., 2015).

Cross-clamping without adequate atrial protection, bicaval venous cannulation, metabolic imbalances, fluid and electrolyte shifts, cardioplegia, the surgical incision, and the surgical procedure itself have also been implicated (Peretto et al., 2014; Zakker et al., 2015). Patients who underwent OPCABG were reported to have a lower incidence of POAF. This is thought to be related to CPB-associated systemic inflammatory effect (Alawani, Chatfield, Ghashi, & Walker, 2018). Inflammation is the most common hypothesized cause of POAF secondary to handling of the heart and use of CPB. Other possible alternative causes include oxidative stress, electrical remodeling, atrial incision, and ischemia (Alawani et al., 2018).

Postoperative factors that have been implicated in the development of POAF include hemodynamic compromise (e.g., secondary to heart failure, myocardial infarction [MI], venous thrombotic events [VTEs], bleeding from anticoagulation), administration of $beta_1$ agonists (e.g., dopamine, dobutamine [Dobutrex®]), hypomagnesemia, extubation, increased sympathetic and parasympathetic tone, and an exaggerated inflammatory response (Lee, 2016).

Complications of POAF

A number of consequences of POAF following cardiac surgery have been reported. Development of POAF has been reported to result in increased LOS in the ICU (Omer et al., 2016; Steinberg et al., 2014); postoperative mortality (LaPar et al., 2014); increased 30-day mortality (Omer et al., 2016); hemodynamic instability (Steinberg et al., 2014); increased risk of stroke (Ha, Mazer, Verma,

Yanagawa, & Verma, 2016; Stephens & Whitman, 2015); and increased costs (LaPar et al., 2014).

Prevention of POAF

Prevention of POAF is essential to help decrease LOS and overall mortality (Steinberg et al., 2014). The individual patient scenario, potential adverse events, and cost should be considered when deciding on the appropriate intervention to prevent POAF. No single agent or combination of agents has entirely eradicated POAF. Use of prophylaxis for POAF is supported in the literature especially in those patients with risk factors (Peretto et al., 2014).

Pharmacotherapy

Patients who are at high risk for the development of POAF may receive preventive antiarrhythmic therapy. Consideration should be given to renal function and the side effects of the agents when deciding if preventive strategies are warranted.

Beta Blockers

The use of beta blockers to prevent POAF is supported by international guidelines (Alawami et al., 2018). Data demonstrate that beta blockers are efficacious in helping to prevent POAF. Beta blockers decrease oxygen demand and ischemic events. The latter results from blunting of catecholamine surge effects. By decreasing ischemic events, the risk of POAF is decreased (Turagam et al., 2015).

Beta blockers are considered the first choice to prevent POAF and should be used unless contraindicated (Alawami et al., 2015; Stephens & Whitman, 2015). Their use has also been shown to decrease postoperative complication rate and costs (Alawami et al., 2018). Contraindications to beta blocker use include hemodynamic compromise, use of inotropes, bradycardia, conduction disturbances, and presence of heart block (i.e., first-degree AV block with a PR interval >0.24 sec, second- or third-degree AV block) (Stephens & Whitman, 2015).

Sotalol

Sotalol (Betapace®) is a class III agent (potassium channel blocker), which causes an increase in repolarization time. It also has beta blocker properties. Sotalol may be more effective in reducing the incidence of POAF with fewer associated side effects than beta blockers. Administration should begin 1 to 2 days preoperatively or within 4 hours postoperatively (Peretto et al., 2014). However, because there is a potential for proarrhythmic effects with sotalol, beta blockers have been reported as safer to administer for the prevention of POAF (Turagam et al., 2015). Administration of sotalol may prolong the QT interval. Sotalol is contraindicated in patients with heart failure (Giardina, 2018).

Amiodarone

Amiodarone (Cordarone®) prolongs both the duration and the refractory period of the myocardial cell action potential. It possesses mild alpha, beta, and calcium channel blocking effects. Because of the wide range of effects, amiodarone has been shown to be effective in decreasing the incidence of AF (Clark, Hodge, Ressler, & Lee, 2011). Amiodarone may be useful when use of beta blockers is not feasible (Turagam et al., 2015). Amiodarone has been shown to be effective to decrease the incidence of POAF by up to 50% (Peretto et al., 2014). A variety of administration schedules and routes of administration are reported. It is unclear if amiodarone is more effective than a beta blocker to prevent POAF (Peretto et al., 2014). An infusion may be started if the patient is at high risk for POAF (e.g., age >65 years, history of COPD or heart failure, or prolonged CPB time) (Raiten, Patel, & Gutsche, 2015). Beta blockers and amiodarone may also be used in combination for this purpose. Because amiodarone has properties from all four classes of cardiac medications, hypotension and bradycardia are possible (Giardina, 2018).

Magnesium

Hypomagnesemia is a risk factor for the development of POAF. Low magnesium levels may last up to 4 days after cardiac surgery. As such, administration of magnesium for prophylaxis has been evaluated. Some data suggest statistically significant differences in the incidence of POAF in patients who received prophylactic magnesium administration (Kotecha, 2016). The data are not consistent (Turagam et al., 2015).

Corticosteroids

Administration of corticosteroids has been evaluated to determine if there is an associated decrease in the incidence of POAF following a CABG procedure or valve replacement surgery. Recent data suggest there is short-term efficacy to prevent POAF in these patients (Al-Shawabkeh et al., 2016). Data from randomized trials, however, do not support its use to prevent POAF (Ha et al., 2016). If used, nurses should consider the impact of corticosteroids on an increase in hyperglycemia and a potential for postoperative infection.

N-acetylcysteine

Administration of N-acetylcysteine (NAC) has been demonstrated to be effective in reducing the incidence of POAF in patients undergoing CABG, valve surgery, or a combination of these procedures (Turagam et al., 2015). As described earlier, a consequence of CPB is ischemia that results in oxidative stress. An increasing body of evidence demonstrates that oxidative stress and inflammatory reaction play an important role in the pathophysiology of POAF. N-acetylcysteine has shown to decrease serum levels of molecular markers of cellular oxidative stress in patients undergoing heart surgery. Administration of NAC, which has antioxidant properties, may decrease the incidence of POAF. The duration of NAC administration should be until postoperative day 2 to 3 when the inflammatory cytokine levels are the highest, corresponding to the day of the highest incidence of POAF (Liu, Xu, & Fan 2014). The data regarding NAC are not consistent (Turagam et al., 2015).

Statins

It has been suggested that preoperative administration of a statin may decrease the incidence of POAF. These data are not consistent. Statins are felt to decrease the development of POAF by decreasing hyperlipidemia and through its anti-inflammatory, antioxidant, cardioprotective, and neurohormonal modulatory effects (Turagam et al., 2015).

Electrical Therapy: Atrial Pacing

Some data suggest that right atrial pacing decreases the incidence of POAF. These data, however, are inconsistent (Lee, 2016). Some data also suggest that biatrial pacing was effective in preventing POAF following CABG and following a Maze procedure (Benjo et al., 2015). The mechanism of action of biatrial pacing has not been fully interpreted.

Atrial Dysrhythmias Following Cardiac Transplant

In the cardiac transplant patient, there is a reported lower incidence of PODs than with other cardiac surgeries. Factors that have been implicated in the development of POAF include ischemia, denervation, pericardial inflammation, potential drug interactions with immunosuppression, autonomic hypersensitivity, primary graft failure, early rejection, administration of inotropes, ventricular dysfunction, valve regurgitation, systemic inflammation, allograft vasculopathy, and a focal trigger from superior or inferior vena cava or coronary sinus. Atrial flutter is reported to be the most common dysrhythmia noted on patient follow-up. It may be due to rejection or graft vasculopathy (Avellana et al., 2015).

Treatment of POAF

Treatment of AF focuses on control of rate and rhythm. Several treatment strategies for the management of AF have been reported. Ultimately, intervention to bring about a conversion from AF to NSR is most desirable. Management strategies of POAF include heart rate control with either medications or electricity (e.g., synchronized cardioversion [SCV]). The latter may not be necessary given the percentage of patients who convert to NSR on their own (Peretto et al., 2014). Knowing the factors that predispose the patient to developing AF, the nurse should attempt to anticipate the occurrence of this complication and be prepared to quickly respond to the dysrhythmias and convert the patient to NSR. A detailed preoperative history is important in preventing postoperative dysrhythmias. Analysis of the electrocardiogram will reveal the presence of preexisting conditions such as LV hypertrophy.

A rapid assessment of the patient's hemodynamic status is essential to help determine the appropriate treatment strategy. If the patient is stable, pharmacotherapy may be attempted. If unstable (e.g., presence of hypotension, mental status changes, chest pain, shortness of breath, heart failure symptoms, or cold and clammy skin), SCV is indicated (Raiten et al., 2015).

Development of POAF becomes clinically significant due to the resultant decreases in diastolic filling and CO. Hypotension and ischemia result from the associated increase in myocardial oxygen consumption. Patients typically become symptomatic when they develop POAF with a rapid ventricular response (Peretto et al., 2014). When a cardiac surgery patient develops POAF, hemodynamic stability status, possible underlying causes, and goals of treatment are all key considerations that need to be identified promptly. Antiarrhythmic therapy and consideration of antithrombotic therapy to prevent a VTE are the mainstays of therapy (Peretto et al., 2014).

Establishment of hemodynamic stability should be the principal goal of therapy. Hemodynamic stability may need to be attained by controlling rate, rhythm, or both; the former is usually all that is required. The pharmacologic agents used to prevent or treat postoperative dysrhythmias are discussed in detail in Chapter 12.

Agents recommended by the American College of Cardiology, European Society of Cardiology, and the American Heart Association that are used to control heart rate associated with POAF include beta blockers and amiodarone. The use of beta blockers has been reported to decrease the incidence of POAF (from 30%–40% to 12%–16%) in patients who underwent CABG. Similarly, a decrease (from 37%–50% to 15%–20%) is reported in patients who have undergone valve procedures. Beta blockers also decrease the ventricular response rate when POAF develops. Patients seem to derive the most benefit when beta blocker therapy is initiated preoperatively or in the immediate postoperative period (Peretto et al., 2014).

The optimal ventricular rate should be established in patients with new POAF. This rate will typically be less than 110 beats per minute (bpm). If the rate is controlled, no SCV should be performed within 24 hours of the POAF development. Synchronized cardioversion may be indicated in patients who are not hemodynamically stable or if the rate is not well controlled. It may also be indicated in asymptomatic patients when hospital discharge is approaching or if the rhythm does not spontaneously convert within 24 to 48 hours so that anticoagulation can be circumvented (Lee, 2016; Raiten et al., 2015).

Patients who are beta blocker naïve will typically remain on therapy at least until their first postoperative ambulatory visit. Those who were on beta blockers in the past (e.g., for MI, heart failure, hypertension) should remain on long-term therapy (Peretto et al., 2014). Amiodarone may also be used to decrease the ventricular response rate of POAF (Alawami et al., 2017).

Anticoagulation

Patients who develop POAF that lasts more than 48 hours are at risk for a VTE (Lee, 2016). The risk increases further in patients with mitral valve disease secondary to rheumatic fever, previous VTE, hypertension, or heart failure. Use of warfarin (Coumadin®), dabigatran (Pradaxa®), rivaroxaban (Xarelto®), apixaban (Eliquis®), or edoxaban (Savaysa®, Lixiana®) decreases the risk of systemic embolization by approximately 70% and should be considered in patients with AF not related to valve problems. The risk of bleeding must be considered when implementing anticoagulation therapy. Data suggest that anticoagulation should be initiated and continued for at least 1 year following the development of POAF following cardiac surgery (Meldun et al., 2015). Data are not consistent regarding the usefulness of anticoagulation in preventing stroke in these patients. Conversion to NSR may be challenging in patients with valve disease (Peretto et al., 2014).

Administration of anticoagulants in the post-operative cardiac surgery period carries the risk of increased bleeding and cardiac tamponade. Given that POAF is typically self-limiting, the provider should weigh the risks and benefits of anticoagulation (Manning, Singer, & Lip, 2018; Peretto et al., 2014). Up to 80% of patients who develop POAF after cardiac surgery convert to NSR within 24 hours; that percentage increases to 90% in 6 to 8 weeks (Peretto et al., 2014). If the patient has normal LV function, long-term therapy is usually not required. However, if the patient has POAF that has lasted more than 48 hours and anticoagulation is deemed necessary, a heparin infusion followed by oral anticoagulants is recommended. Patients with POAF following cardiac surgery may be discharged on oral anticoagulants and antiarrhythmic therapy (Peretto et al., 2014).

Rhythm Control

If patients are asymptomatic, conversion to NSR may not be necessary (Lee, 2016). If patients have a low LVEF, rhythm control may be advantageous. If patients are symptomatic following rate control for POAF, rate control cannot be accomplished; or based on patient preference, attempts to eradicate POAF should be considered. This may be accomplished with either use of pharmacotherapy or electricity.

Rate control is usually accomplished with beta blockers since there is an increased sympathetic state postoperatively. Esmolol (Brevibloc®) is a short-acting beta blocker. The goal rate is individualized to the patient. Typically a heart rate less than 110 will prevent palpitations and will result in optimal heart function (Lee, 2016). Calcium channel blockers and digoxin (Lanoxin®) are shown not to be as effective as beta blockers. If rate control is not achieved with other agents, intravenous amiodarone (Cordorone®) may be used to slow ventricular rate associated with POAF (Lee, 2016).

Ibutilide (Corvert®) is a class III antiarrhythmic (potassium channel blocker). It may be used to convert patients with POAF following cardiac surgery. Ibutilide is administered as an IV bolus and may be repeated once. The ICU nurse must monitor the patient for development of torsade de pointes if ibutilide is used, because QT prolongation is possible (Bhargava, 2016). Data suggest that ibutilide is as effective as amiodarone in converting a patient out of POAF, but the amount of time it took to convert was lower in patients who received ibutilide. Further, there are fewer hemodynamic effects with ibutilide; more patients who received amiodarone developed hypotension (Bhargava, 2016).

In addition to pharmacotherapy, a number of other approaches have been employed, including SCV and surgical interventions (e.g., Cox-Maze III, Ex-Maze procedure, or cryoablation). It is recommended to be performed concomitantly with mitral valve procedures or other cardiac procedures (Badhivar et al., 2017).

Ablative techniques that electrically separate the pulmonary veins from the atria have been used to ensure that impulses are not conducted. Single radiofrequency ablation (RFA) may be tried in patients who did not successfully convert to NSR with one or two drugs. Efficacy of single RFA is reported as high as 45% to 95% in patients (Loardi et al., 2015). This procedure may also be performed concomitantly with cardiac surgery in patients with preoperative AF. Surgical treatment of AF is discussed in more detail in Chapter 3.

▶ Ventricular Dysrhythmias

Three dysrhythmias of ventricular origin have been reported in the postoperative cardiac surgery patient: premature ventricular contractions (PVCs), ventricular tachycardia (VT), and ventricular fibrillation (VF). A number of risk factors for the development of postoperative ventricular arrhythmias (POVAs) have been cited in the literature. Presence of ventricular dysrhythmias should suggest ongoing ischemia (Stephens & Whitman, 2015).

Ventricular dysrhythmias are less common than dysrhythmias of atrial origin in patients having undergone cardiac surgery and may be indicative of myocardial dysfunction. Current data suggest the incidence of postoperative VT/VF in 15.3% of patients (Cheng, Goo, Wang, Yang, & Zhang, 2018). The incidence of nonsustained VT is reported at 17% to 97%. Its development is felt to be related to reperfusion. Sustained polymorphic VT or VF occurs in 1% to 3% of patients within the first week of CABG surgery.

Risk factors include age less than 65 years, female gender, body mass index (BMI) less than 25 kg/m^2, unstable angina, ejection fraction (EF) 50% or less, pulmonary or systemic hypertension, renal failure, lower preoperative EF (<30%), prolonged CPB time, inotrope, or intra-aortic balloon pump therapy requirement. There is an increased risk of postoperative mortality in these patients (24.6% versus 1.5%) (Aranki & Cutlip, 2018; Cheng et al., 2018).

Polymorphic VT is associated with perioperative hemodynamic instability, increased sympathetic activity, and metabolic derangements. Sustained monomorphic VT is associated with a history of MI, heart failure, and decreased LVEF. There is a 30% increased risk of development of monomorphic VT when these three risk factors are present (Aranki & Cutlip, 2018).

Ventricular dysrhythmias are of clinical concern because of the potential for associated hemodynamic instability. Loss of the atrial kick may decrease CO. Further, their presence can impact patient outcomes. Postoperative ventricular arrhythmias are associated with a higher mortality rate prior to hospital discharge and within 1 year following cardiac surgery.

Premature Ventricular Contractions

Premature ventricular contractions can be considered clinically insignificant unless they become frequent (>30/min), are multifocal, or the patient is close to developing R on T. In this case, ventricular function may be impacted (Peretto et al., 2014). Premature ventricular contractions usually do not require intervention if the patient has normal LV function and normal metabolic and electrolyte levels. Any of these etiologies require correction if present. For example, alterations in potassium level may be the underlying cause of PVCs and would require optimization (Peretto et al., 2014).

In addition to treating the underlying cause, treatment of clinically significant PVCs may include pharmacotherapy. While lidocaine (Xylocaine®)

has been effective in decreasing the number of PVCs that cause hemodynamic instability, no improvement in mortality has been reported and it is considered potentially harmful. Nonetheless, lidocaine is still used in clinical practice despite not being endorsed by the American Heart Association Guidelines. Use of overdrive pacing, dual chamber pacing, and implantable cardioverter defibrillators (ICDs) has not impacted patient prognosis. Development of postoperative PVCs does not seem to impact patient outcome (Peretto et al., 2014).

Ventricular Tachycardia and Ventricular Fibrillation

In one report, predictors of postoperative VT or VF included age greater than 30, increased BMI, valve surgery, and male gender (Amatya, Sharma, Pokharel, Amatya, & Shrestha, 2015). Other patients at risk are reported to include those with LV dysfunction, structural heart disease, heart failure, hemodynamic instability, electrolyte imbalance, decreased oxygen levels, hypovolemia, ischemia, MI, reperfusion after CPB, use of inotropes or antiarrhythmics, and acute graft closure. In the immediate postoperative period, hemodynamic instability, acid–base imbalance, hypoxia, anemia, or new ischemia put the patient at risk for VT or VF (Peretto et al., 2014). In a case report, undersensing of epicardial pacing wires induced R on T phenomenon, which resulted in VF (Nakamori, Maeda, & Ohnishi, 2016).

Management of Postoperative Ventricular Dysrhythmias

Patients who develop paroxysmal VT who remain hemodynamically stable and who are otherwise asymptomatic do not necessarily need to be treated aside from treating the underlying cause. Patients who develop sustained VT should be treated with either medication (if asymptomatic) or SCV if symptomatic. Medication management is with amiodarone (Stephens & Whitman, 2015).

In patients with a VT and a pulse, amiodarone is indicated as the first line therapy. A bolus of 150 mg over 10 to 15 min is recommended (American Heart Association [AHA], 2015). Additional doses of 150 mg may be administered. The nurse should observe for hypotension and bradycardia. Amiodarone is reported to be better tolerated than other antiarrhythmic therapies in patients with systolic dysfunction (Peretto et al., 2014).

Procainamide may be used as a second line therapy. A loading dose of 20 to 50 mg/min up to 17 mg/kg can be followed by a continuous infusion of 1 to 4 mg/min. Patients with renal dysfunction may be excluded from this therapy due to an associated buildup of a toxic metabolite, N-acetyl procainamide (Peretto et al., 2014). The nurse should observe the patient for development of hypotension and for QRS widening while the patient is receiving procainamide. Therapy should be stopped if the QRS widens by 50%, hypotension develops, or the maximum dose has been received (AHA, 2015).

Sotalol may also be used to treat VT with a pulse if the patient is stable. Because sotalol has proarrhythmic effects, the nurse should observe the patient for development of torsade de pointes.

Sustained VT may also be treated with electricity. Patients with epicardial pacing wires still in place may be treated with pacing if they develop VT with a slower rate. It is possible for a patient's condition to worsen to a VT with a more rapid ventricular response or VF. Because of this, equipment should be readily available in case SCV (for unstable VT) or defibrillation (for VF or pulseless VT) is required (Peretto et al., 2014). Placement of an internal cardioverter defibrillator should be considered in patients with a low LVEF in whom ventricular dysrhythmias persist (Stephens & Whitman, 2015).

Implantation of an ICD should be considered in patients requiring long-term therapy. These may include patients who do not have a reversible cause such as those with paroxysmal VT, history of MI, LVEF less than 40%, or those who have induced ventricular arrhythmias with electrophysiology studies (Peretto et al., 2014).

Ventricular fibrillation should be treated with immediate defibrillation per advanced cardiac life support (ACLS) protocol, cardiopulmonary resuscitation, administration of epinephrine and antiarrhythmic agents, and eradication of the underlying cause. The amount of energy used for defibrillation is initially 120 joules; this should be followed by 150 joules and then 200 joules in 2-min increments (AHA, 2015).

Amiodarone is indicated as first line therapy for pulseless VT and VF. A bolus of 300 mg may be followed by a continuous infusion of 1 mg/min for the first 6 hours postresuscitation and 0.5 mg/min for the next 18 hours. Additional boluses of 150 mg may be administered as indicated (AHA, 2015; Peretto et al., 2014).

The Society of Thoracic Surgeons has specific recommendations for the resuscitation of patients who develop cardiac arrest following cardiac surgery (The Society of Thoracic Surgeons Task Force on Resuscitation after Cardiac Surgery, 2017). The website is located in web references at the end of this chapter.

▶ Bradyarrhythmias

Following cardiac surgery, development of bradyarrhythmias is common. These rhythms may include second-degree AV block type II, sinus pauses, sinus bradycardia, or complete heart block (Peretto et al., 2014). The most common abnormalities are complete heart block with a narrow or wide escape rhythm, sinus node dysfunction, and junctional rhythm (Aranki & Cutlip, 2018). Bradyarrhythmias are most common in patients who have undergone valve surgery. It may also occur following CABG. Development of this complication is believed to be related to surgical injury and edema (Peretto et al., 2014).

The overall incidence of bradyarrhythmias following CABG is 0.8% to 4% of patients who require implantation of a permanent pacemaker (Aranki & Cutlip, 2018). This is most often seen following valvular surgery. It is felt to be related to surgical injury and local inflammation. Temporary or permanent pacing may be required (Silvestry, 2018). The development of symptomatic bradycardia is higher in patients who undergo tricuspid or aortic valve procedures.

Up to 50% of patients who undergo a heart transplant may develop dysfunction of the sinoatrial (SA) node and 4% to 5% may develop AV block. Its development may be due to surgical trauma to the SA node or blood supply (Eisen & Kusmirek, 2017).

Sinus node dysfunction typically occurs within the first several weeks postoperatively.

Bradycardias can impact morbidity from decreased cardiac output, but do not appear to impact mortality rates. Other potential causes include older age, ischemia during intraoperative hypothermia, surgical trauma to the SA node or perinodal atrial tissue, history of left bundle branch block, calcification of a valve, removal of left ventricular aneurysm, stenosis of the left main coronary artery, larger number of vessels bypassed, CPB time, increased vagal tone during the surgical procedure, type of anesthesia, and presence of postoperative pain (Eisen & Kusmirek, 2017; Peretto et al., 2014). Other factors include medications (e.g., digoxin, amiodarone, calcium channel blockers, and beta blockers) and certain surgical approaches. Patients undergoing procedures involving some specific approaches experienced second-degree AV block type II or complete heart block. Some additional patients developed persistent sinus bradycardia or junctional rhythm (Peretto et al., 2014).

Following a heart transplant, development of sick sinus syndrome (SSS) is common. Up to 21% of these patients require insertion of a permanent pacemaker. Patients at risk for development of bradyarrhythmias following a heart transplant include the donor being of older age, higher donor ischemic time, patients who have undergone biatrial (versus bicaval) transplant, and increased cross-clamp time (Peretto et al., 2014).

Management of Bradyarrhythmias

Treatment of the underlying cause of the bradyarrhythmia is essential. This may include discontinuing the medications that may cause AV block. Referral to a current Advanced Cardiovascular Life Support (ACLS) manual is suggested. Management of bradyarrhythmias usually entails use of a temporary pacemaker. The epicardial wires that are oftentimes left in place following the initial cardiac surgery are used for this purpose. It is suggested that atrial pacing is preferred because of the increase in stroke volume associated with electrical impulses that originate from above the AV node. If AV block occurs, dual chamber pacing is the next best option.

Ventricular pacing should be used as a rescue mode in case of cardiopulmonary arrest or failure to capture atrial leads (Stephens & Whitman, 2015).

If the bradyarrhythmias are clinically significant or if the patient has persistent AV block or SA node dysfunction, permanent pacemaker insertion is indicated (Peretto et al., 2014). Of the patients who develop complete heart block, up to 100% will require insertion of a permanent pacemaker. It is typical for patients with persistent SSS or complete heart block lasting more than 5 to 7 days to receive a permanent pacemaker (Eisen & Kusmirek, 2017). A permanent pacemaker has been required in up to 24% of patients following cardiac surgery (Peretto et al., 2014). Until a permanent pacemaker can be inserted, transcutaneous or transvenous pacing or a pulmonary artery catheter with a pacing port may also be used.

Management of Bradyarrhythmias Following Cardiac Transplant

A significant difference exists in the pharmacologic management of bradydysrhythmias following cardiac transplant and the approaches used in patients who undergo other cardiac surgical procedures and develop postoperative dysrhythmias. Patients may develop bradycardia following a heart transplant due to sympathetic denervation, SA node ischemia, ischemia of the graft, and medications used during surgery (Eisen & Kusmirek, 2017). Bradycardia may develop as a consequence of the incision made in the SA node during surgery. Atropine will not be effective in this instance because of the severing of the vagus nerve.

Management with a pacemaker should be the primary treatment. Pacemakers also give the patient the needed atrial kick and augment CO. Intravenous inotropic support may be used in asymptomatic patients. Agents such as isoproterenol (Isuprel®), theophylline (Theo-Dur®), or terbutaline (Brethine®) may be used to increase heart rate of the newly implanted heart. If the bradyarrhythmia persists, consideration should be given to implanting a pacemaker. The patient should also be evaluated for rejection with endomyocardial biopsy (Eisen & Kusmirek, 2017).

▶ Epicardial Pacemakers

Placement of epicardial pacing wires facilitates temporary pacing following cardiac surgery. Pacing electrodes are attached directly to the atria, the ventricles, or both during surgery. The wires are inserted in the event that the patient develops bradycardia, second-degree AV block type II, complete heart block, prolonged AV delay, bifascicular block with first-degree AV block, prolonged QT syndrome, junctional tachycardia, supraventricular tachycardia, atrial flutter with a rate less than 320 to 340/min, or junctional rhythm, all of which require better conduction control to resolve. The wires are then secured to the epicardium and brought out through the skin. Depending on the surgeon's preference, the patient may have one or two sets of pacing wires emplaced. Generally, the ventricular and atrial wires exit the skin to the left and right of the sternum, respectively. It is essential for the ICU nurse to secure the leads to the patient's chest or abdomen, have a pacemaker generator with new batteries readily available, and ensure that all wiring and connections are tight and free of fraying. The ends of the pacer wires should be covered, insulated, and protected with a clean, dry dressing. Gloves should be worn when handling the wires, and other electrical appliances should be kept away from the ends to prevent electrical interference (Sullivan, Bartels, & Hamilton, 2016).

▶ Summary

Nurses caring for patients who have undergone cardiac surgery must understand which patients are at risk for the development of dysrhythmias, know how to identify these dysrhythmias, be able to prevent their occurrence, and implement early treatment to correct any irregular rhythm that does arise. While it may be difficult to isolate the underlying cause of a postoperative dysrhythmia, correction of possible etiologies is an essential component of successful management. As part of the clinical patient assessment, the ICU nurse should note the duration of the dysrhythmia as well as any associated hemodynamic effects.

🔍 CASE STUDY

B. W., a 70-year-old male patient, is admitted to the cardiothoracic ICU immediately following heart transplantation. His history includes myocardial infarction, heart failure with an LVEF of 15%, and peripheral vascular disease. He is discharged from the ICU on the second postoperative day and transferred to a cardiac surgery stepdown unit. On postoperative day 3, the patient developed complete heart block. He reported feeling lightheaded since the onset of the bradyarrhythmia.

Critical Thinking Questions

1. Which factors might predispose this patient to complete heart block?
2. What treatment should the nurse anticipate to treat the bradyarrhythmia?
3. If medications are not effective to manage the bradyarrhythmia, for which procedure should the nurse prepare the patient?

Answers to Critical Thinking Questions

1. Factors include ischemia during intraoperative hypothermia, surgical trauma to the SA node, perinodal atrial tissue, or SA artery.
2. Administration of theophylline or terbutaline may be used to increase the rate of the SA node firing.
3. Insertion of a temporary pacemaker with either epicardial pacing wires or transvenous or transcutaneous pacing may be the initial treatment if pharmacotherapy is not effective. If persistent, permanent pacemaker implantation may be required.

Self-Assessment Questions

1. Presence of which places the patient at risk for dysrhythmias following cardiac surgery?
   A. Fever
   B. Dehydration
   C. Hypomagnesemia
   D. Hypoadrenergic state

2. Which rhythm is most commonly encountered following coronary artery bypass graft surgery?
   A. Bradycardia
   B. Asystole
   C. Ventricular tachycardia
   D. Atrial fibrillation

3. Your postoperative valve surgery patient develops atrial fibrillation. For which other complication should the nurse observe?
   A. Seizures
   B. Atelectasis
   C. Acute kidney injury
   D. Hemodynamic instability

4. Which patient is at greatest risk for developing atrial fibrillation following cardiac surgery?
   A. A 50-year-old with decreased adrenergic tone
   B. A 60-year-old with hypermagnesemia
   C. A 72-year-old with pericarditis
   D. A 40-year-old with a postoperative fever

5. Following orthotopic heart transplant, you note presence of two P waves. Which is indicated?
   A. Continue to monitor
   B. Anticipate ventricular pacing
   C. Administer atropine 0.5 mg IV
   D. Evaluate potassium level

6. Which is the initial treatment of postoperative atrial fibrillation?
   A. Digoxin
   B. Ibutilide
   C. Metoprolol
   D. Amiodarone

7. Prophylaxis for postoperative atrial fibrillation with beta blockers may be indicated for which patients?
   A. Patients receiving inotropes
   B. Patients with a PR interval greater than 0.24 sec
   C. Patients with second-degree AV block type II
   D. Patients who underwent valve surgery

8. Your postoperative cardiac surgery patient develops multifocal PVCs. Which should the nurse initially anticipate?
   A. Implantation of a cardioverter defibrillator
   B. Implementation of overdrive pacing
   C. Initiation of dual chamber pacing
   D. Administration of antiarrhythmic therapy

9. Which patient who underwent cardiac surgery is at greatest risk for the development of ventricular tachycardia or ventricular fibrillation?
   A. An 80-year-old with history of HF and LVEF 20%
   B. A 60-year-old with history of bradycardia and hemoglobin 12.6 gm/dL
   C. A 75-year-old with history of hypotension and BMI 18.6 kg/m^2
   D. A 50-year-old with history of left coronary artery stenosis and PaO$_2$ 112 mmHg

10. The patient with which set of hemodynamic parameters is at greatest risk for the development of monomorphic ventricular tachycardia?

	PaO$_2$ (mmHg)	CVP (mmHg)
A.	122	16
B.	58	2
C.	114	1
D.	50	14

Answers to Self-Assessment Questions

1. C. **hypomagnesemia**
   Rationale: Dysrhythmias in postoperative cardiac surgery patients may result from electrolyte imbalances such as hypokalemia, hyperkalemia, or hypomagnesemia. Dysrhythmias can also result from hypothermia, fluid overload, or a hyperadrenergic state.

2. D. **atrial fibrillation**
    Rationale: Atrial fibrillation is the most common dysrhythmia following cardiac surgery, especially CABG procedures and valve replacement. Several preoperative, intraoperative, and postoperative risk factors have been implicated.

3. D. **hemodynamic instability**
    Rationale: Development of atrial fibrillation can result in hemodynamic instability due to loss of the atrial kick, which decreases cardiac output.

4. C. **a 72-year-old with pericarditis**
    Rationale: The 72-year-old patient is at greatest risk due to age-related changes in structure and electrophysiology associated with aging. Other patients at risk are those with a hyperadrenergic state, hypermagnesemia, and patients with postoperative hypothermia.

5. A. **continue to monitor**
    Rationale: With an orthotopic heart transplant, part of the right atrium remains. The new heart is implanted into the patient. The end result is the presence of two SA nodes. Both SA nodes will fire, which can result in a presence of two P waves. This is a normal finding; no intervention is required.

6. C. **metoprolol**
    Rationale: Use of beta blockers is supported by international guidelines and is the first choice to use unless contraindicated (e.g., hemodynamic compromise, use of inotropes, or presence of a heart block). Use of beta blockers has been shown to decrease the incidence of POAF. Beta blockers decrease the ventricular response rate when POAF develops.

7. D. **patients who underwent valve surgery**
    Rationale: Postoperative atrial fibrillation is common following valve surgery. Prophylaxis is indicated. Use of inotrope and the presence of first-degree or second-degree AV block are contraindications for use of beta blockers.

8. D. **administration of antiarrhythmic therapy**
    Rationale: Administration of antiarrhythmic therapy should decrease the number of PVCs that cause hemodynamic instability. The other three interventions are not indicated at this time.

9. A. **an 80-year-old with history of HF and LVEF 20%**
    Rationale: Risk factors for the development of ventricular tachycardia or ventricular fibrillation include increased age (>30 years), obesity, valve surgery, male gender, LV dysfunction, structural heart disease, heart failure, hemodynamic instability, hypoxemia, hypovolemia, ischemia, myocardial infarction, reperfusion following CPB, use of inotropes or antiarrhythmics, acid-base imbalance, or anemia.

10. B. **58 / 2**
    Rationale: Hypoxemia and hypovolemia are risk factors associated with the development of monomorphic ventricular tachycardia.

CLINICAL INQUIRY BOX

Question: What are the current guidelines in the prevention and management of atrial fibrillation following cardiac surgery?

Reference: Alawani, M., Chatfield, A., Ghashi, R., & Walker, L. (2016). Atrial fibrillation after cardiac surgery: Prevention and management: The Australasian experience. *Journal of the Saudi Heart Association, 30*(1), 40–46.

Objective: To determine the current guidelines to prevent atrial fibrillation following cardiac surgery

Methods: Literature review and online questionnaire

Results: Of the 194 studies found, no formal protocols were found. Seven (58%) had a protocol for prevention of POAF. These included repletion of electrolytes and use of amiodarone and beta blockers.

Conclusion: The development of a combined medical and surgical protocol for the prevention of POAF in cardiac surgery patients is a vital aspect of care. Extensive consideration should be given to this aspect of care.

References

Alawami, M., Chatfield, A., Ghashi, R., & Walker, L. (2018). Atrial fibrillation after cardiac surgery: Prevention and management: The Australasian experience. *Journal of the Saudi Heart Association, 30*(1), 40–46.

Al-Sarraf, N., Thalib, L., Hughes, A., Houlihan, M., Tolan, M., Young, V., . . . McGovern, E. (2010). The risk of arrhythmias following coronary artery bypass surgery: Do smokers have a paradox effect? *Interactive Cardiovascular & Thoracic Surgery, 11*(5), 550–555.

Al-Shawabkeh, Z., Al-Nawaesah, K., Anzeh, R. A., Al-Odwan, H., Al-Rawashdeh, W. A. B., & Altaani, H. (2016). Use of short-term steroids in the prophylaxis of atrial fibrillation after cardiac surgery. *Journal of the Saudi Heart Association, 29*(1), 23–25.

Amatya, A., Sharma, A., Pokharel, J. N., Amatya, A., & Shrestha, S. M. (2015). Ventricular tachyarrhythmia after aortic cross clamp release in cardiac surgeries. *Journal of Nepal Health Research Council, 13*(31), 201–204.

American Heart Association (AHA). (2015). *Advanced cardiovascular life support provider manual.* Dallas, TX: Author.

Aranki, S., & Cutlip, D. (2016). *Early complications of coronary artery bypass graft surgery.* Retrieved from https://www.uptodate.com/contents/early-complications-of-coronary-artery-bypass-graft-surgery#H13.

Avellana, P., Hadid, C., Ini, A., Radlovachki, D., Di Toro, D., & Ahualli, L. (2015). Atrial flutter after cardiac transplantation: Electrophysiologic characterization and catheter ablation. *The Journal of Heart and Lung Transplantation, 34*(4), S314. doi:10.1016/jhealun.2015/01/888

Badhivar, V., Rankin, J. S., Damiano Jr., R. J., Gillinov, A. M., Bakaeen, F. G., Edgerton, J. R., . . . Ad, N. (2017). The Society of Thoracic Surgeons 2017 clinical practice guidelines for the surgical treatment of atrial fibrillation. *Annals of Thoracic Surgery.* doi:10.1016/j.athoracicsur.2016.10.076

Benjo, A., Garcia, D., Kumar, S., Garcia, W., Macedo, F. Y., Benjo, C., . . . Aziz, E. F. (2015). Biatrial pacing consistently decreases atrial fibrillation in cardiac surgery: A randomized-controlled trial meta-analysis. *Circulation, 128*, A17324.

Bhargava, K. (2016). Role of ibutilide in atrial fibrillation. *The Journal of the Association of Physicians of India.* Retrieved from http://japi.org/august_2016_special_issue_atrial_fibrillation/06_role_of_ibutilide.pdf.

Cheng, N., Goo, C., Wang, R., Yang, M., & Zhang, L. (2018). New-onset ventricular arrhythmias in patients with left ventricular dysfunction after coronary surgery: Incidence, risk factors, and prognosis. *Heart Surgery Forum, 21*(2). Retrieved from http://journal.hsforum,com/index/php.HSF/article/view/1944.

Clark, T. R., Hodge, D., Ressler, E., & Lee, M. (2011). *Antiarrhythmic agents: Dronedarone (Multaq®) and amiodarone.* Retrieved from http://www.ihs.gov/nptc/documents/NPTC%20Amiodarone-Dronedarone%20Monograph.pdf.

Eisen, H. J., & Kusmirek, L. S. (2017). *Arrhythmias following cardiac transplantation.* Retrieved from https://uptodate.com/contents/arrhythmias-following-cardiac-transplantation#H13.

Giardina, E.- G. (2018). *Therapeutic use and major side effects of sotalol.* Retrieved from https://uptodate.com/contents/therapeutic-use-and-major-side-effects-of-sotalol.

Ha, A. C., Mazer, C. D., Verma, A., Yanagawa, B., & Verma, A. (2016). Management of postoperative atrial fibrillation after cardiac surgery. *Current Opinions in Cardiology, 31*(2), 183–190.

Hashemzadeh, K., Dehdilani, M., & Dehdilani, M. (2013). Postoperative atrial fibrillation following open cardiac surgery: Predisposing factors and complications. *Journal of Cardiovascular and Thoracic Research, 5*(3), 101–107.

Hashimoto, M., Yamauchi, A., & Inoue, S. (2014). Premature atrial contraction as a predicator of postoperative atrial fibrillation. *Asian Cardiovascular and Thoracic Annals, 23*(2), 153–156.

Kotecha, D. (2016). Magnesium for atrial fibrillation, myth or magic? *Circulation: Arrhythmia and Electrophysiology.* doi:10.1161/CIRCEP.116.004521.

LaPar, D. J., Speir, A. M., Crosby, K., Fonner, E., Brown, M., Rich, J. B., . . . Allawadi, G. (2014). Postoperative atrial fibrillation significantly increases hospital readmission, and hospital costs. *Annals of Thoracic Surgery, 98*(2), 527–533.

Lee, R. (2016). *Atrial fibrillation and atrial flutter after cardiac surgery.* Retrieved from https://www.uptodate.com/contents/atrial-fibrillation-and-atrial-flutter-after-cardiac-surgery.

Liu, X.-H., Xu, C.-Y., & Fan, G.-H. (2014). Efficacy of N-acetylcysteine in preventing atrial fibrillation after cardiac surgery: A meta-analysis of published randomized controlled trials. *BMC Cardiovascular Disorders, 14*, 52. doi:10.1186/1471-2261-14-52

Loardi, C., Alamanni, F., Veglia, F., Galli, C., Parolari, A., & Zanobini, M. (2015). Modified Maze procedure for atrial fibrillation as an adjunct to elective surgery: Predictors of mid-term recurrence and echocardiographic follow-up. *Texas Heart Institute Journal, 42*(4), 341–347.

Manning, W. J., Singer, D. E., & Lip, G. Y. H. (2018). *Atrial fibrillation anticoagulant therapy to prevent embolization.* Retrieved from https://www.uptodate.com/contents/atrial-fibrillation-anticoagulant-therapy-to-prevent-embolization?topicRef=1011&source=see?link.

Meldun, R. M., Schaff, H. V., Bailey, K. R., Cha, S. S., Ammash, N. M., Seward, J. B., . . . Gersh, B. J. (2015). Implications of new-onset atrial fibrillation after cardiac surgery on long-term prognosis: A community-based study. *American Heart Journal, 170*(4), 659–668.

Nakamori, Y., Maeda, T., & Ohnishi, Y. (2016). Reiterative ventricular fibrillation caused by R-on-T during temporary epicardial pacing: A case report. *JA Clinical Reports, 2.* doi:10.1186/s40981-016-0029-6

Omer, S., Cornwell, L. D., Bakshi, A., Rachlin, E., Preventza, O., Rosengart, T. K., . . . Bakaeen, F. G. (2016). Incidence, predictors, and impact of postoperative atrial fibrillation after coronary artery bypass grafting in military veterans. *Texas Heart Institute Journal, 43*(5), 397–403.

Peretto, G., Durante, A., Limite, L. R., & Cianflone, D. (2014). Postoperative arrhythmias after cardiac surgery: Incidence, risk factors, and therapeutic management. *Cardiology Research and Practice, 2014,* 1–15.

Raiten, J., Patel, P. A., & Gutsche, J. (2015). Management of postoperative atrial fibrillation in cardiac surgery patients. *Seminars in Cardiothoracic and Vascular Anesthesia, 19*(2), 122–129.

Silvestry, F. E. (2018). *Postoperative complications among patients undergoing cardiac surgery.* Retrieved from http://www.uptodate.com/contents/postoperative-complications-among-patients-undergoing-cardiac-surgery.

Steinberg, B. A., Zhao, Y., Hernandez, A. F., Fullerton, D. A., Thomas, K. L., Mills, R., . . . Piccini, J. P. (2014). Management of postoperative atrial fibrillation and subsequent outcomes in contemporary patients undergoing cardiac surgery: Insights from the Society of Thoracic Surgeons CAPS-Care Atrial Fibrillation Registry. *Clinical Cardiology, 37*(1), 7–13.

Stephens, R. S., & Whitman, G. J. R. (2015). Postoperative critical care of the adult cardiac surgical patient. Part I: Routine postoperative care. *Critical Care Medicine, 43*(7), 1477–1497.

Sullivan, B. L., Bartels, K., & Hamilton, N. (2016). Insertion and management of temporary pacemakers. *Seminars in Cardiothoracic and Vascular Anesthesia, 20*(1), 52–62.

The Society of Thoracic Surgeons Task Force on Resuscitation after Cardiac Surgery. (2017). The Society of Thoracic Surgeons Expert Consensus for the resuscitation of patient who arrest after cardiac surgery. *The Annals o Thoracic Surgery, 103*(3), 1005-1020. doi. 10.1016/j.athoracsur.2016.10.033

Turagam, M. K., Downey, F., Kress, D., Sra, J., Tajik, J., & Jahangir, A. (2015). Pharmacological strategies for prevention of postoperative atrial fibrillation. *Expert Review of Clinical Pharmacology, 8*(2), 233–250.

Zakker, M., Ascione, R., James, A. F., Angelini, G. O., & Suleiman, M. S. (2015). Inflammation, oxidative stress and postoperative atrial fibrillation in cardiac surgery. *Pharmacology & Therapeutics, 154,* 13–20.

Web Resources

A guideline for management of post arrest after cardiac surgery: www.sts.org

Catheter ablation—treatment of atrial fibrillation: http://www.youtube.com/watch?v=lP1hPiE_2y8

ECG interpretation and clinical significance: http://www.google.com/url?sa=t&rct=j&q=&esrc=s&frm=1&source=web&cd=7&ved=0CE4QFjAG&url=http%3A%2F%2Fhighered.mheducation.com%2Fsites%2Fdl%2Ffree%2F007351098x%2F451682%2Fsample_ch05.pdf&ei=dR7UU8KSBOfksATZlILgCw&usg=AFQjCNH2pEAxSwRh3gyW58JB3hMRIdb4yg

Watch a live case of AFib ablation: How to fix long-standing persistent AFib: http://www.youtube.com/watch?v=pnO2oNXa9-s

CHAPTER 16

Neurologic Complications

Malissa Mulkey

▶ Introduction

Neurologic complications have been attributed to patient factors, emboli, hypoperfusion, and metabolic derangements. Types of neurologic complications include stroke, seizures (focal or tonic-clonic), postoperative delirium, and postoperative cognitive dysfunction (POCD) (Hood, Budd, Sorond, & Hogue, 2018). These complications impact upwards of 70% of patients (Caldas, Haunton, Panerai, Hajjar, & Robinson, 2018). Because more patients are surviving cardiac surgery, there has been an increase in complications, particularly neurologic complications (Hood et al., 2018). These complications are a strong predictor of mortality and are associated with significant increases in length of hospitalization and overall cost of care as well as reductions in quality of life (Mehta et al., 2017). With a projected proportional growth of the U.S. population 65 years of age and older expected to double over the next 30 years, neurologic complications are and will continue to be a growing concern.

Although surgical procedures and techniques utilized during cardiac surgery have advanced, allowing older adults to be considered for surgery, with many returning to preoperative functional levels, they continue to be at higher risk for complications than younger patients. Availability of better primary care and technological advances with cardiopulmonary bypass (CPB) have allowed cardiac surgery to be offered to older patients with more comorbidities (Neupane, Arora, & Rudolph, 2017). Variability in outcomes is attributed to differences in patient populations, surgical procedure, and study data collection methods. Increased rates of stroke and encephalopathy are attributed to increased numbers of high-risk patients undergoing cardiac surgery (Caldas et al., 2018). This chapter will discuss the incidence and extent of neurologic complications following cardiac operations, offer evidence-based strategies for prevention, and describe nursing management of patients with adverse neurologic outcomes.

▶ Risk Factors for Neurologic Complications

A number of risk factors have been implicated in adverse neurologic outcomes. These include a combination of patient risk factors, intraoperative variables, and postoperative events. It is important to note that the additive effect of variables significantly

---

Oringal contributed by Myra Ellis

TABLE 16.1 Significant Risk Factors for Cerebral Outcomes

Risk Factors

Advanced age (especially >70 years)
History of pulmonary disease
History of hypertension
Existing hypertension
Moderate to severe atherosclerosis
History of neurologic deficit
Diabetes mellitus
History of unstable angina
Use of left ventricular assist device
Use of intra-aortic balloon pump
History of excessive alcohol consumption
Postoperative dysrhythmias
Prior heart surgery

Data from Haider, Jalal, Alamgir, & Rasheed, 2018; Hood et al., 2018.

increases a patient's risk. Identification of risk factors has led to predictive models that allow stroke probability to be calculated for individual patients. Risk factors are summarized in **TABLE 16.1**.

Underlying Pathophysiology

The precise mechanisms of cerebral injury following cardiac surgery are not fully understood. There are numerous factors inherent to cardiac surgery that play a role in adverse neurologic outcomes. These complications were previously thought to be attributed primarily to the effects of CPB. However, more recent research has pointed to patient independent factors rather than surgical technique (on-pump versus off-pump) (Stewart et al., 2018). In fact, Stewart and colleagues (2018) found equal life expectancy and health-related quality of life. Mechanisms of injury are embolism, inadequate cerebral perfusion, and large fluctuations in hemodynamic parameters (Haider, Jalal, Alamgir, & Rasheed, 2018; Hood et al., 2018).

It was previously thought that providing off-pump coronary artery bypass (OPCAB) would be associated with a lower incidence of neurologic complications. Unfortunately, evidence has not supported this concept. Other factors that have been considered as a potential cause for neurologic complications are handling of the aorta and partial clamping. One of the effects of the systemic inflammatory response is related to the development of clots. Patients undergoing cardiac surgery experience a profound systemic inflammatory response and are at risk for hypoperfusion and microembolism regardless of pump use (Haider et al., 2018). To date, data for these theories have been inconclusive. Improvement in CPB, development of modern cardioplegia solutions, and paucity of evidence continue to support this approach. Further studies regarding single versus multiple clamp techniques have been suggested, but due to the small incidence of complications a very large number of patients would need to be enrolled to determine significance (Haider et al., 2018).

Avoiding Injury

Nurses caring for cardiac surgery patients need to understand neurologic complications and identify patients at higher risk. The astute cardiac surgery nurse provides comprehensive care that includes assessment of neurologic function and individualizes the plan of care to prevent and enhance neurologic recovery. Many strategies to reduce complications during cardiac surgery are related to avoiding injury.

Description and Incidence of Neurologic Complications

There are five types of neurologic complications seen after cardiac surgery. These include stroke, encephalopathy, cognitive dysfunction, seizure, and peripheral nerve injury (Jellish & Oftadeh, 2018). All five types are caused by one of two mechanisms: embolization or hypoperfusion.

Stroke

The incidence of stroke following cardiac surgery ranges from 0.4% to 6% (McGarvey, 2017). Stroke after cardiac surgery increases intensive care unit

(ICU) and hospital length of stay (LOS). The risk for secondary complications increases significantly, including five- to tenfold increased mortality risk (Messé et al., 2014). Perioperative stroke increases odds by 2.34 times and has been found to be the strongest risk factor for postoperative mortality. Mortality rates of 14% to 30% are reported in hospitalized patients (Messé et al., 2014; Udesh, Mehta, Gleason, Wechsler, & Thirumala, 2017).

Patients at increased risk for stroke are those with a preexisting history of hypertension, diabetes, prior stroke, and older age (>65 years), or a combination of these. Perioperative risk is 4.5 times higher in adults age 65 to 75 years, and 5.2 times higher for those older than 75 years. Additionally, women are at higher risk for stroke as well as postoperative mortality, even after considering disease severity. Other predictors can play a significant role as well, such as aortic atherosclerosis or calcification, carotid stenosis and genetic predisposition, duration of CPB, redo surgery, aortic or valve surgery, critical preoperative state, renal failure, low cardiac output syndrome (LCOS), postoperative atrial fibrillation (AF), poor ventricular function, peripheral vascular disease, unstable angina, pulmonary hypertension, recent myocardial infarction (MI), left ventricular dysfunction, and smoking (see Table 16.1).

Patients who develop postoperative AF have a two to five times increased risk of having a stroke (Megens, Churilov, & Thijs, 2017; Udesh et al., 2017). Patients with LCOS are at greater risk as a result of blood pressure variability that increases the risk of thrombus formation and cerebral hypoperfusion (Jefferson et al., 2017).

Carotid stenosis increases the risk of neurologic sequela intraoperatively and postoperatively. Carotid stenosis, particularly when symptomatic, increases the stroke risk by two mechanisms. First, the risk for hypoperfusion related to narrowing of the arteries ultimately reduces cerebral blood flow. Second is the risk of artery–artery embolization (mechanisms described later in the chapter).

Genetic predisposition can increase the risk as it relates to activation of C-reactive protein and interleukin-6. Additionally, some genetic variances have been associated with the presence of apolipoproteins and cognitive dysfunction.

Atherosclerosis is an important predictor of stroke. Surgeons have used techniques to identify patients at high risk of intraoperative stroke, including palpation and manipulation of the aorta, use of epiaortic ultrasound, or transesophageal echocardiogram (TEE) to modify cannulation sites and avoid atheroma (fatty deposits in arteries) (Ikram et al., 2018).

However, epiaortic ultrasound scanning (EAS) has shown superiority over both palpation and TEE for intraoperative evaluation of the aorta. Current recommendations to reduce the incidence of atheroembolic complications include routine use of epiaortic ultrasound scanning to evaluate the ascending aorta for plaque (Ikram et al., 2018). In patients with severe atherosclerosis, other options for surgery may be employed, such as OPCAB grafting or replacement of the ascending aorta under deep hypothermic circulatory arrest.

Off-pump coronary artery bypass grafting has been proposed as a means of decreasing adverse neurologic outcomes following cardiac surgery. It seems logical that avoiding CPB—the proposed etiology for much of the damage—would improve outcomes. While there are conflicting data, the most recent systematic review suggests CBP may have superior long-term outcomes as opposed to OPCAB (Smart, Dieberg, & King, 2018). Current recommendations from the American College of Cardiology continue to recommend on-pump CPB as the gold standard (Adams & Chikwe, 2018).

Neuroprotective techniques to reduce risk for thromboembolism, hypoperfusion of watershed regions, and inflammatory processes are still a matter of interest in cardiac surgery. Current neuroprotective approaches include nonpharmacologic and pharmacologic strategies. Thus besides anticoagulation, filters, bubble traps, and hypothermia have been employed to avoid thromboembolic stroke (Salameh, Dhein, Dahnert, & Klein, 2016). Prospective studies assessing long-term neurophysiologic follow-up are still rare, making recommendations on neuroprotective efficacy difficult. The quest for effective neuroprotective drugs during CPB is not at its end but still at the beginning. Hyperglycemia, hypotension, and hyperthermia during rewarming have all been linked to adverse neurologic outcomes and should be avoided (Stewart et al., 2018).

Early Identification and Minimizing Injury.

The majority of strokes related to cardiac surgery are evident in the first 24 to 48 hours after surgery (Haider et al., 2018; Hood et al., 2018). According to Mehta and colleagues (2017) the majority (77.2%) of perioperative strokes occur greater than 24 hours after the procedure, but those that occur within the first 24 hours are the most lethal. Assessment is often difficult in the immediate postoperative period and is confounded by the emergence of anesthesia and postoperative medications. Initial postoperative signs of possible stroke may appear as not waking up, depressed level of consciousness or awareness, inability to follow commands, weakness or paralysis of the face or extremities, or any combination of these.

Because stroke symptoms are dependent on location, it is important to assess for and report focal findings such as facial droop, hemiparesis, aphasia, visual disturbances, as well as balance and gait disturbances. Because of the high risk for intraoperative stroke, it is particularly important to assess for new deficits in the first 6 hours after surgery as the effects of anesthesia and sedation dissipate (Hood et al., 2018). Awareness of high postoperative stroke risk allows the ICU nurse to provide frequent assessment, report changes, and prompt intervention to minimize complications and impact on long-term outcomes.

In addition to early identification, other strategies to reduce neurologic complications are focused on minimizing injury and secondary complications. These include rapid treatment of AF and hypotension. Permissive hypertension increases cerebral blood flow and is therefore one of the mainstays to minimize infarction size (Caldas et al., 2018). Interventions to prevent common secondary complications such as aspiration, pneumonia, venous thrombotic events, urinary tract infections, and skin breakdown are also important (Hood et al., 2018; Udesh et al., 2017).

Diagnosis and Treatment of Central Nervous System Injury.

Diagnosis of potential post-cardiac surgery stroke should be approached in the same manner as diagnosing stroke in any other setting. Post-cardiac surgery strokes are almost exclusively ischemic with intracerebral hemorrhage and thrombotic stroke being extremely rare (Chen, Lin, & Hsu, 2015). Infarct pattern is determined by the mechanism of injury. Ischemia in the setting of hypoperfusion risk is increased by 10% for every 1% drop in hemoglobin at nadir. Patients with postoperative stroke often have multiple small embolic or watershed territories (between major cerebral arteries) infarcts that are not as easily detected by computed tomography (CT) scan.

Magnetic resonance imaging in the initial postoperative period is often impractical due to surgical metal (e.g., epicardial pacing wires). Therefore, an initial head CT is often obtained. The diffusion and perfusion weighted MRI is able to detect microemboli-related events (Lansky et al., 2017). Therefore, it is considered the most accurate neuroimaging technique available. Due to this sensitivity to new ischemic injury, postoperative patients with concern for stroke may benefit from diffusion and perfusion weighted MRI. Because MRI is helpful in determining prognosis, there is a benefit to scanning up to 10 days post-stroke. If stroke occurs bilaterally in the watershed territories, in-hospital mortality risk increases 20 times. Should the patients survive, they are 12 times more likely to require long-term care.

Multiple organizations have published evidence-based guidelines for the management of stroke patients (Dönmez, Adademir, Sacli, Koksal, & Alp, 2016; McDonagh et al., 2014). Management of postoperative stroke is primarily supportive in the immediate phase and is aimed at preventing secondary complications (Hood et al., 2018). Monitoring of neurologic, hematologic, and respiratory status is essential. Nursing care is guided by specific neurologic deficits.

Support oxygenation. Pneumonia is among the leading complications of stroke (Mehta et al., 2017). To support adequate cerebral oxygenation, an oxygen saturation level of at least 94% should be maintained. Acute stroke patients may have abnormal breathing patterns and may need increased support to prevent hypoxia, which can worsen brain injury. Hypoxia may be caused by airway obstruction, aspiration, pneumonia, or atelectasis. Therefore, supporting adequate tissue oxygenation is important in patients experiencing cerebral ischemia. Endotracheal intubation may be necessary if there are concerns about airway protection or the patient's ability to maintain adequate oxygenation. Optimal nursing management includes maintaining airway suction equipment at the bedside and measures to prevent hospital acquired pneumonia (Slater, Stanik-Hutt, & Davidson, 2017).

Temperature Management. Increased body temperature increases morbidity and mortality risk in acute stroke patients (Haider et al., 2018). Hyperthermia can be the result of brain injury or secondary infection. A brain temperature 1.3°C lower or higher is equivalent to living or dying (Zaretsky, Romanovsky, Zaretskaia, & Molkov, 2018). For every 1°C increase in brain temperature, there is an associated 6% to 8% increase in cerebral metabolic rate (Bain, Morrison, & Ainslie, 2014). As a result, even a mild increase in brain temperature (1° to 2°C) can be harmful (Haider et al., 2018). Lowering temperatures below 38.0°C is important to reduce metabolic needs of an already injured brain. Primary interventions should be the administration of antipyretics. Application of cooling devices can be used as adjunct therapy, but never a primary intervention (Skafida et al., 2018).

Hypothermia protects against cerebral ischemia. Mild neurologic hypothermia (33°C), has demonstrated improved neurologic outcomes for patients with global cerebral ischemia secondary to cardiac arrest and neonatal hypoxic-ischemic encephalopathy. Mild hypothermia is currently being investigated as an acute stroke therapy, with trials to date supporting the feasibility of this approach (Baron, 2018).

Hemodynamic status. The body's compensatory mechanism to increase cerebral blood flow, and ultimately, oxygenation and glucose availability, is to increase blood pressure in the acute phase of stroke. These elevations can be higher than a systolic blood pressure (SBP) over 200 mmHg in some patients. American Heart Association (AHA) guidelines suggest postponing BP lowering in acute stroke for days or even weeks unless BP is grossly elevated (greater than 220/120 mmHg), or greater than 200/100 with concomitant evidence of acute kidney injury, aortic dissection, cardiac ischemia, hypertensive encephalopathy, or pulmonary edema (Appleton, Sprigg, & Bath, 2016). Increased BP following an embolic stroke can improve cerebral blood flow and limit ischemic effects. As such, aggressive treatment of hypertension may disrupt autoregulation. Care should be taken to gradually decrease BP to a specified target, since hypotension worsens neurologic outcome. Constant meticulous BP management is crucial. Blood pressure should be maintained within a range to maintain cerebral perfusion and yet not exacerbate further damage. Deleterious effects of hypertension may include vasogenic edema (permeation of intravascular fluid and proteins into the cerebral tissue), disruption of the blood-brain barrier, and an increase in myocardial oxygen consumption (Vranken et al., 2017). Periods of hypotension should be similarly avoided to maintain cerebral perfusion. This can be accomplished by maintaining euvolemia and use of vasoactive agents to maintain a balance between adequate cerebral perfusion and prevention of complications (McGarvey, 2017).

Glycemic Control. Both hypoglycemia and hyperglycemia can have deleterious effects on the brain. At any time there is a change in neurologic presentation, glucose measurement and correction are important. Hypoglycemia may mimic symptoms of stroke and may exacerbate brain injury. In addition, hyperglycemia is associated with poorer outcomes following stroke and should be avoided (McGarvey, 2017). It is suggested that hyperglycemia increases infarct size of a stroke and cerebral lactate levels, which results in acidosis of brain tissue and decreases the function of the mitochondria of the penumbra (an ischemic area that is still viable, adjacent to the area affected by the stroke). Hyperglycemia is also reported to disrupt the blood-brain barrier, which puts the patient at risk to develop cerebral edema, increasing the amount of brain cell death in the stroke-affected area.

Current AHA guidelines for acute ischemic stroke recommend blood glucose between 140 and 180 mg/dL in the acute phase. However, recent studies suggest better functional outcome when the blood sugar is maintained below 140 mg/dL without significantly increased risk of hypoglycemia. The validation of achieving targets below 140 mg/dL in clinical practice require additional research (Nair, Sylaja, Sreedharan, & Sarma, 2017). Careful titration and control of glucose levels are key nursing measures, and are usually best accomplished with an insulin infusion.

Aspirin. In patients with atherosclerotic cardiovascular disease, aspirin is a linchpin of management. Continuing aspirin in patients with acute coronary syndrome up to the time of surgery is recommended. In addition, all patients undergoing CABG should receive aspirin postoperatively—typically within 6 to 12 hours of surgery unless hemostasis has not been successfully achieved (Kayse & Becker, 2016).

Prevent Secondary Complications. Diagnosis of stroke is determined based on the presence of focal neurologic deficits and brain imaging (Lansky et al., 2017). Therefore, all patient suspected of having a stroke should be evaluated by a neurologist and undergo brain imaging. Cerebral swelling can result from acute stroke, therefore, close monitoring and assessment over the first 72 hours is needed. Clinically, symptoms of increased intracranial pressure (ICP) include headache, nausea and vomiting, or altered mental status. Patients with increased ICP may demonstrate physical signs of hypertension, bradycardia, and irregular respirations or apnea (Cushing's triad) although the concurrence of all three signs is an uncommon and often late finding (Cadena, Shoykhet, & Ratcliff, 2017).

Neurologic assessments at regular intervals in the postoperative period are extremely important. This includes assessment of level of consciousness (LOC), pupil reactivity, eye movements, and motor movement. Medications given during the intraoperative period can make accurate assessment more difficult. If deficits are suspected, a full neurologic assessment should be performed. The National Institutes of Health Stroke Scale (NIHSS) is a standardized stroke assessment tool. The scale is 42 points with a higher score indicating worse outcomes. The NIHSS has been shown to be a predictor of both short- and long-term outcome of stroke patients (score over 25 equates to a 90% mortality risk). Additionally, the stroke scale serves as a data collection tool for planning patient care and provides a common language for information exchanges among healthcare providers.

Use of the NIHSS includes LOC, best gaze, visual fields, facial palsy, motor function of arms and legs, limb ataxia, sensory, best language, dysarthria, extinction, and inattention (Wouters, Nysten, Thijs, & Lemmens, 2018).

Cognitive Impairment

Incidence. Postoperative cardiac surgery patients are at greater risk for not only a stroke, but also cognitive impairment. Delirium is the most common neurologic complication after cardiac surgery and frequently the most difficult to manage (Waked, Gordon, Whiteson, & Baron, 2015). This condition can emerge postoperatively or at any time during acute care hospitalization. When it does occur, it represents a neurologic crisis that has been associated with long-term harm and risk of death. Such warrant early identification and immediate medical intervention.

The incidence of postoperative delirium in patients undergoing CABG surgery is estimated to range from 3% to 78% (DELIRIUM-CS Investigators, 2017). The rates of postoperative neurocognitive impairment are comparable between patients who underwent conventional on-pump and off-pump surgery.

There are three distinct subtypes for delirium: Hyperactive, hypoactive, and mixed. Hyperactive delirium presents with agitation, hypervigilance, restlessness, hallucinations, and paranoia. The most prevalent and most overlooked subtype is hypoactive delirium or "quiet" delirium. The hypoactive subtype accounts for about 50% of the cases and presents as lethargic, reduced motivation, and emotional lability. Mixed delirium accounts for the remaining 25% and presents as a fluctuation between hyperactive and hypoactive delirium with behaviors fluctuating between both types. It is important to remember all three subtypes are the result of overwhelming stress from an underlying etiology and not due to a preexisting cognitive impairment such as dementia (American Psychiatric Association, 2013).

Patients who develop postoperative delirium have worse outcomes, increased LOS, and up to 3 times higher mortality rates (Hood et al., 2018). Presence of delirium places increased demands on hospital staff, increases medical morbidity, and significantly reduces quality of life (Waked et al., 2015). When delirium occurs following cardiac surgery, there is often limited improvement in quality of life at 6 months and at 1 year (Hood et al., 2018). At 6 months, 24% of patients exhibit persistent cognitive impairment and approximately 60% have an increased risk of mortality at 1 year (Hood et al., 2018).

Pathophysiology. The terms *encephalopathy* and *delirium* are related but are somewhat different. Delirium represents the behavioral manifestation while encephalopathy identifies the underlying pathophysiologic process. Encephalopathy literally means brain pathology or disease and is used to describe any diffuse disease of the brain that alters brain function or structure. The pathophysiology can be the result of one or more disturbances in the metabolic and physiologic systems including electrolyte imbalances, cerebral edema, amino acid imbalance, and metabolic substrates. Mental status alterations can be because of altered blood flow, body temperature, pH levels, and osmolality. Specific to postoperative cardiac surgery, the pathophysiologic causes of delirium are slowly coming to light, though predictive efforts remain challenging. However, there are a number of predisposing and precipitating factors hypothesized to increase susceptibility such as advanced age, preexisting cognitive impairment, major depression, anemia, AF, prolonged intubation, and postoperative hypoxia (Neupane et al., 2017).

Hypoxic and toxic-metabolic are the two commonly occurring forms of encephalopathy found in cardiac surgery patients. Hypoxic encephalopathy generally occurs because of impaired function or complete organ failure of the heart, lungs, or circulatory system, or any combination of these. Toxic-metabolic encephalopathy is often the result of impaired function or complete organ failure of the kidneys, liver, and lungs. Regardless of the underlying pathophysiology, an interruption and disruption of the reticular activating system, cortex, and hippocampus contribute to a global alteration in arousal, consciousness, responsivity, and altered sleep/wake cycles. Increases in dopamine, decreases in acetylcholine, and reduced GABAergic input mediate sensory input and interactions with other regions of the brain. This is why the American Psychiatric Association's *Diagnostic and Statistical Manual of Mental Disorders, 5th Edition (DSM-5)* classifies acute toxic and metabolic encephalopathic states as delirium and does not use encephalopathy in its definitions.

Delirium is a significant acute change in cognition that develops over a very short period of time—usually hours or days. These changes include disorientation, difficulty learning and retaining information, and language disturbance including disorganized, illogical, or incoherent speech. Some patients have an alteration in perceptions, delusions, or hallucinations, or a combination of these that can change throughout the day or night. Patients can appear oriented and appropriate at one moment then confused and disoriented the next.

Preexisting Conditions, Risk Factors, and Precipitating Factors. There have been multiple attempts to delineate risk factors for the development of postoperative delirium. Risk factors for postoperative delirium include age and history of stroke, hypertension, diabetes, or carotid bruit. Postoperative delirium may be related to the development of microemboli, cerebral edema secondary to the inflammatory response, inadequate temperature regulation, or cerebral hypoperfusion (Neupane et al., 2017).

Signs and symptoms usually become apparent after extubation has taken place (Waked et al., 2015). Patients with preexisting cognitive deficits, cerebrovascular disease, and poor nutritional status have limited physiologic reserve and are more likely to manifest signs of brain end-organ dysfunction. Patients at higher risk include those with advanced age (>65 years), preexisting psychological disorders, history of stroke or transient ischemic attack, a lower baseline Mini-Mental

Status Exam score, high scores on a geriatric depression screening tool, abnormal serum albumin levels, current or prior drug or alcohol abuse or both, left ventricular ejection fraction less than 30%, preoperative intra-arterial balloon pump support, cerebral artery disease, or those who undergo an emergent procedure (Neupane et al., 2017). These findings highlight the role of preoperative systemic disease in the development of postoperative delirium. Additional factors include preexisting cognitive disorders such as brain injury, stroke, mild cognitive impairment, and Alzheimer's disease. Medical comorbidities include alcoholism, uncontrolled hypertension, chronic pain syndrome, and diabetes. Sensory loss affecting vision or hearing, polypharmacy, and acute illnesses (e.g., sepsis, dehydration, malnutrition) have been implicated (Waked, 2015).

Risk Factors. Intraoperative anesthesia, sedation, time in circulatory arrest greater than 30 minutes, and intraoperative hypothermia ($<25°C$) are associated with an increased delirium incidence. Postoperative risk factors include sleep deprivation, renal or hepatic failure, cardiogenic shock, AF, massive blood transfusions (>1 L), bilirubin greater than 2 mg/dL, hypoalbuminemia, low hematocrit, acute infection, dehydration, and thyroid disorders.

Because delirium is a diffuse brain issue, focal neurologic findings are not present. Symptoms of delirium are acute and include an inability to maintain attention, disturbance of consciousness, cognitive deficits, memory impairment, disorientation, inappropriate speech, and perceptual changes not associated with preexisting psychiatric disorders (Neupane et al., 2017). Differentiating delirium and encephalopathy from other conditions such as depression/anxiety and dementia can be difficult (Waked et al., 2015). Hypoactive delirium marked by slowed thinking, diminished concentration, and memory impairment may be mistaken for major depression. Similarly, hyperactive delirium may be mistaken for an agitated depression or mania, marked by diminished attention, agitation, rapid fluctuations, and psychosis. Early detection and treatment are important aspects of postoperative

cardiac surgery patients' nursing care and may limit its severity or prevent it altogether.

Differentiating Delirium and Encephalopathy from Dementia. Dementia is slow to develop over a number of years and does not present with fluctuating symptoms or a sudden onset of mental status change. While distinctly different than delirium or dementia, electroencephalogram (EEG) recordings may be atypical and reflect slowing (Oh, Fong, Hshieh, & Inouye, 2017). Delirium or encephalopathy can cause patients with preexisting dementia to appear more disorganized or confused than usual. If this occurs, the patient may have delirium superimposed on dementia. This warrants prompt attention and investigation. Like dementia, major depression and mania do not present with an acute onset of disorientation or a fluctuating course.

Evaluation of Encephalopathy and Delirium. Identification of mental status changes may be observed by any clinician. Screening positive for delirium or acute mental status changes warrant evaluation and medical attention (Waked et al., 2015). It is important to review medications including all those that have been recently initiated and discontinued, especially sedative-hypnotic agents, narcotics, antidepressants, and immunosuppressive agents. A routine EEG will typically reveal distinct changes including slowing of electrical activity (Oh et al., 2017). Blood tests, urinalysis, and toxicology screens are important to rule out other causes and determine potential causes. A brain CT scan and MRI may be ordered. A clinical assessment to determine mental status is critical as well as a thorough review of the patient's history to determine premorbid cognitive, social, and emotional functioning that may identify co-existing conditions and rule out dementia and other psychiatric conditions (Oh et al., 2017). This includes any altered state of orientation or consciousness that is marked by vigilance (hyperalert), lethargy (drowsy, but easily aroused), stupor (difficult to arouse), or coma (unresponsive and unarousable). Stupor and comatose states are rarely, if ever, seen in patients receiving inpatient cardiopulmonary rehabilitation services.

Agitation often accompanies postoperative delirium. It is defined as extreme motor or vocal behavior that is disruptive, unsafe to patient and staff, or interferes with the delivery of patient care and medical therapies. Some examples of agitation in hospitalized patients may include screaming, shouting, moaning, combativeness (e.g., biting, kicking, hitting, scratching), pulling out tubes, disconnecting monitoring devices, and getting out of bed. Delirium and agitation are often present together and may be difficult to distinguish.

Delirium monitoring instruments such as the Confusion Assessment Method (CAM), the CAM-ICU, and the Intensive Care Delirium Screening Checklist (ICDSC) have provided clinicians with the ability to monitor for delirium without having to rely on a psychiatrist. These delirium assessments can also be performed with patients who are mechanically ventilated. Given that the majority of delirium is missed even when using a monitoring tool, hospitals should make delirium monitoring a standard of practice as recommended by the Society of Critical Care Medicine (SCCM) pain, agitation/sedation, delirium, immobility, and sleep disruption (PAD-IS) guidelines (Devlin et al., 2018).

Interventions and Considerations

Intraoperative Management. There have been several large studies looking at the impact of anesthesia on the development of delirium. These studies have led researchers to similar findings in that use of bispectral index monitoring (BIS) guided anesthesia resulted in a lower incidence of delirium (Wildes et al., 2016). Interestingly, patients whose anesthesia was guided by adding BIS monitoring to current practices resulted in higher anesthetic doses. It remains unclear whether an increased anesthetic dose is protective or simply a marker of severity of illness. As a result, many large academic centers have incorporated intraoperative use of BIS monitoring to assist with guiding the use of anesthetics based on patient drug response.

Anemia. Low hemoglobin (less than 6.0 mmol or 9.7 gm/dL) has been implicated as a risk factor in the development of delirium. It is presumed anemia evokes delirium because it leads to decreased cerebral oxygenation. This likely contributes to abnormal neurotransmitter synthesis, metabolism and release, and failure to eliminate neurotoxic by-products effectively, which all can lead to delirium. Risk adjusted studies have had similar findings, patients who received blood transfusions to maintain hemoglobin levels greater than 6.0 mmol or 9.7 gm/dL have had a lower incidence of delirium (van der Zanden et al., 2016).

Treatment of Delirium. There are four main aspects of managing delirium: (1) identify and treat underlying causes; (2) provide environmental and support measures; (3) drug therapy aimed at treating symptoms, however, pharmacologic management remains controversial; and (4) regular evaluations of the effectiveness of treatment (Oh et al., 2017).

Identify. There are currently more than 30 available screening tools, however, many are not well validated. Despite these significant limitations, standardized tools do improve delirium recognition over no screening. In patients experiencing postoperative delirium, a thorough assessment to correct possible causes is essential. Delirium after cardiac surgery is common and multifactorial, therefore, it is important for ICU nurses to recognize patients at risk and adjust care to reduce or prevent postoperative delirium.

When using a screening tool, it is important to understand the limitations of that particular tool. For example, some tools are better in one population than another and some are better at detecting hypoactive delirium most commonly seen in older adults. Many of the screening tools are able to differentiate delirium from other pathologies. When patients screen positive for delirium, the findings should not be dismissed as due to dementia, depression, or some other cause.

Depending on the selected screening tool, patients can be screened in 3 to 15 minutes; most tools take 3 to 5 minutes. Research has shown consistency in assessment between caregivers is a significant limitation when using standardized screening tools. Therefore, prior to using these tools, appropriate education and training should be provided. Additionally, ongoing education is needed to maintain accuracy.

Two screening tools have been developed for use in non-verbal mechanically intubated patients and are recommended by SCCM. In 2013, SCCM published their Pain, Agitation and Delirium Guidelines recommending patient management begin with standardized assessments including the Critical Care Pain Observation Tool (CPOT) or Behavioral Pain Scale (BPS), Richmond Agitation-Sedation Scale (RASS) or Sedation-Agitation Scale (SAS), and the CAM-ICU or ICDSC. Most recently, SCCM published the pain, agitation/sedation, delirium, immobility, and sleep disruption guidelines (Devlin et al., 2018).

Treat the Underlying Cause. The underlying causes of delirium may be metabolic derangements including electrolyte disorders, drug or alcohol withdrawal, nutritional deficiencies, or medications. Several drugs frequently prescribed for cardiac patients are associated with neuropsychiatric changes including beta blockers, calcium channel blockers, angiotensin converting enzyme (ACE) inhibitors, diuretics, antiarrhythmics, and lipid-lowering agents (Maldonado, 2017; Shapiro, 2017). Careful review of medications should include a review of home medications that were discontinued after surgery and new medications administered while in the hospital setting. Home medications such as antidepressants, medications with central nervous system or anticholinergic effects should be resumed. Drugs that interrupt sleep-wake cycles such as benzodiazepines should be avoided (Oh et al., 2017). Analgesics are associated with mental status changes, however, undertreating pain can exacerbate postoperative delirium by contributing to increased stress and sleep deprivation. While addressing pain is important, special care should be given to administering narcotics in the elderly population. With advanced age, the ability to metabolize and excrete medications decreases as a result of reductions in glomerular filtration rate with age (Boesen, Andersen, Bendtsen, & Jennum, 2016; Oh et al., 2017). The ICU nurse should closely monitor patients to avoid adverse effects.

Environmental and Supportive Measures. To reduce the likelihood of developing delirium, implementing prevention strategies is the primary step. The goals of prevention strategies are to promote sleep-wake cycles, optimize pain levels, and reduce the use of sedatives and narcotics to the smallest dose required to obtain pain and sedation goals. In the ICU, patients are exposed to interruptions in sleep patterns, noise, and environmental stimulation (Oh et al., 2017). Maintaining an environment that promotes sleep-wake cycles and reducing sensory overload are key to delirium treatment. Improving sleep hygiene has been shown to reduce delirium duration. Managing the patient's environment, such as turning on lights during the day and off at night, providing glasses or hearing aids, and reorientation to the surroundings have been frequently advocated for their simplicity and have been shown to be effective prevention strategies. This should include creating an environment to promote sleep so the patient's sleep cycle can be reestablished, if possible (Arumugam et al., 2017). Strategies such as uninterrupted sleep and promotion of quiet time from 2 to 4 AM and PM based on circadian rhythms are critical to the resolution of delirium. Additionally, transferring patients to a progressive care unit often results in an abatement of symptoms. Therefore, transferring the patient out of the ICU should be done as soon as medically feasible.

Care should be taken to reduce sensory impairment. Applying glasses or hearing aids as soon as practical is recommended. It is important to provide patients with reorientation and reassurance. The presence of family (or a significant caregiver) usually has a beneficial impact in helping confused patients regain their cognitive bearings. Family contact during the day and accompaniment at night may provide a sense of security and familiarity. Education regarding the confusion and potential causes for the condition typically leads to a reduction in patient and family distress, as does encouraging words regarding the likelihood of improvement over time. Family members, in particular a spouse, may become especially anxious and worried that restoration of role functioning and family life as it was may not occur. This may lead to the development of new tensions between the couple if improvement is slower than expected. It is also possible that one or the other, or both, may experience significant depression if the cognitive state does not improve or there is a progressive deterioration in cognitive abilities and functional independence.

Early mobilization is another important intervention. Early mobilization and physical therapy have been shown to be effective in reducing the duration of delirium. Minimizing physical restraints is also important. These devices have been associated with increased delirium in the 24 hours following use and should be utilized only when absolutely necessary for patient safety. There are occasions, however, when family members can increase the patient's level of agitation, anxiety, and confusion, warranting added intervention. Attendance at the bedside by family members or sitters is preferable to the use of physical restraints. Sitters may participate in orienting activities by talking to the patient, frequent touch, and eye contact. In extreme cases of agitation, restraints may be needed to ensure the patient's safety.

Promoting an understanding by all members of the team that a high degree of structure, simplified instructions, slower pace, frequent rest periods, repetition, and cuing with return demonstration and immediate concrete feedback are needed to facilitate optimal learning and retention of skills. This applies to patient teaching and education, verbal instructions to follow a routine or learn a new breathing strategy, and when attempting to enhance the patient's awareness of cognitive issues. For example, verbal learning of instructions and names of medications may be very slow to improve if at all. This, in turn, leads to reliance on external aids (e.g., lists, timers, scheduled reminders) and likely the added help and training of informal caregivers. In contrast, procedural learning of motor skills (e.g., dressing, bathing, toileting, and cooking) may be partially spared or relearned with the help of repetition and cuing with return demonstration over several days. Safety awareness and practices, however, may not improve even with repetition and return demonstration by the nursing staff and treating therapists. As a result, the patient may require varying levels of supervision.

Pharmacologic Considerations. The final step in delirium management is pharmacotherapy. Ensuring effective pain management using pharmacologic and non-pharmacologic methods prior to addressing sedation or agitation and avoiding use of medications such as benzodiazepines, which may promote development of delirium (Arumugam et al., 2017). Sedatives and hypnotics such as benzodiazepines and Propofol (Diprivan®) are γ-aminobutyric acid GABAergic medications that act on $GABA_A$ receptors in the brain. While these medications produce a sleep-like state, they actually prevent the patient from achieving rapid eye movement (REM) sleep otherwise known as restorative sleep. As such, they interrupt circadian rhythms and increase the risk for delirium as early as the first postoperative day and should be minimized in the operating room and ICU setting. Alternative sedatives such as dexmedetomidine (Precedex®) should, therefore, be considered as first-line sedatives after pain is controlled (Skrobik, Duprey, Hill, & Devlin, 2018).

Pharmacologic interventions may be indicated when agitation is present. Despite the prevalence of postoperative delirium, a limited number of agents have been studied. The most commonly used drugs are antipsychotics. Most notably haloperidol (Haldol®) is a first-generation high-potency neuroleptic and has long been used in the ICU to control agitated delirium. Despite their frequent use, there is little evidence for use in critically ill patients and, therefore, they are not included in professional guidelines. Implementation of treatment protocols using haloperidol in cardiac surgical patients has not been shown to impact the resolution of delirium. Additionally, haloperidol has been linked to cardiac dysrhythmias including torsades de pointes (Shen, Peng, Zhang, Meng, & Ji, 2018). Patients receiving antipsychotic therapy should have ECG monitoring, including the measurement of the corrected QT interval. A QTc interval of greater than 500 msec warrants close monitoring and possibly psychiatric consultation to evaluate the individual risk of haloperidol or other antipsychotic medications, although QT prolongation may not precede dysrhythmias (Beach et al., 2018).

Atypical antipsychotics have been increasingly used to prevent and treat postoperative delirium. Many of the drugs in this class have been evaluated, including ziprasidone (Geodon®), quetiapine (Seroquel®), and risperidone (Risperdal®).

Studies have shown that atypical antipsychotics are safe and effective in critically ill patients though large placebo controlled trials are needed to assess the risk and benefit ratio of the administration of antipsychotic medications. They may be considered for symptomatic relief of agitated/hyperactive delirium but should be administered at the lowest dose required to maintain patient safety. There continues to be little evidence to suggest any beneficial role in patients with hypoactive delirium. While newer antipsychotics may have fewer extrapyramidal complications, they are not without risk. For example, risperidone has been associated with an increased risk of ventricular arrhythmias and sudden cardiac death. Few studies have evaluated their use in cardiac surgery patients (Beach et al., 2018).

Benzodiazepines and high-potency anticholinergic drug exposure in the preceding 48 hours were found to be associated with delirium (Egberts et al., 2017). Treatment of delirium with benzodiazepines is reserved for patients with withdrawal of alcohol or sedative-hypnotics and those who are unable to tolerate high doses of antipsychotic medications (Sutton & Jutel, 2016).

Multivitamin replacement should be implemented for patients with a deficiency in vitamin B. In extreme cases of delirium and agitation with hypercatabolic conditions, paralysis, sedation, intubation, and mechanical ventilation may be required (Sutton & Jutel, 2016).

Given the recent attention to the short- and long-term effects of postoperative and ICU delirium and encephalopathy and its possible relation to increased risk of dementia in the geriatric population, studies are now beginning to examine specific medications and treatment protocols to help reduce the incidence. So far, no such drug or treatment protocol has been identified, and it may take years before new innovations in surgery lead to substantial reductions in the incidence of postoperative confusion and toxic-metabolic encephalopathy in the cardiac surgery patient population. Meanwhile, early identification and individually tailored in-patient rehabilitation interventions may substantially benefit affected patients. The ABCDEF bundle is recommended for appropriate care of patients requiring mechanical ventilation

and, therefore, sedation in ICU patients. The ABCDEF bundle strategies help reduce sedation, liberate patients from mechanical ventilation, and reduce the burden of delirium. The individual elements of the bundle are daily Awakening and Breathing (AB) coordinated trials, Choosing (C) the right sedative, Delirium monitoring (D), Early mobility (E). and integrating family (F). This framework has been shown to reduce the duration of mechanical ventilation and delirium in critically ill patients and should be considered a standard of care in the management of critically ill patients (Society of Critical Care Medicine, n.d.).

When there are persisting deficits, follow-up neurocognitive assessment and a course of outpatient individual or group cognitive remediation treatment, or both may be indicated. Further, in some cases, referral to a neurologist should be considered, particularly for patients with more widespread cognitive deficits who are at high risk of developing dementia. Systematic mental status screening for delirium or encephalopathy on arrival to the cardiopulmonary inpatient rehabilitation unit may lead to better identification of affected individuals, earlier psychological and neuropsychological intervention, and greater continuity of follow-up aftercare services.

Finally, for persisting neurocognitive deficits that do not change in response to participation in a cardiopulmonary rehabilitation program, counseling and psychoeducation for the patient and caregiver(s) will need to address the emotional, cognitive, and behavioral issues. Specifically, these efforts may help the patient adjust to the new reality and the psychological implications this has on self-esteem, identity, and altered role functioning. Sometimes, acute depression and anxiety may exacerbate cognitive problems, in which case a psychiatric consult may be indicated. Psychological treatment also may help enhance self-awareness of areas of difficulty, may prevent or minimize untoward secondary psychological effects such as avoidant behaviors, acute depression, or anxiety symptoms, and address adaptive coping and flexible problem solving that could lead to an improvement in mental health, interpersonal functioning, and quality of life, and indirectly, aid the psychological and interpersonal adjustment of the family and caregivers alike (Waked et al., 2015).

Postoperative Cognitive Decline

Postoperative cognitive decline (POCD) was first described in 1955 and is now considered a significant risk factor of cardiac surgery (Benson, Ozdemir, Matthews, & Loftus, 2017). It is described as an ongoing persistent problem with memory, language, attention, and learning that was not present prior to surgery (Benson et al., 2017). Cognitive decline has been linked to surgeries other than cardiac, although at a lower rate.

Exposure to general anesthetic agents likely contribute to cognitive decline. Delirium has been linked to an increased risk of POCD. Recent evidence shows that its prevalence is higher in patients who have undergone open aortic surgery when compared with other major vascular surgeries (Benson et al., 2017).

Prevalence and Risk Factors. Cognitive decline is common following cardiac surgery, with reported incidence ranging from 45% to 80% (Benson et al., 2017; Cropsey, Kennedy, Han, & Pandharipande, 2015). Soon after the advent of CPB, concerns were raised about the associated effects on patients' cognition in the postoperative setting period. Patients and caregivers observed a noticeable decline in cognitive performance following cardiac surgery in a significant number of patients. These anecdotal concerns were subsequently confirmed via observational cohort studies. It was concluded that CPB was likely responsible for these increased disabilities. Most of the neuropsychological deficits appeared to persist beyond hospital discharge for up to 5 years. However, subsequent studies have cast doubts on the role of CPB on POCD. Recent studies have shown no significant differences in cognitive decline between those receiving CPB and those who did not at 1 year after surgery and attributed the decline to factors such as the patient's prior cognitive score, age, education, and ethnicity. Perhaps the most striking aspect of POCD is the abundance of conflicting data. This is ultimately a reflection of the uncertainty surrounding the diagnosis itself. Early investigators realized the importance of standardized criteria for evaluation. More recent publications do not all use the same set of cognitive assessment measures, nor is there universal agreement about the timing of assessment. These criteria generally (but not always) include neuropsychological testing to assess executive function, memory, and learning, with POCD defined as a decline in one or more domains of cognitive function.

In a comparison between patients receiving medical management, undergoing off-pump CABG, CABG with CPB, or percutaneous coronary interventions, all groups displayed similar cognitive outcomes at 6 and 7.5 years following the procedure suggesting that patient-specific factors, rather than surgical intervention play the most important role in the development of cognitive decline. These data are complemented by data from patients who survive critical illness, whether it is after a surgical procedure or after being admitted to the medical ICU. In these patients cognitive impairment is common, but again prior cognitive status, education, and then duration of delirium in the ICU were the main drivers associated with the decline in cognitive scores. With the plethora of conflicting data, the clinician is left with few answers with regard to optimal management of cardiac surgery patients to reduce the risk of cognitive decline. Detailed preoperative neurocognitive testing is complex, time-consuming, and requires specialized training.

Evaluation and Management. While the available evidence does not allow for strong or very specific recommendations, clinicians in the OR and in the ICU should focus on those patients who may be deemed at high risk (i.e., the elderly, those with prior cognitive impairments or lower levels of education, and those who are at risk for delirium postoperatively.) In these patients, close attention to the basic tenets of management should be employed, including optimal hemodynamic management, prevention of hypoxemia, reduction of sedatives (especially benzodiazepines) and analgesic medications that might predispose to delirium, and implementation of strategies that have been shown to decrease delirium burden (non-pharmacological and pharmacological as outlined in the delirium section).

Hypoxemia has been a target for intervention. Measuring and optimizing cerebral oximetric saturations may improve cognitive outcomes. Patients who maintain higher cerebral oxygen saturation had a decreased risk of developing early POCD. Conversely, time spent below 50% cerebral oxygen saturations is a risk factor for POCD. Techniques used to optimize cerebral oxygen delivery include increased pump flows, increased mean arterial pressure, and transfusion. Providing surplus oxygen to maintain arterial hyperoxia has not been shown to have a positive impact on cognitive function following cardiac surgery. There is a concern for providing excess oxygen delivery since oxygen free radicals have been implicated as part of the inflammatory milieu responsible for POCD, though in at least one study hyperoxia was not associated with significant cognitive decline (Vacas, Degos, Feng, & Maze, 2013).

Postoperative hyperthermia and cerebral edema have been linked to poor neurologic outcomes, although these may be a result of processes that resulted in cerebral injury itself, rather than directly responsible (Haider et al., 2018). Typical cognitive disturbances reported include mild difficulty with memory, problem solving, attention, and ability to learn. Most patients report improvement of symptoms in one or two months.

Anxiety and Depression

Postoperative depression occurs commonly and may last two to three months following cardiac surgery. The majority of depression is mild and will resolve without intervention. Interestingly, patients who reported a higher level of satisfaction with discharge teaching and those who participated in cardiac rehabilitation were less likely to experience postoperative depression (Hweidi, Gharaibeh, Al-Obeisat, & Al-Smadi, 2018).

Early studies of postoperative cardiac surgery patients suggest the presence of anxiety and depression may have a negative impact on outcomes. There is positive correlation between presence of depressive symptoms six months after surgery and cardiac-related hospital readmission. Aside from the physiologic impact,

persistent symptoms often have a negative effect on long-term quality of life and may increase the risk of mortality (Neupane et al., 2017). Patients who continue to have depressive symptoms one year after surgery have been found to have higher mortality rates. It is, therefore, important to identify and treat psychiatric symptoms in patients undergoing cardiac surgery (Geulayov, Novikov, Dankner, & Dankner, 2018).

Approximately 50% of cardiac surgery patients will experience anxiety. Patients with persistent anxiety (>6 months) tend to have at least one of the following traits: preoperative anxiety, hypertension, pessimism, decreased social support, lower self-rated health scores, or use of avoidance to cope with preoperative anxiety. Preoperative anxiety is considered to be one of the strongest predictors for anxiety 6 months after surgery (Joseph, Whitcomb, & Taylor, 2015). Anxiety has been associated with worse outcomes because of the effects on BP, myocardial oxygen consumption, and coronary perfusion that can lead to hyperventilation, arrhythmias, coronary artery spasm, and fatal cardiac events and can mask neurocognitive impairment.

Poor postoperative psychological functioning is associated with an increase in health care utilization and overall worse outcomes including an increased risk for developing AF and acute myocardial infarction, an increase in LOS, unplanned readmissions, and mortality. Addressing anxiety in patients improves outcomes after CABG and is an essential part of the nurse's role in providing patient-centered care (Joseph et al., 2015; Neupane et al., 2017).

Anxiety and depression occur more commonly in patients with a history of psychiatric disorders. Careful preemptive management may result in decreased LOS, analgesic use, and postoperative morbidity. Use of benzodiazepines should be done prudently and minimized to lowest required dose due to the increased risk of delirium. Tricyclic antidepressants and monoamine oxidase inhibitors are contraindicated in patients with coronary artery disease because of their pro-arrhythmic and cardiotoxic effects. While selective serotonin reuptake inhibitors have been considered safe in cardiac surgery patients, caution should also be taken as some of these agents may interact with cardiac medications (Neupane et al., 2017). The ICU nurse should collaborate with members of the multidisciplinary team to help assure early recognition and prompt management of anxiety and depression.

Seizures

Seizures are a rare neurologic complication following cardiac surgery, occurring in 0.5% to 3.5% of patients following CABG (Sheth & Nourollahzadeh, 2017). There is little consensus regarding etiology and prognosis. Causes are thought to be variable and multifocal including a prior history of epilepsy with subtherapeutic antiepileptic medications, new or old structural brain lesion (stroke or tumor), hypoxic-ischemic encephalopathy, metabolic derangements such as hyponatremia or hypoglycemia or medications such as transexamic acid (TXA, Cyklokapron®) (Sheth & Nourollahzadeh, 2017).

Similar to stroke, early detections and management of seizures are time sensitive. Delays in identifying and treating seizures can significantly impact morbidity and mortality. Preoperative and postoperative focused neurologic examinations are required. For all patients, neurologic exams should include LOC, motor examination, cranial nerve and brainstem evaluation. Finally, inspection for twitches of face, mouth, and extremities as well as gaze deviation should also be completed. In conscious patients, additional assessment should include mental status, (orientation, attention, and concentration), language, and visual fields (Sheth & Nourollahzadeh, 2017). Any patient with an acute neurologic deficit should undergo a CT scan. Subsequent neurodiagnostic testing would then be tailored to the patient's history and neurologic examination. Specifically related to seizure, this may include EEG, MRI, or both. If rhythmic tonic-clonic activity was observed, continuous EEG monitoring (12 to 48 hours depending on the patient status) and treatment with an antiepileptic would be warranted. First-line agents to stop the current seizure are benzodiazepines. To prevent subsequent seizure activity, a second-line drug would then be tailored to the patient according to their side effect profile. Phenytoin (Dilantin®) and lacosamide (Vimpat®) are usually avoided in cardiac surgery patients as they may cause arrhythmias. Because valproate (Depakote®) and levetiracetam (Keppra®) can be given intravenously, these may be viable alternatives (Sheth & Nourollahzadeh, 2017).

▶ Other Neurologic Injuries

Although central neurologic complications receive more attention, several other neurologic complications associated with cardiac surgery bear mentioning. These include, but are not limited to, injury to the brachial plexus, phrenic nerve, and recurrent laryngeal nerve.

The rate of nerve injury from cardiac surgery varies widely and depends heavily on the thoroughness of the postoperative neurologic evaluation. Recent reviews describe peripheral nerve injury complication rates after cardiac surgery to be between 2% and 15% (McGarvey, 2017). Up to 30% of patients may experience diaphragmatic paralysis due to phrenic nerve injury following cardiac surgery. Data suggest diabetes as the sole medical risk factor for its development. Age, gender, and duration of surgery did not play a role (Jellish & Oftadeh, 2018).

Peripheral Nerve Injury

Recent reviews have put the incidence of peripheral nerve injury after cardiac surgery between 7% and 61% for patients with temporary deficits and 1.6% to 23% for those with permanent deficits (Jellish & Oftadeh, 2018). Thin patients are believed to be at particularly increased risk (He et al., 2016). Predisposing factors for the development of neurologic injury have been associated with diabetes, preexisting peripheral neuropathy, peripheral vascular disease, or a combination of these (McGarvey, 2017). Reports on open heart surgery patients have described a correlation between the use of intraoperative hypothermia and the development of nervous system injuries.

Potential causes for peripheral nerve injury during cardiac surgery include lateral decubitus positioning, arm position, use of asymmetrical sternal retractors and vessel cannulation. Peripheral nerve injuries can vary widely from temporary short-term interruption of blood supply from compression causing reversible conduction block to severe stretching that tears intraneural vessels causing ischemia to tears in connective tissue resulting in necrosis. Once significant loss of neurons occurs, denervation changes in the muscle will appear on an electromyelogram. Recovery requires regrowth of axons down the degenerated segments. Although regrowth is variable, the typical rate of regrowth is approximately 1 mm of growth/day.

Phrenic Nerve Neuropathy

Phrenic nerve injury is a known sequelae from open heart surgery that occurs anywhere from 1% to 60% (Jellish & Oftadeh, 2018). Multiple confounding factors have resulted in an unclear etiology. Potential causes are thought to be primarily the result of hypothermic injury from the use of ice slush, surgical injury, or ligation of the blood supply during internal thoracic artery (ITA) dissection.

The close anatomic relationship between the phrenic nerves and the pericardium make these nerves vulnerable to hypothermic injury during topical cooling, when either ice slush or cold saline is applied in the pericardium. Blood supply to the phrenic nerve comes from the pericardiophrenic artery, an upper branch of the ITA. This anatomic location in relation to the IMA is inconsistent increasing risk for injury with dissection of the ITA at or above the first rib.

Injury to the phrenic nerve frequently results in diaphragmatic dysfunction and therefore has important potential implications postoperatively (Jellish & Oftadeh, 2018). Paralysis of the left diaphragm occurs more frequently than right diaphragm paralysis. Even though the left phrenic nerve is more often affected due to the ice slush commonly being applied around the left ventricle, there have been reports of bilateral diaphragmatic paralysis. Paralysis of the diaphragm

results in immobility or paradoxical movement of the affected side. Unilateral phrenic nerve palsy is usually associated with minimal symptoms because of the recruitment of accessory muscles. The most common complaints include nocturnal orthopnea or dyspnea on exertion. However, bilateral phrenic nerve injury results in prolonged mechanical ventilation until nerve function improves. Bilateral phrenic nerve paralysis is rare but carries a significant associated mortality risk. The first indication may be difficulty in weaning the patient with normal lung function from mechanical ventilation. These patients may compensate with accessory muscle use during the day, but experience respiratory insufficiency at night. Prolonged ventilatory support may be necessary.

Aside from surgical factors, pulmonary comorbidities have been shown to be a significant risk factor for phrenic nerve injury. Patients experiencing chronic pulmonary disease are not only at higher risk to experience a phrenic nerve injury but also have been found to have more morbidity and mortality related to concomitant phrenic nerve injury. While postoperative atelectasis makes diagnosis more difficult, diagnosis of phrenic nerve damage may be made by chest radiograph, fluoroscopy, spirometry, ultrasound, or nerve conduction studies.

Phrenic nerve dysfunction typically resolves with conservative management over the course of a year. Bilateral phrenic neuropathy has a much longer recovery time.

Brachial Plexus Injury

The brachial plexus is one of the major peripheral nerve bundles that has the greatest chance of injury during cardiac surgery. Three factors make the brachial plexus particularly susceptible to injury during cardiac surgery. The superficial location makes these nerves susceptible to direct pressure damage. Second, the nerve roots of the brachial plexus are fixed both proximally at their site of origin and distally where they are tethered to the investing fascia, muscle, and tissue (Gavazzi, de Rino, Boveri, Picozzi, & Franceschi, 2016; Jellish & Oftadeh, 2018). Force applied between these points could have a high probability of stretching the nerves. Finally, the space between the first rib and clavicle is limited; thus, fracture or displacement of the first rib from downward traction could directly damage the brachial plexus. Asymmetric sternal retractors used for ITA harvest have the potential to increase plexus injury by the mechanism in which they lift the chest wall and push the clavicle head into the nerve bundle at the shoulder, increasing the stretch of the nerves over the humeral head (Cassarla & Lee, 2014).

Arm position also may affect nerve injury during cardiac procedures. In addition, adduction of the arms at the side of the patient can increase the development of ulnar neuropathy. Radial artery harvest for cardiopulmonary grafting is associated with sensory abnormalities. The incidence of these abnormalities is reported at 3% to 15% (Balkoussis, Papakonstantinou, & Apostolakis, 2018).

A brachial plexus injury usually involves mechanical traction on the nerves, usually related to the sternal retractors, or reduced blood flow from compression directly on the nerve related to arm positioning (Gavazzi et al., 2016; Jellish & Oftadeh, 2018). Sternal retractors rotate the first rib superiorly, pushing the clavicles posteriorly, compressing the plexus, and typically injuring the medial cord and its major branch, the ulnar nerve. Force applied along the nerve pathway has a high probability of stretching the nerves. Fracture or displacement of the first rib from downward traction could directly damage the brachial plexus. Risk may be reduced by using a chest roll to elevate the axilla from the OR table, which reduces the amount of weight exerted on the plexus. However, malpositioning of this roll may predispose to axillary nerve injury. Radial artery harvesting, in lieu of the saphenous vein, may result in sensory abnormalities that typically resolve, however, permanent thumb weakness with decreased grip strength and dexterity have been reported.

The majority of these injuries are sensory, and any observed weakness usually resolves quickly. However, sensory and motor symptoms can vary, depending on the affected site. The most common presentation for brachial plexus injury is paresthesia of the fourth and fifth digits on the affected side, loss of coordination in the upper extremity, and may also cause pain and weakness. Patients often report symptoms several days postoperatively. These subtle injuries may be overlooked in the immediate postoperative period. If a brachial plexus injury is suspected, a full assessment of motor and sensory function in both upper extremities should be performed.

The symptoms of brachial plexus injuries may persist for several months, but generally resolve without treatment. It is important to reassure patients that a brachial plexus injury is generally temporary. Collaboration with physical therapy is indicated to augment strength and flexibility. Overall prognosis for brachial plexus injuries after cardiac surgery is good in most cases with close to 100% recovery after one year. The duration of symptoms from brachial plexus injury varies, but most studies have shown that radial sensory abnormalities lessen with time. An average of 2 to 12 months has been reported (Rubin, 2016).

Recurrent Laryngeal Nerve Neuropathy

The left recurrent laryngeal nerve lies in close proximity to the parietal pleura as it encircles the aortic arch (Gavazzi et al., 2016). Vocal cord paralysis as a result of injury to this nerve is less common than injury to the brachial plexus or phrenic nerve, with a reported incidence at 1% to 2% (Jellish & Oftadeh, 2018). The left recurrent laryngeal nerve may be injured during cardiac surgery if the pleura is opened and large amounts of ice slush are placed in the pleural cavity. Other sources of injury to the left recurrent laryngeal nerve include tracheal intubation, central line placement, surgical dissection, or trauma from the TEE probe (Jellish & Oftadeh, 2018).

It is important for the nurse caring for the postoperative cardiac surgery patient to observe for patients with a weak or ineffective cough, respiratory insufficiency, or hoarseness following extubation, as these may be indications of recurrent laryngeal nerve neuropathy and not laryngeal edema. Dysphagia, change in voice quality, inefficient cough, and throat clearing are often associated with vocal cord paralysis. Other considerations regarding swallowing deficit, the loss of taste and gag reflex may be due to the injury of the glossopharyngeal nerve while restricted movement of the tongue may be due to an injury to the hypoglossal nerve (Jellish & Oftadeh, 2018). Suspicious patients should remain NPO until further evaluation is performed as these patients are at risk for aspiration and pneumonia (Jellish & Oftadeh, 2018).

Patients with unilateral vocal cord paralysis may manifest respiratory insufficiency, stridor, and signs of airway obstruction. Postoperative cardiac surgery patients often have these symptoms attributed to cardiac or respiratory dysfunction. It is essential to promptly recognize and address these symptoms promptly to avoid patient decompensation and reintubation (Gavazzi et al., 2016; Jellish & Oftadeh, 2018).

Diagnosis is made be laryngoscopy in a spontaneously breathing patient. Recovery following unilateral vocal cord paralysis usually takes 8 to 12 months. Most patients recover with conservative treatment, but occasionally patients require reintubation, tracheostomy, vocal cord medialization (an implant to provide bulk to the vocal cord), or any combination of these (Jellish & Oftadeh, 2018).

Intercostal Nerve Injury

Internal thoracic artery harvesting may cause injury to the anterior intercostal nerves. Symptoms that may be reported include numbness, tenderness, pain with light touch, or persistent burning pain over the sternum or left anterolateral aspect of the chest wall (Jellish & Oftadeh, 2018). Typical symptom resolution is reported at 4 months, but symptoms may last up to 28 months (Gavazzi et al., 2016; Jellish & Oftadeh, 2018).

Other Peripheral Neuropathies

The ulnar nerves also can be damaged at the edge of the supinator muscle below the elbow, the ulnar groove at the elbow, cubital tunnel, and the medial base of the palm. The frequency of ulnar neuropathy, the most common form of brachial plexus damage, is 1.9% to 18.3%. In many instances, these procedures use the arm at side position, which is affected by the different sternal in addition, adduction of the arms at the side of the patient could increase the development of ulnar neuropathy. Peroneal nerve injury causing foot drop may occur on the dependent side if the fibular head is compressed into the table. The sciatic nerve also may be at risk, particularly when semilateral positioning is used due to compression between the ischial tuberosity and the operating table.

Other less common peripheral neuropathies have been reported. Horner's syndrome, characterized by miosis, ptosis, and anhidrosis (inability to sweat), is thought to result from damage to the cervical sympathetic chain by first rib fracture. Injury to the saphenous nerve during saphenous vein harvest may result in neuralgia that presents as anesthesia, hyperesthesia, and pain along the medial side of the operative leg and foot. Endoscopic vein harvesting has reduced the incidence of this injury (Gavazzi et al., 2016).

▶ Summary

Nurses in the ICU who are caring for the postoperative cardiac surgery patient should be able to recognize patients at risk for these complications and plan care to prevent these complications from occurring, minimize the associated detrimental effects, and provide symptom management. Preventive strategies may include maintaining adequate blood pressure, avoiding development of shock, preventing infection, and administering albumin. While management of neurologic complications is primarily supportive in nature, early recognition and prompt intervention may minimize complications (Haider et al., 2018; Hood et al., 2018).

🔍 *CASE STUDY*

A 78-year-old patient is admitted for elective 3-vessel CABG and mitral valve replacement for mitral regurgitation. Her medical history was significant for intermittent AF, diabetes, hypertension, and transient ischemic attacks. Her intraoperative course was uneventful and she was extubated and weaned off inotropic therapy on the day of surgery. She was transferred to the progressive care unit on postoperative day (POD) #1. Her medications included metoprolol 25 mg PO q12h (hold for systolic BP <90 or HR <50), furosemide 40 mg PO q12h, and atorvastatin 20 mg qHS.

On POD #2, the patient reported feeling "funny." The nurse detected several subtle neurologic changes from the morning assessment. She was less responsive, had some difficulty with speech, and a slight right facial droop. Her BP and blood glucose were checked to rule out hypotension or hypoglycemia as causes and found both to be within the patient's normal limits. The nurse initiated a "stroke code" and notified the provider. The members of the team quickly responded to offer rapid assessment and recommendations for care. The patient's neurologic status was assessed utilizing the NIHSS. She was alert and oriented, had normal pupil function, normal motor and sensory function, slight right facial droop with normal sensation, and dysarthria. She was transferred to the ICU for further evaluation and treatment.

The patient was hemodynamically stable and experiencing no respiratory difficulty. She was transported to the radiology department for a non-contrast CT scan. The CT scan showed no evidence of new infarct or hemorrhage. Her recent surgery made her ineligible for fibrinolytic therapy.

The patient returned to the ICU and a dopamine infusion was started to increase her BP and cerebral perfusion. The patient had a BP of 110/70 mmHg, which was lower than her admission BP of 170/80. A goal BP of 160 mmHg was achieved with a dopamine infusion rate of 5 mcg/kg/min. The patient's neurologic changes resolved after initiation of the dopamine. She was made NPO until her ability to swallow could be assessed and a small-bore feeding tube was inserted for enteral feedings. Her blood glucose was 210 mg/dL; an insulin infusion was started and the cardiac surgery insulin protocol initiated.

On POD #5, the patient's dopamine infusion was weaned off without any changes in neurologic function and she was subsequently transferred to the progressive care unit. Her clinical status continued to improve and she was discharged home on POD #8.

Critical Thinking Questions

1. What risk factors did the patient have that put her at risk for a postoperative stroke?
2. What factors contributed to the patient's outcome?
3. Why was an insulin infusion an important aspect in the patient's plan of care?

Answers to Critical Thinking Questions

1. The patient underwent a CABG procedure. Intraoperative cerebral microembolization during CABG is felt to be the most common etiology. Other factors that put the patient at risk include her female gender, age greater than 65 years, atrial fibrillation, and diabetes.
2. The patient recognized a change in her clinical status and alerted the nurse, who immediately summoned the stroke team. A stroke team is a multidisciplinary group with training and experience in stroke care. The physicians on a stroke team have typically received additional preparation to care for patients with a stroke. Patients who are managed by a stroke team have experienced better outcomes.
3. Hypoglycemia may mimic symptoms of stroke and may exacerbate brain injury. Initial assessment at the presentation of stroke symptoms should include measurement of glucose and correction of hypoglycemia. In addition, hyperglycemia is associated with poorer outcomes following stroke and should be avoided. It is suggested that hyperglycemia increases infarct size of a stroke and increases cerebral lactate levels, which results in acidosis of brain tissue and decreases the function of the mitochondria of the penumbra (an ischemic area that is still viable, adjacent to the area affected by the stroke). Hyperglycemia is also reported to disrupt the blood-brain barrier, which puts the patient at risk to develop cerebral edema, increasing the amount of brain cell death in the stroke-affected area. All of these factors impact morbidity and mortality following a stroke.

Self-Assessment Questions

1. Which is a risk factor for neurologic complications following cardiac surgery?
   A. Advanced age
   B. Preoperative premature ventricular contractions
   C. Stable angina
   D. Acute respiratory failure

2. Which patient is at increased risk of stroke following cardiac surgery? A patient:
   A. aged 63 years old
   B. with BP 112/68
   C. with HbA_{1c} 5.3
   D. with serum creatinine 2.3 mg/dL

3. For which should the nurse monitor when caring for a patient receiving haloperidol for delirium?
   A. QTc prolongation
   B. 1° AV block
   C. Atrial dysrhythmia
   D. Ischemic changes

4. Which increases the risk of mortality in patients with a stroke following cardiac surgery? A patient with:
   A. temperature 37.9°C
   B. heart rate 100 BPM
   C. SBP 170 mmHg
   D. blood glucose 160 mg/dL

5. A postoperative cardiac surgery patient manifests lethargy and emotional lability. Which should the nurse suspect?
   A. Transient ischemic attack (TIA)
   B. Hypoactive delirium
   C. Dementia
   D. Postoperative cognitive decline

6. Which patient is at greatest risk for development of postoperative delirium following cardiac surgery? A patient:
   A. with hemoglobin 14.2 g/dL
   B. aged 58 years
   C. with preoperative anxiety
   D. postoperative PaO_2 55 mmHg

7. Administration of which medication places the patient at risk for neuropsychiatric changes?
   A. Metoprolol (Lopressor®)
   B. Levofloxacin (Levoquin®)

   C. Midazolam (Versed®)
   D. Haloperidol (Haldol®)

8. Management of postoperative stroke includes:
   A. systemic hypothermia
   B. glycemic control
   C. maintenance of SBP greater than 180 mmHg
   D. thrombolytic therapy

9. Patients report a lower incidence of postoperative depression with what intervention?
   A. Antidepressant therapy with selective serotonin reuptake inhibitors
   B. Discharge teaching that includes realistic expectations of recovery
   C. Discharge to a long-term facility
   D. Preoperative administration of haloperidol

10. Which is a sequela of postoperative anxiety following cardiac surgery?
    A. Decreased myocardial oxygen consumption
    B. Angina
    C. $PaCO_2$ 32
    D. SBP 80 mmHg

Answers to Self-Assessment Questions

1. A. **Advanced age.**
   Rationale: Advanced age is a recognized risk factor for development of neurologic complications following cardiac surgery. Other risk factors include postoperative dysrhythmias and unstable angina. Acute respiratory failure is not a reported risk factor

2. D. **with serum creatinine 2.3 mg/dL**
   Rationale: A patient with renal failure is at risk for development of a stroke following cardiac surgery. Other risk factors include age greater than 65 years, hypertension, and diabetes mellitus.

3. A. **QTc prolongation**
   Rationale: QTc prolongation is a known complication of haloperidol. Ongoing monitoring with electrocardiogram is essential to mitigate patient harm. First-degree AV block, atrial dysrhythmias, and ischemic changes are not known side effects of haloperidol therapy.

4. D. **blood glucose 160 mg/dL**
    Rationale: Recent data suggest that blood glucose 140 mg/dL or less puts the patient at less risk for complications following cardiac surgery. A temperature less than 38°C is needed to decrease metabolic needs. Heart rate is not a risk factor for development of a stroke following cardiac surgery. A BP greater than 220/120 or 200/100 with concomitant acute kidney injury, aortic dissection, ischemia, pulmonary edema or hypertensive encephalopathy is a risk factor for development of a stroke following cardiac surgery.

5. B. **Hypoactive delirium**
    Rationale: This patient has symptoms of hypoactive delirium. The symptoms reported are not consistent with a diagnosis of TIA, dementia, or postoperative cognitive decline.

6. D. **postoperative PaO2 55 mgHg.**
    Rationale: Hypoxemia is a risk factor for the development of postoperative delirium. Other risk factors include anemia (hemoglobin less than 9.7 g/dL), advanced age, and major depression.

7. A. **Metoprolol (Lopressor®)**
    Rationale: Beta blockers can put the patient at risk for neuropsychiatric changes following cardiac surgery. Antibiotics, benzodiazepines, and haloperidol are not medications that place the patient at increased risk for this complication.

8. B. **glycemic control**
    Rationale: A blood glucose of less than 140 mg/dL is suggested to be effective in postoperative stroke management. Systemic hypothermia is being investigated as a possible therapy; more data are needed. A systolic BP greater than 180 mmHg places the patient at risk for a stroke. Use of thrombolytic therapy depends on timing and type of stroke. Their use may be contraindicated postoperatively.

9. B. **Discharge teaching that includes realistic expections of recovery**
    Rationale: Discharge teaching that includes realistic expectations of recovery has been shown to decrease the incidence of postoperative depression. The other options are not effective strategies.

10. C. **PaCO$_2$ 32**
    Rationale: Hyperventilation is a sequela of postoperative anxiety. There is also an associated increase in myocardial oxygen consumption, hypertension, and acute myocardial infarction.

CLINICAL INQUIRY BOX

Question: Does preexisting depression (versus perioperative variables) predict postoperative reactive or persistent depression?

Reference: Patron, E., Benvenuti, S. M., & Palomba D. (2014). Preoperative and perioperative predicators of reactive and persistent depression after cardiac surgery: A three-month follow-up study. *Psychosomatics, 55,* 261–271.

Objective: The purpose of this study was to determine whether preexisting depression or perioperative variables predict postoperative reactive or persistent depression.

Methods: Longitudinal study (preoperative cardiac surgery and at 3 months postoperatively). Ninety-six patients completed a psychiatric evaluation, including the Center for Epidemiologic Studies Depression Scale and State and Trait Anxiety Inventory.

Results: In this study, 28% of the patients had preoperative depression; 25% had depression at the 3-month follow-up. Postoperative depression was predicted by the Center for Epidemiologic Studies of Depression Scale and European System for Cardiac Operative Risk Evaluation.

Discussion: Degree of preexisting depression and biomedical risk factors can be markers of depression-related risk at 3 months postoperatively in patients with persistent and reactive depression. A combined psychologic and biomedical evaluation is pivotal to help predict which patients may manifest depressive symptoms after cardiac surgery.

References

Adams, D. H., & Chikwe, J. (2018). On-pump CABG in 2018. Still the gold standard, *Journal of the American College of Cardiology, 71*(9), 992–993.

American Psychiatric Society (2013). *Diagnostic and statistical manual of mental disorders: DSM-5.* Washington, DC: Author.

Appleton, J. P., Sprigg, N., & Bath, P. M. (2016). Blood pressure management in acute stroke. *Stroke and Vascular Neurology, 1*(2), 72–82.

Arumugam, S., El-Menyar, A., Al-Hassani, A., Strandvik, G., Asim, M., Mekkodithal, A., . . . Al-Thani, H. (2017). Delirium in the intensive care unit. *Journal of Emergencies, Trauma, and Shock, 10*(1), 37–46.

Bain, A. R., Morrison, S. A., & Ainslie, P. N. (2014). Cerebral oxygenation and hyperthermia. *Frontiers in Physiology, 5.* doi:10.3389/fphys.2014.00092

Balkoussis, N. G., Papakonstantinou, N. A., & Apostolakis, E. (2018). Radial artery as graft for coronary artery bypass surgery: Advantages and disadvantages for its usage focused on structural and biological characteristics. *Journal of Cardiology, 63*(5), 321–328.

Baron, J.-C. (2018). Protecting the ischaemic penumbra as an adjunct to thrombectomy for acute stroke. *Nature Reviews Neurology, 14*(6), 325–337.

Beach, S. R., Celano, C. M., Sugrue, A. M., Adams, C., Ackerman, M. J., Noseworthy, P. A., . . . Huffman, J. C. (2018). QT prolongation, torsades de pointes, and psychotropic medications: A 5-year update. *Psychosomatics, 59*(2), 105–122.

Benson, R. A., Ozdemir, B. A., Matthews, D., & Loftus, I. M. (2017). A systematic review of postoperative cognitive decline following open and endovascular aortic aneurysm surgery. *Annals of the Royal College of Surgeons of England, 99*(2), 97–100.

Boesen, H. C., Andersen, J. H., Bendtsen, A. O., & Jennum, P. J. (2016). Sleep and delirium in unsedated patients in the intensive care unit. *Acta Anaesthesiologica Scandinavica, 60*(1), 59–68.

Cadena, R., Shoykhet, M., & Ratcliff, J. J. (2017). Emergency neurological life support: Intracranial hypertension and herniation. *Neurocritical Care, 27*(1), 82–88.

Caldas, J. R., Haunton, V. J., Panerai, R. B., Hajjar, L. A., & Robinson, T. G. (2018). Cerebral autoregulation in cardiopulmonary bypass surgery: A systematic review. *Interactive Cardiovascular and Thoracic Surgery, 26*(3), 494–503.

Cassarla, L., & Lee, J.-W. (2014). Patient positioning and associated risks. In R. D. Miller (Ed.) *Miller's Anesthesia* (8th ed., pp. 1240–1265). Philadelphia, PA: Elsevier.

Chen, J. W., Lin, C. H., & Hsu, R. B. (2015). Mechanisms of early and delayed stroke after systematic off-pump coronary artery bypass. *Journal of the Formosan Medical Association, 114*(10), 988–994.

Cropsey, C., Kennedy, J., Han, J., & Pandharipande, P. (2015). Cognitive dysfunction, delirium, and stroke in cardiac surgery patients. *Seminars in Cardiothoracic and Vascular Anesthesia, 19*(4), 309–317.

DELIRIUM-CS Investigators. (2017). Incidence of delirium after cardiac surgery: Protocol for the DELIRIUM-CS Canada cross-sectional cohort study. *Canadian Medical Association Journal, 5*(3), E565–E569.

Dönmez, A. A., Adademir, T., Sacli, H., Koksal, C., & Alp, M. (2016). Comparison of early outcomes with three approaches for combined coronary revascularization and carotid endarterectomy. *Brazilian Journal of Cardiovascular Surgery, 31*(5), 365–370.

Egberts, A., van der Craats, S. T., van Wijk, M. D., Alkilabe, S., van den Bemt, P. M. L. A., & Mattace-Raso, F. U. S. (2017). Anticholinergic drug exposure is associated with delirium and postdischarge institutionalization in acutely ill hospitalized older patients. *Pharmacology Research & Perspectives, 5*(3), e00310. Retrieved from https://www.ncbi.nlm.nih.gov/pmc/articles/PMC5464339/

Gavazzi, A., de Rino, F., Boveri, M. C., Picozzi, A., & Franceschi, M. (2016). Prevalence of peripheral nervous system complications after major heart surgery. *Neurological Sciences, 37*(2), 205–209.

Geulayov, G., Novikov, I., Dankner, D., & Dankner, R. (2018). Symptoms of depression and anxiety and 11-year all-cause mortality in men and women undergoing coronary artery bypass graft (CABG) surgery. *Journal of Psychosomatic Research, 105*, 106–114.

Haider, Z., Jalal, A., Alamgir, A. R., & Rasheed, I. (2018). Neurological complications are avoidable during CABG. *Pakistan Journal of Medical Sciences, 34*(1), 5–9.

He, C., Zhang, Q., Zhu, X., Qian, T., FuguiRuan, Sun, X., . . . Wang, H. (2016). Peripheral nerve injuries following cardiac surgery: A neglected side effect. *Scholars Journal of Applied Medical Sciences, 4*(6), 2229–2233.

Hood, R., Budd, A., Sorond, F. A., & Hogue, C. W. (2018). Peri-operative neurological complications. *Anaesthesia, 73* Suppl 1, 67–75.

Hweidi, I. M., Gharaibeh, B. A., Al-Obeisat, S. M., & Al-Smadi, A. M. (2018). Prevalence of depression and its associated factors in patients post-coronary artery bypass graft surgery. *Journal of Research in Nursing, 23*(1), 76–88.

Ikram, A., Mohiuddin, H., Zia, A., Siddiqui, H. U., Javadikasgari, H., Koprivanac, M., . . . Zafar, A. (2018). Does epiaortic ultrasound screening reduce perioperative stroke in patients undergoing coronary surgery? A topical review. *Journal of Clinical Neuroscience, 50*, 30–34.

Jefferson, A. L., Liu, D., Gupta, D. K., Pechman, K. R., Watchmaker, J. M., Gordon, E. A., . . . Donahue, M. J. (2017). Lower cardiac index levels relate to lower cerebral blood flow in older adults. *Neurology, 89*(23), 2327–2334.

Jellish, W. S., & Oftadeh, M. (2018). Peripheral nerve injury in cardiac surgery. *Journal of Cardiothoracic and Vascular Anesthesia, 32*(1), 495–511.

Joseph, H. K., Whitcomb, J., & Taylor, W. (2015). Effect of anxiety on individuals and caregivers after coronary artery bypass grafting surgery: A review of the literature. *Dimensions of Critical Care Nursing, 34*(5), 285–288.

Kayse, R., & Becker, R. C. (2016). The case for preoperative aspirin administration in patients undergoing elective CABG: Is it open or closed? *Annals of Translational Medicine, 4*(Suppl 1), S26. doi:10.21037/atm.2016.10.31

Lansky, A. J., Messe, S. R., Brickman, A. M., Dwyer, M., van der Worp, H. B., Lazar, R. M., . . . Baumbach, A. (2017). Proposed standardized neurological endpoints for cardiovascular clinical trials: An academic research consortium initiative. *Journal of the American College of Cardiology, 69*(6), 679–691.

Maldonado, J. R. (2017). Psychiatric aspects of critical care medicine: Update. *Critical Care Clinics, 33*(3), i. doi:10.1016/S0749-0704(17)30032-5

McDonagh, D. L., Berger, M., Mathew, J. P., Graffagnino, C., Milano, C. A., & Newman, M. F. (2014). Neurological complications of cardiac surgery. *Lancet, Neurology, 13*(5), 490–502.

McGarvey, M. L. (2017). *Neurologic complications of cardiac surgery.* Retrieved from https://www.uptodate.com/contents/neurologic-complications-of-cardiac-surgery

Megens, M. R., Churilov, L., & Thijs, V. (2017). New-onset atrial fibrillation after coronary artery bypass graft and long-term risk of stroke: A meta-analysis. *Journal of the American Heart Association, 6*(12). doi:10.1161/jaha.117.007558

Mehta, A., Gleason, T., Wechsler, L., Winger, D., Wang, L., & Thirumala, P. D. (2017). Perioperative stroke as a predictor of mortality and morbidity in patients undergoing CABG. *Journal of Clinical Neuroscience, 44*, 175–179.

Messé, S. R., Acker, M. A., Kasner, S. E., Fanning, M., Giovannetti, T., Ratcliffe, S. J., . . . Floyd, T. F. (2014). Stroke after aortic valve surgery: Results from a prospective cohort. *Circulation, 129*(22), 2253–2261.

Nair, S. S., Sylaja, P. N., Sreedharan, S. E., & Sarma, S. (2017). Maintenance of normoglycemia may improve outcome in acute ischemic stroke. *Annals of Indian Academy of Neurology, 20*(2), 122–126.

Neupane, I., Arora, R. C., & Rudolph, J. L. (2017). Cardiac surgery as a stressor and the response of the vulnerable older adult. *Experimental Gerontology, 87*, 168–174.

Oh, E. S., Fong, T. G., Hshieh, T. T., & Inouye, S. K. (2017). Delirium in older persons: Advances in diagnosis and treatment. *Journal of the American Medical Association, 318*(12), 1161–1174.

Rubin, M. (2016). *Peripheral nerve disorders after cardiac surgery.* Retrieved from https://www.ahcmedia.com/articles/137527-peripheral-nerve-disorders-after-cardiac-surgery

Salameh, A., Dhein, S., Dahnert, I., & Klein, N. (2016). Neuroprotective strategies during cardiac surgery with cardiopulmonary bypass. *International Journal of Molecular Sciences, 17*(11). doi:10.3390/ijms17111945

Shapiro, P. A. (2017). Psychiatric aspects of heart disease (and cardiac aspects of psychiatric disease) in critical care. *Critical Care Clinics, 33*(3), 619–634.

Shen, Y. Z., Peng, K., Zhang, J., Meng, X. W., & Ji, F. (2018). Effects of haloperidol on delirium in adult patients: A systematic review and meta-analysis. *Medical Principles and Practice, 27*(3), 250–259.

Sheth, K. N., & Nourollahzadeh, E. (2017). Neurologic complications of cardiac and vascular surgery. In E. F. M. Wijdicks & A. H. Kramer (Eds.), *Handbook of Clinical Neurology*, (Vol. 141, pp. 573–592). Philadelphia, PA: Elsevier.

Skafida, A., Mitrakou, A., Georgiopoulos, G., Alevizaki, M., Spengos, K., Takis, K., . . . Vemmos, K. (2018). In-hospital dynamics of glucose, blood pressure and temperature predict outcome in patients with acute ischaemic stroke. *European Stroke Journal, 3*(2), 174–184.

Skrobik, Y., Duprey, M. S., Hill, N. S., & Devlin, J. W. (2018). Low-dose nocturnal dexmedetomidine prevents ICU delirium. A randomized, placebo-controlled trial. *American Journal of Respiratory and Critical Care Medicine, 197*(9), 1147–1156.

Slater, T., Stanik-Hutt, J., & Davidson, P. (2017). Cerebral perfusion monitoring in adult patients following cardiac surgery: An observational study. *Contemporary Nurse, 53*(6), 669–680.

Smart, N. A., Dieberg, G., & King, N. (2018). Long-term outcomes of on- versus off-pump coronary artery bypass grafting. *Journal of the American College of Cardiology, 71*(9), 983–991.

Society of Critical Care Medicine (n.d.). *ABCDEF bundle.* Retrieved from http://www.sccm.org/ICULiberation/ABCDEF-Bundles

Stewart, J. A., Ilkka, V. H., Jokinen, J. J., Vakkuri, A. P., Suojaranta, R. T., Wennervirta, J., . . . Salminen, U. S. (2018). Long-term survival and quality of life after hypothermic circulatory arrest in aortic surgery. *Scandinavian Journal of Surgery.* doi:10.1177/1457496918766719

Sutton, L. J., & Jutel, A. (2016). Alcohol withdrawal syndrome in critically ill patients: Identification, assessment, and management. *Critical Care Nurse, 36*(1), 28–38.

Udesh, R., Mehta, A., Gleason, T. G., Wechsler, L., & Thirumala, P. D. (2017). Perioperative strokes and early outcomes in mitral valve surgery: A nationwide analysis. *Journal of Cardiothoracic and Vascular Anesthesia, 31*(2), 529–536.

Vacas, S., Degos, V., Feng, X, & Maze, M. (2013). The neuroinflammatory response of postoperative cognitive decline. *British Medical Bulletin, 106*(91), 161–178.

van der Zanden, V. B., Beishuizen, S. J. M. D., Scholtens, R. M. M. D., de Jonghe, A. M. D. P., de Rooij, S. E. M. D. P., & van Munster, B. C. M. D. P. (2016). The effects of blood transfusion on delirium incidence. *Journal of the American Medical Directors Association, 17*(8), 748–753.

Vranken, N. P. A., Weerwind, P. W., Sutedja, N. A., Severdija, E. E., Barenbrug, P. J. C., & Maessen, J. G. (2017). Cerebral oximetry and autoregulation during cardiopulmonary bypass: A review. *The Journal of Extra Corporeal Technology, 49*(3), 182–191.

Waked, W. J., Gordon, R. M., Whiteson, J. H., & Baron, E. M. (2015). Recognizing encephalopathy and delirium in the cardiopulmonary rehabilitation setting. *Rehabilitation Psychology, 60*(2), 201–210.

Wildes, T. S., Winter, A. C., Maybrier, H. R., Mickle, A. M., Lenze, E. J., Stark, S., . . . Avidan, M. S. (2016). Protocol for the electroencephalography guidance of anesthesia to alleviate geriatric syndromes (ENGAGES) study: A pragmatic, randomised clinical trial. *British Medical Journal Open, 6*(6), e011505. doi:10.1136/bmjopen-2016-011505

Wouters, A., Nysten, C., Thijs, V., & Lemmens, R. (2018). Prediction of outcome in patients with acute ischemic stroke based on initial severity and improvement in the first 24 h. *Frontiers in Neurology, 9*(308). doi:10.3389/fneur.2018.00308

Zaretsky, D. V., Romanovsky, A. A., Zaretskaia, M. V., & Molkov, Y. I. (2018). Tissue oxidative metabolism can increase the difference between local temperature and arterial blood temperature by up to 1.3°C: Implications for brain, brown adipose tissue, and muscle physiology. *Temperature, 5*(1), 22–35.

Web Resource

Devlin, J. W., Skrobik, Y., Gélinas, C., Needham, D., Slooter, A, J. C., Pandharipande, P. P., . . . Alhazzani, W. (2018). Clinical practice guidelines for the prevention and management of pain, agitation/sedation, delirium, immobility, and sleep disruption in adult patients in the ICU. *Critical Care Medicine, 46*(9), e825–e873.

CHAPTER 17

Fluid and Electrolyte Imbalances Following Cardiac Surgery

Vicki Morelock

▶ Introduction

Numerous factors increase the cardiac surgery patient's predisposition for postoperative fluid and electrolyte imbalances. These include anesthesia, induced hypothermia, physiologic effects of cardiopulmonary bypass (CPB) techniques, cardioplegia, hemodilution, and rapid fluid and electrolyte shifts across fluid compartments following CPB. A systemic inflammatory response post bypass (vasoplegia), postoperative myocardial stunning, ischemia or infarct, shocklike syndrome resulting in potential renal insult, use of positive and negative inotropic agents, degree of oxygenation and oxygen delivery to the tissues, and third spacing are additional factors affecting the hemodynamic, fluid, and electrolyte indices. Peripheral vascular tone, intraoperative and postoperative volume repletion, the rewarming process that follows hypothermia, stress associated with surgery (including sympathetic stimulation from pain and anxiety), and rhythm conduction changes such as bradycardia, tachycardia, or dysrhythmias

also affect fluid balance and electrolyte shifting. Comorbidities such as diabetes, hypertension, smoking, chronic obstructive pulmonary disease (COPD), chronic kidney disease changes, and normal aging (elderly) must be taken into account when treating cardiac surgery patients (Yazdchi & Rawn, 2018).

This chapter provides an overview of some of the common acid–base and fluid and electrolyte imbalances, treatments for these alterations, and the intensive care unit (ICU) nurse's role in caring for these patients in the immediate postoperative period. The chapter concludes with a brief look at acute kidney injury (AKI) and its treatment implications as they relate to the patient who has undergone cardiac surgery.

▶ Fluid and Electrolyte Distribution

Slightly more than half of the average adult's body weight is made up of fluid—55% to 60% of body weight in men, 50% to 55% of body weight in women, and slightly less in older adults (Shires, 2015). The term *fluid* refers to both water and substances such as electrolytes that are dissolved in it. Electrolytes are substances that develop a positive (cation) or negative (anion) electrical charge when dissolved in body fluid (Huether, 2017a).

Fluids are found in both the intracellular and extracellular compartments of the body. Intracellular fluid (ICF) accounts for approximately two-thirds of all body fluids. It is located primarily in skeletal muscle mass and provides nutrients for daily cellular metabolism. Intracellular fluid contains high levels of potassium and phosphorus, and has a moderate amount of magnesium and proteins (Huether, 2017a). Extracellular fluid (ECF) is further divided into intravascular fluid (plasma) and interstitial fluid (between the cells). Extracellular fluid is more easily lost than ICF because of its location. Electrolyte values that are reported reflect plasma levels and represent ECF.

▶ Factors Affecting Fluid Volume Distribution

Fluid balance and homeostasis are maintained by several body systems, including the heart, lungs, endocrine system, and renal system. Additionally, the pituitary, adrenal, and parathyroid glands all play important roles in maintaining fluid balance and composition. Without a properly functioning cardiovascular system, blood could not be pumped to the kidneys. The renal system requires approximately 25% of cardiac output (CO) for adequate function to occur. The goals for patients are to maintain adequate oxygen delivery to all the tissues and minimize stress on the body. This is accomplished with maintaining a mixed venous O_2 greater than 60%, a mean arterial pressure (MAP) greater than 65 mmHg, and a cardiac index (CI) greater than 2 L/min/m^2 for most patients (Yazdchi & Rawn, 2018).

Without proper lung function, blood is inadequately oxygenated, carbon dioxide is not removed through exhalation, and insensible water loss does not occur. The lungs act as the first line of defense against acid–base imbalances. Without all three body systems functioning in harmony, acid–base, fluid, and electrolyte disturbances will occur.

Fluid exchange takes place between the intracellular and extracellular compartments according to differences in hydrostatic pressure and colloid osmotic pressure (COP). Surgery causes a decrease in COP by causing increased capillary permeability, which results in fluid shifts from the vasculature to the interstitium (Huether, 2017a).

The endocrine system causes sodium and water retention and potassium excretion by stimulating production of antidiuretic hormone (ADH) in response to surgical trauma. Antidiuretic hormone secretion causes the kidneys to reabsorb water with a subsequent decrease in diuresis and serum sodium concentration in the postoperative period. Increased production of renin and aldosterone leads to sodium retention and potassium excretion (Huether, 2017a). Cortisol, which is secreted in response to stress, inhibits production of stress-related mediators (e.g., tumor necrosis factor 1, cytokines, growth factors), contributing to postoperative fluid homeostasis by maintaining capillary integrity and decreasing fluid shifts seen with the inflammatory process (Clayton, McCance, & Takahashi, 2017).

During and following CPB, the body experiences an increase in interstitial volume, sodium retention, and potassium excretion. Plasma COP decreases over this same period. Depending on the length of the case, the interstitial compartment may swell 8% to 33% (Hammon & Hines, 2018).

▶ Acid–Base Imbalances

Acid–base balance is determined by the arterial blood pH (hydrogen ion concentration; normal range 7.35–7.45), arterial carbon dioxide (pCO$_2$; normal range 35–45 mmHg), partial pressure of oxygen (pO$_2$) in arterial blood (normal range 80–100 mmHg), and bicarbonate (HCO$_3$) value (normal range 22–26 mEq/L). **TABLE 17.1** provides a brief overview of arterial blood gas (ABG) values and their interpretive implications.

TABLE 17.1 Arterial Blood Gas Values and Interpretation		
Lab Parameter	**Normal Value**	**Results and Implications**
pH	7.35–7.45	Less than 7.35 = acidosis Greater than 7.45 = alkalosis If compensation is suspected and the pH is within normal limits, look at the "end" where the pH falls: Is it closer to the acidosis side or the alkalosis side?
HCO_3	22–26 mEq/L	Less than 22 = metabolic acidosis Greater than 26 = metabolic alkalosis
pCO_2	35–45 mmHg	Less than 35 = respiratory alkalosis Greater than 45 = respiratory acidosis
pO_2	80–100 mmHg	Less than 80 = possible hypoxemia

The human body desires to maintain a state of homeostasis at all times. When changes in pH occur, buffer systems are activated to assist the body to normalize pH. As changes in pH occur, cellular responses are stimulated immediately. When the cellular responses are inadequate to handle the resultant change in pH, the respiratory system will provide compensation; if needed, the renal system will activate its compensatory mechanisms as well. Arterial blood gas (ABG) changes that are primarily driven by the kidneys may take days to appear, whereas changes caused by the respiratory system will occur in a matter of minutes.

Acidosis

Respiratory Acidosis

Respiratory acidosis may occur in the immediate postoperative period following cardiac surgery and is a direct result of inadequate ventilation or sedation causing hypoventilation and hypercarbia (Ginwalla, Faraday, & Whitman, 2014; Huether, 2017a). **BOX 17.1** lists common causes of respiratory acidosis in the postoperative cardiac surgery patient. Evaluation of ABG results and observation for signs and symptoms are essential roles of the ICU nurse. Early signs and symptoms of respiratory acidosis

may include headache, restlessness, blurred vision, and anxiety. If the condition continues, the patient may develop dizziness, confusion, weakness, palpitations, tetany, convulsions, coma, or ventricular fibrillation (Huether, 2017a).

Treatment of respiratory acidosis will vary according to the cause, but generally focuses on improving the patient's ventilation/perfusion (V/Q) status. Conventional interventions performed by the ICU nurse include frequent pulmonary hygiene; use of incentive spirometry; and encouraging turning, coughing, and deep breathing. Titration of sedation may be indicated if it will not cause excessive patient discomfort. If the patient is on mechanical ventilation, respiratory acidosis can be corrected by increasing the patient's minute ventilation; this goal can be accomplished by increasing the preset rate or tidal volume. If the patient is not on mechanical ventilation and conventional interventions are not successful in correcting the respiratory acidosis, depending on the patient's clinical status and ABG results, intubation and mechanical support may be required.

Metabolic Acidosis

Because a state of electrical neutrality must be maintained within the body at all times, patients

BOX 17.1 Common Causes of Respiratory Acidosis in the Postoperative Cardiac Surgery Patient

Central Respiratory Depression
- Cardiac arrest with resultant cerebral hypoxia
- Obesity
- Use of opiates, sedatives, or anesthesia

Pulmonary Issues
- Acute respiratory distress syndrome
- Aspiration, pneumonia, airway obstruction, or any combination of these
- Asthma
- Atelectasis
- Bronchospasm or laryngospasm
- Pneumothorax
- Pulmonary edema
- Pulmonary embolism
- Restrictive lung diseases

Increased CO_2 Production
- Shivering
- Sepsis

Hypoventilation Secondary to the Following Conditions
- Pain
- Sternal incision
- Residual anesthesia
- Awakening with inadequate analgesia and impaired respiratory mechanics
- Side effects of opiates

Other
- Inadequate mechanical ventilation (user error)
- Inadequate ventilation/perfusion ratio (decreased ventilation)
- Neuromuscular blocking agents

Data from Huether, 2017a; Shires, 2015.

BOX 17.2 Common Causes of Metabolic Acidosis in the Postoperative Cardiac Surgery Patient

Hemodynamics
- Decreased cardiac output
- Inadequate systemic perfusion
- Decreased cardiac function
- Decreased peripheral perfusion
- Hypotension
- Hypovolemia
- Vasoconstriction from hypothermia

Physiologic Conditions (Increasing Acids)
- Sepsis
- Renal failure
- Renal tubular acidosis
- Regional ischemia
- Diabetic ketoacidosis
- Splanchnic ischemia
- Anaerobic metabolism

Data from Huether, 2017a; Shires, 2015.

with a metabolic acidosis must retain a positive ion (cation) to adjust for the increasing bicarbonate. This goal is accomplished by the renal system, which accumulates positively charged potassium ions. Hyperkalemia frequently accompanies a metabolic acidosis (unless the metabolic acidosis is caused by lactic acidosis or diarrhea). It has been suggested that when acid (hydrogen ion) levels are high in the blood, the body attempts to compensate by causing muscles to take up the excess hydrogen. To maintain neutrality, in exchange for the hydrogen ions, potassium is transferred into the blood. Signs and symptoms of metabolic acidosis may include headache and lethargy, followed by confusion and drowsiness leading to coma. Other symptoms include nausea, vomiting, or both; abdominal discomfort; and warm, flushed skin from peripheral vasodilation. Cardiac output may decrease as myocardial contractility is depressed. Hypotension and dysrhythmias may occur (Huether, 2017a). Because of the contractility issues commonly associated with metabolic acidosis and the potential for hyperkalemia, the ICU nurse should monitor for dysrhythmias in patients who develop this imbalance. **BOX 17.2** lists common causes of metabolic acidosis seen in the postoperative cardiac surgery patient.

Metabolic acidosis is generally classified as having either a high or normal anion gap. Bicarbonate and chloride are considered the major anions in the body. To calculate the plasma anion gap, subtract chloride and bicarbonate from sodium (Pollock & Funk, 2013). In cases where a metabolic acidosis is accompanied by a loss of bicarbonate with retention of chloride to maintain balance, a normal anion gap metabolic acidosis state is present. The most common causes of normal anion gap acidosis include renal tubular acidosis, excessive administration of isotonic solutions, and diarrhea. In cases where the concentration of anions (other than chloride) increases (thereby destroying the electrical neutrality of the body), a high anion gap acidosis is said to exist (Huether, 2017a). Lactic acidosis, renal failure, and diabetic ketoacidosis (DKA) are the most common causes of high anion gap acidosis.

Alkalosis

Respiratory Alkalosis

Respiratory alkalosis occurs when there is alveolar hyperventilation causing hypocapnia (Huether, 2017a; Shires, 2015). **BOX 17.3** lists common causes of respiratory alkalosis seen in the postoperative cardiac surgery patient. When respiratory alkalosis is seen early in the postoperative period, it is related to ventilator-induced hyperventilation, pain, or anxiety (Shires, 2015). When it is seen later in the postoperative course, respiratory alkalosis is arising as a compensatory mechanism (e.g., in response to diuretic therapy) (Huether, 2017a).

Signs and symptoms of respiratory alkalosis may include lightheadedness, inability to concentrate, dizziness, confusion, headache, numbness and tingling of the extremities (paresthesias), tinnitus, palpitations, dry mouth, sweating, chest pain, or nausea and vomiting. Late-stage signs and symptoms may include loss of consciousness or seizures. The most notable signs are rapid and deep respirations (Huether, 2017a). The neurologic symptoms may be caused by a hypocalcemic state, which is commonly seen with a respiratory alkalosis. This acid–base disturbance can cause an increase in protein binding of ionized calcium (the amount of calcium not bound to protein and

> **BOX 17.3** Common Causes of Respiratory Alkalosis in the Postoperative Cardiac Surgery Patient
>
> **Hyperventilation Secondary to the Following Conditions**
> - Anxiety or fear
> - Pain or generalized discomfort
>
> **Increased Oxygen Demand as a Result of the Following Conditions**
> - Fever
> - Bacteremia (especially with gram-negative organisms)
> - Sepsis
>
> **Pulmonary Disorders**
> - Pneumonia
> - Pulmonary edema
> - Pulmonary embolism
> - V/Q mismatch (increased ventilation, decreased perfusion)
>
> **Medications: Respiratory Stimulants**
> - User error
> - Inappropriate ventilator settings
> - Hyperventilation during transfer from operating room

Data from Huether, 2017a; Shires, 2015.

available for use by the body). Treatment is aimed at correcting the underlying cause.

Metabolic Alkalosis

Common causes of metabolic alkalosis in the postoperative cardiac surgery patient are presented in **BOX 17.4**. Like respiratory alkalosis, metabolic alkalosis is usually seen later in the postoperative cardiac surgery patient. It is likely related to citrate in banked blood (Kouchoukos, Blackstone, Hanley, & Kirklin, 2013). Patients often have concomitant hypokalemia and hypocalcemia;

BOX 17.4 Common Causes of Metabolic Alkalosis in the Postoperative Cardiac Surgery Patient

Adrenal disorders: hyperaldosteronism
Hypokalemia
Hypochloremia
Excessive diuretic administration
Nasogastric suctioning
Overuse of potassium-wasting drugs (e.g., increased use of thiazide diuretics)
Vomiting
Massive transfusions (from citrate)

Data from Huether, 2017a; Shires, 2015.

TABLE 17.2 Electrolyte Reference Values

Electrolyte	Normal Value
Potassium	3.5–5.0 mEq/L
Sodium	135–145 mEq/L
Magnesium	1.8–2.4 mg/dL[†]
Phosphorus	2.5–4.5 mg/dL
Calcium	8.5–10.5 mg/dL[‡]

[*]Normal value markers may vary according to facility. Always check with your local laboratory if unsure of the normal values for any laboratory finding.
[†]Serum magnesium may also be reported in millimoles per liter (mmol/L). In these cases, normal values would be in the range of 0.65–1.1 mmol/L.
[‡]Serum calcium can be reported as total calcium, ionized calcium, or nonionized calcium. The value provided in the table is for the total calcium. A normal ionized calcium value is in the range of 4.4–5.3 mg/dL.

---

these underlying conditions must be simultaneously corrected. With a metabolic alkalosis, as the hydrogen ion concentration increases in the blood, potassium ions move into the cells to maintain neutrality. This results in a hypokalemic state. Signs and symptoms of metabolic alkalosis include poor skin turgor (from fluid loss). Treatment is aimed at restoring fluid balance and correcting the underlying disorder.

▶ Electrolyte Imbalances

Electrolyte imbalances are frequently seen in postoperative cardiac surgery patients. The ICU nurse should recognize normal values, signs, and symptoms associated with these imbalances, and implement appropriate interventions to correct them. **TABLE 17.2** lists the common electrolytes and their associated normal values.

Potassium

Fluctuations in potassium levels are common following cardiac surgery and can affect cardiac automaticity and conduction (Yazdchi & Rawn, 2018). Potassium works with sodium to help maintain fluid balance within the body, with kidney regulation being the mechanism that governs the balance. The potassium found in the extracellular fluid is responsible for neuromuscular function

and plays a major role in myocardial contractility, function, and rhythm (Rhee & Joseph, 2017). Cardiac rhythm often has depressed T waves and U waves. Arrhythmias commonly seen include atrial tachyarrhythmias, ventricular tachycardia (VT), or ventricular fibrillation (VF). Treatment requires potassium replacement whether via oral or intravenous (IV) routes of administration. Intravenous replacement, if using central line, can occur with higher concentrations (up to 40 mEq/hr) in emergent situations (Rhee & Joseph, 2017).

Hyperkalemia

Patients with progressive hyperkalemia will present with ventricular dysrhythmias and may develop nausea, intestinal cramping, diarrhea, paresthesias, muscle weakness, or paralysis (muscle weakness first appears in the larger muscles and the myocardium). These symptoms are directly related to the effect of the elevated potassium on the cellular membrane potential. Respiratory failure secondary to muscle weakness and paralysis may also occur as a result of hyperkalemia. Peaked T waves are noted with cardiac monitoring.

Cardiac arrest will occur if left untreated (Rhee & Joseph, 2017).

Treatment of moderately elevated serum potassium levels may include sodium polystyrene sulfonate (Kayexalate®). Kayexalate acts by exchanging sodium ions for potassium ions in the gastrointestinal (GI) tract, thereby allowing for elimination of excess potassium in the stool. Before Kayexalate is administered, however, it must be known if a patient can tolerate an increase in serum sodium (Shires, 2015).

Emergent renal replacement therapy is an option to lower serum potassium levels in those patients who do not respond to conservative therapy. With severe hyperkalemia, 10 units of regular insulin with one ampule of $D_{50}W$, calcium gluconate, a beta agonist, or sodium bicarbonate may be administered. These interventions are temporary in nature, but will provide almost immediate lowering of potassium levels and allow time for the patient to be prepared for dialysis therapy (Rhee & Joseph, 2017; Shires, 2015).

The major causes of hyperkalemia in the postoperative cardiac surgery patient are decreased urinary output, cardioplegia, decreased insulin levels, metabolic acidosis, diabetes, and hemolysis of red blood cells (Yazdchi & Rawn, 2018). Acute kidney injury or failure to excrete and metabolize potassium through the kidneys may occur postoperatively. Many cardiac medications can cause hyperkalemia (e.g., angiotensin-converting enzyme [ACE] inhibitors, potassium-sparing diuretics, beta blockers, unfractionated heparin, and digoxin). Massive blood transfusions are also associated with higher levels of potassium. Age-related renal changes with distal renal tubular function decline and reduced renin-aldosterone response can exacerbate hyperkalemia in the elderly patients (El-Sharkawy, Sahota, Maughan, & Lobo, 2014).

Evidence of hyperkalemia may be noted in the electrocardiogram (ECG). Peaked T waves (**FIGURE 17.1**), a widening QRS complex, a prolonged PR interval, and atrioventricular (AV) block may be noted (Rhee & Joseph, 2017). Cardiac arrest may occur at any point if potassium levels continue to increase. Treatment needs to begin at a level of 6.5 mEq/L even if there are no ECG changes.

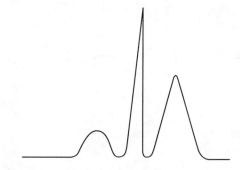

FIGURE 17.1 Hyperkalemia—peaked T wave.
Illustrated by James R. Perron

Hypokalemia

The major causes of hypokalemia in cardiac surgery patients include brisk diuresis, rapid correction of hyperglycemia with insulin, adrenal hyperreactivity, vomiting, alkalosis, and hypothermia (Shires, 2015).

Hypokalemia is associated with increased dysrhythmias by delay in ventricular repolarization with a prolonged PR interval, prolonged QT interval, U-wave development as the T wave flattens, and ST segment depression. Sinus bradycardia, AV blocks, premature atrial contractions, paroxysmal atrial tachycardia, ventricular ectopy, VT, and VF may result. Depending on rapidity of potassium loss, skeletal muscle weakness, smooth muscle atony, and respiratory weakness that can lead to respiratory arrest may result if left untreated (Huether, 2017a). **FIGURE 17.2** illustrates the development of U waves in the hypokalemic patient.

Hypokalemia can manifest as muscle weakness, fatigue, postural hypotension, absent or diminished bowel sounds, distended abdomen, constipation, and flaccid paralysis (Shires, 2015). Cardiac dysrhythmias that may develop include atrial ectopy, supraventricular tachycardias and atrial flutter, ventricular ectopy, VT, VF, and torsades de pointes. Patients may be more susceptible to digitalis toxicity. Hypokalemia is frequently accompanied by metabolic alkalosis and hypomagnesemia (Rhee & Joseph, 2017; Shires, 2015).

Treatment of hypokalemia involves replacement of potassium, either orally or intravenously. If concomitant hypomagnesemia exists,

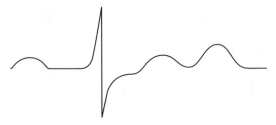

FIGURE 17.2 Hypokalemia—U wave.

Illustrated by James R. Perron

correction of magnesium levels is required before or simultaneously with potassium correction (Rhee & Joseph, 2017; Shires, 2015).

Sodium

Sodium is the major extracellular ion found in the body; its concentration normally ranges between 135 and 145 mEq/L. Sodium is directly responsible for maintaining the fluid balance in the body, ensuring appropriate water distribution and maintaining the ECF volume status. The serum sodium concentration parallels with the osmolality of the blood. Antidiuretic hormone is the primary regulator of osmolality (Shires, 2015).

Hypernatremia

Hypernatremia is a relatively uncommon phenomenon, but is associated with a 40% to 60% (or greater) mortality rate. This imbalance occurs when there is a gain of sodium in excess of water or a loss of water in excess of sodium. In the postoperative cardiac surgery patient, it is most commonly seen in conjunction with hyperventilation. Hypernatremia may also develop secondary to dehydration from fever, diabetes, or use of osmotic diuretics. Usually, the patient's blood urea nitrogen (BUN) and creatinine will be elevated as well (Lindner & Funk, 2013).

Signs and symptoms of hypernatremia may include thirst, fever, restlessness, irritability, ataxia, seizures, weakness, dry oral mucosa or tongue, poor skin turgor, and disorientation with possible progression to lethargy, stupor, or coma (Rhee & Joseph, 2017; Shires, 2015). The majority of patients exhibiting this are also hypovolemic

and hyperosmolar. Depending on the cause, treatment will focus on either increasing water within the body or removing sodium from it (Shires, 2015). Rhee and Joseph (2017) recommend that if treating with free water, do so at a rate that corrects the serum sodium by less than 1 to 2 mEq/hr or 8 mEq/day.

Postoperative cardiac surgery patients with a severe hypernatremia (>150 mEq/L) may experience an acid–base imbalance that is difficult to correct. In this situation, use of tromethamine or tris(hydroxymethyl)aminomethane (Tham®) to treat metabolic acidosis is recommended instead of sodium bicarbonate, because the latter therapy may increase sodium levels further, worsen intracellular acidosis, reduce ionized calcium, create hyperosmolality, and cause central nervous system effects. Tham buffers without creating CO_2; patients will need intact kidneys, dialysis, or continuous renal replacement therapy (CRRT). Potassium and acid–base levels must be monitored regularly when using Tham (Rhee & Joseph, 2017).

Hyponatremia

Hyponatremia is the most common electrolyte abnormality in hospitalized patients and is associated with increased mortality, increased hospital length of stay (LOS), gait imbalance, falls, rhabdomyolysis, bone fractures, and increased health care costs (Crestanello et al., 2013; El-Sharkawy et al., 2014). Up to 21% of preoperative cardiac surgery patients are known to have hyponatremia (Crestanello et al., 2013). Hyponatremia commonly arises when cells swell as water enters them. This swelling can progress to the point that it eventually leads to cellular rupture. Common causes of hyponatremia include use of certain medications (e.g., thiazide diuretics, nonsteroidal anti-inflammatory drugs, ACE inhibitors), pneumonia, acute respiratory failure, and hyperglycemia. Excess fluid volume and the stressors from cardiac surgery (e.g., nausea, pain, anesthesia) can stimulate the release of ADH, causing hyponatremia for the first few days after surgery. Severe hyperglycemia increases osmolality of extracellular fluid pulling water from the cells; this will

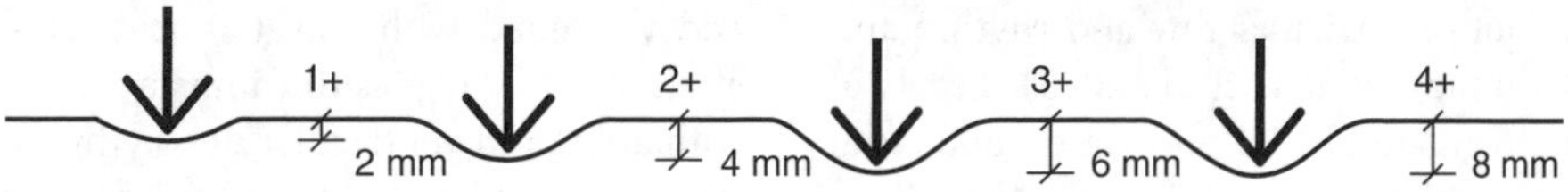

FIGURE 17.3 Pitting edema.

Illustrated by James R. Perron

normalize when glucose levels return to normal (Rhee & Joseph, 2017). It also occurs in patients with congestive heart failure, with diminished CO stimulating the release of ADH. Signs and symptoms may include headache, confusion, nausea and vomiting, generalized muscle weakness, fatigue, and seizures and coma if severe. Symptoms vary according to the severity of hyponatremia and how quickly it occurs (Moritz & Ayus, 2015; Shires, 2015). Cheyne-Stokes respirations and respiratory failure may accompany severe hyponatremia (Moritz & Ayus, 2015; Thomas, 2014). Common characteristics of patients with hyponatremia include lower left ventricular function, higher pulmonary artery pressures, lower glomerular filtration rates, and higher rates of comorbidities such as diabetes, hypertension, previous myocardial infarction (MI), COPD, peripheral vascular diseases, and previous cardiac surgical procedures (Crestanello et al., 2013).

Hyponatremia may be seen in patients who are either hypovolemic, normovolemic, or hypervolemic. Most often, this type of sodium imbalance is seen in patients with severe heart failure, in whom a decrease in CO triggers the release of ADH, which in turn causes hypervolemia. Patients who are hypovolemic may develop hyponatremia secondary to brisk diuresis, excess insensible loss from the skin or GI tract, or glucocorticoid deficiency. Those who are normovolemic may develop hyponatremia secondary to hypokalemia, medications, or hypothyroidism. Patients with hypervolemia may also develop hyponatremia secondary to renal failure or heart failure and increased total body water accumulation (Huether, 2017b; Rhee & Joseph, 2017). Postoperative use of hypotonic solutions should be avoided to lower the risk of the patient developing hyponatremia (Moritz & Ayus, 2015).

The patient with hypervolemia-associated hyponatremia will present with changes in mental status, restlessness, anxiety, decreased urinary output, weight gain, peripheral and dependent edema (including pitting edema; **FIGURE 17.3**), hypertension, jugular vein distention, shortness of breath, diffuse crackles, and muffled heart sounds. Because of their fluid volume status, these patients also present with low hematocrit levels (Shires, 2015).

Treatment of hyponatremia includes replacement of fluid in patients with hypovolemic hyponatremia, water restriction in hypervolemic or normovolemic hyponatremia, and management of associated adrenal and ADH imbalances, as appropriate. For those patients with volume overload, treatment includes a loop diuretic agent and moderate fluid restriction (Dynamed Plus, 2017). During treatment, close monitoring and accurate intake and output records should be maintained, and the nurse should monitor the patient's vital signs closely to assess for rapid fluid changes. In case of severe hyponatremia (<120 mEq/L) or if the patient is symptomatic, infusions of 3% to 5% sodium may be indicated. Patients must be closely monitored while receiving this infusion (Rhee & Joseph, 2017). Rapid changes in level of consciousness indicate a worsening cerebral edema.

Magnesium

Magnesium is an electrolyte that plays a key role in cellular function and is a major intracellular cation. Magnesium helps maintain cellular permeability, promotes ion transport across the cellular membranes, and increases neuromuscular excitability. Magnesium is intrinsically involved with potassium, sodium, and adenosine triphosphatase (ATPase)—the enzyme that helps regulate potassium concentration, especially in the myocardium (Huether, 2017a). Several studies have been done in the last few years looking at the efficacy of magnesium supplementation to control atrial and ventricular arrhythmias. Its use has been found to be of benefit in controlling and preventing both ventricular rate and rhythm and atrial arrhythmias (Raiten et al., 2015). Levels of this ion are regulated by GI absorption and renal excretion; the normal range is 1.8 to 2.4 mg/dL.

Hypermagnesemia

Hypermagnesemia (>2.5 mEq/L) is rare and is most likely to occur in patients with decreased renal function. The patient with an elevated magnesium level will present with flushing, warmth, lethargy, muscle weakness, diminished deep tendon reflexes, dilated pupils, vomiting, diarrhea, anorexia, muscle weakness, decreased or absent bowel sounds, hypotension, and respiratory depression (Huether, 2017a). Ventricular dysrhythmias, bradycardia, a prolonged PR interval, widened QRS, complete heart block, and cardiac arrest are not uncommon in patients whose magnesium levels exceed 2.5 mg/dL (Shires, 2015).

Magnesium levels greater than 10 mg/dL (particularly 15 mg/dL) are usually fatal. Treatment for symptomatic hypermagnesemia includes an infusion of insulin and glucose as well as IV calcium gluconate, which acts as a magnesium antagonist. Calcium gluconate rapidly reverses cardiac dysrhythmias or respiratory depression directly related to hypermagnesemia. The ICU nurse should prepare to administer 10 to 20 mEq of calcium gluconate over 10 min or follow facility policy in cases of life-threatening hypermagnesemia. Patients who develop this electrolyte imbalance will also require fluid resuscitation and loop diuretics. Mechanical ventilation may be required for those individuals with severe respiratory depression. A temporary pacemaker may be required in patients who experience severe bradycardia. Hemodialysis may be required if the patient's renal function is inadequate (Shires, 2015).

Hypomagnesemia

Hypomagnesemia is a common clinical problem in postoperative cardiac surgery patients, especially in those individuals who develop hemodilution following CPB or who receive diuretics (Shires, 2015). It is also a common problem associated with normal aging and is commonly thought to arise from decreased dietary intake and worsened with elevated acids (El-Sharkawy et al., 2014). Magnesium imbalance is associated with atrial and ventricular dysrhythmias. Patients are more apt to develop atrial fibrillation (AF) in the postoperative phase with hypomagnesemia. A meta-analysis revealed that 2,988 patients receiving magnesium therapy had a 10% reduced chance of AF postoperatively (Tokmaji, McClure, Kaneko, & Aranki, 2013). In addition, affected patients may present with depression, muscle weakness, coronary spasm, confusion, irritability, hyperactive reflexes, positive Chvostek's sign, leg and foot cramping, twitches and tremors, tetany, delirium, and seizures (Shires, 2015). Vascular effects include an increased peripheral vascular resistance with hypertension resulting and potential for vasospasms.

Hypomagnesemia is often accompanied by hypophosphatemia, hypocalcemia, and hypokalemia. This can lead to osteoporosis, arrhythmias, and MI (El-Sharkawy et al., 2014). Changes will appear on the ECG tracing, including nonspecific T-wave changes, appearance of U waves, prolonged QT intervals, widened QRS complex, ST segment depression, peaked T waves, and torsades de pointes. Ventricular ectopy, paroxysmal supraventricular tachycardia, premature ventricular contractions, and AF and VF are likely to occur as well (Shires, 2015). Finally, insulin resistance may occur in patients with severe hypomagnesemia, making serum glucose levels hard to control (Chhabra, Chhabra, Chhabra, & Ramessur, 2012).

Treatment entails magnesium repletion. If magnesium is to be administered intravenously, the patient's renal function should be determined prior to its administration to help avoid hypermagnesemia. Additionally, during infusions of magnesium, urinary output should be closely monitored. If urinary output decreases to less than 100 mL over 4 hours, the infusion of magnesium should be discontinued and the surgeon notified.

Protection of the patient's overall condition remains a high priority in a hypomagnesemic patient. Seizure precautions should be implemented, the airway and respiratory status should be continually monitored, and fall precautions should be implemented for those individuals who have an altered mental status.

Calcium

The majority (>99%) of the body's calcium is found in the skeletal system. Most of the remaining calcium is found inside cells. The serum calcium is found bound to protein, bound or complexed with anions, and ionized (free) (Huether, 2017a; Shires, 2015). A normal serum calcium level is in the range of 8.5 to 10.5 mg/dL in individuals with a normal pH and normal serum albumin levels. Assessment of total calcium level requires pH and serum albumin evaluation.

In cases of protein malnutrition or other issues affecting serum albumin, an ionized calcium level is a more accurate indicator of calcium status than total calcium level. Ionized calcium is the calcium that is not bound to protein; its normal range is from 4.4 to 5.3 mg/dL. Adequate levels of ionized calcium are essential for cardiac performance; treatment is recommended if levels are less than 4.0 mg/dL (Shires, 2015; Song, 2017; Yazdchi & Rawn, 2018).

Hypercalcemia

Three basic causes exist for hypercalcemia: increased intestinal absorption, increased bone resorption, and decreased elimination. Decreased elimination of calcium is seen generally with medication use, or when decreased availability of physiologic calcium is present (such as with acidosis). Medications that increase serum calcium levels include thiazide diuretics and lithium carbonate, both of which decrease renal calcium excretion. Some estrogens also increase calcium levels. Immobilization, rhabdomyolysis, and excess vitamin D can also lead to this condition (Gurrado et al., 2012).

Patients with hypercalcemia will present with altered mental status, fatigue, muscle weakness, lethargy, anorexia, nausea, vomiting, constipation, abdominal pain, decreased renal function or AKI, polyuria, polydipsia, shortened QT segments, and depressed T waves. Nonspecific dysrhythmias, bradycardia, and first-, second-, or third-degree AV block may develop. Bundle branch blocks may also be seen. The patient with severe hypercalcemia may develop confusion, personality change,

BOX 17.5 Corrected Calcium Formula
Corrected calcium = (4 − serum albumin in g/dL) × 0.8 + serum calcium

Data from Agraharkar, 2018.

psychosis, or lethargy that can lead to coma (Green, 2017).

Goals for treatment are to restore urinary calcium excretion and inhibit bone resorption. Prior to treating hypercalcemia, it is important to determine if serum albumin is low. Because calcium binds to albumin, it is important to correct an elevated calcium before treatment begins; once a corrected calcium is calculated, the patient may no longer have hypercalcemia. A corrected calcium can be calculated using the formula in **BOX 17.5**.

Calcitonin is able to meet both goals and may be given intravenously as a treatment for hypercalcemia; it may also be given intramuscularly or subcutaneously (Agraharkar, 2018). Hydration with saline to promote urine output can be utilized depending on a patient's age and comorbidities (congestive heart failure, renal failure). Glucocorticoids have also been used successfully in cases of hypercalcemia; however, results will not be seen for 5 to 7 days with this therapy. If no positive results are seen within 10 days, this treatment should be stopped. Patients may develop increased risks for hyperglycemia and sodium and water retention while being treated with glucocorticoids such as methylprednisolone (Medrol®) or prednisone (Tamez-Pérez, Quintanilla-Flores, Rodriguez-Gutiérrez, González-González, & Tamez-Peña, 2015).

Hypocalcemia

Hypocalcemia occurs when serum calcium is less than 8.5 mg/dL. At a minimum, measurement of ionized calcium level is needed to confirm a diagnosis of hypocalcemia, and these data should always be reviewed in conjunction with the acid–base status of the patient. A patient with a low serum calcium but normal ionized calcium is typically asymptomatic, and is referred to as having pseudohypocalcemia.

Development of hypocalcemia is expected following CPB, hemodilution, low CO, or administration of citrated blood (Yazdchi & Rawn, 2018). Packed red blood cells, for example, are conditioned with citrate to prevent their coagulation. When citrate combines with calcium, hypocalcemia can occur. This effect generally does not occur during normal blood transfusions, because citrate has adequate time to metabolize in the liver; only in cases of faster than normal blood transfusions or cases of liver dysfunction does this citrate–calcium binding become a potential problem. Vitamin D deficiency, malnourishment, renal failure, or parathyroidism are other reasons that a patient may become hypocalcemic. Altered magnesium levels, elevated phosphorus, and alkalosis can lead to hypocalcemia. Hyperphosphatemia is noted with rhabdomyolysis as hypocalcemia is seen in early stages of this disease process (Song, 2017).

Patients with hypocalcemia may report numbness or tingling of the fingers and toes. Muscle cramps, spasms, tremors, twitching, and abdominal and intestinal cramps are common. Bowel sounds are hyperactive. Because of the increased neuromuscular activity, hypocalcemic patients who are left untreated may develop tetany, seizures, laryngospasm, and bronchospasm. These spasms may lead to laryngeal stridor, which will eventually necessitate intubation if the calcium level is not adequately treated (Shires, 2015; Song, 2017). Auscultation of breath sounds may reveal inspiratory and expiratory wheezing. In approximately 70% of patients with hypocalcemia, positive Trousseau's and Chvostek's signs are present. Trousseau's sign is considered positive when an inflated blood pressure cuff elicits a carpopedal spasm (**FIGURE 17.4**). Chvostek's sign is considered positive when tapping of the facial nerve elicits facial muscle movement (Shires, 2015).

Cardiac complications associated with hypocalcemia include a decrease in myocardial contractility and CO. Symptoms of hypocalcemia will likely include hypotension, a prolonged QT interval, shortness of breath, and dysrhythmias ranging from bradycardia to asystole. Heart sounds may be muffled (Yazdchi & Rawn, 2018).

Acute hypocalcemia should be promptly corrected with administration of 10% calcium

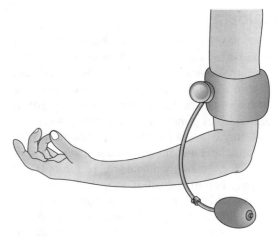

FIGURE 17.4 Test for hypocalcemia.
Illustrated by James R. Perron

gluconate. This medication may be given either as an intravenous push over 5 to 10 minutes or mixed in 0.9% normal saline (NS) for infusion according to facility policy.

Phosphorus

Phosphate is located primarily in bone, with the rest located in intracellular and extracellular compartments. These ions play integral roles in the repair of cells and tissues, and are crucial ions in the production of adenosine triphosphate (ATP) (Huether, 2017a). Phosphorus is excreted through the kidneys; as kidney function declines, phosphorus levels are likely to increase (Shires, 2015; Song, 2017). As is the case with calcium, hormonal regulation is provided through the parathyroid gland (Song, 2017). A normal serum phosphorus is in the range of 2.5 to 4.5 mg/dL.

Hyperphosphatemia

Hyperphosphatemia is defined as a serum phosphorus level greater than 4.5 mg/dL, but becomes clinically significant when phosphorus levels exceed 5.0 mg/dL (Lederer, Ouseph, & Nayak, 2014). Almost all cases of hyperphosphatemia are a direct result of decreased renal function. When the glomerular filtration rate (GFR) falls below 50 mL/min, the kidneys are no longer able to adequately metabolize phosphorus (Song, 2017). Respiratory acidosis and DKA may also lead to hyperphosphatemia. It is suggested that the relationship between a respiratory acidosis and hyperphosphatemia is twofold. First, a sudden rise in carbon dioxide levels can lead to an elevation in phosphorus levels. Second, presence of a respiratory acidosis causes phosphorus to move from the intracellular to extracellular fluid compartment. Presence of a metabolic acidosis, as seen in DKA, is associated with hyperphosphatemia (Song, 2017).

Signs and symptoms of hyperphosphatemia may include altered mental status, delirium, seizures, paresthesias (especially around the mouth or in the fingers and toes), and tetany. Positive Trousseau's and Chvostek's signs, hypotension, and cardiac dysrhythmias may also be present. Heart sounds may be muffled, and a pericardial friction rub may be present, indicative of potential heart failure. The QT interval is often prolonged.

A low phosphate diet, calcium-based binders, and non-calcium-based binders such as sevelamer (Renagel®) are being used with chronic kidney disease to block the ingestion of phosphorus (Nguyen, Bose, & Finkelstein, 2016). If kidney function is adequate, an NS infusion may help return the serum phosphorus levels to baseline. If the patient is symptomatic, emergent renal replacement therapy may be indicated (Lederer et al., 2014).

Hypophosphatemia

Patients with a serum phosphorus level less than 1.5 mg/dL are considered severely compromised. Because of the key role that phosphorus plays with ATP, a sharp decrease in phosphorus levels results in cell energy depletion (Song, 2017). Garazi, Bridge, Caffarelli, Ruoss, and Van der Starre (2015) related cellular insulin resistance, increasing hyperglycemia, and hypophosphatemia during the early postoperative phase post cardiac surgery. Causes for hypophosphatemia include chronic alcoholism, hyperparathyroidism, excessive antacid use, malnutrition or malabsorptive conditions, intravenous glucose or bicarbonate infusions, use of inotropes, emesis, dialysis, and respiratory alkalosis or hyperventilation (Garazi et al., 2015; Song, 2017).

Signs and symptoms of severe hypophosphatemia include paresthesias; severe, profound, and progressive muscle weakness; tremors; muscle pain and tenderness; lethargy; confusion; anxiety; and apprehension. If this condition is left untreated, the patient will develop hypoxia and bradycardia. Hypotension will be present, and stroke volume will be decreased. Muscle weakness will eventually lead to acute respiratory failure from decreased contraction of the diaphragm (Garazi et al., 2015; Song, 2017). Seizures and coma may also be present. Hypophosphatemia may cause eventual rhabdomyolysis secondary to the muscle cell's inability to maintain cell membrane integrity with the overall ATP depletion. Hemolytic anemia as well as leukocyte and platelet dysfunction will be noted. Respiratory rate decreases as phosphorus levels decrease. However, if the hypophosphatemia is related to the presence of respiratory alkalosis, tachypnea will be present. Hypomagnesemia and hypercalcemia are oftentimes present in conjunction with hypophosphatemia (Garazi et al., 2015; Song, 2017).

Treatment for severe hypophosphatemia requires IV replacement of phosphorus. The precise therapy employed depends on the patient's renal status, because one phosphorus preparation is built on sodium and the other relies on potassium. For the patient with adequate renal function, potassium phosphate may be administered; sodium phosphate should be administered to those patients with decreased renal function.

Should a heart block or flaccid paralysis develop, the infusion of phosphorus should be immediately discontinued, as these symptoms indicate rebound hyperphosphatemia. A patient with severe hypophosphatemia may also be more prone to infection. Consequently, a complete blood count should be performed on the postoperative cardiac surgery patient to provide information about the presence of bleeding and possible infection.

▸ Fluid Balance and Volume Management

Fluids shift on an as-needed basis between compartments to maintain homeostasis. This fluid exchange is partly affected by osmolarity, and hence by electrolyte concentrations (Huether, 2017a). Shifts between compartments occur as the body seeks to maintain an appropriate cation and anion distribution as well as optimal fluid levels in each compartment. Frequently, alterations in fluid volume status accompany electrolyte imbalances. For the nurse caring for the postoperative cardiac surgery patient, either hypovolemia or hypervolemia may represent worsening of a preexisting medical condition or may be related to the surgical procedure and associated interventions. In either case, it is important to recognize the implications of alterations in fluid volume status and to determine appropriate courses of treatment.

Hypovolemia

Hypovolemia, which is also known as fluid volume deficit (FVD), results when both water and electrolytes are lost together. This condition is not the same as dehydration, which results from water loss alone (and, therefore, leads to hypernatremia). An isotonic FVD indicates that electrolyte levels remain essentially unchanged (Huether, 2017a). Common causes of fluid losses in the postoperative cardiac surgery patient include blood loss, fever, and third spacing of fluid. Hypovolemic shock results when circulating blood volume falls to such a level that vital organs are not perfused adequately, causing potential damage to these organs.

Assessment

Hypovolemia is common postoperatively, but often proves difficult to assess. Signs and symptoms of FVD and hypovolemia include decreased capillary refill time, central venous pressure (CVP), and urinary output; dizziness; increased osmolality, specific gravity, thirst sensation in conscious patients, hematocrit, and BUN to serum creatinine ratio (usually >30:1); postural or prolonged hypotension; tachycardia; weak and thready pulse; and decreased vein filling. A urinary output rate that is less than 0.5 mL/kg/hr is indicative of severe FVD and inadequate renal perfusion. Assessment of skin turgor reveals skin that does

not "spring" back, but remains in the tented position; dry mucous membranes; reduced sweating in axillae (especially in the elderly); and a tongue that appears shrunken, with fissures. Severe FVD is also accompanied by confusion, upper body weakness, and speech difficulties. Shock develops when FVD is left untreated. In such cases, hypotension becomes severe and perfusion to vital organs is compromised (Weinstein, 2014).

Treatment

Treatment of hypovolemia depends on the cause of the FVD. The goal of FVD treatment is to expand plasma volume until a desired MAP has been attained and sustained. When planning for delivery of replacement fluids, daily insensible fluid losses and intraoperative fluid loss must also be accounted for and added into the replacement. A fever greater than 38.3°C (101°F) increases the daily fluid requirement. If the patient is not severely hypotensive, the fluid replacement plan may be based on an assumption that 50% to 80% of the fluid loss will be replaced over 12 to 24 hours; in cases where severe hypotension or shock exists, volume repletion must take place much more quickly. The vasodilation that occurs with rewarming following CPB may necessitate administration of additional fluid to maintain adequate CO.

Fluid Challenge

For the patient who has developed oliguria, has a urinary output of less than 0.5 mL/kg/hr with symptomatic hypotension, and has had fluid losses (e.g., blood, urine, preoperative fasting), a fluid challenge should be anticipated (Ricci, Romagnoli, & Ronco, 2012). The goal of a fluid challenge is to replenish the intravascular volume. A supplemental dose of fluid (e.g., 250 mL) is administered over a short period of time (e.g., 15 min). Using pulse contour systems to provide dynamic indices can reflect intravascular volume status when mechanical ventilation is used and the patient is in normal sinus rhythm. Measurements of stroke volume variation and pulse pressure variation can give a positive reflection of response to fluid challenges/treatment. Parameters such as CVP, pulmonary artery occlusive pressure, MAP, and even urinary output are not as reliable in identifying a response to fluid challenges in improving cardiac function (Shaw, 2012).

Instead of liberal use or restricted use of fluid therapy, many now prefer to use a goal-directed fluid therapy approach with a combination of inotropic therapy when needed (Schortgen & Schetz, 2017). Fluid needs will differ for patients based on their history, comorbidities, and the surgical procedure performed. In addition, patients' hemodynamic profiles and tolerance to fluid will vary. For example, postoperative patients who underwent valve repair for aortic stenosis will initially continue to have left ventricular hypertrophy following surgery. This condition may result in outflow obstruction and subsequent postoperative hemodynamic instability from preload reduction. Treatment will include volume repletion. Conversely, postoperative patients who underwent repair for aortic regurgitation will likely require vasodilator therapy. Patients who underwent repair for mitral stenosis will likely need prudent fluid administration in combination with inotropic support to augment CO. Finally, patients who underwent repair for mitral regurgitation may develop postoperative right ventricular failure and therefore require inotropic administration (Yazdchi & Rawn, 2018).

Crystalloid Therapy

Crystalloid solutions contain solutes that dissolve and crystallize easily, such as dextrose and sodium. *Isotonic* refers to the osmolality (normal total body water is 295 mOsm/kg) and helps control distribution of water across the cell membrane (endothelial glycocalyx layer) of the ICF and ECF with oncotic pressure from their solutes (Annane et al., 2013; Shaw, 2012).

Commonly used isotonic replacement fluids include 0.9% NS, lactated Ringer's (LR), Ringer's acetate (RA), and Plasma-Lyte. Normal saline is a nonbuffered solution (a simple salt solution). Lactated Ringer's and Plasma-Lyte are buffered solutions, because they are balanced with acids and bases similar to the balance in the body. Buffered solutions do not have the problem with hyperchloremic acidosis and, hence, metabolic acidosis (Shires, 2015). The balanced/buffered crystalloids have

become preferred solutions for volume replacement in the European community (Protsyk et al., 2017). It has been reported that use of Plasma-Lyte may be associated with an increased need for blood transfusions; further studies will be needed (Reddy et al., 2017). Normal saline is excreted more slowly than LR, increasing the volume effect for a longer period of time (Hahn, 2011). Lactated Ringer's and RA can increase blood sugar levels, which may affect patients with diabetes, slightly increase oxygen consumption secondary to the lactate and acetate, and have vasodilator (lactate and acetate) properties with rapid administration (Hahn, 2011). Patients who received RA versus hydroxyethyl starch (HES) had a decreased risk of death and were less likely to require renal replacement therapy (RRT) (Perner et al., 2012). Factors driving the use of crystalloid therapy include the solutions' ready availability in the ICU and their low cost. Other considerations with crystalloid administration for volume repletion include crystalloids' tendency to cause decreased blood viscosity, increased urinary output with associated sodium and potassium excretion, and increased peripheral blood flow, thereby improving tissue perfusion.

A negative aspect of isotonic crystalloid administration is that approximately 75% of the volume moves out of the vascular space, with half being lost to the circulating volume shortly after crystalloid administration. Further, one of the components of crystalloids used for fluid repletion in postoperative cardiac surgery patients is sodium. If excessive amounts of sodium are administered, the patient's osmolarity may become elevated and water may be drawn from cells, resulting in cellular dehydration and reduction in renal blood flow secondary to accumulation of chloride (Protsyk et al., 2017). In addition, infusion of 2 L or more of NS can cause hyperchloremic metabolic acidosis, renal vasoconstriction, and an increased incidence of AKI because this fluid has chloride ions in it and is not buffered (Moritz & Ayus, 2015; Rhee & Joseph, 2017). Some providers prefer to alternate administration of 0.9% NS with administration of LR in an effort to avoid this excessive sodium load.

Administration of hypotonic crystalloids may occasionally result in cerebral edema or seizures and can worsen cerebral damage in the event of cardiac arrest, acute stroke, or in cardiac surgery secondary to high risk of cerebral ischemia (Hahn, 2011). Administration of glucose-containing solutions for volume repletion (e.g., D_5W) can cause dilutional hyponatremia or hyperglycemia with hyperosmolarity, and a shift of water from intracellular to extracellular compartments with resultant osmotic diuresis (Shires, 2015).

Colloid Therapy

Following CPB, patients develop a low colloid osmotic pressure secondary to a systemic inflammatory response. Colloids such as albumin, plasma protein fraction, fresh frozen plasma, gelatins, HES, or dextran solutions can raise COP. Unlike crystalloids, colloids remain in the intravascular space for an extended period of time, allowing for the osmotic force to promote movement of water back into the intravascular space from the interstitium. They do, however, carry a risk for allergic reactions not seen with crystalloids (Sheikh, Platts-Mills, & Worth, 2013).

Although they are more expensive than crystalloids, colloids were traditionally preferred following cardiac surgery, because crystalloid therapy may decrease COP and increase the risk of pulmonary edema. In some patients, colloid administration may improve the patient's hemodynamic profile and improve balance between oxygen supply and demand through enhancement of microvascular blood flow (Kara, Akin, & Ince, 2016). The CRISTAL trial determined that those who received colloids had more days without mechanical ventilation, less use of inotropic agents, less use of RRT, and decreased mortality at 90 days (Annane et al., 2013). The update of the Cochrane review (Mutter, Ruth, & Dart, 2013) after investigating 42 randomized clinical trials concluded that HES products compared to other fluid therapies increased the risk of AKI by 59% and had a 32% increased risk of needing dialysis. Their recommendation was to avoid the use of HES products and use alternative therapies instead. Similar results were found in the CHEST trial when HES use was compared to NS (Myburgh et al, 2012). In another study, patients receiving a chloride-restrictive fluid strategy (Plasma-Lyte or chloride-poor albumin)

had a reduced risk for developing AKI in comparison to other fluids with higher levels of chloride such as NS and 4% albumin, no change in LOS for ICU or hospital, or mortality (Yunos et al., 2012). Dextrans can be used as volume expanders and to prevent thromboemboli, decrease blood viscosity, and improve microcirculatory flow. They do have a risk for anaphylaxis in patients who have antibodies to dextran. There is a risk for bleeding if large doses are administered (Vogel & Comerota, 2014).

A recent large cohort study (17,742 patients from 2004–2014) compared three groups: HES versus crystalloid, albumin versus crystalloid, and HES versus albumin. There was a significant increase in mortality parameters (30 days and 6 months) and in new onset dialysis with the use of albumin in comparison to HES and to crystalloids. This study did not see the magnitude of problem with HES that other studies reported (Ryhammer et al., 2017). Raiman, Mitchell, Biccard, and Rodseth (2016) in a meta-analysis of 13 small (n=20–200) random controlled studies determined that there were insufficient data to identify differences in outcomes between the use of HES and crystalloids in planned surgeries.

Health care providers should remember that colloids do not contain clotting factors or contribute to oxygen-carrying capacity. In addition, some of the protein molecules do eventually leak into the interstitium when the endothelial glycocalyx layer has been disrupted secondary to systemic inflammatory states such as diabetes, hyperglycemia, surgery, trauma, and sepsis. When this phenomenon occurs, the oncotic pull may promote third spacing of fluid as the COP equalizes in ICF and ECF (Ricci et al., 2012).

The efficacy of fluid challenges is traditionally assessed based on improvements in the patient's hemodynamic profile and physical assessment findings. Completing a passive leg raise maneuver is a quick assessment to see if the patient will respond to a fluid bolus before actually giving volume (Shaw, 2012).

Third Spacing

Third spacing refers to the movement of fluids from the vascular space to a part of the body where exchange with the rest of ECF is decreased, resulting in alterations of capillary membrane permeability (Yazdchi & Rawn, 2018). Symptoms of third spacing will mimic those associated with FVD, except that either weight gain may occur or weight may remain stable.

Third spacing occurs in two phases. The first phase mimics FVD (except for the weight loss), and the second (recovery) phase mimics hypervolemia. In the postoperative cardiac surgery patient, third spacing is most likely to arise as a result of vasodilation, hypothermia, or hyperemia (increased amount of blood) to the tissue bed (Yazdchi & Rawn, 2018). Treatment is aimed at moving the fluid from the third space to the cellular compartments as well as forcing diuresis. During the initial stage, treatment with LR is generally considered appropriate unless other alterations in electrolyte balance are present. The goal remains to provide adequate circulating volume to maintain an optimal blood pressure and urinary output until the recovery phase begins (Hammon & Hines, 2018).

Hypervolemia

Fluid weight gain with subsequent diuresis should be anticipated following CPB. Hypervolemia, which is also known as fluid volume excess (FVE), occurs when water and serum sodium are proportionately increased in the body. Common causes of FVE include excessive intake of fluids that cannot be removed (e.g., as occurs in renal failure or heart failure, or following administration of fluids at an excessive rate), excessive sodium intake, or inadequate sodium and water elimination (e.g., secondary to heart, renal, or liver failure). In the postoperative cardiac surgery patient, hypervolemia is most commonly related to excessive fluid administration intraoperatively, most notably in patients with either preexisting renal dysfunction, heart failure, or hypoalbuminemia (Shires, 2015).

Assessment

Patients with FVE will manifest weight gain, peripheral edema, distended peripheral veins, jugular venous distention, increased CVP, crackles, decreased dilutional BUN and hematocrit, and bounding pulses. Patients may also develop hypertension, cough, heart murmur, and dependent edema. In cases of severe FVE, pulmonary edema, ascites, or pleural effusion may develop (Huether, 2017a; Shires, 2015).

Treatment

For patients who do not have preexisting renal dysfunction, diuresis is attempted to normalize volume status when hypervolemia occurs, usually with loop diuretics either through continuous infusion or intermittent boluses (Shaw, 2012). Electrolyte balance must be carefully monitored during this time to avoid potentially life-threatening complications of rapid diuretic therapy. For the patient with AKI, RRT (usually through hemodialysis or CRRT) will be necessary to maintain an appropriate fluid volume state. Fluid restriction to less than 1,000 mL/day is typically implemented as well.

Glycemic Issues

Postoperative cardiac surgery patients may have comorbidities that include either type 1 or 2 diabetes mellitus. During times of increased stress, serum glucose levels become more labile, and the patient with or without a history of diabetes is more likely to exhibit hyperglycemia (>110 mg/dL) or hypoglycemia (Hargraves, 2014). Fluctuations in blood glucose levels will also result in alterations in fluid and electrolyte status. Insulin resistance may be noted with utilization of inotropic agents (e.g., epinephrine, norepinephrine), glucocorticoids, or both (Klinkner & Murray, 2014). Tight glycemic control (blood sugars <180 mg/dL) is essential to optimize patient outcomes (Ginwalla et al., 2014; Hargraves, 2014).

In 2009, the Society of Thoracic Surgery published blood glucose guidelines for cardiac surgery patients that recommended the use of continuous insulin infusions during the perioperative phase, up to 24 hours after surgery to maintain blood glucoses at a target of less than 180 mg/dL (Lazar et al., 2009). In 2012, the Society of Critical Care Medicine published a glycemic control guideline recommending starting insulin infusion therapy for a blood glucose greater than 150 mg/dL to maintain a range of 110 to 150 mg/dL and keep below a target of 180 mg/dL for critically ill patients (Jacobi et al., 2012). Since January 2014, the Surgical Care Improvement Plan Inf-4 measure was changed to maintain blood glucose levels less than 180 mg/dL between 18 and 24 hours after anesthesia end time (Klinkner & Murray, 2014).

▶ Acute Kidney Injury and Renal Insufficiency

Unfortunately, some postoperative cardiac surgery patients may have sustained renal damage from ischemia or decreased blood flow. Cardiopulmonary bypass causes an increased secretion of catecholamines, renin, angiotensin II, aldosterone, vasopressin, atrial natriuretic peptide, and proinflammatory mediators. Release of these substances leads to decreases in renal blood flow and GFR (Yazdchi & Rawn, 2018). During CPB, attempts to protect the kidneys focus on ensuring hemodilution, returning to a pulsatile flow as soon as possible, and reestablishing a normal body temperature as quickly as possible (Hammon & Hines, 2018). Monitoring of serum creatinine levels post surgery usually conveys a 0.1- to 0.2-mg/dL decrease for most patients; when it does not, patients need close monitoring for potential in worsening kidney function (Shaw, 2012). Up to 50% of patients post cardiac surgery will experience up to a 25% reduction in creatinine clearance (Ginwalla et al., 2014).

The incidence of AKI in patients undergoing cardiac surgery is approximately 25% to 30%. Of these patients, 1% to 5% may require dialysis therapy (Ginwalla et al., 2014). Patients who had a myocardial infarction may have resultant renal impairment or acute tubular necrosis (ATN) from the ischemia. Patients who are older, have diabetes mellitus, or who have a history of heart failure are more likely to develop AKI following a cardiovascular event (Ricci et al., 2012). Other individuals at higher risk include those with poor underlying cardiac performance, advanced atherosclerosis, and preexisting decreased GFR. The amount of

time spent on CPB and intraoperative instability are also predictors of the development of postoperative renal impairment (Hammon & Hines, 2018).

Renal perfusion must be maintained in all patients. Urinary output should be at least 0.5 mL/kg/hr. For these goals to be met, satisfactory CO and blood pressure are essential. Maintaining them at appropriate levels can be accomplished by delivering volume repletion to keep up with urinary output, which is typically 200 to 300 mL/hr following CPB. If urinary output is maintained with the use of diuretics, renal perfusion is considered adequate (Yazdchi & Rawn, 2018).

Azotemia

Azotemia is the buildup of nitrogenous waste products from protein metabolism; these wastes are normally eliminated by urination (Huether, 2017b). The patient with azotemia will demonstrate increasing serum creatinine and BUN levels, and GFR will decrease. As GFR continues to decline, FVE will develop. Sodium retention with a urine sodium concentration less than 20 mEq/L is a common finding. In this state, a fluid challenge to correct hypovolemia will correct the early renal failure with the exceptions of heart failure or liver failure (Remer et al., 2013).

Acute Kidney Injury

Formerly known as acute renal failure, AKI may be recognized by a sudden, rapid deterioration in renal function. Despite new treatment strategies and improved surveillance methods, the number of patients who develop AKI after cardiac surgery varies in studies from 4% to 9%. The incidence of patients requiring RRT is 2% to 6% with cardiac surgery AKI (Thiele, Isbell, & Rosner, 2015). This is dependent on preoperative renal function and the complexity of the surgical procedure. An increase in serum creatinine of 0.3 mg/dL within 48 hours of surgery signifies Stage I injury according to the Acute Kidney Injury Network (Shaw, 2012).

Elderly patients (>70 years), African Americans, or those with diabetes mellitus, obesity, metabolic syndrome, peripheral vascular disease, preoperative hyperglycemia (>300 mg/dL), preoperative serum creatinine in the range of 1.4 to 2.0 mg/dL, or heart failure prior to admission are at greater risk for development of AKI (Yazdchi & Rawn, 2018). In addition, emergency, aortic, redo, or revision surgeries; prolonged bypass runs (>3 hours); ventricular dysfunction; hypothermia; exposure to nephrotoxic drugs such as contrast media and antibiotics; transfusions; and poor intraoperative blood pressure control contribute to the development of AKI postoperatively (Thiele et al., 2015).

In 2012 the Kidney Disease Improving Global Outcomes (KDIGO) published clinical practice guidelines for AKI. These guidelines build off of Risk, Injury, and Failure; and Loss; and End-stage kidney disease (RIFLE) criteria (Hughes, 2018). More information can be found in web resources at the end of the chapter.

Three types of AKI exist, and diagnosis is based on the point of initial renal insult:

- Prerenal: injury occurring before the kidney
- Intrarenal: intrinsic to the kidney
- Postrenal: injury occurring after the kidney

Acute kidney injury results in alterations in electrolyte balance, acid–base and fluid volume status, nitrogenous waste accumulation, and decreased production of erythropoietin. In the majority of cases, an insult occurs, resulting in multiple organ damage and affecting the ability of the kidneys to function appropriately. Management of AKI will vary based on the etiology and the degree of renal injury.

The predominant cause of AKI in postoperative cardiac surgery patients is ATN. What leads to the cardiac surgery patient developing ATN? Decreased perfusion (MAP <50 mmHg), extremes in anemia, and use of transfusions when hemoglobin is greater than 8 g/dL have been identified as precursors to AKI with cardiac surgery patients (Haase et al., 2012). A meta-analysis showed that timing of coronary angiography, if less than 1 day to time of surgery, significantly increased the incidence of AKI postoperatively (Thiele et al., 2015). A study comparing a higher MAP (75–85 mmHg) while on normothermic CPB versus a control group with a MAP of 50 to 60 mmHg on normothermic CPB did not reduce the incidence of postoperative AKI (Azau et al., 2014). Though these do not answer the question specifically, they are helping to identify ways to prevent ATN and AKI and focus research questions for the future. Prevention of hypotension, hypovolemia, and nephrotoxic agents are key to preventing AKI (Huether, 2017b).

The majority of cases of ATN result in suppression of bone marrow, endocrine disturbance, coagulopathy, and cardiovascular dysfunction as normal homeostasis can no longer be maintained. Acute tubular necrosis can be postischemic, nephrotoxic, or both (Dynamed Plus, 2017). Prolonged hypotension and hypovolemic shock are the most common causes of postischemic ATN. Renal cellular death begins to occur when MAP falls below 75 mmHg. The extent of the renal damage may be estimated by determining the length of time of renal ischemia, with ischemia of 25 min or less generally causing reversible mild injury, ischemia of 40 to 60 min causing damage that will take the kidneys 2 to 3 weeks to recover from, and ischemia lasting longer than 1 to 1.5 hours causing irreversible damage (Dynamed Plus, 2017). As ischemia progresses, the renal tubular cells swell, become injured, and eventually become necrotic (Huether, 2017b).

Assessment

The patient with ATN will present with oliguria or anuria, elevated BUN and serum creatinine, and isosthenuria (a condition in which urinary osmolality approximates plasma osmolality). Oliguria is generally defined as urinary output less than 500 mL over a period of 24 hours; anuria is defined as urinary output less than 50 mL in 24 hours. Patients should be closely monitored for life-threatening alterations in electrolyte levels. Frequent laboratory testing will be necessary to monitor serum electrolytes and complete blood count. Fluid volume excess will develop, and the patient will present with its associated signs and symptoms.

The patient with ATN will progress through the four stages of AKI in a relatively predictable pattern. Initiation is the first stage; it is followed by oliguria, diuresis, and then recovery. The last two stages will typically not be managed in the ICU and therefore are not within the scope of this chapter. The total length of time from onset of renal damage to recovery can last from months to 1 year.

Initiation Stage

The initiation stage of AKI begins when the renal insult occurs and lasts from a few hours to a few days. Initial signs and symptoms of renal impairment are noticed (increase in serum creatinine by ≥0.3 mg/dL within 48 hours, or increase to at least 1.5 times baseline occurring within previous week, or urine output <0.5 mL/kg/hr for 6 hours). The cause of AKI is investigated. Initial signs and symptoms generally include a decrease in urinary output, crackles, muffled heart sounds, development of a new heart murmur or S_3 gallop, and an increase in body weight indicating FVE (Huether, 2017b). Three new biomarkers can be measured through plasma or urine—neutrophil gelatinase-associated lipocalin, kidney injury molecule-1, and cystatin C—which may be indicative of early kidney ischemia/injury in as little as 2 to 24 hours after surgery (Shaw, 2012). In addition, urine interleukin-18 is another promising biomarker being studied to identify early kidney injury (Mao et al., 2013). The earlier that injury can be identified, the earlier treatment can begin.

Oliguric Stage

Oliguria is a decrease in urinary volume to less than 500 mL/24 hours or less than 0.5 mL/kg/hr for more than 6 hours. The diminished urinary output seen with ATN occurs when shock or dehydration leads to inadequate perfusion of the kidneys. The oliguric stage generally lasts from 1 to 3 weeks and is potentially reversible (Huether, 2017b).

Laboratory data will indicate a decrease in GFR, an increase in serum creatinine and BUN, and an elevation in the electrolytes excreted by the renal system (potassium, sodium, and phosphorus). Laboratory data must be closely monitored, because these patients are susceptible to developing hyperkalemia and hyperphosphatemia from apoptosis (cellular death and breakdown). A frequent cause of death during the oliguric stage is cardiac arrest secondary to hyperkalemia.

Symptoms of heart failure may occur as FVE increases. Potential for infection, particularly pulmonary, and delay in incisional wound healing may occur. Anuria is rare in ATN and involves injury to both kidneys. Nonoliguria is evidenced in 10% to 20% of cases and is less severe with fewer complications (Huether, 2017b).

During the oliguric or anuric phase, the patient needs to be closely monitored for alterations in electrolyte status and prepared for RRT to remove waste products and excess fluid, and to return electrolytes to near normal levels.

Treatment

Morbidity and mortality rates are significantly increased in postoperative cardiac surgery patients who develop renal dysfunction (Yazdchi & Rawn, 2018). The most essential prevention measure and treatment intervention for AKI is maintaining adequate renal perfusion monitoring CO, stroke volume, and degree of responsiveness to fluid (Thiele et al., 2015). Normal autoregulation in healthy individuals maintains a MAP of 60 to 120 mmHg (Shaw, 2012). Nursing interventions focus on maintaining strict intake and output and monitoring oxygen saturation, vital signs, and fluid volume status. Prevention of further ischemia is necessary to prevent additional renal damage from occurring. Because third spacing and significant diuresis are common following CPB, a fluid challenge will likely be initiated. Urinary output should be maintained at a rate of at least 0.5 mL/kg/hr. The patient's hemodynamic profile must be optimized, and use of nephrotoxic agents should be avoided (Yazdchi & Rawn, 2018). If the patient progresses to oliguria or anuria, RRT will be required.

Both hemodialysis and CRRT act via the principles of osmosis, diffusion, and filtration. Continuous renal replacement therapy has the added advantage of being able to slowly and safely provide for ultrafiltration and thereby help remove excess fluid over a slower period of time. This gradual action is beneficial when cardiac performance is compromised and the patient cannot tolerate rapid fluctuations in fluid volume status. Cardiac failure intrinsically leads to hemodynamic instability, making CRRT an optimal choice for the postoperative cardiac surgery patient with AKI (Brownback, Fletcher, Pierce, & Klaus, 2014). Zou, Hong, and Xu (2017), in a meta-analysis looking at 1,597 cases in 15 studies, concluded that early initiation of CRRT decreased 28-day mortality, particularly if therapy was started within the first 24 hours.

While receiving CRRT, the patient must be closely monitored for alterations in fluid and electrolyte status, as well as cardiac, respiratory, GI, and neurologic function. Successful CRRT results in removal of fluid and toxins, clearer breath sounds, improved CO, and stabilization in vital signs.

▶ Summary

Caring for postoperative cardiac surgery patients requires extensive knowledge, skill, and sound critical thinking that allow the critical care nurse to perform patient assessment and management in a rapidly changing environment. Life-threatening alterations in fluid and electrolyte balances may be present from previous surgery, previous comorbid conditions, or a combination of these factors.

Nurses caring for postoperative cardiac surgery patients should also be aware of the manifestations of AKI and its treatment options. The primary methods of prevention and treatment of AKI for cardiac surgery patients entail interventions that optimize perfusion and oxygen delivery to all tissues. Patients usually receive diuretic therapy starting on the first postoperative day for postoperative fluid overload and redistribution when a patient is nonoliguric. This therapy typically continues until the patient's preoperative weight has been reestablished. The ICU nurse plays a pivotal role in assessing, attaining, and maintaining fluid and electrolyte balance and optimizing patient outcomes.

🔍 CASE STUDY

W. G., a 67-year-old patient with a history of angina, hypertension, and hyperlipidemia, is admitted through the emergency department with chest pain. An ECG revealed ST segment elevation; an echocardiogram revealed an ejection fraction of 25%. The patient underwent cardiac catheterization, which revealed triple-vessel disease. He is taken to the operating room for an on-pump coronary artery bypass grafting (CABG) procedure. During the procedure, he underwent cardioplegic arrest. He was cooled to 28°C during the procedure and gradually rewarmed. Bypass time was 94 min. A total of 2,400 mL of crystalloids and colloids were administered. He is admitted to the ICU postoperatively.

Critical Thinking Questions

1. Based on this patient's clinical course, for which electrolyte abnormalities should the nurse observe?
2. What risk factors put the patient at risk for electrolyte disturbances postoperatively?
3. For which dysrhythmias should the nurse assess if the patient has hypomagnesemia?

Answers to Critical Thinking Questions

1. This patient is at particular risk for depleted levels of potassium, magnesium, calcium, and phosphorus. Extracorporeal circulation leads to the depletion of multiple electrolytes.
2. Patients who receive CPB are at risk for electrolyte depletion. These depletions are likely related to intracellular ion shift and increased urinary elimination of electrolytes from the bypass circuitry and from intraoperative hypothermia. Cardioplegia, decreased urinary output, hemolysis from the extracorporeal circuit, and decreased insulin levels may result in hyperkalemia. Conversely, aggressive diuresis, presence of an alkalosis, or increased insulin levels may lead to hypokalemia. Following CPB and hemodilution, hypomagnesemia is common. Hypocalcemia is common following CPB as well.
3. Patients with hypomagnesemia should be observed for atrial fibrillation and torsades de pointes.

Self-Assessment Questions

1. Which of the following consequences affecting fluid exchange should the nurse anticipate following cardiac surgery?
   A. Increased hydrostatic pressure
   B. Increased colloid osmotic pressure
   C. Decreased hydrostatic pressure
   D. Decreased colloid osmotic pressure

2. Which of the following should the nurse anticipate following cardiopulmonary bypass?
   A. Sodium excretion
   B. Potassium retention
   C. Increased cortisol levels
   D. Decreased extracellular volume

3. A patient with a body mass index of 35 kg/m² immediately following cardiac surgery has pain and shivering and develops dizziness, weakness, confusion, and tetany. Which of the following ABG results should the nurse suspect?

	pH	pCO₂	HCO₃
A.	7.30	50	25
B.	7.49	42	31
C.	7.51	31	22
D.	7.31	35	18

4. A postoperative cardiac surgery patient has the following ABG values: pH 7.24, pCO₂ 30, pO₂ 65, HCO₃ 16. For which of the following should the nurse assess?
   A. Serum calcium 12.2 mg/dL
   B. Serum potassium 5.9 mEq/L
   C. Serum calcium 8.0 mg/dL
   D. Serum potassium 3.6 mEq/L

5. A postoperative cardiac surgery patient develops the following ABG values: pH 7.50, pCO₂ 30, pO₂ 68, HCO₃ 23. For which of the following should the nurse assess?
   A. Pain
   B. Hypothermia
   C. Atelectasis
   D. Hyperkalemia

6. A patient following cardiac surgery has the following ABG results: pH 7.51, pCO₂ 45, pO₂ 80, HCO₃ 30. For which of the following electrolyte abnormalities should the nurse observe?
   A. Serum calcium 8.1 mg/dL

   B. Serum potassium 5.0 mEq/L
   C. Serum sodium 132 mEq/L
   D. Serum phosphorus 4.9 mg/dL

7. A postoperative cardiac surgery patient has the following laboratory results: Na 137 mEq/L, K 2.9 mEq/L, Mg 1.4 mg/dL, pH 7.50, pCO₂ 39, pO₂ 78, HCO₃ 30. For which of the following should the nurse observe?
   A. Shortened PR interval
   B. Peaked T waves
   C. ST segment elevation
   D. U wave

8. A postoperative cardiac surgery patient presents with lethargy, muscle weakness, and dilated pupils. A magnesium level of 3.2 mg/dL is noted. For which of the following should the nurse observe?
   A. Shortened PR interval
   B. Tachycardia
   C. Atrial arrhythmias
   D. Complete heart block

9. A patient following CPB who received multiple transfusions intraoperatively and postoperatively develops tremors, muscle cramps, numbness of the fingers, and hyperactive bowel sounds. For which of the following should the nurse observe?
   A. Shortened QT interval
   B. Asystole
   C. Tachycardia
   D. Bundle branch block

10. A patient is receiving 0.45% NS. For which of the following should the nurse observe?
    A. Hyperosmolarity
    B. Hyponatremia
    C. Osmotic diuresis
    D. Cerebral edema

Answers to Self-Assessment Questions

1. D. **decreased colloid osmotic pressure**
   Rationale: During and following cardiopulmonary bypass, the body experiences an increase in interstitial volume, sodium retention, and potassium excretion. Plasma

colloid osmotic pressure decreases over the same time. A decrease in colloid osmotic pressure from surgery causes an increase in capillary permeability. This results in fluid shifts from the vascular space to the interstitium.

2. C. **increased cortisol levels**
   Rationale: Cortisol is secreted in response to stress.

3. A. **7.30 / 50 / 25**
   Rationale: This patient has obesity, as evidenced by the body mass index. Obesity is a cause of a respiratory acidosis in the postoperative cardiac surgery patient. This ABG reveals a respiratory acidosis.

4. B. **serum potassium 5.9 mEq/L**
   Rationale: This patient has an uncompensated (compensating) metabolic acidosis. Hyperkalemia frequently accompanies a metabolic acidosis.

5. A. **pain**
   Rationale: This patient has a respiratory alkalosis. Pain is a common cause of a respiratory alkalosis postoperatively as it can cause hyperventilation.

6. A. **serum calcium 8.1 mg/dL**
   Rationale: This patient has a metabolic alkalosis. These patients oftentimes have a concomitant hypokalemia and hypocalcemia.

7. D. **U wave**
   Rationale: This patient has a metabolic alkalosis. These patients oftentimes have a concomitant hypokalemia. Patients with hypokalemia often have depressed T waves and the presence of a U wave.

8. D. **complete heart block**
   Rationale: It is not uncommon for patients with a magnesium level higher than 2.5 mg/dL to experience ventricular dysrhythmias, bradycardia, prolonged PR interval, widened QRS, complete heart block, or cardiac arrest.

9. B. **asystole**
   Rationale: This patient is demonstrating symptoms of hypocalcemia. It is likely related to the multiple transfusions received during surgery. Packed red blood cells are conditioned with citrate to prevent clotting. When citrate combines with calcium, hypocalcemia can occur. Signs and symptoms of hypocalcemia include QT prolongation, shortness of breath, and dysrhythmias ranging from bradycardia to asystole.

10. D. **cerebral edema**
    Rationale: 0.45% saline is a hypotonic solution. Administration of hypotonic crystalloids may result in cerebral edema or seizures.

CLINICAL INQUIRY BOX

Question: Does the conventional model on the distribution of electrolyte infusion hold true in patients undergoing cardiac surgery?

Reference: Hessels, L., Lansink, A. O., Renes, M. H., van der Horst, I. C., Hoekstra, M., Touw, D. J., . . . Nijsten, M. W. (2016). Postoperative fluid retention after heart surgery is accompanied by a strongly positive sodium balance and a negative potassium balance. *Physiological Reports, 4*(1). doi:10.14814/phy2.12807

Objective: To determine if the conventional model on the distribution of fluid and electrolytes over the extracellular and intracellular spaces holds true after cardiac surgery.

Method: Complementary balance studies in 39 patients over 4 days.

Results: Over a 4-day period, 14 ± 0.6 of fluid, 1,465 ± 79 mm sodium, 196 ± 11 mmol potassium, and 1,408 ± 69 mmol chloride were administered. Cumulative balance of fluid 4.0 ± 0.6 L was seen with positive 8.14 ± 75 and 569 ± 83 potassium and chloride. Net potassium balance of −101 ± 14 mmol and new extracellular fluid volume balance of −1.1 ± 0.2 L.

Conclusion: There was rapid and extreme volume expansion of extracellular volume, while intracellular fluid volume did not expand.

References

Agraharkar, M. (2018). *Hypercalcemia treatment and management*. Retrieved from https://emedicine.medscape.com/article/240681-treatment

Annane, D., Siami, S., Jaber, S., Martin, C., Elatrous S., Declere, A. D., . . . Chevret, S. (2013). Effects of fluid resuscitation with colloids vs crystalloids on mortality in critically ill patients presenting with hypovolemic shock: The CRISTAL randomized trial. *Journal of the American Medical Association, 310*(17), 1809–1817.

Azau, A., Markowicz, P., Corbeau, J. J., Cottineau, C., Moreau, X., Baufreton, C., . . . Beydon, L. (2014). Increasing mean arterial pressure during cardiac surgery does not reduce the rate of postoperative acute kidney injury. *Perfusion, 29*(6), 496–504.

Brownback, C. A., Fletcher, P., Pierce, L. N., & Klaus, S. (2014). Early mobility activities during continuous renal replacement therapy. *American Journal of Critical Care, 23*(4), 348–351.

Chhabra, S., Chhabra, S., Ramessure, K. & Chhabra S. (2012). *Hypomagnesemia and its implications in type 2 diabetes mellitus—A review article*. Retrieved from https://www.webmedcentral.com/article_view/3878

Clayton, M. F., McCance, K. L., & Takahashi, L. K. (2017). Stress and disease. In S. E. Huether, K. L. McCance, V. L. Brashers, & N. S. Rote (Eds.), *Understanding pathophysiology* (6th ed, pp. 214–232). St. Louis, MO: Elsevier.

Crestanello, J. A., Philllips, G., Firstenberg, M. S., Sai-Sudhakar, C., Sirak, J., Higgins, R., . . . Abraham, W. T. (2013). Postoperative hyponatremia predicts an increase in mortality and in-hospital complications after cardiac surgery. *Journal of the American College of Surgeons, 216*(6), 1135–1143.

Dynamed Plus. (2017). *Acute kidney injury*. Ipswich, MA: EBSCO Information Services. Retrieved from https://www.dynamed.com/resultlist?q=acute+kidney+injury&filter=all

El-Sharkawy, A. M., Sahota, O., Maughan, R. J., & Lobo, D. N. (2014). The pathophysiology of fluid and electrolyte balance in the older adult surgical patient. *Clinical Nutrition, 33*(1), 6–13.

Garazi, E., Bridge, S., Caffarelli, A., Ruoss, S., & Van der Starre, P. (2015). Acute cellular insulin resistance and hyperglycemia associated with hypophosphatemia after cardiac surgery. *Anesthesia & Analgesia Case Reports, 4*(2),22–25.

Ginwalla, R., Faraday, N., & Whitman, G. (2014). Postoperative management of the cardiac surgical patient. In D. D. Yuh, L. A. Vricella, S. C. Yang, & J. R. Doty (Eds.), *Johns Hopkins textbook of cardiothoracic surgery* (2nd ed., pp. 371–386). New York, NY: McGraw-Hill.

Green, T. E. (2017). *Hypercalcemia in emergency medicine*. Retrieved from https://emedicine.medscape.com/article/766373-overview?pa=1Pa8pwUDbUzFuzy7OYkP55meDedEBzMwk3NNnvC1zBjCQ%2Fdu6OjMTqjH1JpfhKob

Gurrado, A., Piccinni, G., Lissidini, G., Di Fronzo, P., Vittore, F., & Testini, M. (2012). Hypercalcaemic crisis due to primary hyperparathyroidism—A systematic literature review and case report. *Endokrynologia Polska, 63*(6), 494–502.

Haase, M., Bellomo, R., Story, D., Letis, A., Klemz, K., Matalanis, G., . . . Haase-Fielitz, A. (2012). Effect of mean arterial pressure, haemoglobin and blood transfusion during cardiopulmonary bypass on post-operative acute kidney injury. *Nephrology Dialysis Transplantation, 27*(1) 153–160.

Hahn, R. G. (2011). Crystalloid fluids. In R. G. Hahn (Ed.), *Clinical fluid therapy in the perioperative setting* (pp. 1–10). New York, NY: Cambridge University Press.

Hammon, J. W., & Hines, M. H. (2018). Extracorporeal circulation. In L. H. Cohn & D. Adams (Eds.), *Cardiac surgery in the adult* (5th ed., pp. 299–346). New York, NY: McGraw-Hill.

Hargraves, J. D. (2014). Glycemic control in cardiac surgery: Implementing an evidence-based insulin infusion protocol. *American Journal of Critical Care, 23*(3), 250–258.

Huether, S. E. (2017a). Fluids and electrolytes, acids and bases. In S. E. Huether, K. L. McCance, V. L. Brashers, & N. S. Rote (Eds.), *Understanding pathophysiology* (6th ed., pp. 114–132). St. Louis, MO: Elsevier Inc.

Hughes, P. J. (2018). *Classification systems for acute kidney injury*. Retrieved from www.emedicine.medscape.com/article/1925597-overview

Huether, S. E. (2017b). Alterations of renal and urinary tract function. In S. E. Huether, K. L. McCance, V. L. Brashers, & N. S. Rote (Eds.), *Understanding pathophysiology* (6th ed., pp. 747–769). St. Louis, MO: Elsevier Inc.

Jacobi, J., Bircher, N., Krinsley, J., Agus, M., Braithwaite, S. S., Deutschman, C., . . . Schunemann, H. (2012). Guidelines for the use of an insulin infusion for the management of hyperglycemia in critically ill patients. *Critical Care Medicine, 40*(12), 3251–3276.

Kara, A., Akin, S., & Ince, C. (2016). The response of the microcirculation to cardiac surgery. *Current Opinion in Anaesthesiology, 29*(1), 85–93.

Klinkner, G., & Murray, M. (2014). Clinical nurse specialists lead teams to impact glycemic control after cardiac surgery. *Clinical Nurse Specialist, 28*(4), 240–246.

Kouchoukos, N. T., Blackstone, E. H., Hanley, F. L., & Kirklin, J. K. (2013). Postoperative care. In N. T. Kouchoukos, E. H. Blackstone, F. L. Hanley, & J. K. Kirklin (Eds.), *Kirklin/Barratt-Boyes cardiac surgery* (4th ed., pp. 189–250). Philadelphia, PA: Elsevier Saunders.

Lazar, H. L., McDonnell, M., Chipkin, S. R., Furnary, A. P., Engelman, R. M., Sadhu, A. R., . . . Shemin, R. J. (2009). The Society of Thoracic Surgeons practice guideline series: Blood glucose management during adult cardiac surgery. *Annals of Thoracic Surgery, 87*, 663–669.

Lederer, E., Ouseph, R., & Nayak, V. (2014). *Hyperphosphatemia*. eMedicine Update. Retrieved from http://emedicine.medscape.com/article/241185-overview

Lindner, G., & Funk, G.-C. (2013). Hypernatremia in critically ill patients. *Journal of Critical Care, 28*, 216, e11–e20.

Mao, H., Katz, N., Ariyanon, W., Blanca-Martos, L., Adybelli, Z., Giuliani, A., . . . Ronco, C. (2013). Cardiac surgery-associated acute kidney injury. *Cardiorenal Medicine, 3*(3), 178–199.

Moritz, M. L., & Ayus, J. C. (2015). Maintenance intravenous fluids in acutely ill patients. *The New England Journal of Medicine, 373*(14), 1350–1360.

Mutter, T. C., Ruth, C. A., & Dart, A. B. (2013). Hydroxyethyl starch (HES) versus other fluid therapies: Effects on kidney function. *Cochrane Database of Systematic Reviews, 7*, Art. No.: CD007594. doi:10.1002/14651858.CD007594.pub3

Myburgh, J. A., Finfer, S., Bellomo, R., Billot, L., Cass, A., Gattas, D., . . . Webb, S. A. R. (2012). Hydroxyethyl starch or saline for fluid resuscitation in intensive care. *The New England Journal of Medicine, 367*(20), 1901–1911.

Nguyen, H. V., Bose, S., & Finkelstein, E. (2016). Incremental cost-utility of sevelamer relative to calcium carbonate for treatment of hyperphosphatemia among pre-dialysis chronic kidney disease patients. *BMC Nephrology, 17*, 1–9.

Perner, A., Haase, N., Guttormsen, A. B., Tenhunen, J., Klemenzson, G., Aneman, A., . . . Wetterslev, J. (2012). Hydroxyethyl starch 130/0.42 versus Ringer's acetate in severe sepsis. *The New England Journal of Medicine, 367*(2), 124–134.

Pollock, F., & Funk, D. C. (2013). Acute diabetes management: Adult patients with hyperglycemic crises and hypoglycemia. *AACN Advanced Critical Care, 24*(3), 314–324.

Protsyk, V., Rasmussen, B. S., Guarracino, F., Erb, J., Turton, E., & Ender, J. (2017). Fluid management in cardiac surgery: Results of a survey in European cardiac anesthesia departments. *Journal of Cardiothoracic and Vascular Anesthesia, 31*, 1624–1629.

Raiman, M., Mitchell, C. G., Biccard, B. M., & Rodseth, R. N. (2016). Comparison of hydroxyethyl starch colloids with crystalloids for surgical patients—a systemic review and meta-analysis. *European Journal of Anesthesiology, 33*, 42–48.

Raiten, J. M., Ghadimi, K., Augoustides, J. G. T., Ramakrishna, H., Patel, P. A., Weiss, S. J., . . . Gutsche, J. T. (2015). Atrial fibrillation after cardiac surgery: Clinical update on mechanisms and prophylactic strategies. *Journal of Cardiothoracic and Vascular Anesthesia, 29*(3), 806–816.

Reddy, S. K., Bailey, M. J., Beasley, R. W., Bellomo, R., Mackle, D. M., Psirides, A. J., . . . Young, P. J. (2017). Effect of 0.9% saline or Plasma-Lyte 148 as crystalloid fluid therapy in the intensive care unit on blood product use and postoperative bleeding after cardiac surgery. *Journal of Cardiovascular and Vascular Anesthesia, 31*(5), 1630–1638.

Remer, E. M., Papanicolaou, N., Casalino, D. D., Bishoff, J. T., Blaufox, M. D., Coursey, C. A., . . . Weinfeld, R. M. (2013). *ACR Appropriateness Criteria®: Renal failure.* Retrieved from http://www.guideline.gov/content.aspx?id=47681

Rhee, P., & Joseph, B. (2017). Shock, electrolytes, and fluid. In C. M. Townsend Jr., R. D. Beauchamp, B. M. Evers, & K. L. Mattox (Eds.), *Sabiston textbook of surgery* (20th ed., pp. 44–97). St. Louis, MO: Elsevier.

Ricci, Z., Romagnoli, S., & Ronco, C. (2012). Perioperative intravascular volume replacement and kidney insufficiency. *Best Practice & Research Clinical Anaesthesiology, 26*, 463–474.

Ryhammer, P. K., Tang, M., Hoffmann-Petersen, J., Leonaviciute, D., Greisen, M. S., & Jakobsen, C.-J. (2017). Colloids in cardiac surgery—friend or foe? *Journal of Cardiothoracic and Vascular Anesthesia, 31*, 1639–1648.

Schortgen, F., & Schetz, M. (2017). Does this critically ill patient with oliguria need more fluids, a vasopressor, or neither? *Intensive Care Medicine, 43*, 907–910.

Shaw, A. (2012). Update on acute kidney injury after cardiac surgery. *The Journal of Thoracic and Cardiovascular Surgery, 143*(3), 676–681.

Sheikh, A., Platts-Mills, T., & Worth, A. (2013). Allergic reactions to colloid infusions—another chapter in the colloid debate. *Oxford Medicine Online.* doi:10.1093/med/9780199651559.001.0001

Shires III, G. T. (2015). Fluid and electrolyte management of the surgical patient. In F. Brunicardi, D. K. Andersen, T. R. Billiar, D. L. Dunn, J. G. Hunter, J. B. Matthews, R. E. Pollock (Eds.), *Schwartz's principles of surgery* (10th ed., pp. 65–84). New York, NY: McGraw-Hill.

Song, L. (2017). Calcium and bone metabolism indices. *Advances in Clinical Chemistry, 82*, 1–46.

Tamez-Pérez, H. E., Quintanilla-Flores, D. L., Rodriguez-Gutiérrez, R., González-González, J. G., & Tamez-Peña, A. L. (2015). Steroid hyperglycemia: Prevalence, early detection and therapeutic recommendations: A narrative review. *World Journal of Diabetes, 6*(8), 1073–1081.

Thiele, R. H., Isbell, J. M., & Rosner, M. H. (2015). AKI associated with cardiac surgery. *Clinical Journal of American Society of Nephrology, 10*, 500–514.

Thomas, C. P. (2014). *Syndrome of inappropriate antidiuretic hormone secretion.* Retrieved from http://emedicine.medscape.com/article/246650-overview

Tokmaji, G., McClure, R. S., Kaneko, T., & Aranki, S. F. (2013). Management strategies in cardiac surgery for postoperative atrial fibrillation: Contemporary prophylaxis and futuristic anticoagulant possibilities. *Cardiology Research and Practice, 2013*, 1–16. http://dx.doi.org/10.1155/2013/637482

Vogel, D., & Comerota, A. J. (2014). Role of antithrombotic drugs in maintaining graft patency. In J. C. Stanley, F. Veith, & T. W. Wakefield (Eds.), *Current therapy in vascular and endovascular surgery* (5th ed., pp. 620–621). Philadelphia, PA: Elsevier Saunders.

Weinstein, S. M. (2014). Fluid and electrolyte balance. In S. M. Weinstein & M. E. Hagle (Eds.), *Plumer's principles and practices of infusion therapy* (9th ed., pp. 142–172). Philadelphia, PA: Lippincott Williams & Wilkins.

Yazdchi, F., & Rawn, J. D. (2018). Postoperative care of cardiac surgery patients. In L. H. Cohn, & D. Adams (Eds.), *Cardiac surgery in the adult* (5th ed., pp. 405–428). New York, NY: McGraw-Hill.

Yunos, N. M., Bellomo, R., Hegarty, C., Story, D., Ho, L., & Bailey, M. (2012). Association between a chloride-liberal vs chloride-restrictive intravenous fluid administration strategy and kidney injury in critically ill adults. *Journal of American Medical Association, 308*(15), 1566–1572.

Zou, H., Hong, Q., & Xu, G. (2017). Early versus late initiation of renal replacement therapy impacts mortality in patients with acute kidney injury post cardiac surgery: A meta-analysis. *Critical Care, 21*(150), 1–10.

Web Resource

Guidelines for AKI management from Kidney International Supplements: https://www.kdigo.org/clinical_practice_guideline/pdf/KDIGO%20AKI%20Guideline.pdf

Water and electrolyte balance: http://www.youtube.com/watch?v=vvGyHBWcQQU

CHAPTER 18

Wound Care

Vicki Morelock, Mary Zellinger

▶ Introduction

Assessment and care of postoperative surgical sites will have a profound impact on patient outcomes after cardiac surgery. Surgical site infections (SSIs) of the sternum and underlying mediastinum occur in up to 5% of patients who undergo such procedures (Bryan & Yarbrough, 2013; Lazar, Salm, Engelman, Orgill, & Gordon, 2016; Lemaignen et al., 2015; Sexton, 2016). The incidence of superficial SSIs is approximately 3% (Stephens & Whitman, 2015).

Infections can lead to significant morbidity, warranting an increased length of hospitalization due to complications, pain and stress, higher costs of care, and patient mortality. In the past, patients with a deep sternal wound infection (DSWI) had an expected mortality rate of 20% to 45%. This rate has dramatically decreased to 1% to 14% with the advent of superior surgical techniques (Gudbjartsson et al., 2016). Care must include preventive measures. Observant practitioners must routinely assess for factors that may potentially slow surgical wound healing and follow strict and consistent protocols in caring for these incisions. This chapter describes the wound care that is required for the postoperative cardiac surgery patient and explores the pivotal role the intensive care unit

(ICU) nurse plays in preventing potentially fatal complications associated with SSIs.

▶ Incision Sites

Surgical access options in cardiac surgery patients have greatly increased in the past several years. Midline sternotomy access is still the most common access and is used for patients who are operated on with or without the aid of cardiopulmonary bypass (CPB). The lengths of these incisions can range from 6 to 10 inches. Mini-thoracotomy incisions of approximately 2 inches are also used in cardiac surgery. Alternative approaches to the traditional midsternal incision include submammary incisions (can be full or partial sternotomies), the anterolateral or posterolateral thoracotomies, and the clamshell incision, also known as a transverse sternotomy. All of these have an improved cosmetic appeal. A right mini-thoracotomy approach may also be used to reach the aortic area to repair congenital heart defects such as ventricular septal defects in adults (An, Zhang, Zheng, Wang, & Ma, 2017; Bowdish et al., 2015). Right vertical infra-axillary and totally thorascopic approaches can be used for atrial septal defects in adults and children (Luo et al., 2014). Port access and robotic surgeries approach the heart through the left chest wall in the case of coronary artery bypass and through the right chest wall for mitral valve repair or replacement.

In minimally invasive bypass, ports for the left internal mammary artery (IMA), also known as the internal thoracic artery (ITA), are placed in the third, fifth, and seventh intercostal spaces (ICSs), with a fourth slightly larger working port (2–3 inches) for the anastomosis located in the fourth or fifth ICS. Minimally invasive valve procedures may utilize a mini–right thoracotomy (third ICS for aortic valve and fourth ICS for mitral valve) or a hemisternotomy (upper for aortic valve procedures and lower for mitral valve procedures) (Bowdish et al., 2015; Kaneda et al., 2013). Each of these procedures has the potential to result in the complication of infection.

▶ Conduits

The internal thoracic artery is an ideal conduit to use for bypass grafting, although other conduits may be used as well. The ITA does not have valves as vein grafts do, so there is no obstruction to flow. In addition, arteries are more vasoresponsive than veins. The IMA also lends distal protection to atherosclerosis. The ITA is taken down from the chest wall during on-pump, off-pump, and minimally invasive surgery and does not require a separate incision for removal.

The radial artery is another frequently used conduit. It can be removed without fear of diminishing blood flow to the hand if the ulnar artery is functioning adequately. Removal of the radial artery typically requires a 2- to 4-inch incision. Because of its visibility, it may be easily monitored in the postoperative period. Due to its potential for spasm, typically diltiazem (Cardizem®) is started for the first postoperative day. The gastroepiploic artery is rarely used as a conduit during cardiac surgery because of the high chance of contamination that may occur when the abdominal cavity is open at the same time as the sternum.

The saphenous vein is often removed from the leg when other arteries are not available or when additional grafts are needed. The saphenous vein may be removed utilizing an open vein harvest procedure or through an endoscopic procedure—endoscopic vein harvesting (EVH) using two or three small (1.5–3 cm) incisions via endoscope (Raja & Sarang, 2013; Santo et al., 2014). The saphenous vein is the most commonly used graft, even though within 1 year, 10% to 20% fail, an additional 5% to 10% fail in 1 to 5 years, and an additional 20% to 25% fail in 6 to 10 years. At 10 years, only about half of saphenous vein grafts are patent, and of those, only half are free of angiographic arteriosclerosis (Sabik, 2011). Patients who undergo EVH experience less swelling and discomfort when walking, which is an early postoperative goal. However, patients who undergo EVH may develop a myocardial infarction (MI). Revascularization may need to be repeated. Increased mortality rates are also associated with EVH (Hess et al., 2014).

Wound complication incidence with open vein harvest procedures ranges from 2% to 25%. It is well documented through multiple studies and meta-analyses that EVH has significantly reduced infection rates. In addition, with the increased use of EVH, noninfective wound derangements have lessened (e.g., wound drainage, edema, erythema, dehiscence) (Raja & Sarang, 2013; Santo et al., 2014). Although wound complications are reduced, reported endoscopic harvested vein graft failure has heightened the need for further randomized clinical trials (Hess et al., 2014).

When comparing a preoperative microbial skin sealant on the skin versus bare skin in a randomized control study, Falk-Brynhildsen, Soderquist, Friberg, and Nilsson (2014) found no significant difference in infection or dehiscence rates. They observed a 16.8% infection rate with *Staphyloccous aureus* as the pathogen 62% of the time. This was thought to be contamination from the hands and nares of the patient, health care workers, environment, or any combination of these.

While saphenous veins are the most commonly utilized grafts, arterial grafts are the preferred conduits. Arterial grafts have better long-term patency, but are short in length, have a small diameter, and have limited availability, resulting in the need for multiple grafts.

▸ Risk Factors for Wound Complications

Several factors put patients at greater risk for developing postoperative wound complications. These risk factors can be categorized as preoperative, intraoperative, or postoperative.

Preoperative Risk Factors

Preoperative assessment of risk factors for wound complications is imperative. Early and sustained attention to these risk factors is mandatory. **BOX 18.1** lists the most common preoperative risk factors.

The presence of diabetes may impede wound healing by leading to a compromised immune system. Both chemotaxis and phagocytosis play a role in the wound healing process. If serum glucose levels remain elevated, both of these processes will be compromised (Ahmed & Antonsen, 2016). Chemotaxis is the oriented movement toward or away from a chemical stimulus—in this case, the process by which white cells are attracted to the site of an infection. Phagocytosis is the ingestion of bacteria by white cells. Delayed macrophage introduction and diminished leukocyte migration, which cause a prolonged inflammatory phase, interfere in the wound healing process (Ahmed & Antonsen, 2016; Xuan et al., 2014). Unfortunately, a large number of patients presenting for surgery are unaware of their diabetes status and thus may have an uncontrolled serum glucose level preoperatively. It is becoming common practice for HbA_{1c} to be tested preoperatively because it is a high predictor of adverse outcomes (Subramaniam et al., 2014). Faritous and colleagues (2014) found that patients with elevated HbA_{1c} and elevated fasting blood sugars had significantly higher rates of wound infection, sepsis, and postoperative reintubation. Controlling blood glucose levels preoperatively and addressing them immediately in the perioperative period help mitigate complications such as impaired wound healing in the postoperative period.

Advanced age may also diminish wound healing. There are age-related changes affecting

BOX 18.1 Preoperative Risk Factors for Wound Complications

Diabetes
Elevated HbA_{1c}
Advanced age
Obesity
Diabetes or perioperative hyperglycemia
Peripheral artery disease
Tobacco use
Previous cardiac surgery
Large breast size
COPD (e.g., emphysema)
Urgent or emergent CABG repeat operations
Steroids
Preoperative hospital stay of greater than 5 days
Poor nutrition
Venous impairment
Renal failure
Certain medications
Jaundice
Decreased mobility/activity
Dehydration
Respiratory disease
Infection
Anemia
Smoking
Pain
Decreased immunity

CABG, coronary artery bypass grafting; COPD, chronic obstructive pulmonary disease; HbA_{1c}, hemoglobin A_{1c}
Data from Bryan & Yarbrough, 2013; Cotogni, Barbero, & Rinaldi, 2015; Musallam 2014, Sexton 2016; Stephens & Whitman, 2015; Subramaniam et al., 2014.

all aspects of wound healing. Evidence suggests that inherent diminished phagocytic activity may impair tissue repair and regeneration in older patients (Sgonc & Gruber 2013). Comorbidities are more common among the elderly (e.g., those with peripheral vascular disease, pneumonia, or heart disease); any of these may affect wound healing (Greenhalgh, 2015). Osteoporosis, decreased bone tissue, and increased fragility of bone tissue can contribute to a poorly healing sternum, sternal dehiscence, and increased potential for mediastinitis (Feron & Maupriez, 2016).

Obesity is a risk for sternal infections because of the increased force applied to the line of closure in these patients. The increased force affects the quantity, aggregation, and orientation of collagen fibers. This may be the result of ischemia or possible relative hypoperfusion that may occur in the subcutaneous adipose tissue (Pierpont et al., 2014). In addition, undue pressure on the wound, venous insufficiency, chronic inflammation with release of inflammatory mediators, and edema contribute to poor oxygenation, which may lead to ischemia of the surrounding tissues (Pierpont et al., 2014). Increased tension on wound edges contributes to wound dehiscence. Wound tension increases pressure on tissues. Perfusion to the microcirculation is reduced, thereby decreasing oxygen delivery to the wound (Pierpont et al., 2014). Pharmacokinetics of drugs can be altered in the obese, requiring dosage adjustments based on body weight and a need for redosing intraoperatively (Bratzler et al., 2013; Sankaralingam, Kim, & Padwal 2015). Antibiotics may be inadequately distributed in the adipose tissue secondary to the impaired vascularity. Obesity along with poor nutrition and osteoporosis may exacerbate poor bone healing, increasing the likelihood of sternal dehiscence (Pierpont et al., 2014). Skin folds make it more difficult to maintain sterility intraoperatively. There is difficulty in suturing, whether the patient is in the sitting position (skin edges forced apart in an inframammary fold) or in the supine position (the weight of the mammaries tends to pull apart skin edges) (Grauhan et al., 2013).

Chronic obstructive pulmonary disease, pneumonia, and anemia may present problems because effective wound healing requires adequate oxygenation, hemoglobin for oxygen transport, and adequate tissue perfusion (Allegranzi, Zayed, et al., 2016; Sgonc & Gruber, 2013). Oxygen supply must meet the increased tissue demand for wound healing to occur. Protein–calorie malnutrition and the resultant body composition changes are additional considerations that may delay wound healing. The local ability to supply oxygen to the healing wound process is inhibited by peripheral vascular disease, previous radiation, chronic inflammation with elevated inflammatory mediators, chronic edema states, or any combination of these conditions (Pierpont et al., 2014). Carbohydrates, fats, protein, and vitamins all provide energy needed for wound healing; iron deficiency may impair collagen production (Stopher & Jansen, 2017).

Prior ventricular assist device insertion and preoperative inotropic support have been identified as risk factors for orthotopic heart transplants (Héquet et al., 2016). In a retrospective, nonrandomized study, Kim and colleagues (2013) found a 2% deep sternal wound infection rate for the 239 adult patients enrolled undergoing heart transplantation between 1999 and 2011.

Intraoperative Risk Factors

Intraoperative risk factors also affect the potential for postoperative problems related to wound healing (**BOX 18.2**). Use of both ITAs is associated with increased chance of infection because these arteries provide the major source of blood supply to the sternum (Taggart et al., 2016). The removal of the ITA significantly devascularizes the sternal half from which it is taken. Surgical technique and adherence to sterile technique have critical implications for incision and mediastinum status (Allegranzi, Bischoff, et al., 2016; Allegranzi, Zayed, et al., 2016; Bryan & Yarbrough, 2013; Sgonc & Gruber, 2013).

An increase in the number of coronary artery grafts, which can prolong surgical time, increases the likelihood of infection. Long CPB pump runs and long surgical procedure times (>4 hours) are known to increase the risk for infection (Bryan & Yarbrough, 2013; Diaz & Newman, 2015; Gelijns et al., 2014). Hypothermia, which is used for cardiac protection during surgery, needs to be corrected quickly in the immediate postoperative period, because prolonged hypothermia increases the risk for infection. Hypothermia impairs neutrophil function and indirectly may cause tissue hypoxia through vasoconstriction of the subcutaneous tissue layer. Maintaining warmth preoperatively and intraoperatively with a warming blanket and forced air warming helps minimize the effects (Anderson et al., 2014). Rewarming immediately postoperatively can be carried out using warming blankets, fluid warmers, and radiant heat lamps. Occasionally, patients have periods of ischemia leading to the development of myocardial or

BOX 18.2 Intraoperative Risk Factors

Use of both internal thoracic arteries
Surgical technique and adherence
Number of grafts
Electrocautery use
Bone wax
Prolonged operative time
Blood transfusions
Mobilization of the internal thoracic arteries
Surgery longer than 5 hours
Transfusion of PRBCs
Long cardiopulmonary pump runs
Infractions in sterile technique
Hypothermia
Periods of ischemia
Improper preoperative prep
Improper antimicrobial prophylaxis
Hypoxia
Inadequate ventilation in the OR
Increased traffic in the OR
Improper use of flash sterilization of instruments

OR, operating room; PRBCs, packed red blood cells.
Data from Ahsan, 2015; Allegranzi, Bischoff et al., 2016; Anderson et al., 2014; Bryan & Yarbrough, 2013; Sexton, 2016; Stephens & Whitman, 2015.

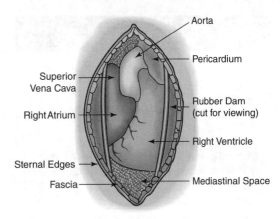

FIGURE 18.1 Rubber dam.
Data from Zellinger, M. & Lienberger, T. (1991). Use of the rubber dam after open heart surgery. *Critical Care Nurse, 11*(8), 24–27.

pulmonary edema, hemodynamic instability, recurrent dysrhythmias, a pressure tamponade, or any combination of these (Allegranzi, Zayed, et al., 2016; Diaz & Newman, 2015). A pressure tamponade may result from an edematous organ, subsequently resulting in a significant decrease in cardiac index (the amount of blood ejected by the heart per minute in relation to the body surface area) and possibly prohibiting closure of the chest wall. This complication may warrant leaving the chest cavity open after the procedure for a period of several days to allow cardiac edema, pulmonary edema, or both to decrease, thus enhancing cardiac recovery. During this time, the sternal opening is covered by one of a variety of methods, including a plastic film, silicone membrane, sterile drape, or an impermeable piece of rubber latex called a "rubber dam" (Calafiore et al., 2017; Spiliopoulos, Autschbach, Koefer, & Tenderich, 2015) (**FIGURE 18.1**).

While the mediastinum is left open in such cases, it does not remain exposed. The rubber dam is securely sutured to the skin edges, covered with gauze that has been soaked in povidone-iodine, and then covered with a sterile dressing. The initial dressing change should be performed with the surgeon in attendance so that the site can be assessed and evaluated together with the ICU nurse, thereby preventing unnecessary additional site exposures. All dressing changes are done with strict aseptic technique using full barrier precautions. The use of delayed sternal closure does not increase the risk of sternal infection (Spiliopoulos et al., 2015; Yost, Pappas, Tatooles, & Bhat, 2015).

Postoperative Risk Factors

In the immediate postoperative period, risk factors for wound infection (**BOX 18.3**) include chest reexploration, need for transfusion of multiple units of blood (Cutrell et al., 2016), hypothermia, periods of impaired oxygenation and/or tissue perfusion, and prolonged mechanical ventilation time (Gelijns et al., 2014). Other postoperative risk factors include autotransfusion of mediastinal blood, low cardiac index or cardiac output (CO; the amount of blood ejected by the heart each minute), prolonged periods of cardiopulmonary resuscitation, sternal instability, and infections arising from sites other than the sternal incision. For example, a patient with a tracheostomy is at greater risk for poor wound healing because of

BOX 18.3 Postoperative Risk Factors

Chest reexploration
Blood transfusions
Hypothermia (<36.0°C)
Prolonged mechanical ventilation time
Prolonged ICU length of stay
Impaired oxygenation
Impaired perfusion
Prolonged cardiopulmonary resuscitation
Autotransfusions
Low cardiac output
Sternal instability
Infections from other sites or sources (e.g., central
    line–associated bloodstream infections,
    pneumonia)

ICU, intensive care unit.
Data from Allegranzi, Zayed, et al., 2016; Bryan & Yarbrough, 2013;
Cutrell et al., 2016; Gelijns et al., 2014; Pierpont et al., 2014; Stephens &
Whitman, 2015.

the close proximity of the surgical incision to the tracheal stoma, which is colonized by bacteria. In such a case, the sternal wound should be protected from the tracheostomy by dressings. Another example is if a patient develops a central line–associated bloodstream infection, the risk for an SSI increases fivefold (Cove, Spelman, & MacLaren, 2012).

▶ Wound Infections Classification

An infection that occurs within 30 days of a surgical procedure is considered an SSI, according to the definition established by the Centers for Disease Control and Prevention (CDC) National Healthcare Safety Network (NHSN) (Anderson et al., 2014; CDC, 2014) (**BOX 18.4**). Numerous

BOX 18.4 Criteria for Defining Surgical Site Infections

Superficial Incisional SSI

Infection occurs within 30 days after surgery
- Involvement of only the skin and subcutaneous tissue of the incision
- Dehiscence of superficial incision
- Stable sternum
- At least one of the following:
  - Purulent drainage from the incision
  - Organisms isolated from an aseptically obtained culture of superficial incision's tissue or fluid
  - Presence of signs and symptoms of infection of incision (e.g., pain, tenderness, localized swelling, redness, heat) *and* superficial incision deliberately opened by surgeon or affiliate and is culture positive or not cultured (negative culture is not an SSI)
  - Diagnosis of superficial SSI made by a health care provider
- Note that there are two specific types of superficial SSIs:
  1. *Superficial incisional primary*—infection identified in the primary or chest incision
  2. *Superficial incisional secondary*—infection identified in the secondary or donor site such as leg (saphenous vein grafts) or arm incision (radial grafts)

Deep Incisional SSI

- Infection occurs within 30 days after surgery (if no implant was left in place) or within 1 year (if an implant was left in place and infection appears to be related to surgery)
- Involves fascia and muscle layers of incision

- Presence of at least one of the following:
  - Purulent drainage from the deep incision (e.g., mediastinum)
  - Dehiscence of deep incision, spontaneous or opened by surgeon, and culture positive or not cultured when the patient has at least one of the following symptoms: fever (>38.0°C), localized pain, or tenderness
  - Presence of an abscess or other signs of deep incision infection found on direct exam, reoperation, or via radiography/histology
  - Diagnosis of deep SSI made by a health care provider
- Please note that there are two specific types of deep SSIs:
  1. *Deep incisional primary*—infection identified in the primary or chest incision
  2. *Deep incisional secondary*—infection identified in the secondary or donor site such as leg (saphenous vein grafts) or arm incision (radial grafts)

Notes:

1. If there is presence of both superficial and deep SSIs, it should be reported as a deep incisional SSI.
2. If there is an infection with drainage to an organ/space related to the surgery, it should be reported as a deep incisional SSI.

Organ/Space SSI

- Infection occurs within 30 days after surgery (if no implant was left in place) or 1 year (if an implant was left in place and infection appears to be related to surgery)
- Infection entails any anatomical structure (e.g., organ, space) aside from the skin incision, fascia, or muscle layers
- Presence of at least one of the following:
  - Purulent drainage from a drain placed through a stab wound or incision in the organ/space
  - Organisms isolated from an aseptically obtained culture of tissue or fluid from the organ/space
  - Abscess or other evidence of infection in organ/space found on direct exam, reoperation, or via radiology/histology
  - Diagnosis of organ/space SSI made by a health care provider

Note: Report mediastinitis following cardiac surgery that is accompanied by osteomyelitis as SSI-MED rather than SSI-BONE.
Data from Anderson et al., 2014; CDC, 2014; Diaz & Newman, 2015.

classifications of SSIs have been developed. Most often, they are classified as either superficial, deep, or organ/space.

Superficial Wound Infections

Superficial wound infections are classified as Type 1. These wound infections involve only the skin or subcutaneous tissue around the incision and occur within 30 days of surgery. They may be identified by purulent drainage; isolated organisms upon culture; signs and symptoms of purulent infection such as pain, tenderness, swelling, redness, or heat; or by any combination of these. Such infections are usually identified and treated in an outpatient setting (Anderson et al., 2014).

Sternal Wound Dehiscence

Sternal wound dehiscence is associated with a Type 2 infection. A Type 2 infection is further classified into one of three subcategories:

- Type 2A: a sterile viable bone
- Type 2B: a nonviable bone in the presence of sternal osteitis (inflammation) in the upper two-thirds of the sternum
- Type 2C: a nonviable bone in the presence of sternal osteitis in the lower third of the sternum

A Type 2 sternal wound infection could require any number of interventions, ranging from debridement and rewiring to flap surgery (Shi, Qi, & Zhang, 2014).

Mediastinitis

Deep wound infections that occur within 30 days of a procedure and involve the deep soft tissue (i.e., the fascia and muscle) warrant a diagnosis of mediastinitis, which is considered a Type 3 sternal wound infection. Typically, there is purulent drainage, dehiscence of the surgical site, fever, pain, tenderness at the site, possible sternal instability, and evidence of infection (Anderson et al., 2014). Treatment of a Type 3 sternal wound infection, deep or organ space, may require a sternectomy. There may be a single advanced flap of the pectoralis major, the latissimus dorsi, or the rectus abdominis, or these can be used in combination (Allegranzi, Bischoff, et al., 2016; Berg & Jaakkola, 2013; Hillis et al., 2012; Pancholy & Raman, 2015; Shi et al., 2014).

Septicemia

A Type 4 infection is characterized by the presence of a Type 2 or 3 wound infection along with septicemia. Treatment of such an infection involves radical debridement, delayed closure, and aggressive intravenous antibiotic therapy (Lazar et al., 2016; Shi et al., 2014).

▶ Prevention of Surgical Site Infection

Appropriate incisional care must be initiated in the preoperative phase and includes a variety of necessary interventions. The CDC and Healthcare Infection Control Practices Advisory Committee updated the 1999 guidelines for prevention of SSIs in 2014 in the compendium addressing all hospital-acquired infections (Yokoe et al., 2014). Preoperative prevention of SSIs begins with meticulous handwashing by all surgical team members and appropriate preparation of the operative site (Allegranzi, Bischoff, et al., 2016; Yokoe et al., 2014). In addition, a multitude of preventive strategies (**BOX 18.5**) are incorporated into any cardiac surgical program to decrease the risk of postoperative complications.

BOX 18.5 Strategies for Preventing Surgical Site Infections

- Identify and treat infections before the patient undergoes an elective operation.
- Minimize hair removal at or around the incision site. Use clipping instead of shaving when hair removal is needed.
- Bathe the patient with an antiseptic solution at least the night before surgery.
- Clean the incision site of any gross contaminants and then prep the skin with chlorhexidine gluconate, povidone-iodine, or alcohol-containing products prior to making the incision.
- Use local collagen-gentamicin.
- Use additional fixation wires at the lower sternum.
- Use the vertical interrupted mattress suture technique with cyanoacrylate sealant in high-risk groups (e.g., obese patients).

Data from Allegranzi, Bischoff et al., 2016; Bryan & Yarbrough, 2013; Diaz & Newman, 2015; Goh, 2017; Kowalewski et al., 2015; Mishra et al., 2014.

Local Collagen-Gentamicin

The use of local collagen-gentamicin sponges has been found to reduce the incidence of sternal wound infections caused by all major clinically important microbiologic agents, including coagulase-negative *Staphylococcus* (CoNS) (Formanek, Herwaldt, Perencevich, & Schweizer, 2014; Kowalewski, 2015; Mishra et al., 2014). Godbole, Pai, Kolvekar, & Wilson (2012) noted that two of four randomized controlled trials (RCTs) showed benefits when used in both routine and emergent surgeries. One RCT showed sternal rebleeding occurring when gentamicin sponges were used in double layers. Another RCT showed that there was no significant difference between the gentamicin arm and the control arm when treating patients at high risk for SWIs (diabetics, obesity of body mass index [BMI] >30, or both). This latter study had a few patients with methicillin-resistant *Staphylococcus aureus* (MRSA), which gentamicin does not affect

(Bennett-Guerrero et al., 2010). If a patient has a suspected infection prior to an elective operation, the infection source and site need to be identified and treated before the patient undergoes surgery. Elective surgery should be postponed until the infection has resolved.

Hair Removal

It is recommended not to remove hair preoperatively unless the hair at or around the incision site might interfere with the surgical procedure. If hair removal is necessary, hair should be removed with electrical clippers or a depilatory agent rather than the traditional shaving method. Clipping is recommended to be performed immediately prior to the operation—but completed outside of the operating room (OR) (Anderson et al., 2014).

Preoperative Skin Cleansing

Cleansing the patient's skin at least the night before surgery is imperative. In particular, removing gross contaminants by showering or bathing, and then cleansing the skin with a preparation that lowers microbial skin burden, has been shown to be effective in lowering the incidence of SSIs (Allegranzi, Bischoff, et al., 2016; Anderson et al., 2014; Diaz & Newman, 2015; Edmiston et al., 2013; George, Leasure, & Horstmanshot, 2016; Graling & Vasaly, 2013).

Several antimicrobial preparations are currently available: chlorhexidine gluconate (CHG), povidone-iodine, and alcohol. Reports suggest that CHG is the superior product in terms of its ability to remove the microbial burden on the skin and to maintain a greater residual activity hours after the skin is prepared (Allegranzi, Bischoff, et al., 2016; Anderson et al., 2014; Chien, Lin, & Hsu, 2014; Edmiston et al., 2013; Mimoz et al., 2015; Privitera et al., 2017). In addition, CHG no-rinse reduces MRSA and vancomycin-resistant *Enterococcus* (VRE) counts and reduces risk for central line infections. *Acinetobacter* counts did not decrease (Allen, Kohan, & Smith 2015; George et al., 2016; Mimoz et al., 2015).

Two methods are currently used to prepare patients' skin:

- The rinse-off method that uses a CHG 4% solution or presoaked scrub packets
- The no-rinse method that uses CHG 2% presoaked preparation cloths, allowing a residual barrier layer once skin dries

To lower the microbial count, it is recommended to apply the antiseptic several times. Studies comparing these two methods have shown some positive results with the no-rinse method (Allen et al., 2015; Edmiston & Spencer, 2014; Edmiston et al., 2013; Morrison et al., 2016; Privitera et al., 2017). With this method, the patient takes an initial shower to wash any gross contaminants off the skin and to enhance comfort. After a minimum of 1 hour, the no-rinse method cloth is used to prepare the skin. It is recommended that the no-rinse method be used at least once the evening before and again the morning of surgery. It is then followed by skin preparation in the OR (Allen et al., 2015; Morrison et al., 2016).

Skin preparation in the OR before surgery begins is standard practice. An ideal surgical skin antiseptic has the ability to significantly reduce microorganisms, has a rapid and persistent effect, has broad spectrum activity, and is easy to use. Ayoub, Quirke, Conroy, and Hill (2015) conducted a systematic review and meta-analysis on use of CHG and povidone-iodine as preoperative skin preparation. Chlorhexidine gluconate was more protective against SSIs (6.8% versus 11%).

MRSA Prophylaxis

Staphylococcus aureus is a frequent offender in sternal wound infections. The nares are known to be colonized with *S. aureus* in approximately 20% to 80% of the healthy population (Brown, Leech, Rogers, & McLoughlin, 2013). Infections post coronary artery bypass surgery are due to *S. aureus*, including resistant strains, 40% to 50% of the time (Bryan & Yarbrough, 2013; Gelijns et al., 2014; Musallam, 2014). Mupirocin (Bactroban®) ointment, a topical antibiotic, is effective in treating nasal colonization, including some resistant strains of this pathogen (Allegranzi, Bischoff, et al., 2016; George et al., 2016). Mupirocin, given intranasally, is recommended preoperatively for all cardiac surgical patients in the absence of documented *S. aureus* colonization testing (Bryan & Yarbrough, 2013; Gelijns et al., 2014; George et al., 2016; Stephens & Whitman, 2015). It is administered by the patient for a period up to 5 days to reduce any nasal colonization involving *S. aureus*. Treatment should begin at least 1 day preoperatively and may extend into the postoperative period until the treatment is complete (George et al., 2016).

Phillips and colleagues (2014) conducted an investigator-initiated, open-label randomized study comparing use of mupirocin for 5 days twice daily versus two applications of povidone-iodine solution in each nostril 2 hours prior to incision. Both treatments were found effective. The povidone-iodine may be a viable alternative treatment, and it is slated for future studies in multiple centers. This is worth considering in light of the potential for mupirocin resistance and costs (povidone-iodine treatment is less expensive).

Preoperative Antibiotic Administration

Preoperative antibiotic administration should be performed for all cardiac surgical patients to reduce their risk of postoperative infection (Bryan & Yarbrough, 2013; Diaz & Newman, 2015; Gelijns et al., 2014; Hillis et al., 2012). This measure reduces the incidence of infection fivefold; *S. aureus* has been identified as the infective organism in more than 50% of all SSIs (Musallam, 2014). A cephalosporin is the preferred prophylactic agent of choice for cardiac surgery procedures in populations that do not have a high incidence of MRSA (Diaz & Newman, 2015; Gelijns et al., 2014; Hillis et al., 2012). Data suggest that prophylaxis with glycopeptides, such as vancomycin (Vancocin®), is more effective in preventing infection by methicillin-resistant organisms, but is less effective in countering methicillin-sensitive organisms (Diaz & Newman, 2015; Gelijns et al., 2014; Hillis et al., 2012). Use of a first or second generation cephalosporin is recommended for patients without MRSA colonization. Vancomycin is recommended for patients with MRSA or for those patients who have an allergy to penicillin. Antibiotic therapy should continue for up to 48 hours postoperatively (Stephens & Whitman, 2015). If a patient is allergic to cephalosporins, a glycopeptide should not be used as a sole agent because it does not provide any coverage for gram-negative organisms. In such a case, it is recommended that an aminoglycoside be used in addition to the glycopeptide.

Prophylaxis is accomplished by administering one preoperative dose and one postoperative dose (Allegranzi, Bischoff, et al., 2016). Correctly timing the preoperative antibiotic dose is essential so that a bactericidal concentration of the drug is present in the patient's serum and tissues by the time the skin incision is made (Allegranzi, Bischoff, et al., 2016; Bratzler et al., 2013; Diaz & Newman, 2015; Gelijns et al., 2014). With cephalosporins, the dose needs to be administered within 30 to 60 min of the time the incision is made. It is best accomplished by the anesthesiologist after induction of anesthesia and may be included in the call to order and OR checklist processes. The surgeon should confirm that the antibiotic dosing has occurred prior to the scalpel being in hand. If the length of the operative procedure exceeds 3 hours, redosing is mandated based on cephalosporin pharmacokinetics. Redosing should occur at intervals of 2 half-lives (measured from the time the preoperative dose was administered) (Anderson et al., 2014). If the combination of a glycopeptide and an aminoglycoside is used, the medications are usually administered over a 60- to 90-minute period (dependent on dosage) to avoid red-man syndrome and impairing renal function. There is no associated benefit to administering prophylactic antibiotics beyond 48 hours (Aldea et al., 2016; Anderson, 2014; Diaz & Newman, 2015; Gelijns et al., 2014).

Glycemic Control

According to the 2009 consensus statement by the American Association of Clinical Endocrinologists and American Diabetes Association, for patients who are not critically ill (e.g., cardiac surgery patients who are preparing for discharge and are healing at home), it is recommended that preprandial serum glucose should be 110 mg/dL, up to a maximum of 180 mg/dL (Goh, 2017). Attaining these goals reduces mortality, reduces length of stay (LOS) in the hospital, improves healing potential, and lessens the risk of mediastinitis (Berrios-Torres et al., 2017; Hillis et al., 2012; Umpierrez et al., 2015). As of January 2014, the Surgical Care Improvement Project (SCIP)—Infection Prevention 4 (SCIP-Inf 4) measure changed. Blood glucose levels must be maintained less than 180 mg/dL between 18 and 24 hours after anesthesia end time (Klinkner & Murray, 2014; Goh, 2017). Pezzella, Holmes, Pritchard, Speir, and Ad (2014) compared a tight target (90–120 mg/dL) versus a liberal target (121–180 mg/dL) in diabetic and nondiabetic patients and found that the liberal target was easier to maintain and stay within the target levels, avoiding hypoglycemic events. These patients were contacted at 6 months and 40 (±4.4) months after surgery; the survival rate was the same in both groups (diabetics included), and physical health–related quality of life was improved in the liberal group.

Appropriate glycemic control is accomplished by assessing the patient preoperatively for elevated HbA$_{1c}$ levels, noting any history of diabetes and checking for any elevated serum glucose. If a patient's HbA$_{1c}$ level is greater than 7.0%, the risk for morbidity and mortality is known to be significantly increased. The patient should begin insulin therapy at least 1 day before surgery. Ideally, achieving adequate glycemic control before the patient's admission for surgery will lower the risk for infection (Martin et al., 2016).

If patients have elevated serum glucose levels, they should be treated with a continuous intravenous insulin infusion immediately prior to, during, and immediately following surgery in the postanesthesia care unit and the ICU. Hargraves (2014) describes use of an insulin infusion protocol post cardiac surgery. She found that educating the nursing team on glycemic control and implementing an insulin infusion protocol developed by an interdisciplinary team improved overall glycemic control and minimized hypoglycemic episodes. Klinkner and Murray (2014) found that improving access of insulin orders, using an insulin infusion protocol, developing a nursing protocol to initiate the insulin infusions, and increasing frequency/regularity of glucose monitoring improved postoperative glycemic protocol in cardiac surgery patients. It is suggested that published protocols in the literature be reviewed, and that one be selected that is appropriate for the respective facility. Regardless of which protocol is followed, serum glucose levels should be checked frequently (e.g., every 1–2 hours during this time frame) to adjust the insulin infusion.

Once the patient is being advanced on a diet, serum glucose targets should be adjusted to 150 mg/dL as a mean target (100–140 mg/dL preprandial; 180 mg/dL maximum serum glucose) (McDonnell, Alexanian, White, & Lazar, 2012). While it is considered safe to maintain a patient's blood glucose in the 140 to 180 mg/dL range, it is better to maintain the level less than 150 mg/dL (Girish et al., 2014). The patient is then transitioned from the intravenous insulin to a combination of subcutaneous injections: basal, nutritional, and a supplemental corrective dosing (McDonnell et al., 2012; Umpierrez et al., 2012). Noninsulin agents have limited use in the hospital secondary to irregular meal intake. Caution must be used with the oral agents to prevent complications (Umpierrez et al., 2012). Sulfonylureas can be started slowly based on the patient's dietary intake. Patients must have a documented return to normal or baseline renal function before restarting metformin (McDonnell et al., 2012). If serum glucose levels remain elevated, consultation with an endocrinologist to attain tighter glycemic control is advisable.

Avoiding Potentially Contaminated Sources

Reestablishing the skin barrier can prevent the onset of superficial infections. Diabetes, obesity, and renal failure are all conditions that can delay wound closure. Dressings are not the only way to protect the incision site. Electrocardiogram wires are known to be a source of infection;

disposable lead wires are available and should be considered for SSI prevention. Of note, this recommendation is not consistent as data vary regarding SSI prevention between disposable and nondisposable lead wires (Albert et al., 2014). Reusable blood pressure cuffs have also been noted to be infection sources; disposable cuffs are now available. Individual stethoscopes should be cleansed with alcohol after each individual patient assessment. It is imperative that the nurse assess the incision regularly and protect the incision as it heals.

Postoperative Dressings

Postoperative incisional dressing assessment should be performed upon admission and every 4 hours thereafter until the patient is transferred out of the ICU. To minimize the risk of infection, most cardiac surgical centers opt to keep the initial dressing on the incision for 24 to 48 hours, as per CDC recommendations (Goh, 2017).

If the patient is experiencing a coagulopathy, a small amount of blood or blood-tinged fluid may drain from the incisional site. The dressing should be changed using sterile technique when it becomes saturated. Dumville, Gray, Walter, Sharp, and Page (2014) reviewed 16 RCTs comparing use of different types of dressings or no dressing. They reported no difference in healing, degree of infection, comfort, or amount of scarring. Silver-impregnated dressings need a large controlled study to determine effects on wound healing, infection prevention, and a cost–benefit analysis (Staveski et al., 2016). Negative pressure incision management systems have been utilized in some centers over closed incisions for the first 6 to 10 days on high-risk patients (e.g., patients with obesity or diabetes) with good success (Cotogni, Barbaro, & Rinaldi, 2015; Grauhan et al., 2013; Pierpont et al., 2014; Tarzia et al., 2014). Optimal dressing characteristics are permeable to allow for gas exchange, impermeable to prevent microorganism and exogenous sources of contamination, and the ability to provide an insulating effect. Dressing decisions should be based on cost and managing specific conditions, such as drainage absorption (Dumville et al., 2014).

Evaluation of the Incision Site: Phases of Incision Healing

An incision goes through three major phases as it heals. During the inflammatory phase, after the incision is made, a cascade of clotting and immune responses produces inflammation at the incision site. After incisional closure, neutrophils migrate toward the fibrin clot at the margins of the incision and fill in the incisional space. During the proliferative phase, new capillaries are formed, and fibrin, collagen, and growth factors spread across the wound bed. Basophils (a type of white blood cells) migrate to the incision borders and multiply. During the maturation phase, collagen matrix development furthers wound closure. As keratinization occurs, the skin thickness returns to normal (Greenhalgh, 2015; Sgonc & Gruber, 2013). Recent studies have found that placement of additional fixation wires at the lower sternum, along with prophylaxis with a local collagen-gentamicin, decreases the incidence of deep sternal wound infections (Formanek et al., 2014; Godbole et al., 2012; Kowalewski et al., 2015).

After waiting the designated time stated in the institution's protocol, performing appropriate hand hygiene, and donning clean gloves, the nurse should remove and discard the dressing. Initially, the incision site may appear slightly red around the edges. The edges should be well approximated, with minimal tension evident. The surrounding tissue should display no inflammation, hematoma, swelling, erythema, skin discoloration, or warmth, and it should not cause pain when palpated. Several variables, if present, need to be documented and brought to the attention of the surgeon; the variables indicative of an infection are listed in **BOX 18.6**.

Saphenous vein graft infections occur more frequently in patients with obesity, diabetes, extracardiac arteriopathy, decreased glomerular filtration rate, or any combination of these (Turtiainen, Hakala, Hakkarainen, & Karhukorpi, 2014). Staples versus suture closure of leg wounds after vein harvest have no statistically significant difference in complications based on three trial reviews (Sandy-Hodgetts, Carville, & Leslie,

BOX 18.6 Variables Indicative of Infection

Nonapproximated incision
Excessive pain and tenderness
Redness, odor, or swelling
Wound breakdown
Exudate (Note the amount—none, minimal,
     moderate, heavy leakage through the
     bandage—and type—serous/straw-colored
     fluid or serosanguineous/red fluid, as well
     as any frank blood or pus [creamy yellow or
     green])
Sternal instability
Fever (>38.0°C)

2015). Drainage of noninfected serosanguineous fluid from leg incisions is common. Oftentimes, the drainage results from an underlying hematoma that has liquefied and is draining out of the neighboring skin incision. The presence of erythema, induration, and undue tenderness to palpation indicate infection. In such cases, the patient may require a dilation and curettage procedure, followed by open packing of the wound and administration of antibiotics.

If unresolved, these infections, late lower limb ischemia, or both can lead to the need for further interventions, including skin grafts, vascular procedures, or even amputations (Santo et al., 2014).

▶ Nursing Responsibilities to Enhance Wound Healing

The radial artery site is easy to assess because of its visibility. Regular assessments (minimum every 2 hours) should always include color, capillary refill time, temperature, and presence of an ulnar artery pulse. Assessment for an underlying incision hematoma is imperative, because its presence may impede blood flow to the hand and lead to loss of function. Elevation of the arm

and affected hand on pillows will help decrease any edema.

The multitude of factors that may potentially affect wound healing should be examined for each individual patient. Providing for optimal wound healing, eliminating any underlying causative or contributory factors, and stimulating positive physiologic factors required for the healing process are essential ICU nursing interventions. Optimizing the patient's nutritional status, including assuring that the patient is consuming a diet with adequate intake of protein and calories, trace metals, and vitamins, is equally essential. Collaboration with a dietitian is recommended.

The ICU nurse should also assess the patient's emotional and psychosocial status. Depression makes it difficult for a patient to be fully compliant with treatment regimens, which may potentially inhibit wound healing. Assuring adequate pain control helps enhance the patient's willingness to be active and ability to adhere to treatment regimens. If the patient has an elevated serum glucose level, close monitoring to maintain tight glycemic control to promote wound healing is required. Renal or liver insufficiency also requires correction, because both of these conditions will impede healing. Finally, ICU nurses must implement measures to optimize perfusion and oxygenation and promote early ambulation, as soon as feasible. Early goal-directed mobilization helps minimize complications of immobility and delirium and decreases LOS both in the ICU and hospital (Barr et al., 2013; Dong et al., 2016; Hashem, Nelliot, & Needham, 2016; Meyer et al., 2013; Patel, Pohlman, Hall, & Kress 2014; Reade, Phil, & Finter, 2014).

▶ Wound Infection Sequelae

When wound infections occur, they can be devastating. Most SSIs are identified on a posthospitalization basis. They can require frequent outpatient and emergency department (ED) visits, radiology services, lab work, home health services, hospital readmissions for treatment, and, possibly, further surgery. In addition, the patient and family will deal with the consequences of a loss in the patient's productivity. In particular, the patient may be out of work for an extended period of time. The patient's functional status may be decreased, such that the individual requires assistance to complete activities of daily living, including transportation to and from the many visits for health care.

Impact of Postoperative Infection

There are more than 230 million operations worldwide annually. Infections are estimated to occur in approximately 5% of the patients. This is a significant health care issue both economically and as a potential detriment to patient morbidity and mortality (Schimmer et al., 2017). Surgical site infections can add an additional 10 hospital days to a patient's LOS (Chen et al., 2012). Hospital costs can range from $40,000 to $53,000 higher with SSIs, particularly MRSA (Lipke & Hyott, 2010). Mortality rate can be 30% higher in those with mediastinitis than those without infection (Schimmer et al., 2017).

Reducing the potential for any SSI to occur is a paramount concern with any surgical procedure. Approximately 300,000 to 400,000 SSIs occur in conjunction with the estimated 45 million surgical procedures performed in the United States annually (Lobdell, Stamou, & Sanchez , 2012). The Deficit Reduction Act, passed in 2005, allows the Centers for Medicare and Medicaid Services (CMS) to adjust payments downward for patients experiencing hospital-acquired infections; this provision took effect in October 2008. As of October 1, 2008, the CMS no longer reimburses for hospital-acquired conditions such as SSIs— specifically, mediastinitis after coronary artery bypass grafting (CABG) surgery (Richter, Jarrett, & LaBresh, 2014) or flap surgery due to an SSI. Hospitals are now paid at the "with complications rate" when such SSI-related events occur, instead of the "without complications" higher rate that they had been receiving in the past (Richter et al., 2014). The impact of this change in billing practice on hospitals' financial status can be considerable.

The general trend is toward surgical patients who are increasingly sicker and have more complex comorbidities. Many of these patients are elderly (>80 years). When these patients develop SSIs, increasing numbers of them are infected with resistant strains of microbes (e.g., MRSA and VRE).

▶ Wound Infection Prediction

The CDC's NHSN, formerly the National Nosocomial Infection Surveillance system, predicts the risk of SSI based on three factors: length of surgery, wound class, and the patient's American Society of Anesthesiology (ASA) score (Maragakis et al., 2009). This system has not been adapted specifically for cardiac surgery.

The first scale to predict surgical wound infections in CABG patients was developed in 1998 (Hussey, Leeper, & Hynan, 1998; Troutman, Hussey, Hynan, & Lucisano, 2001). This scale, known as the Sternal Wound Infection Predictor Scale (SWIPS), consists of weighted predictors related to the preoperative, intraoperative, and postoperative phases of care (**TABLE 18–1**).

In 1986, the Society of Thoracic Surgeons (STS) developed their first risk scoring system for patients undergoing CABG procedures. This has been updated several times with the latest update published in 2009 (Shahian et al, 2009a). The STS has created two additional scoring systems predicting risk for infection following valve surgery (O'Brien et al., 2009) and one for combination valve surgery plus CABG (Shahian et al., 2009b), which includes both preoperative and intraoperative scores and takes several variables into account.

Currently, mediastinitis occurs in 0.25% to 4.0% of cardiac surgical patients, with more than 50% of these infections involving *S. aureus* and *S. epidermidis*. Those with a major infection in the hospital had potential for higher mortality (1.1%– 19%) and were more likely to have a prolonged hospital LOS, often exceeding 14 days (Bryan & Yarbrough, 2013; Goh, 2017).

TABLE 18.1 Sternal Wound Infection Predictor Scale (SWIPS)

Variable	Weight
Preoperative	
Smoking	9
Diabetes mellitus	
IDDM	7
NIDDM	5
COPD	8
Preoperative ICU stay	4
Obesity (>30 kg/m²)	4
Advanced age (>70 years)	3
Sex (male)	1
Impaired immune response	8
Intraoperative	
Bilateral ITA	6
Single ITA	3
Long operative time (>4 hours)	7
Reexploration for bleeding	6
Long cardiopulmonary bypass time (>2 hours)	6
Postoperative	
Hypoperfusion/hypotension	8
Ventilator support (>48 hours)	6
Pharmacologic support	
Dopamine/dobutamine only	2
All others	6
Postoperative CPR	7
Hypoxemia	5
Banked blood transfusions	3

COPD, chronic obstructive pulmonary disease; CPR, cardiopulmonary resuscitation; ICU, intensive care unit; IDDM, insulin-dependent diabetes mellitus; ITA, internal thoracic artery; NIDDM, noninsulin-dependent diabetes mellitus.
Data from Hussey, Leeper, & Hynan, 1998.

▶ Management of Wound Infections

Sternal Wound Infections

Sternal wound infections may be superficial, involving only the skin and subcutaneous fat, or they may be deep, involving the sternum and underlying structures. Superficial infections are characterized by drainage from the wound and local inflammation, even as the underlying sternum remains stable (see Table 18–1). In this instance, removal of the overlying skin sutures, culture of the drainage, administration of antibiotics, and local dressings are often effective interventions. Reconstructive surgery can be avoided in clinically stable patients with the use of vacuum-assisted closure (Lo Torto et al., 2017).

Mediastinitis

Bacterial mediastinitis starts when the invasion of a pathogen causes an inflammatory response. The invading bacteria proliferate and the body forms a thick layer of fibrin in an attempt to encapsulate the foreign agents. An area of dead space forms underneath the sternum as the infection expands through sinus tracts that have formed. The patient develops fever, and the systemic inflammatory response causes production of leukocytes and proinflammatory mediators. Staphylococci, including CoNS (usually *S. epidermidis* or *S. aureus*), have been identified as the most common causative agents of SWIs (Goh, 2017; Mishra et al., 2014).

Mediastinitis can develop as early as 7 to 10 days following a cardiac surgical procedure. Patients have often been discharged home before any sign of this infection occurs. Oftentimes, the first sign is significant serous drainage that appears 4 to 5 days postoperatively. Patients experience fever, chills, pain, and leukocytosis within 2 to 5 days after the onset of infection. Erythema may form on the outside borders of the incision and is often first seen at the xiphoid process. Occasionally, a section of the incision may dehisce and purulent drainage will exude from the site.

More commonly, mediastinitis becomes evident later in the postoperative course, usually within 30 days after surgery. Patients often develop sternal pain, become lethargic, and demonstrate an unwillingness to do many activities that they were doing previously. The incision then begins to drain purulent fluid and will separate. Upon assessment, the nurse often finds that the sternum is unstable, with the borders rubbing against each other. Pain will be worse with respiration. Fever, chills, and leukocytosis are evident.

Treatment of mediastinitis depends on the stage of the infectious process at the time of diagnosis. If identified early (i.e., the sternum is not destroyed), success may be achieved with prompt surgical intervention, debridement of the sternal edges, copious irrigation of the mediastinum, placement of retrosternal irrigation and drainage catheters, rewiring of the sternum, and closure of the fascia and skin. Appropriate intravenous antibiotic therapy is given for a minimum of 7 days. The results of a Gram stain are utilized to identify the appropriate antibiotic to infuse through an irrigating catheter, with the fluid being directed to exit via drainage catheters. The irrigation continues for 3 to 5 days, until the drainage is sterile as confirmed by culture. Although frequently successful, this treatment method can have serious complications (e.g., erosion of the catheters into mediastinal structures and systemic toxicity from absorption of the irrigating antibiotic). For these reasons, this procedure is reserved for specific groups of patients (Shi et al., 2014).

More long-standing, advanced infections are associated with large amounts of suppurative fluid in the mediastinum, loss of integrity of the sternum, and diffuse cellulitis of the skin and subcutaneous tissue. Patients with such infections may require opening of the sternum and debridement of necrotic tissue, exposure and draining of the mediastinum, and packing of the wound with moist gauze. Vacuum-assisted closure therapy can be used as a bridge between debridement and closure of the wound. It can assist in decreasing overall wound edema, reduce bacterial counts in the wound, and reduce the time to closing the wound

(Deniz et al., 2012; Goh, 2017; Hillis et al., 2012; Lo Torto et al., 2017; Shi et al., 2014). After control of the infection is achieved and a healthy-appearing bed of granulation tissue forms, secondary closure is performed with or without a muscle flap. The treatment plan depends on severity of the infection and may involve a combination of debridement, packing, closure delay, reconstruction, rewiring, and irrigation with antibiotics (Deniz et al., 2012).

The most frequently used approach to treating serious mediastinitis is a single-stage procedure in which radical debridement of the sternum and cartilage is performed with advanced muscle flaps, using the pectoralis major or rectus muscle, or both (Lo Torto et al., 2017). Depending on the degree of sternal resection required, the remaining bone tissue may or may not be approximated. Soft silastic drains are placed beneath the muscle flaps and connected to gentle suction. Often performed by a plastic surgeon, this procedure may be associated with decreased morbidity and mortality and a decreased LOS. The patient may be discharged home with drains in place. The drains remain in place until the daily drainage volume becomes small; they may then be removed in the health care provider's office. Early aggressive use of debridement and muscle flaps in serious mediastinitis is considered the optimal approach (Goh, 2017; Hillis et al., 2012; Lo Torto et al., 2017).

Several long-term complications are associated with mediastinitis. Notably, patients have a significant increase in mortality during the first year and subsequent 4 years. The potential for other nosocomial infections, including systemic infections, is increased as well. Patients may develop sepsis and organ system failure. Identifying mediastinitis early allows for earlier treatment and is associated with a better prognosis (Goh, 2017).

For patients who have a relatively uneventful postoperative course, discharge may occur on the third or fourth postoperative day. Many infections do not become evident until after the patient has been discharged, which makes early diagnosis of sternal infection and mediastinitis

---

BOX 18.7 Patient/Family Discharge Education Regarding Incision Care

Emphasize the following points when explaining wound care at home:
- Shower daily with soap and water.
- Avoid sitting in the bathtub.
- A dressing is needed only if drainage is present.
- Remove any dressings applied during hospitalization on the day after going home.
- Inspect the wound daily using a mirror. If you see any redness, irritation, swelling, tenderness, or unusual drainage, contact the surgeon or surgeon on call.

Optimal Patient Outcomes
- Patient can perform appropriate incision care.
- Patient has no signs and symptoms of infection.
- Patient can list signs and symptoms of infection.
- Patient modifies lifestyle to reduce risk factors that may impede wound healing.

---

after cardiac surgery difficult. In some patients, fever, leukocytosis, and a positive blood culture will be the first manifestations of a hidden infection that will become obvious only later. The most common early sign is fluid drainage from the wound; sternal instability usually develops subsequently.

Clear and thorough patient education reviewing the appearance of a normally healing incision is of utmost importance in recognizing postoperative wound infections. The patient and family members must be instructed to frequently observe the incision for any changes in status and to call the surgeon's office if changes or questions arise (**BOX 18.7**). Given the trend toward earlier hospital discharge following cardiac surgery, fewer SSIs will be detected prior to patient discharge. Without careful supervision and intervention, the physical and financial costs of these infections will increase.

Effective wound infection prevention strategies and opportunities for group review of data are essential for all cardiac surgical programs. Members of the interdisciplinary team must continuously review the literature and revise practices and guidelines based on the latest evidence. Process measures and compliance must be assessed, and education must be initiated whenever deviations are noted.

▶ Summary

Sternal wound infections occur in a small percentage of patients who undergo cardiac surgery. There is a high associated cost in terms of morbidity, mortality, LOS, time away from work, and financial costs if an infection develops. Infected patients have increased potential for pain and delirium, often seen as complications of immobility and prolonged ICU and hospital stays. Delirium can have deleterious long-term effects post hospitalization (Barr et al., 2013; Jenks, Laurent, McQuarry, & Watkins, 2014; Vasunilashorn et al., 2017).

A number of predictive variables have been identified that put the patient at greater risk for development of an SWI, and a number of preventive strategies must be implemented to avoid development of this potentially catastrophic complication. A strong team approach utilizing evidenced-based practices is statistically significant in minimizing sternal infections (Goh, 2017). Although an SWI is not likely to develop while the patient is in the ICU postoperatively, initiation of preventive measures must begin while the patient is in the early phase of recovery. The ICU nurse has a pivotal role in preventing SWIs and beginning the essential patient and family education that must be accomplished to help ensure optimal postoperative outcomes are attained.

🔍 *CASE STUDY*

B. F., a 50-year-old obese male patient with a history of hypertension, diabetes mellitus (elevated HbA$_{1c}$), obesity, hypoalbuminemia (serum albumin 2.2g/mL), and end-stage renal disease and receiving hemodialysis three times weekly, underwent CABG surgery for two-vessel heart disease. Bilateral internal thoracic arteries were used for the procedure. Preoperatively, the patient had hemodynamic instability that was managed in the ICU. The patient had purulent drainage noted from the sternotomy wound. He was noted to be febrile (38.6°C) and had an increasing white blood cell count. The surgical site was tender to palpation. He returned to the OR for reexploration of his sternotomy wound. Surgical debridement with open wound packing was performed. He was started on broad spectrum antibiotic therapy. His postoperative course was otherwise uncomplicated. He was ultimately successfully discharged home after a prolonged ICU and hospital stay.

Critical Thinking Questions

1. What should the nurse suspect as being the underlying cause of this patient's condition?
2. What risk factors did the patient have for this complication?
3. What are some possible intraoperative risk factors that might have contributed to this patient's condition?

Answers to Critical Thinking Questions

1. This patient is manifesting signs and symptoms of mediastinitis.
2. Patient's age, gender (male), use of bilateral internal thoracic arteries, diabetes mellitus, and preoperative hemodynamic instability are risk factors. Use of bilateral internal thoracic arteries is a risk factor because the sternum loses more than 90% of its blood supply when the associated internal thoracic artery is mobilized. The decrease in blood supply will affect wound healing (Lazar et al., 2016; Sajja, 2015).
3. Possible intraoperative risk factors include improper preoperative prep, improper antimicrobial prophylaxis, perioperative hypothermia, hypoxia, or both, inadequate ventilation in the OR, increased traffic in the OR, or improper use of flash sterilization of instruments (Ahsan, 2015).

Self-Assessment Questions

1. Which patient is at greatest risk for wound complications following cardiac surgery?
   A. A 68-year-old with BMI 24 kg/m^2
   B. A 65-year-old with chronic bronchitis
   C. A 50-year-old with HbA$_{1c}$ 5.5%
   D. A 60-year-old with albumin level 2.5 mg/dL

2. Use of which vessel for grafts puts the patient at increased risk of postoperative infection?
   A. Internal thoracic artery
   B. Radial artery
   C. Saphenous vein
   D. Gastroepiploic artery

3. Which intraoperative condition puts the patient at increased risk for postoperative infections?
   A. Need for fewer coronary artery grafts
   B. Shorter pump runs
   C. Shortened hypothermia time
   D. Decreased cardiac index

4. Which patient is at greatest risk for a postoperative wound infection following cardiac surgery? A patient:
   A. with a rubber dam.
   B. needing autotransfusion of mediastinal blood.
   C. with peripheral edema.
   D. with an elevated cardiac output.

5. Which patient should be suspected as having a deep incisional surgical site infection? A patient with:
   A. an infection and drainage to an organ related to surgery.
   B. dehiscence of a superficial incision.
   C. organisms aseptically obtained from tissue of an incision.
   D. purulent drainage from an incision of a sterile sternum.

6. Which dressing characteristic should be considered to promote surgical site healing?
   A. Permeable to allow for gas exchange
   B. Permeable to only select microorganisms
   C. Inability to insulate the wound
   D. Limited absorptive properties

7. Which is a target blood glucose level for a postoperative cardiac surgery patient who is advancing on a diet?
   A. 80 mg/dL preprandial
   B. 110 mg/dL preprandial
   C. 140 mg/dL maximum
   D. 150 mg/dL maximum

8. Which should cause the nurse to suspect the presence of an infection?
   A. Approximated wound
   B. Induration
   C. Minimal wound tension
   D. Incision site slightly red at edges

9. A patient with a BMI of 31 kg/m^2 has a saphenous vein graft. Erythema and induration are noted. For which should the nurse anticipate preparing the patient?
   A. Wound irrigation and closure with packing
   B. Dilation and curettage
   C. Open sternotomy and evacuation of any hematomas
   D. Use of no-rinse CHG 2% twice daily

10. Nursing responsibilities to enhance wound healing following cardiac surgery may include
    A. limiting ambulation until the wound is approximated.
    B. encouraging consumption of a high-carbohydrate diet for energy.
    C. discouraging resuming use of antidepressants until discharge.
    D. administering pain medication as needed.

Answers to Self-Assessment Questions

1. B. a **65-year-old with chronic bronchitis**
   Rationale: Chronic obstructive pulmonary disease, diabetes, hypoalbuminemia, and obesity are risk factors for wound complications. The patients in options A, C, and D do not meet those criteria. The patient in option B has COPD.

2. A. **internal thoracic artery**
   Rationale: Use of the ITA decreases blood supply by 90%. The decrease in blood supply will delay wound healing and put the patient at risk for a postoperative SSI.

3. D. **decreased cardiac index**
   Rationale: Decreased perfusion, as evidenced by a decrease in cardiac index, can increase risk for development of surgical site infections. Increased number of grafts, longer CPB runs, and hypothermia place patients at risk as well.

4. B. **needing autotransfusion of mediastinal blood**
   Rationale: Autotransfusion of mediastinal blood is a documented risk factor for the development of postoperative surgical site infections. Presence of a rubber dam decreases the risk of a surgical site infection. Peripheral edema is not a risk factor. Increased cardiac output will likely increase perfusion to the surgical site, which will decrease the risk of development of a surgical site infection.

5. A. **an infection and drainage to an organ related to surgery**
   Rationale: Infection with drainage to organ or space related to surgery should be reported as a deep incisional surgical site infection. The other three options describe a superficial surgical site infection.

6.   A. **permeable to allow for gas exchange**
     Rationale: Optimal dressing characteristics are permeable to allow for gas exchange, impermeable to prevent microorganism and exogenous sources of contamination, and the ability to provide an insulating effect. Dressing decisions should be based on cost and managing specific conditions such as drainage absorption.

7.   B. **110 mg/dL preprandial**
     Rationale: According to the consensus statement by the American Association of Clinical Endocrinologists and the American Diabetes Association, for patients who are not critically ill, it is recommended that preprandial serum glucose levels be 100 mg/dL up to a maximum of 180 mg/dL.

8.   B. **induration**
     Rationale: Presence of induration may indicate presence of infection. An approximated wound and minimal wound tension indicate wound healing. Slight redness at the edges of the incision site is an expected finding during the healing process.

9.   B. **dilation and curettage**
     Rationale: Saphenous vein graft infections occur more frequently in patients with obesity. Dilation and curettage followed by open packing of the wound may be required.

10. D. **administering pain medication as needed**
     Rationale: Assuring adequate pain control helps enhance the patient's willingness to be active and the ability to adhere to treatment regimens.

CLINICAL INQUIRY BOX

Question: What are the outcomes of patients with sternal wound infections who are treated with Redon drains (RD) and antibiotic therapy?

Reference: Dubert, M., Pourbaix, A., Alkhoder, S., Mabileau, G., Lescure, F.-X., Ghodhbane, W., . . . Lucet, J.-C. (2015). Sternal wound infection after cardiac surgery: Management and outcome. *PLOS ONE*. doi:10.1371/journal.pone.0139122

Objective: To determine the effectiveness of treatment of sternal wound infections with Redon drains and antibiotic therapy.

Method: Single-center analysis of consecutive patients who underwent reexploration surgery for surgical wound infection over a 3-year period.

Results: 160 patients developed a surgical wound infection. Of these 64% met CDC criteria. Similar surgical procedures were performed on the CDC+ and CDC− criteria groups. Patients with CDC+ surgical wound infections had longer antibiotic therapy; there was a 17% mortality rate in that group of patients. This compared with a mortality rate of 3% in the CDC− criteria group. Death or redo operations were associated with female gender, higher EuroSCORE, and longer ICU length of stay.

Conclusion: Patients who developed a surgical wound infection and who underwent one-stage debridement with Redon drains had a favorable outcome. The CDC+ criteria group of patients had a less favorable outcome.

References

Ahmed, A. S., & Antonsen, E. L. (2016). Immune and vascular dysfunction in diabetic wound healing. *Journal of Wound Healing, 25*(Suppl7), S35–S46.

Ahsan, S. (2015). A delayed case of surgical wound infection after coronary artery bypass graft surgery. *Clinical Microbiology & Case Reports, 1*(3). Retrieved from http://scientonline.org/open-access/a-delayed-case-of-surgical -wound-infection-after-coronary-artery-bypass-graft- surgery.pdf

Albert, N. M., Slifcak, E., Roach, J. D., Bena, J. F., Hoevath, G., Wilson, S., . . . Murray, T. (2014). Infection rates in intensive care units by electrocardiographic lead wire type: Disposable vs reusable. *American Journal of Critical Care, 23*(6), 460–468.

Aldea, G. S., Bakaeen, F. G., Pal, J., Fremes, S., Head, S. J., Sabik, J., . . . Mitchell, J. D. (2016). The Society of Thoracic Surgeons clinical practice guidelines on arterial conduits for coronary artery bypass grafting. *The Annals of Thoracic Surgery, 101*(2), 801–809.

Allegranzi, B., Bischoff, P., de Jonge, S., Kubilay, Z., Zayed, B., Gomes, S. M., . . . Solomkin, J. S. (2016). New WHO recommendations on preoperative measures for surgical site infection prevention: An evidence-based global perspective. *The Lancet Infectious Diseases, 16*(12), e276–e287. doi:10.1016/S1473-3099(16)30398-X

Allegranzi, B., Zayed, B., Bischoff, P., Kubilay, N. Z., de Jonge, S., & de Vries, F. (2016). New WHO recommendations on intraoperative and postoperative measures for surgical site infection prevention: An evidence-based global perspective. *The Lancet Infectious Diseases, 16*(12), e288–e303. doi:10.1016/S

Allen, V. G., Kohan, C., & Smith, B. A. (2015). CHG crosswalk: Critical guideline review. *Prevention Strategist, Winter,* 56–64. Retrieved from http://www.apic.org/Member-Services/Prevention-Strategist

An, G., Zhang, H., Zheng, S., Wang, W., & Ma, L. (2017). Mid-term outcomes of common congenital heart defects through a right subaxillary thoracotomy. *Heart, Lung, and Circulation, 26*(4), 376–382. doi:10.1016/j.hlc.2015.05.028

Anderson, D. J., Podgorny, K., Berrios-Torres, S. I., Bratzler, D. W., Dellinger E. P., Greene, L., . . . Kaye, K. S. (2014). Strategies to prevent surgical site infections in acute care hospitals: 2014 update. *Infection Control and Hospital Epidemiology, 35*(6), 605–627.

Ayoub, F., Quirke, M., Conroy, R., & Hill, A. (2015). Chlorhexidine-alcohol versus povidine-iodine for pre-operative skin preparation: A systematic review and meta-analysis. *International Journal of Surgery Open, 1,* 41–46.

Barr, J., Fraser, G. L., Puntillo, K., Ely, E. W., Gélinas, C., Dasta, J. F., . . . Jaeschke, R. (2013). Clinical practice guidelines for the management of pain, agitation, and delirium in adult patients in the intensive care unit. *Critical Care Medicine, 41*(1), 263–306.

Bennett-Guerrero, E., Ferguson T. B., Lin, M., Garg, J., Mark, D. B., Scavo, V. A., . . . Corey, G. R. (2010). Effect of an implantable gentamicin-collagen sponge on sternal wound infections following cardiac surgery: A randomized trial. *Journal of the American Medical Association, 304*(7), 755–762.

Berg, L. T., & Jaakkola, P. (2013). Kuopio treatment strategy after deep sternal wound infection. *Scandinavian Journal of Surgery, 102*(1), 3–8.

Berrios-Torres, S. I., Umscheld, C. A., Bratzkerm, D. W., Leas, B., Stone, E. C., Kelz, R. R., . . . Schedter, W. P. (2017). Centers for Disease Control and Prevention guidelines for the prevention of surgical site infection. *Journal of the American Medical Association Surgery, 152*(8), 784–791.

Bowdish, M. E., Hui, D. S., Cleveland, J. D., Mack, W. J., Sinha, R., Ranjan, R., . . . Starnes, V. A. (2015). A comparison of aortic valve replacement via an anterior right minithoracotomy with standard sternotomy: A prospective score analysis of 492 patients. *European Journal of Cardio-Thoracic Surgery, 49*(2), 456–463.

Bratzler, D., Dellinger, E. P., Olsen, K., Perl, T., Auwaerter, P., Bolon, M., . . . Weinstein, R. A. (2013). Clinical practice guidelines for antimicrobial prophylaxis in surgery. *American Journal of Health-System Pharmacy, 70*(3), 195–283.

Brown, A. F., Leech, J. M., Rogers, T. R., & McLoughlin, R. M. (2013). Staphylococcus aureus colonization: Modulation of host immune response and impact on human vaccine design. *Frontiers in Immunology, 4.* doi:10.3389/fimmu2013.00507

Bryan, C. S., & Yarbrough, W. M. (2013). Preventing deep wound infections after coronary artery bypass grafting. *Texas Heart Institute Journal, 40*(2), 125–139.

Calafiore, A. M., Sheikh, A. A., Alfonso, J. J., Tantawi, T., Maklouf, B., Shawki, A., . . . DiMauro, M. (2017). Elective primary or secondary delayed sternal closure improves outcome in severely compromised patients. *The Thoracic and Cardiovascular Surgeon.* doi:10.1055/s-0037-1599132

Centers for Disease Control and Prevention. (2014). CDC/NHSN surveillance definitions for specific types of infections. Retrieved from http://www.cdc.gov/nhsn/PDFs/pscManual/17pscNosInfDef_current.pdf

Chen, L. F., Arduino, J. M., Sheng, S., Muhlbaier, L. H., Kanafani, Z. A., Harris, A. D., . . . Fowler, V. G. (2012). Epidemiology and outcome of major postoperative infections following cardiac surgery: Risk factors and impact of pathogen type. *American Journal of Infection Control, 40*(10), 963–968.

Chien, C. Y., Lin, C. H., & Hsu, R. B. (2014). Care bundle to prevent methicillin-resistant *Staphylococcus aureus* sternal wound infection after off-pump coronary artery bypass. *American Journal of Infection Control, 42*(5), 562–564.

Cotogni, P., Barbero, C., & Rinaldi, M. (2015). Deep sternal wound infection after cardiac surgery: Evidences and controversies. *World Journal of Critical Care Medicine, 4*(4), 265–273.

Cove, M. E., Spelman, D. W., & MacLaren, G. (2012). Infectious complications of cardiac surgery: A clinical review. *Journal of Cardiothoracic Anesthesiology, 26*(6), 1094–1100.

Cutrell, J. B., Barros, N., McBroom, M., Luby, J., Minhajuddin, A., Ring, S., . . . Grelich, P. (2016). Risk factors for deep sternal wound infection after cardiac surgery: Influence of red blood cell transfusions and chronic infection. *American Journal of Infection Control, 44*(11), 1302–1309.

Deniz, H., Gokaslan, G., Arslanoglu, Y., Ozcaliskan, O., Guzel, G., Yasim, A., . . . Ustunsoy, H. (2012). Treatment outcomes of postoperative mediastinitis in cardiac surgery; negative pressure wound therapy versus conventional treatment. *Journal of Cardiothoracic Surgery, 7.* Retrieved from http://www.cardiothoracicsurgery.org/content/7/1/67

Diaz, V., & Newman, J. (2015). Surgical site infection and prevention guidelines: A primer for certified registered nurse anesthetists. *AANA Journal, 83*(1), 63–68.

Dong, Z., Yu, B., Zhang, Q., Pei, H., Xing, J., & Song, Z. (2016). Early rehabilitation therapy is beneficial for patients with prolonged mechanical ventilation after coronary bypass surgery. *International Heart Journal, 57*(2), 241–246.

Dumville, J. C., Gray, T. A., Walter, C. J., Sharp, C. A., & Page, T. (2014). Dressings for the prevention of surgical site infection. *Cochrane Database of Systematic Reviews, 9,* CD003091.

Edmiston, C. E., Bruden, B., Rucinski, M. C., Henen, C., Graham, M. B., & Lewis, B. L. (2013). Reducing the risk of surgical site infections: Does chlorhexidine gluconate provide a risk reduction benefit? *American Journal of Infection Control, 41*(5), S49–S55.

Edmiston, C. E., & Spencer, M. (2014). Patient care interventions to help reduce the risk of surgical site infections. *AORN Journal, 100*(6), 590–602.

Falk-Brynhildsen, K., Soderquist, B., Friberg, O., & Nilsson, U. (2014). Bacterial growth and wound infection following saphenous vein harvesting in cardiac surgery: A randomized control trial of the impact of microbial skin sealant. *European Journal of Clinical Microbiology & Infectious Diseases, 33*(11), 1981–1987.

Faritous, Z., Ardeshiri, M., Yazdanian, F., Jalali, A., Totonchi, Z., & Azarfarin, R. (2014). Hyperglycemia or high hemoglobin A1C: Which one is more associated with morbidity and mortality after coronary artery bypass graft surgery? *Annals of Thoracic and Cardiovascular Surgery, 20*(3), 223–228.

Feron, J. M., & Maupriez, R. (2016). Fracture repair: General aspects and influence of osteoporosis and anti-osteoporosis treatment. *Injury, 47*(Suppl 1), S10–S14.

Formanek, M. B., Herwaldt, L. A., Perencevich, E. N., & Schweizer, M. L. (2014). Gentamicin/collagen sponge use may reduce the risk of surgical site infections for patients undergoing cardiac operations: A meta-analysis. *Surgical Infection, 15*(3), 244–255.

Gelijns, A. C., Moskowitz, A. J., Acker, M. A., Argenziano, M., Geller, N. L., Puskas, J. D., . . . Blackstone, E. H. (2014). Management practices and major infections after cardiac surgery. *Journal of the American College of Cardiology, 64*(4). doi:10.1016/j.jacc.2014.04.052

George, S., Leasure, A. R., & Horstmanshot, D. (2016). Effectiveness of decolonization with chlorhexidine and mupirocin in reducing surgical site infections: A systematic review. *Dimensions of Critical Care Nursing, 35*(4), 204–222.

Girish, G., Agarwal, S., Satang, D. K., Tempe, D., Dutta, N., & Pratap, H. (2014). Glycemic control in cardiac surgery: Rationale and current evidence. *Annals of Cardiac Anaesthesia, 17*(3), 222–228.

Godbole, G., Pai, V., Kolvekar, S., & Wilson A. (2012). Use of gentamicin-collagen sponges in closure of sternal wounds in cardiothoracic surgery to reduce wound infection. *Interactive Cardiovascular and Thoracic Surgery 14*(4), 390–394.

Goh, S. S. C. (2017). Post-sternotomy mediastinitis in the modern era. *Journal of Cardiac Surgery, 32,* 556–566.

Graling, P. R., & Vasaly, F. W. (2013). Effectiveness of 2% CHG cloth bathing for reducing surgical site infections. *AORN Journal, 97*(5), 547–551.

Grauhan, O., Navasardyan, A., Hofmann, M., Muller, P., Stein, J., & Hetzer, R. (2013). Prevention of poststernotomy

wound infections in obese patients by negative pressure wound therapy. *The Journal of Thoracic and Cardiovascular Surgery, 145*(5), 1387–1392.

Greenhalgh, D. G. (2015). Management of the skin and soft tissue in the geriatric surgical patient. *Surgical Clinics of North America, 95*(1), 103–114.

Gudbjartsson, T., Jeppsson, A., Sjögren, J., Steingrimsson, S., Geirsson, A., Friberg, O., . . . Dunning, J. (2016). Surgical wound infections following open heart surgery—a review. *Scandinavian Cardiovascular Journal, 50*(5/6). doi:10.1080/14017431.2016.1180427

Hargraves, J. D. (2014). Glycemic control in cardiac surgery: Implementing an evidence-based insulin infusion protocol. *American Journal of Critical Care, 23*(3), 250–258.

Hashem, M., Nelliot, A., & Needham, D. M. (2016). Early mobilization and rehabilitation in the ICU: Moving back to the future. *Respiratory Care, 61*(7), 971–979.

Héquet, D., Kralidis, G., Carrel, T., Cusini, A., Garzoni, C., Hullin, R., . . . Manuel, O. (2016). Ventricular assist devices as bridge to heart transplantation: Impact on post-transplant infections. *BMC Infectious Disease, 16*(321). doi:10.1186/s12879-016-1658-0

Hess, C. N., Lopes, R. D., Gibson, C. M., Hager, R., Wojdyla, D. M., Englum, B. R., . . . Alexander, J. H. (2014). Saphenous vein graft failure after coronary artery bypass surgery: Insights from PREVENT IV. *Circulation, 130*(17), 1445–1451.

Hillis, L. D., Smith, P., Anderson, J., Bittl, J., Bridges, C., Byrne, J., . . . Winniford, M. D. (2012). 2011 ACCF/AHA guideline for coronary artery bypass graft surgery: Executive summary. A report of the American College of Cardiology Foundation/American Heart Association task force on practice guidelines. *Anesthesia & Analgesia, 114*(1), 11–45.

Hussey, L. C., Leeper, B., & Hynan, L. S. (1998). Development of the sternal wound infection prediction scale. *Heart & Lung, 27*(5), 326–336.

Jenks, P. J., Laurent, M., McQuarry, S., & Watkins, R. (2014). Clinical and economic burden of surgical site infection (SSI) and predicted financial consequences of elimination of SSI from an English hospital. *Journal of Hospital Infection, 86*(1), 24–33.

Kaneda, T., Nishino, T., Saga, T., Nakamoto, S., Ogawa, T., & Satsu, T. (2013). Small right vertical infra-axillary incision for minimally invasive port-access cardiac surgery: A moving window method. *Interactive CardioVascular and Thoracic Surgery, 16*(4), 544–546.

Kim, H. J., Jung, S. H., Kim, J. B., Choo, S. J., Yun, T. J., Chung, C. H., . . . Lee, J. W. (2013). Early postoperative complications after heart transplantation in adult recipients: Asan Medical Center experience. *The Korean Journal of Thoracic and Cardiovascular Surgery, 46*(6), 426–432.

Klinkner, G., & Murray, M. (2014). Clinical nurse specialists lead teams to impact glycemic control after cardiac surgery. *Clinical Nurse Specialist, 28*(4), 240–246.

Kowalewski, M., Pawliszak, W., Zaborowska, K., Navarese, E. P., Szwed, K., & Kowalkowska, M. E. (2015).

Gentamicin-collagen sponge reduces the risk of sternal wound infections after heart surgery: Meta-analysis. *The Journal of Thoracic and Cardiovascular Surgery, 149*(6), 1631–1640. doi:10.1016/jtcvs.2015.01.034

Lazar, H. L., Salm, T. V., Engelman, R., Orgill, D., & Gordon, S. (2016). Prevention and management of surgical wound infections. *The Journal of Thoracic and Cardiovascular Surgery, 152*(4), 962–972.

Lemaignen, A., Birgand, G., Ghodhbane, W., Alihoder, S., Lonom, I., Belorgey, S., . . . Lucet, J. C. (2015). Surgical wound infection after cardiac surgery: Incidence and risk factors according to clinical presentation. *Clinical Microbiology & Infection, 2*(7), e11–e18.

Lipke, V. L., & Hyott, A. S. (2010). Reducing surgical site infections by bundling multiple risk reduction strategies and active surveillance. *AORN Journal, 92*(3), 288–296.

Lobdell, K. W., Stamou, S., & Sanchez, J. A. (2012). Hospital-acquired infections. *The Surgical Clinics of North America, 92*(1), 65–77.

Lo Torto, F., Monfrecola, A., Kaciulyte, J., Ciudad, P., Casella, D., Ribuffo, D., . . . Carlesimo, B. (2017). Preliminary result with incisional negative pressure wound therapy and pectoralis major muscle flap for median sternotomy wound infection in a high-risk patient population. *International Wound Journal, 4*(6), 1335–1339.

Luo, H., Wang, J., Qiao, C., Zhang, X., Zhang, W., & Song, L. (2014). Evaluation of different minimally invasive techniques in the surgical treatment of atrial septal defect. *The Journal of Thoracic and Cardiovascular Surgery, 148*(1), 188–193.

Maragakis, L. L., Cosgrove, S. E., Martinez, E. A., Tucker, M. G., Cohen, D. B., & Perl, T. M. (2009). Intraoperative fraction of inspired oxygen is a modifiable risk factor for surgical site infection after spinal surgery. *Anesthesiology, 110*(3), 556–562.

Martin, E. T., Kaye, K. S., Knott, C., Nguyen, H., Santarossa, M., Evans, R., . . . Jaber, L. (2016). Diabetes and risk of surgical site infection: A systematic review and meta-analysis. *Infection Control Hospital Epidemiology, 37*(1), 88–99.

McDonnell, M., Alexanian, S., White, L., & Lazar, H. (2012). A primer for achieving glycemic control in the cardiac surgical patient. *Journal of Cardiac Surgery, 27*(4), 470–477.

Meyer, M. J., Stanislaus, A. B., Lee, J., Waak, K., Ryan, C., Saxena, R., . . . Eikermann, M. (2013). Surgical intensive care unit mobilisation score (SOMS) trial: A protocol for an international, multicentre, randomised controlled trial focused on goal-directed early mobilization of surgical ICU patients. *BMJ, 3*(8). Retrieved from http://bmjopen.bmj.com/content/3/8/e003262.full

Mimoz, O., Lucet, J. C., Kerforne, T., Pascal, J., Souweine, B., Goudet, V., . . . Timsit, J. F. (2015). Skin antisepsis with chlorhexidine-alcohol versus povidone iodine-alcohol, with and without skin scrubbing, for prevention of intravascular-catheter-related infection (CLEAN): An open-label, multicenter, randomised, controlled, two-by factorial trial. *The Lancet, 386*(10008), 2069–2077.

Mishra, P. K., Ashoub, A., Sallayeh, K., Aktuerk, D., Ohri, S., Raja, S. G., . . . Luckraz, H. (2014). Role of topical application of gentamicin containing collagen implants in cardiac surgery. *Journal of Cardiothoracic Surgery, 9*(122), 1–20.

Morrison, T. N., Chen, A. F., Taneja, M., Kucukdurmaz, F., Rothman, R. H., & Parvizi, J. (2016). Single vs repeat surgical skin preparations for reducing surgical site infection after total joint arthroplasty: A prospective, randomized, double-blinded study. *The Journal of Arthroplasty, 31*(6), 1289–1294.

Musallam, E. (2014). The predictors of surgical site infection post cardiac surgery: A systematic review. *Journal of Vascular Nursing, 32*(3), 105–118. doi:10.1016/j.jvn2014.01.003

O'Brien, S. M., Shahian, D. M., Filardo, G., Ferraris, V. A., Haan, C. K., Rich, J. B., . . . Anderson, R. P. (2009). The Society of Thoracic Surgeons 2008 cardiac surgery risk models: Part 2—isolated valve surgery. *Annals of Thoracic Surgery, 94*(6), 2166–2171.

Pancholy, B., & Raman, J. (2015). Chest wall reconstruction using sternal plating in patients with complex sternal dehiscence. *Annals of Thoracic Surgery, 99*, 2228–2230.

Patel, B. K., Pohlman, A. S., Hall, J. B., & Kress, J. P. (2014). Impact of early mobilization on glycemic control and ICU-acquired weakness in critically ill patients who are mechanically ventilated. *Chest, 143*(3), 583–589.

Pezzella, A. T., Holmes, S. D., Pritchard, G., Speir, A. M., & Ad, N. (2014). Impact of perioperative glycemic control strategy on patient survival after coronary bypass surgery. *Annals of Thoracic Surgery, 98*(4), 1281–1285.

Phillips, M., Rosenberg, A., Shopsin, B., Cuff, G., Skeete, F., Foti, A., . . . Bosco. J. (2014). Preventing surgical site infections: A randomized, open-label trial of nasal mupirocin ointment and nasal povidone-iodine solution. *Infection Control and Hospital Epidemiology, 35*(7), 826–832.

Pierpont, Y. N., Dinh, T. P., Salas, R. E., Johnson, E. L., Wright, T. G., Robson, M. C., . . . Payne, W. G. (2014). Obesity and surgical wound healing: A current review. *International Scholarly Research Notices, Obesity, 2014*. Retrieved from http://www.hindawi.com/journals/isrn/2014/638936/

Privitera, G. P., Costa, A. L., Brusaferro, S., Chirletti, P., Corsasso, P., Masimetti, G., . . . Viale, P. (2017). Skin antisepsis with chlorhexidine versus iodine for the prevention of surgical site infection: A systematic review and meta-analysis. *American Journal of Infection Control, 45*(2), 180–189.

Raja, S. G., & Sarang, Z. (2013). Endoscopic vein harvesting: Technique, outcomes, concerns & controversies. *Journal of Thoracic Disease, 5*(Suppl 6), S630–S637.

Reade, M. C., Phil, D., & Finter, S. (2014). Sedation and delirium in the intensive care unit. *The New England Journal of Medicine, 370*, 444–454.

Richter, J. H., Jarrett, N. M., & LaBresh, K. A. (2014). *Evidence-Based Guidelines for Selected, Candidate, and Previously Considered Hospital Acquired Conditions: Final Report.* Retrieved from http://www.cms.gov/Medicare/Medicare

-Fee-for-Service-Payment/HospitalAcqCond/Downloads/Evidence-Based-Guidelines.pdf

Sabik, J. F. (2011). Understanding saphenous vein graft patency. *Circulation,124*(3), 273–275.

Sajja, L. R. (2015). Strategies to reduce deep sternal wound infection after bilateral internal mammary artery grafting. *International Journal of Surgery, 16,* 171–178.

Sandy-Hodgetts, K., Carville, K., & Leslie, G. D. (2015). Determining risk factors for surgical wound dehiscence: A literature review. *International Wound Journal, 12*(3), 265–275.

Sankaralingam, S., Kim, R. B., & Padwal, R. S. (2015). The impact of obesity on the pharmacology of medications used for cardiovascular risk factor control. *Canadian Journal of Cardiology, 31*(2), 167–176.

Santo, V. J., Dargon, P. T., Azarbal, A. F., Liem, T. K., Mitchell, E. L., Monetta, G. L., . . . Landry, G. J. (2014). Open versus endoscopic great saphenous vein harvest for lower extremity revascularization of critical limb ischemia. *Journal of Vascular Surgery, 59,* 427–437.

Schimmer, C., Gross, J., Ramm, E., Morfeld, B. C., Hoffmann, G., Panholzer, B., . . . Petzina, R. (2017). Prevention of surgical site infections in cardiac surgery: A two-centre prospective randomized controlled study. *European Journal of Cardiothoracic Surgery, 51,* 67–72.

Sexton, D. J. (2016). *Postoperative mediastinitis after cardiac surgery.* Retrieved from http://www.uptodate.com/contents/postoperative-mediastinitis-after-cardiac-surgery

Sgonc, R., & Gruber, J. (2013). Age-related aspects of cutaneous wound healing: A mini-review. *Gerontology, 59,* 159–164.

Shahian, D. M., O'Brien, S. M., Filardo, G., Ferraris, V. A., Haan, C. K., Rich, J. B., . . . Anderson, R. P. (2009a). The Society of Thoracic Surgeons 2008 cardiac surgery risk models: Part 1—coronary artery bypass grafting surgery. *Annals of Thoracic Surgery, 88*(1 suppl), S2–S22.

Shahian, D. M., O'Brien, S. M., Filardo, G., Ferraris, V. A., Haan, C. K., Rich, J. B., . . . Anderson, R. P. (2009b). The Society of Thoracic Surgeons 2008 cardiac surgery risk models: Part 3—valve plus coronary artery bypass grafting surgery. *Annals of Thoracic Surgery, 88*(1 suppl), S43–S62.

Shi, Y.-D., Qi, F. Z., & Zhang, Y. (2014). Treatment of sternal wound infections after open-heart surgery. *Asian Journal of Surgery, 37*(1), 24–29.

Spiliopoulos, S., Autschbach, R., Koefer, R., & Tenderich, G. (2015). Delayed sternal closure after total artificial heart implantation. *The Journal of Thoracic and Cardiovascular Surgery, 150,* 417–418.

Staveski, S., Arajano, C., Casazza, M., Bair, E., Quan, H., Dong, E., . . . Roth, S. J. (2016). Silver-impregnated dressings for sternotomy incisions to prevent surgical site infections in children. *American Journal of Critical Care, 25*(5), 402–408.

Stephens, R. S., & Whitman, G. (2015). Postoperative critical care of the adult cardiac surgery patient: Part II: Procedure-specific considerations, management of complications, and quality improvement. *Critical Care Medicine, 43*(9), 1995–2014.

Stopher, L., & Jansen, S. (2017). Systematic review of the impact and treatment of malnutrition in patients with chronic vascular wounds. *Wound Practice and Research, 25*(2), 71–80.

Subramaniam, B., Lerner, A., Novack, V., Khabbaz, K., Paryente-Wiesmann, M., Hess, P., . . . Talmor, D. (2014). Increased glycemic variability in patients with elevated preoperative HbA$_{1C}$ predicts adverse outcomes following coronary artery bypass grafting surgery. *Anesthesia & Analgesia, 118*(2), 277–287.

Taggart, D. P., Altman, D. G., Gray, A. M., Lees, B., Gerry, S., Benedetto, U., . . . Flather, M. (2016). Randomized trial of bilateral versus single internal-thoracic-artery grafts. *The New England Journal of Medicine, 375,* 2540–2549.

Tarzia, V., Carrozzini, M., Bortolussi, G., Buratto, E., Bejko, J., Comisso, M., . . . Gerosa, G. (2014). Impact of vacuum-assisted closure therapy on outcomes of sternal wound dehiscence. *Interactive CardioVascular and Thoracic Surgery, 19*(1), 70–75.

Troutman, S., Hussey, L. C., Hynan, L., & Lucisano, K. (2001). Sternal wound infection prediction scale: A test of the reliability and validity. *Nursing and Health Sciences, 3*(1), 1–8.

Turtiainen, J., Hakala, T., Hakkarainen, T., & Karhukorpi, J. (2014). The impact of surgical wound bacterial colonization on the incidence of surgical site infection after lower limb vascular surgery: A prospective observational study. *European Journal of Vascular Endovascular Surgery, 47*(4), 411–417.

Umpierrez, G., Cardona, S., Pasquel, F., Jacobs, S., Peng, L., Unigwe, M., . . . Thourani, V. H. (2015). Randomized controlled trial of intensive versus conservative glucose control in patients undergoing coronary artery bypass graft surgery: GLUCO-CABG trial. *Diabetes Care, 38*(9), 1665–1672.

Umpierrez, G. A., Hellman, R., Korytkowski, M. T., Kosiborod, M., Maynard, G. A., Montori, V. M., . . . Van den Berghe, G. (2012). Management of hyperglycemia in hospitalized patients in non-critical care setting: An Endocrine Society clinical practice guideline. *The Journal of Clinical Endocrinology & Metabolism, 97*(1), 16–38.

Vasunilashorn, S., Fong, T., Albuquerque, A., Marcantonio, E., Schmitt, E. M., Tommet, D., . . . Inouye, S. (2017). Delirium severity post-surgery and its relationship with long-term cognitive decline in a cohort of patients without dementia. *Journal of Alzheimer's Disease, 61*(1), 347–358.

Walter, C., Dumville, J., Sharp, C., & Page, T. (2012). Systematic review and meta-analysis of wound dressings in the prevention of surgical-site infections in surgical wounds healing by primary intention. *British Journal of Surgery, 99*(9), 1185–1194.

Xuan, Y., Huang, B., Tian, H., Chi, L., Duan, Y., Wang, X., . . . Jin, L. T. (2014). High-glucose inhibits human fibroblast cell migration in wound healing via repression of bFGF-regulating JNK phosphorylation. *PLoS ONE, 9*(9), e108182. doi:10.1371/journal.pone.0108182

Yokoe, D. S., Anderson, D. J., Berenholtz, S. M., Calfee, D. P., Dubberke, E. R., Ellingson, K. D., . . . Maragakis, L. L. (2014). A compendium of strategies to prevent healthcare associated infections in acute care hospitals: 2014 update. *Infection Control Hospital Epidemiology, 35*(8), 967–977.

Yost, G., Pappas, P., Tatooles, A., & Bhat, G. (2015). Does delayed sternal closure cause increased infection rates after left ventricular assist device implantation? *The Journal of Heart and Lung Transplantation, 34*(4), S68. doi:10.1016/j.healun.2015.01.174

Zellinger, M., & Lienberger, T. (1991). Use of the rubber dam after open heart surgery. *Critical Care Nurse, 11*(8), 24–27.

Web Resources

Centers for Disease Control and Prevention, National Healthcare Safety Network (NHSN): Surveillance for Surgical Site Infection (SSI) Events: http://www.cdc.gov/nhsn/acute-care-hospital/ssi/index.html

Guideline for the Prevention of Surgical Site Infection, 1999: http://www.cdc.gov/HAI/ssi/ssi.html

Medicare Program: Changes to the hospital in-patient prospective payment systems and fiscal year 2008 rates: https://www.cms.gov/Medicare/Medicare-Fee-for-Service-Payment/AcuteInpatientPPS/downloads/CMS-1533-FC.pdf

The Society of Thoracic Surgeons: http://www.sts.org

CHAPTER 19

Bridge to Transplant and Cardiac Transplantation

Dalton Skipper, Carey Mitchell

▶ Introduction

According to the American Heart Association (AHA) Heart Disease and Stroke Statistics, 2018 Update, approximately 6.5 million adult Americans had a diagnosis of heart failure (HF) between 2011 and 2014. In 2015, one in eight deaths in the United States (U.S.) included HF as a contributing cause (Benjamin et al., 2018). Of those people who develop HF, approximately 50% will die within 5 years of diagnosis (Yancey et al., 2013). There are approximately 1 million new cases of HF being diagnosed in the U.S. each year (Benjamin et al., 2018). Total inclusive HF costs (including medications, hospitalizations, missed work days) in the U.S. are estimated to be $32 billion (Go et al., 2013).

Since the early 2000s, medical advances have greatly increased treatment options for people living with HF. In particular, mechanical circulatory support (MCS) technology has emerged as a life-saving option for patients with acute and chronic HF not amenable to maximal therapy.

In the U.S., 254 facilities currently have the ability to perform cardiac transplantation. According to Organ Procurement and Transplantation Network (OPTN) data, 3,422 heart transplants were performed in the U.S. in 2017. Based on OPTN data as of May 29, 2018, 60,679 heart transplants have been performed in the U.S. since 1988. As of May 29, 2018, per OPTN data, there were 4,002 waitlisted candidates for a heart transplant. Waitlist mortality has decreased each year since 2006; in 2013, 7.2% of those in the first year on the waitlist died (Colvin et al., 2018). A new heart allocation system planned for implementation in fall 2018 will change the stratification process for the most urgent candidates, changing from a three-tier to a six-tier system, while taking into account the increased use of MCS and addressing geographical inequalities in access to donors (OPTN, 2018).

This chapter reviews the management of HF as the patient moves through the trajectory of illness toward consideration for MCS, transplantation, or both. The role of the critical care nurse

Original contributions from Tracy Andrews and Roberta Kaplow is discussed during the various phases of illness, including the special decision regarding mechanical assistance devices and transplantation.

▶ Management of Heart Failure

Heart failure is the result of structural or functional impairment to the heart that causes impairment in ventricular filling, ejection, or both of blood from its different chambers. In its advanced stages, HF can produce decreased cardiac output (CO) and fluid overload. It can be a result of impairment to any layer of the heart, including the pericardium, the heart valves, or from vessels feeding the heart (Yancey et al., 2013). Heart failure is separated into two separate categories based on ejection fraction (EF): those with a reduced EF (HFrEF), which is typically an EF of 40% or less, and those with a preserved EF (HFpEF), or an EF greater than 50%. Those with an EF between 40% and 50% are generally treated like patients with HFrEF.

Heart failure is further classified by the American College of Cardiology Foundation and the American Heart Association (ACCF/AHA) into four separate stages, A through D. The ACCF/AHA stages are progressive and unidirectional; once patients move to a higher stage, they cannot regress to a lower stage. Medical management and intervention are specific to each stage.

The New York Heart Association (NYHA) has four functional classifications that gauge severity of symptoms in structural heart disease based on exercise capacity and symptom burden.

Management of HF is tailored to stage. In stage A, those at risk for HF but without symptoms, management includes controlling blood pressure, diabetes, and dyslipidemia and reducing body mass index (BMI) if obese. Smoking cessation should be addressed as well as heavy alcohol use. Stage B heart failure, where there is structural heart disease but no symptoms of HF, uses a regimen of angiotensin-converting enzyme (ACE) inhibitors or angiotensin receptor blockers (ARBs) in addition to beta blockers, as tolerated (Yancey et al, 2013). Patients with stage C HF, those with

both structural heart disease and symptoms of HF, should take an ACE inhibitor, ARB, or angiotensin receptor neprilysin inhibitor (ARNI) in addition to a beta blocker and an aldosterone receptor antagonist such as spironolactone (Aldactone®). Ivabradine (Corlanor®), a medication that inhibits the I_f current in the sinoatrial node, can also help with heart rate reduction (Yancey et al., 2017). Isosorbide dinitrate (Isordil®) and hydralazine (Apresoline®) are also used in stage C HF in addition to implantable cardioverter-defibrillators and cardiac resynchronization therapy.

Unfortunately, despite medical optimization, approximately 5% of all patients with HF progress to stage D (Habal & Garan, 2017). Functional status declines as the disease progresses and patients become refractory to treatment. At this time, options are limited to palliation, ongoing supportive medical management, and advanced therapies such as MCS or transplantation (Chaudhry & Stewart, 2016). The Interagency Registry for Mechanically Assisted Circulatory Support (INTERMACS) classification system was developed in 2009 and divides advanced HF patients considering MCS into seven different profiles: from profile 7, with advanced NYHA class III HF, to profile 1, the "crash and burn" patient who is not stable on maximum inotrope support (Chaudhry & Stewart, 2016).

As a patient's HF progresses, advanced therapies for volume management, including thoracentesis for accumulative pleural effusions or ultrafiltration for overall volume reduction, may be required. When clinical status declines and these measures begin to lose efficacy, end-organ perfusion is compromised. Patients may present to an intensive care unit (ICU) with either a "warm and wet" profile, which means they are volume overloaded but still have compensatory perfusion, or a "cold and wet" profile, which means they are either in or nearing cardiogenic shock. When a patient reaches this point, advancement in therapy will typically include inotropic agents (e.g., dobutamine [Dobutrex®], dopamine [Intropin®], milrinone [Primacor®], or inamrinone [Inocor®]) or intra-aortic balloon pump (IABP) insertion. Intra-aortic balloon pump placement is not feasible in all patients, though. Some patients require even more advanced therapies, including ventricular assist device (VAD) implantation.

Ventricular assist devices can provide left ventricular (LVAD), right ventricular (RVAD), or biventricular (BiVAD) support. The most common scenario involves the use of LVAD to counteract LV dysfunction. Mechanisms for movement of blood vary among the different types of pumps. In general, blood is drained from the apex of the LV to the pump via the inflow cannula. It is returned to the body via an outflow cannula, which is attached to the aorta. The pump is housed in the pre-peritoneal space of the abdomen, near the stomach, or in the pericardial space. The pumps can pump 8 to 10 L of flow based on pump type and speed (Miller & Rogers, 2018). A percutaneous driveline that is tunneled across the pre-peritoneal space to the left side of the body carries the electrical cable and air vent to the electrical controller outside the patient's body. The risk of pump infection is reduced by tunneling the cable across the abdomen, thereby increasing the distance from the pump to the exit site and allowing the body to form a natural seal around the driveline. The controller controls the power and speed of the device and reports operating parameters to the user. It uses batteries or wall power as a power source. More specific information to VAD operation and postoperative nursing care for VADs is discussed later in this section.

FIGURES 19.1, 19.2, and **19.3** show an LVAD, RVAD, and BiVAD, respectively.

Multidisciplinary teams have become an integral part of HF management. These teams include physicians, pharmacists, nutritionists, physical and occupational therapists, and critical care

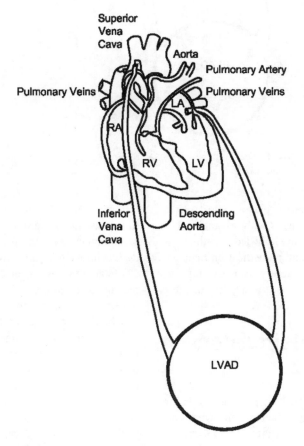

FIGURE 19.1 Left ventricular assist device.
Illustrated by Lydia Lemmond

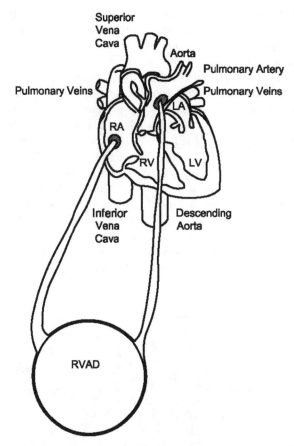

FIGURE 19.2 Right ventricular assist device.

Illustrated by Lydia Lemmond

nurses. Critical care nurses play a major role in the management of patients with advancing HF. Their assessment skills and knowledge of the multiple phases of HF, including medication management and post cardiac surgery recovery, improve patient care and lead to better outcomes in these patients (Paul & Hice, 2014).

▶ Mechanical Circulatory Support

After optimizing medical therapy and treating reversible causes, patients that remain symptomatic progress to advanced HF. At this point, options include a heart transplant, MCS, or palliation. While a heart transplant is the gold standard for

HF treatment, it is not available to all patients due to limitations in the donor pool and strict transplantation criteria. As a result, the number of MCS devices implanted has risen each year. Between June 23, 2006, and the end of 2016, more than 22,000 patients received a U.S. Food and Drug Administration (FDA)–approved MCS (Kirklin et al., 2017).

Mechanical circulatory support has three primary functions: bridge to transplant, bridge to recovery, and destination therapy. For those patients who meet heart transplantation criteria, have NYHA stage 4 HF, and have deterioration of their clinical status to the point where they can no longer live without mechanical support, bridge to transplant is explored. Intermediate- to long-term MCS placement is utilized to provide these patients support until heart transplantation

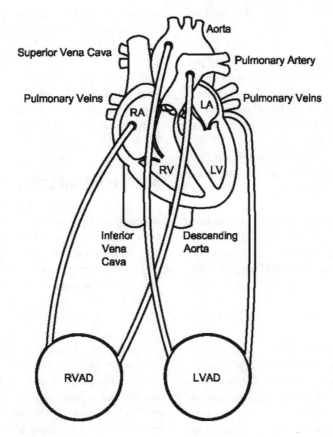

FIGURE 19.3 Biventricular assist device.

Illustrated by Lydia Lemmond

can occur. LVADs were approved for bridge to transplantation in 1994. According to the International Society for Heart and Lung Transplantation Registry (2017a), from 2009 through June 2016, 42.9% of heart transplant recipients were utilizing MCS at the time of transplant, with 40.6% using an LVAD. This is an increase from 23% of recipients using MCS (21.4% using LVAD) from 2003 to 2008. Recent analyses have also shown that an LVAD, used as a bridge to transplantation, did not change survival times or incidence of rejections (Kwak, Majewski, & LeVan, 2018). Of all patients receiving LVADs, 26% were listed as bridge to transplant (Kirklin et al, 2017).

Patients who may have short-term contraindications to heart transplantation, end-organ compromise secondary to advanced HF, or lack of approval for heart transplantation listing are selected for bridge to decision or candidacy. These are the patients who are too unstable to be placed on the transplant list or receive long-term MCS. The short-term MCS that they receive is also known as rescue therapy. From recent INTERMACS data, 23% of patients who received continuous flow LVADs and BiVADs from 2015 to 2016 were listed as bridge to decision or candidacy (Kirklin et al., 2017).

For those patients who are ineligible for heart transplantation but meet MCS criteria, destination therapy (DT) is explored. As of July 2014, there are 173 U.S. centers that have been deemed DT by the Centers for Medicare and Medicaid Services (CMS) (2016). By 2015, almost half of the continuous-flow LVADs and BiVADs listed in the INTERMACS database were implanted as destination therapy (Kirklin et al., 2017). Research supports the use of VADs as DT. In 2001, the Randomization Evaluation of Mechanical Assistance for the Treatment of Congestive Heart Failure (REMATCH) trial compared the outcomes of pulsatile LVAD devices for DT with the outcomes of medical therapy. The survival rates and quality of life at 1 year were better in the LVAD patients than in the medical therapy patients (Desai & Hwang, 2018; Habal & Garan, 2017).

Bridge to recovery therapy is sought for those patients who have had an acute myocardial infarction or cardiogenic shock that has been deemed to be reversible. By LV unloading, these patients have the benefit of most or all of their native heart function, which allows reverse cardiac remodeling. From 2015 to 2016, per INTERMACS data, only 0.2% of continuous flow LVADs and BiVADs were used as bridge to recovery (Kirklin et al., 2017). Approximately 5% to 10% of patients are successfully weaned off VAD support (Subramaniam, 2015).

Contraindications for MCS may include septic shock, prolonged cardiopulmonary resuscitation, renal failure, predicted extremely short-term life expectancy due to comorbidities, patient/family declination of MCS, or clinical judgment against MCS by primary medical team (Takayama, Takeda, Doshi, & Jorde, 2014). Contraindications can also include frailty, which is based on a combination of factors, including functional capabilities, strength, and mood (Hayward & Jansz, 2015; Miller & Rogers, 2018). Individual centers that provide MCS also have algorithms that help decide appropriateness of treatment.

Mechanical circulatory support devices can be classified based on a number of different criteria: duration of support (short, intermediate, or long term), location of pump relative to the body, ventricles supported (left, right, or both), flow characteristics (pulsatile or continuous), pump design (axial or centrifugal), and generation of design.

Regardless of MCS used, anticoagulation is necessary to prevent pump thrombosis and thromboembolic events. Anticoagulation is generally administered per hospital protocol and often includes an antiplatelet agent (normally aspirin) and warfarin (Coumadin®). Clopidogrel (Plavix®) or dipyridamole (Persantine®) can be used if the patient is allergic to aspirin, if the center prefers dual antiplatelet therapy, or if pump thrombosis is a concern. A typical goal international normalized ratio (INR) is 1.5 to 2. Most centers have stopped heparin bridges to warfarin (Toega, Ruel, & Haddad, 2015). The percutaneous VADs generally use a manufacturer-recommended heparinized purge solution in addition to systemic heparin to prevent device thrombosis.

MCS Selection Criteria

Selection criteria for patients requiring any MCS therapy are rigorous. As part of patient evaluation, a battery of laboratory and diagnostic tests are performed to determine eligibility for a device. This process can also help decide which device, if any, is most appropriate for the patient. A VAD medical team is typically comprised of advanced HF-certified cardiologists, social workers, nurses, VAD coordinators, and cardiac surgeons who collaborate to determine the appropriateness of the device for the patient and decide on the plan of care. The surgeon and cardiologist determine the type of support required (i.e., LVAD, RVAD, or BiVAD). Left ventricular assist device recipients must have adequate RV function to achieve a successful outcome, because the LVAD is dependent on blood flow from the right ventricle. If RV failure is present, patients' length of stay, post implantation morbidity/mortality, and costs are increased. In such cases, RV failure must be treated with inotropes, decreasing pulmonary vascular resistance (PVR), and adjusting the flow of the LVAD. Severe RV failure necessitating RVAD implementation occurs in 10% to 25% of LVAD patients and should only be used as a last resort (Desai & Hwang, 2018).

Following placement of a short-term circulatory assist device and a period of hemodynamic stability, the patient's heart function and need for continued support are assessed. Some patients will regain some or most of their previous cardiac function, thus allowing for the removal of the assist device. Patients with acute viral myocarditis, for example, often experience improved cardiac function once the initial inflammatory processes within the cardiac muscle have resolved. Many patients, however, have chronic irreversible HF such that long-term mechanical support, transplant, or both will be necessary.

Recovery of heart function is assessed by briefly decreasing the amount of support provided by the device (e.g., decreasing device blood flow to 2 L/min) and monitoring the patient's hemodynamic parameters. If this brief trial is well tolerated, a transthoracic echocardiogram is obtained during a trial of decreased support to more accurately assess valve and ventricular function. Depending on the results of these trials, plans are made for device removal followed by appropriate medical therapy if there has been adequate recovery of cardiac function, or for transition to a long-term implanted device, heart transplant, or both if poor cardiac function persists.

Short-Term Mechanical Circulatory Support

The goal of short-term MCS is stabilization of acute cardiogenic shock, by decreasing preload and afterload, before employing longer term methods. Short-term MCS includes intra-aortic balloon counterpulsation, extracorporeal membranous oxygenation (ECMO), and the use of percutaneous ventricular assist devices (pVADs). As of 2018, current pVADs available include the TandemHeart PTVA® system (CardiacAssist, Inc., Pittsburgh, PA) and the Impella® system (Abiomed, Pittsburgh, PA). Percutaneous ventricular assist devices are advantageous in management of actively decompensated HF patients because of their ability to be quickly inserted via a less invasive procedure for the already unstable patient (Desai & Hwang, 2018). All of the short-term devices require anticoagulation, generally with heparin. A comparison of mechanical circulatory devices appears in **TABLE 19.1**.

Intra-Aortic Balloon Counterpulsation

Intra-aortic balloon pump placement assists the LV to unload some of the redundant accumulating volume, but it is not feasible in all patients. Those patients with severe aortic insufficiency, peripheral artery disease, or major aortopathies (e.g., dissection, large untreated aortic aneurysms) are not suitable candidates for IABP placement. Intra-aortic balloon pump therapy was initially thought to be an effective mechanical support mechanism for patients with cardiogenic shock and acute myocardial infarction; however, in the IABP-Shock II trial, this was shown not to be true (Takayama et al., 2014). Development of more powerful means of hemodynamic support has been required to manage advanced HF. While not shown to be the most effective means of MCS, more than 50,000 IABPs are implanted annually, making it the most frequently used MCS (Al Musa, Chue, & Lim, 2017). Intra-aortic balloon pump therapy was discussed in Chapter 10.

Extracorporeal Membrane Oxygenation

Extracorporeal membrane oxygenation (ECMO) is a technique of partial cardiopulmonary bypass (CPB) that was initially developed to treat reversible neonatal respiratory failure. There are three types of ECMO: veno-arterial (VA), veno-venous (VV), and arterial-arterial (AA). VV-ECMO is primarily used in respiratory failure, whereas VA-ECMO is used in cardiac collapse. An ECMO system uses standard CPB equipment that has been modified to reduce hemolysis, thrombus formation, and risk of air embolus. Extracorporeal membrane oxygenation can provide support for days or weeks. In VA-ECMO, blood is continuously withdrawn from any large central vein and pumped into a gas exchanger that oxygenates hemoglobin and removes carbon dioxide. The oxygenated blood is then pumped into any large artery (**FIGURE 19.4**). The heart and lungs are bypassed, providing both hemodynamic and respiratory support. VA-ECMO increases left ventricle afterload, necessitating venting of some kind to prevent LV dilation or pulmonary edema. This is often done with the addition of IABP or atrial septostomy. Additionally, VA-ECMO has no venous reservoir; hypervolemia is managed

TABLE 19.1 MCS Device Comparisons

	HeartMate II	HeartMate XVE	Thoratec PVAD	NOVACOR	Total Artificial Heart	ABIOMED (AB5000)	TandemHeart
Type of blood flow	Pulsatile flow	Continuous flow (axial)	Pulsatile flow	Pulsatile flow	Pulsatile flow	Pulsatile flow	Continuous flow (axial)
BSA limitation (m²)	1.5	1.3	Smallest used on 0.73	1.5	1.7	1.2	1.2
Anticoagulation	ASA only	Antiplatelet therapy and initial heparin followed by warfarin	Initial heparin followed by warfarin or ASA	Antiplatelet therapy and initial heparin followed by warfarin	Antiplatelet therapy and initial heparin followed by warfarin	Antiplatelet therapy and initial heparin followed by warfarin	Antiplatelet therapy and heparin
Indications for use	Destination and bridge to transplant	Destination and bridge to transplant	Bridge to transplant	Bridge to transplant	Bridge to transplant	Temporary support and bridge to recovery	Temporary support and bridge to recovery
Positive aspects	Permits non-tethered ambulation Approved for patient discharge No warfarin required	Permits non-tethered ambulation Approved for patient discharge Quiet operation Small percutaneous lead	Permits discharge home Wide range of flow capacities	Three-year durability	Biventricular support	Flexible design for biventricular support	Percutaneous placement by cardiology
Negative aspects	Limited durability Large device Potential for infection and discomfort	Fixed motor speed with risk of LV suction events	Potential for infection due to being paracorporeal	Large size limits application to small people	Large console limits mobility System not designed for hospital discharge	Cannot be discharged Extracorporeal design limits mobility	Patients must remain in bed with no mobility Partial support
Support design	LVAD	LVAD	LVAD, RVAD, or BiVAD	LVAD	Total orthotopic heart	LVAD, RVAD, or BiVAD	LVAD
Internal or Paracorporeal (external)	Internal	Internal	Paracorporeal	Internal	Paracorporeal	Internal	Paracorporeal

Type of blood flow	Continuous flow (axial)	Continuous flow (axial)	Continuous flow (axial)	Continuous flow (axial)	Pulsatile flow
BSA limitation (m²)	1.2	2.3	> 1.4	> 1.2	> 1.5
Anticoagulation	ASA or ASA 1 low dose heparin or ASA 1 warfarin or ASA 1 Aggrenox® 1 extended-release dipyridamole or ASA 1 clopidogrel	Heparin (some proceed without anticoagulation)	Heparin	ASA	Initially heparin, then warfarin
Indications for use	Refractory advanced HF	CHF, bridge to transplant, destination therapy	Cardiogenic Shock	Bridge to transplant	Bridge to transplant
Positive aspects	Designed for in-hospital and out-of-hospital settings, including fixed-wing aircraft and helicopter	Avoids extracorporeal circulation and decreased transfusion requirements; Silent; Lightweight and small size	Delivers high flows; Minimal complications; Less hemolysis	Small size; May be placed in the pericardial space; In-hospital and out-of-hospital use; May be taken on fixed-wing aircraft or helicopter	In-hospital and out of hospital use; May be taken on fixedwing aircraft or helicopter
Negative aspects	Life-threatening adverse events, including stroke	Not for patients in cardiogenic shock; Risk of thrombus formation	Approved for up to 6 hours of support; No rechargeable battery	Several associated risks but these risks are reportedly outweighed by the benefits	Risk of clot formation if blood is not ejected with each beat
Support design	LVAD	LVAD	RVAD	LVAD	LVAD, RVAD, or BiVAD
Internal or Paracorporeal (external)	Internal	Internal	Internal	Internal	Internal

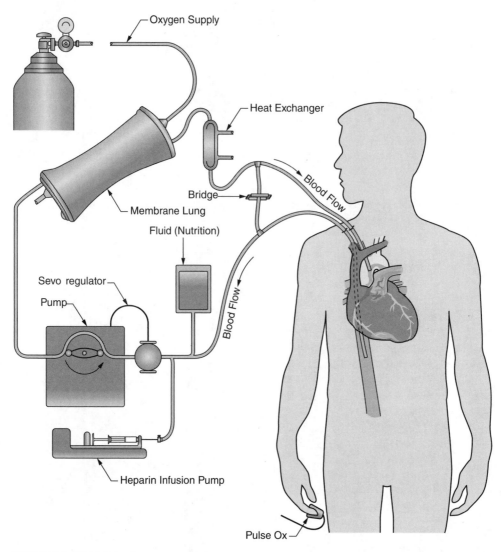

FIGURE 19.4 ECMO Pulse Ox.

Illustrated by James R. Perron

with diuretics or renal replacement therapy (Desai & Hwang, 2018). VA-ECMO has some advantages over other short-term MCS. Cannulation via percutaneous vessels is easy; it provides support for left, right, or both ventricles, and facilitates gas exchange during respiratory dysfunction (Schaheen, Thiele, & Isbell, 2015). Survival to hospital discharge among ECMO patients has increased from 40% in 2012 to 58% in 2016 (Desai & Hwang, 2018).

Percutaneous Ventricular Assist Devices

TandemHeart PTVA. The TandemHeart PTVA system is a continuous-flow pump that can provide up to 4 L/min of flow at 7,500 g (Takayama et al., 2014). The system is inserted via the femoral vein into the left atrium through a transseptal puncture. An added feature of the TandemHeart is that the positioning of the cannulae in the main pulmonary artery and right atrium allows for RVAD configuration (Desai & Hwang, 2018). The pump withdraws oxygenated blood from the left atrium; propels it via a magnetically driven, six-bladed impeller through the outflow port; and returns it to the femoral artery via an arterial cannula. Additional advantages of the TandemHeart are that it has shown improved hemodynamics over the IABP, can be used when an LV thrombus or prosthetic aortic valve is present, or if the patient has aortic stenosis (Ergle, Parto, & Krim, 2016). A disadvantage of the TandemHeart is the technical complexity of transseptal puncture and occasional dislodgement of left atrial cannulae into the right atrium (Takayama et al., 2014). The TandemHeart can also increase afterload and the risk of peripheral limb ischemia; it does require systemic anticoagulation. Contraindications to the TandemHeart include severe aortic insufficiency, peripheral vascular disease, and the presence of ventricular septal defect (Ergle et al., 2016). The TandemHeart is illustrated in **FIGURE 19.5**.

Impella System. The Impella VAD system uses rotary pump technology in a miniaturized form. Hemodynamic support is achieved secondary to decreasing workload of the LV while simultaneously improving CO by augmenting forward flow. Pump size is as small as 12-French, which makes this device amenable to percutaneous insertion. Under both fluoroscopic and echocardiographic guidance, an experienced cardiothoracic surgeon or interventional cardiologist places a catheter-mounted continuous-flow axial pump across the aortic valve with inflow in the LV and outflow in the ascending aorta. Because of this positioning, the Impella device provides active flow and systemic pressure improvement. Inflow of the device draws blood directly from the LV, resulting in decreased left ventricular workload and myocardial oxygen demand. Impella devices include Impella 2.5 (12-Fr, 2.5 L/min of flow; most widely used model), Continuous Power (14-Fr, 3.5 L/min flow), Impella 5.0 (21-Fr, 5 L/min flow), and a right VAD (23-Fr, 5 L/min flow). The larger Impella 5.0 requires a minimally invasive surgical cut-down and device implantation via axillary or femoral artery (Desai & Hwang, 2018).

All pumps are operated through an 11-French catheter (Takayama et al., 2014). In addition to improving access time, the use of smaller cannulae also helps reduce the risk of limb ischemia frequently seen in devices that require larger cannulae insertion (i.e., TandemHeart and ECMO). Disadvantages of the Impella include short duration of support, frequent cannula dislodgement, risk of hemolysis, and mandatory anticoagulation (Al Musa et al., 2017). Contraindications to Impella use include LV thrombus, moderate to severe aortic stenosis or insufficiency, ventricular septal defect, and moderate to severe peripheral arterial disease (Takayama et al., 2014; Ergle et al., 2016).

Surgical Short-Term, Continuous-Flow VADs

Although pVADs are popular, surgical implantation of a VAD may be advantageous. Surgically implanted VADs have notable durability, stability, and generation of excellent forward flow. The CentriMag® VAD (Thoratec Corp., Pleasanton, CA) is one of the most commonly surgically implanted short-term, continuous-flow VADs (Al Musa et al., 2017). CentriMag can generate up to 10 L/min of flow at 5,500 g. The system utilizes a magnetic levitation, bearingless centrifugal pump, which greatly improves CO and reduces myocardial oxygen demand. It is an extracorporeal pump that is designed for left, right, or biventricular support and is commonly used as bridge to recovery or bridge to decision (Desai & Hwang, 2018).

CentriMag implantation requires a surgical cut-down. Traditionally, a sternotomy has been required; however, there have recently been developments to allow for mini-thoracotomy implantation. Postoperative management of CentriMag VADs is often easier for critical care nurses than that seen with pVADs. CentriMag has extracorporeal tubing that facilitates the bedside nurse's ability to quickly identify the need for additional fluid resuscitation. This can be noted when the VAD tubing begins to shake, which is called "chatter." Advantages to CentriMag are potential to ambulate, long-term duration, and effective LV and RV decompression (Al Musa et al., 2017).

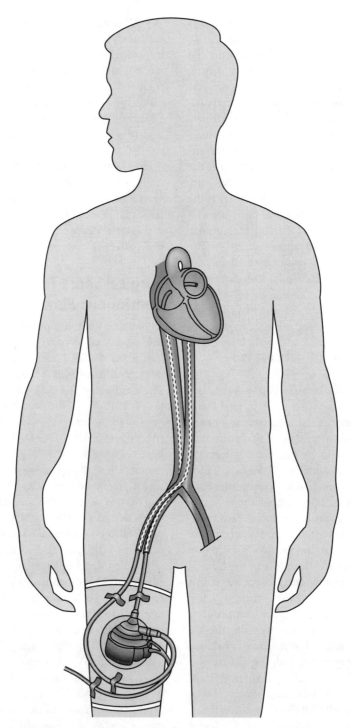

FIGURE 19.5 The TandemHeart PTVA®—this device utilizes a centrifugal pump and is inserted percutaneously.

Illustrated by James R. Perron

Long-Term Mechanical Circulatory Support

As mentioned, patients who are deemed bridge to transplant, bridge to decision, or destination therapy candidates require longer term MCS. For those who are deemed bridge to transplant, intermediate to long-term VAD use provides hemodynamic support until a suitable organ can be located. Ventricular assist device selection is determined by the patient's hemodynamic needs. Since 2008, the overall survival rate for patients with a continuous flow LVAD was 81% at 1 year and 70% at 2 years (Kirklin et al., 2017). Recent INTERMACS data show an improvement in quality of life in the first 3 months through at least the first 2 years after LVAD insertion (Desai & Hwang, 2018; Kirklin et al., 2017).

First Generation Long-Term Mechanical Circulatory Support

Ventricular assist device technology has greatly improved since the mid-1990s. First generation VADs employed pulsatile positive displacement pumps. HeartMate I®, HeartMate XVE, and PVAD™ (paracorporeal ventricular assist device; all from Thoratec) are examples of first generation VADs. Because of improved technology, these types of VADs are rarely used; however, the use of HeartMate I in the REMATCH trial is the basis for the concept of destination therapy.

Second Generation Long-Term Mechanical Circulatory Support

Second generation VADs use nonpulsatile (continuous) axial flow pumps. They are more durable than first generation VADs because they only have one moving part, the rotor. They are also smaller, quieter, and require a less traumatic surgical implantation. They have smaller driveline circumferences, which have been shown to decrease driveline infection rates. At 2 years postimplantation, the continuous-flow LVADs showed a higher survival rate than pulsatile-flow LVADs (Desai & Hwang, 2018). Because of these

vast improvements, the second generation devices have predominantly overtaken VAD implantation.

Upon review of the INTERMACS database, second generation VAD implantation increased from zero in 2007 to 1,145 in 2010, while use of first generation VADs decreased from 219 in 2007 to 6 in 2010 to 2 in 2016 (Kirklin et al., 2017). Examples of second generation VADs include HeartMate II (Thoratec), Jarvik 2000 (Jarvik Heart, Inc., New York, NY), MicroMed DeBakey (MicroMed, Houston, TX), and INCOR (Berlin Heart, Berlin, Germany). The HeartMate II was approved as a bridge to transplantation in 2008 and as destination therapy in 2010 (Kirklin et al., 2017).

HeartMate II. The HeartMate II is a second generation axial (continuous) flow LVAD device that can be used in patients who have smaller frames (body surface area of 1.3 to 2.3 m^2). This device is FDA approved for use as a bridge to transplant and destination therapy. In addition, the HeartMate II generates less noise and has a smaller percutaneous lead than the HeartMate XVE. These features are appreciated by patients. Because the HeartMate II pump requires anticoagulation with heparin/warfarin and antiplatelet therapy, the risk of postoperative bleeding is increased with this device.

Third Generation Long-Term Mechanical Circulatory Support

As VAD technology has improved, there have still been challenges with VAD durability. Ventricular assist device exchange due to device failure is not uncommon; therefore, a third generation of VAD development has begun with the goal of decreasing size, increasing durability, and lowering the risk of adverse effects. Third generation VADs generally use centrifugal continuous-flow pumps. These devices are much smaller than the second generation VADs, allowing for minimally invasive surgical approaches. Examples of third generation VADs include HeartWare® HVAD (HeartWare, Inc., Framingham, MA), HeartMate III (Thoratec), and DuraHeart™ (Terumo

Heart, Inc., Ann Arbor, MI). All are available in the United States. The HeartWare HVAD was approved for bridge to transplantation in 2012 (Kirklin et al., 2017).

HeartMate III and HeartWare HVAD. The HeartMate III is a third generation centrifugal (continuous) flow LVAD that has no mechanical contacts or bearings. The MOMENTUM3 trial found that the HeartMate III had fewer pump failures and required fewer redo surgeries for pump malfunction than the HeartMate II. In the ENDURANCE trial, the HeartMate II showed a higher mechanical failure rate than the HeartWare HVAD while the HeartWare HVAD showed a higher rate of stroke than the HeartMate II (Desai & Hwang, 2018). The HeartMate III is FDA approved for bridge to transplant and bridge to recovery. The HeartWare HVAD is FDA approved for bridge to transplant, destination therapy, and bridge to recovery. Given the small size, biventricular support with both a right and left VAD can be used and the pumps can be placed in the pericardial space (Al Musa et al., 2017; Desai & Hwang, 2018).

Use of second and third generation continuous-flow LVADs increased from 1% of all implanted MCS in 2006 to 97% in 2013 (Hayward & Jansz, 2015). The HeartWare HVAD and the HeartMate II are the two most commonly implanted pumps worldwide (Hayward & Jansz, 2015).

Biventricular Support

In patients with biventricular failure, biventricular support is often required. This support can be provided through a single unit such as the Thoratec BiVAD or through use of more temporary support such as the TandemHeart or CentriMag. It can also be provided by the use of two separate VADs, one in the right ventricle and another in the left ventricle. Biventricular support can be provided until transplantation or can be slowly weaned off as heart function returns. Right ventricular assistance is typically weaned first. This weaning can be done either at the bedside or in the operating room (OR).

Total Artificial Heart

A total artificial heart (TAH) is a treatment alternative for patients with biventricular failure, acute or chronic cardiac rejection, or left ventricular failure with multiple thrombi. The CardioWest™ (SynCardia, Tucson, AZ) was FDA approved as a bridge to transplant in 2004 (Torregrossa, Anyanwu, Zucchetta, & Gerosa, 2014). The AbioCor® (Abiomed, Inc., Pittsburgh, PA) was discontinued several years ago. The TAH replaces the function of both ventricles and the four heart valves. It is implanted in the patient's chest and attached to the atria. Tubes from the SynCardia ventricles continue from the patient's chest to outside the body through holes in the patient's abdomen to a power-generating console. A mobile power console that is used to power the TAH has allowed select patients to discharge home while awaiting transplant.

The TAH can deliver CO as high as 9.5 L/min (SynCardia, 2018). The 12-month survival rate is 53% for patients who received TAH between June 2006 and April 2017 (Arabia et al., 2018). At high-volume MCS centers, the 1-year survival for destination therapy LVADs was 78% compared to 66% for TAH. Arabia and colleagues (2018) also found the most common adverse events to be bleeding, infection, respiratory failure, neurologic events, and device malfunction. Contraindications to the TAH are body size area less than 1.7 m^2 or small anteroposterior diameter (Torregrossa et al., 2014).

Mechanical Circulatory Support Postoperative Complications

Ventricular assist device placement is a major surgical procedure with significant risk for postoperative complications. Approximately 80% of patients receiving an LVAD will have an adverse event in the first year (Miller & Rogers, 2018). The most common complications in the immediate postoperative period are bleeding, dysrhythmias, RV failure, aortic regurgitation, endocarditis, vasoplegia, and infection. Later postoperative complications include gastrointestinal (GI) bleeding, thrombosis, venous thrombotic event, device failure, neurologic events, and psychological problems.

Bleeding

Bleeding in the immediate postinsertion period is the most common adverse event occurring in 31% to 81% of patients (Subramaniam, 2015). Bleeding can be related to a lack of surgical hemostasis or coagulopathies as patients will require long-term anticoagulation with aspirin and warfarin. Surgical bleeding is more common in the first 3 months and GI bleeding occurs more often thereafter (Kirklin et al., 2017). Almost one-third of all continuous-flow LVAD patients will experience GI bleeding (Kirklin et al., 2017; Miller & Rogers, 2018). The high shear forces in the continuous flow LVADs cause all patients to have acquired von Willebrand disease, which increases the incidence of mucosal bleeding (Chmielinski & Koons, 2017; Miller & Rogers, 2018). Second and third generation VADs are also associated with an increased risk of GI bleeding due to arteriovenous malformations in the GI tract. These are possibly related to hypoperfusion of the GI mucosa due to the nonpulsatile nature of the VAD (Birati & Rame, 2014a). The critical care nurse should monitor bleeding at the access site and all surgical incisions. Transfusions should be avoided, if possible, to prevent transfusion-related reactions that could create antibodies that complicate being listed for a heart transplant.

Infection

Infections can either be device related, including the driveline and pump-pocket or sternal wound, or systemic, from a catheter or the respiratory system. Driveline infections are the most common type of infection (Chmielinski & Koons, 2017). Drivelines should be secured with an anchoring device and all dressing changes should be done using sterile technique. Prophylactic antibiotics are given in the OR and continued postoperatively for several days. Infection is the second most common adverse event in the first 3 months (42%) and

---

BOX 19.1 General Infection Control Guidelines

- Dressings over driveline exit sites must be kept clean and dry at all times.
- Sterile dressing changes to the driveline exit site must be performed daily at first then decrease in frequency depending on provider.
- Dressing should be changed more frequently when increased drainage is observed.
- Immobilize the driveline or exit cannulas with abdominal binders or anchoring devices, preventing trauma to the exit site.
- Remove monitoring lines as soon as possible to decrease the risk of infection.
- Notify the physician of a change in the patient's temperature (<36°C [96.9°F] or >38°C [100.4°F]) or other signs and symptoms of driveline infection (e.g., redness, increase in drainage, purulent drainage, foul odor, or skin separation from driveline).
- Ensure adequate nutrition to encourage the healing process (maintain albumin >2.5 g/dL).
- Encourage early mobilization to prevent complications of immobility.

Data from Chmielinski & Koons, 2017.

---

the most common thereafter, with 94% having any kind of infection at 1 year (Kirklin et al., 2017; Subramaniam, 2015).

BOX 19.1 provides general infection control guidelines for VADs.

Right Ventricular Failure

Left ventricular assist device function depends on adequate flow from the right ventricle. Right ventricular failure can be present prior to LVAD implantation due to pulmonary hypertension or ischemia or may develop after LVAD implantation due to volume overload, shift of the interventricular septum from right to left, hypothermia, metabolic acidosis, or sepsis. The risk of RV failure after LVAD insertion is 20% to 50% and RVADs are placed in 10% to 25% of patients who have had an LVAD implanted (Desai & Hwang, 2018).

Patients who suffer from RV failure have longer hospital stays and increased mortality (Subramaniam, 2015). Pulmonary artery catheters are inserted preoperatively for close monitoring of right-sided function (right atrial pressure, central venous pressure). The critical care nurse should monitor LVAD flow, volume status, inotropic and vasoactive drug doses, and arterial blood gases to watch for acidosis (Desai & Hwang, 2018).

Right ventricular failure is treated by optimizing intravascular volume status and LVAD flow, correcting acidosis and electrolyte abnormalities, and using intravenous (IV) diuretics, inotropes, and vasopressors. Nitric oxide (NO) and prostaglandin I2 are inhaled pulmonary vasodilators that have been shown to improve RV function by reducing pulmonary artery pressure, which in turn improves LV filling, CO, and systemic arterial pressure (Desai & Hwang, 2018). Oral pulmonary vasodilators can also help improve RV function.

Pump Thrombosis

Pump thrombosis occurs when a clot forms in one of the components of the VAD. More than 60 days postimplant, the incidence of pump thrombosis is 2% to 9% (Subramaniam, 2015). Risk factors of pump thrombosis include noncompliance to anticoagulation, an inherited coagulopathy, atrial fibrillation (AF), infection, low pump flow, or an incorrectly positioned inflow cannulae. Signs of pump thrombosis vary from mild or nonspecific to cardiogenic shock. An increase in LVAD power usage can be one of the first signs. Tea-colored urine can also be seen due to hemolysis. Treatment for pump thrombosis varies depending on symptom. Inotropes can be employed if the patient is hemodynamically unstable. Antiplatelet dosages can be increased, a second antiplatelet agent can be added, or the INR goal can be increased. If hemolysis continues despite treatment, manufacturers of the HeartMate II recommend pump exchange while manufacturers of the HeartWare HVAD recommend the use of tissue plasminogen activator prior to pump exchange (Birati & Rame, 2014a). The nurse should observe for elevation in lactate dehydrogenase (LDH), a marker for hemolysis, which could indicate pump thrombosis; plasma free hemoglobin levels; and pump power usage.

Neurologic Events

Neurologic events are often seen in the first 30 days post-LVAD implantation. The incidence of stroke, transient ischemic attack, and seizure is 15%, 12%, and 4%, respectively (Subramaniam, 2015). Among strokes, 8% to 10% are ischemic. These are normally due to subtherapeutic INR levels, pump thrombosis, or hypercoagulable states (Chmielinski & Koons, 2017). Hemorrhagic strokes are normally due to infection and supertherapeutic INR. Neurologic events were discussed in detail in Chapter 16.

Dysrhythmias

More than 30% to 60% of LVAD patients experience dysrhythmias in the early postoperative period (<30 days) (Subramaniam, 2015). A suction event (decreased preload) or increased pump speed or poorly positioned inflow cannula can induce arrhythmias. Atrial dysrhythmias can be treated with beta blockers. Ventricular dysrhythmias should be treated with amiodarone (Cordarone®) or lidocaine (Xylocaine®) (Chmielinski & Koons, 2017). Implantable cardioverter-defibrillators should also be considered. Additionally, reversible causes should be fixed by administering IV fluids (for hypovolemia), decreasing the pump speed, or moving the inflow cannula (Birati & Rame, 2014a).

Vasoplegia

Almost one-third of continuous-flow LVAD patients experience vasoplegia, or a lowering of systemic vascular resistance. Vasoplegia is caused by sedatives, vasodilators, sepsis, adrenal insufficiency, anaphylaxis, or neurologic insult. The critical care nurse should monitor for hypotension in post-LVAD implantation patients and avoid excessive patient warming, which can cause a vasodilatory effect. Administration of vasopressors, especially norepinephrine and vasopressin, is the primary treatment for vasoplegia.

Renal Dysfunction

The patient who has undergone LVAD placement may have baseline renal dysfunction. This may be due to renal hypoperfusion. Yoshioka and colleagues (2017) found that renal function improved during the first year postimplantation of a continuous-flow LVAD, but after 1 year renal function gradually declined. Because renal failure or severe renal insufficiency is generally a contraindication to heart transplant, care must be taken to minimize injury to the kidneys. Diligent intake and output surveillance and medication administration are necessary so that the kidneys can recover for the impending heart transplant. The ICU nurse should monitor for improvement in renal function during LVAD therapy.

Postoperative Care of the LVAD Patient

Critical care nurses need to understand various LVAD parameters and how these parameters relate to the patient's condition. The pump speed, how fast the motor spins, is a fixed number set by the VAD team. Pump flow (in L/min) is an approximation of blood flow through the LVAD. Pump power, which changes according to pump speed, pump flow, or physiologic demand, is a measure of voltage and current used by the LVAD. Increases in pump power required could indicate a thrombosis. The pulsatility index (PI) is a measure of the change in flow through the LVAD during the cardiac cycle. A high PI means there is less LVAD support (more native heart functioning). A low PI means less ventricular filling (either due to obstruction or low circulating blood volume or RV dysfunction) and more LVAD support (Chmielinski & Koons, 2017).

Left ventricular assist device output is a function of preload and afterload. Preload is reduced when the patient is dehydrated, overdiuresed, bleeding, or has RV dysfunction. Low pump flow/output is a hemodynamic emergency. Hemodynamics are monitored with an arterial line and pulmonary artery catheter. General mean arterial pressure (MAP) targets are 70 to 80 mmHg but can vary depending on device implanted. Note that if a continuous-flow LVAD is being used,

arterial line waveforms will be dampened. Automatic or manual blood pressure measurements often underestimate the MAP. Pulmonary artery catheters are useful to obtain data on CO and filling pressures. Pulse oximetry can also be unreliable. If numbers displayed do not seem correct, an arterial blood gas (ABG) should be used to confirm oxygen saturation (Birati & Rame, 2014a). In addition to hemodynamic monitoring, the critical care nurse should keep an eye on ABGs, mixed venous blood gases, serum lactate levels, LDH, and results from coagulation panels, complete blood counts, and chemistry panels.

Hemodynamics, including central venous pressure (CVP), pulmonary artery pressure (PAP), pulmonary artery occlusive pressure (PAOP), MAP, and results of an echocardiogram can be used to determine if the low flow is due to hypovolemia, tamponade, right heart failure, or obstruction. Treatments are tailored to etiology of low pump flow and hospital-specific protocols but can vary from administration of blood or volume for suspected hypovolemia to inotropes and inhaled pulmonary vasodilators for right heart failure to emergent surgical intervention if tamponade or obstruction is present (Birati & Rame, 2014a). Monitoring of filling pressures and afterload should also take place. If elevated, the patient can be treated with IV vasodilators and fluids and warmed, to promote vasodilation.

In addition to hemodynamic and laboratory monitoring, a nursing assessment can be invaluable. Critical care nurses should assess a patient's mentation as changes in mentation can signal a neurologic event or possibility of infection. The critical care nurse must also monitor capillary refill and peripheral warmth as an indication of good systemic perfusion and to also check for limp ischemia. The critical care nurse should also monitor urine output to determine if renal function has been impaired.

Requirements for Being Discharged with an LVAD

Patients who return home with an LVAD require extra education to ensure the safety of this therapy.

A grounded, three-pronged outlet near the patient's sleeping site is required for the patient to switch to the power source during sleep. In the event of battery or generator failure, ongoing functioning of the device can be ensured through hand pumping, switching power sources, emergency interventions, or a combination of these. Extra batteries should always be available. Routine care and provisions for emergencies must be addressed. Education should include troubleshooting of alarms, exit site infection prevention, immobilization of the percutaneous lead, and maintaining fluid volume status/dehydration prevention. Additionally, blood pressure monitoring is problematic as continuous-flow LVAD patients do not always have a palpable pulse. Blood pressure is generally measured with Doppler ultrasound to determine a MAP. A MAP goal for continuous flow LVAD patients is 80 mmHg (Lima et al., 2018). **BOX 19.2** lists the safety precautions required of the patient who is discharged to home with an LVAD.

▶ Heart Transplantation

Although many advanced HF patients can be supported with either medical management or a VAD as destination therapy, another cohort of patients would benefit from receiving a heart transplant. After extensive discussions with their HF provider teams, these patients are evaluated for heart transplant and, if indicated, placed on the waiting list for a new heart.

Criteria for Heart Transplantation

A patient may become a candidate for a heart transplant based on specific criteria. Stringent cardiac transplantation screening tools exist with considerable variations in inclusion criteria among transplant centers. Not all patients are deemed transplant candidates regardless of the degree of decompensation. The patient may have terminal HF that has not responded to medical therapy or cardiomyopathy (ischemic, nonischemic, idiopathic, or valvular) in addition to the absence of reversible HF (Khoshbin & Dark, 2017). The ACCF/AHA has guidelines for indications for heart transplantation.

In 2018, United Network for Organ Sharing (UNOS) changed the listing criteria for patients awaiting heart transplant. Patients are now listed in one of six categories. Patients in category one has the highest level of acuity and patients in level six have the lowest level of acuity. There is a web site in web resources that provides more detailed information about each category.

Absolute indications for transplant for patients with HF-related hemodynamic compromise include refractory cardiogenic shock requiring continuous IV inotrope dependence to maintain adequate organ perfusion or circulatory support with IABP or MCS, or persistent NYHA class IV HF refractory to optimized medical therapy; peak oxygen consumption should be at less than 14 mL/kg/min (12 mL/kg/min for patients on

---

BOX 19.2 LVAD Safety Precautions at Discharge

- Maintain a method to obtain a backup generator in case of power failure.
- Notify the local electricity provider of the use of life support equipment.
- Keep backup equipment nearby at all times.
- Clean and inspect the VAD daily.
- Change exit site dressings as instructed.
- Do not bathe or swim (avoid immersion in water).
- Avoid static electricity (e.g., touching a computer screen).
- Never disconnect both batteries simultaneously.
- Connect to a power source while sleeping.
- Do not play contact sports or engage in excessive jumping.
- Do not kink, bend, or pull on the driveline.
- Do not sleep on your stomach.
- Do not let children sit on the patient's chest.
- Do not have an MRI.
- Cardiopulmonary resuscitation varies depending on the model of LVAD used.
- Pregnancy is not permitted.

LVAD, left ventricular assist device; MRI, magnetic resonance imaging.
Data from Martonik, 2017; Smith & Franzwa, 2015.

beta blockers). Indications also include severe ischemia that consistently limits activity and cannot be corrected with coronary artery bypass graft (CABG) surgery or percutaneous coronary intervention (PCI) as well as recurrent symptomatic and refractory arrhythmias, specific patients with restrictive and hypertrophic cardiomyopathies and NYHA class III to IV HF, and congenital heart disease not amenable to palliation or surgery.

Relative indications for heart transplant include a peak oxygen consumption of 13 to 14 mL/kg/min (or <55% predicted) and major limitations to activities of daily living, recurrent unstable ischemia that is not amenable to other interventions, and recurrent fluid balance/renal function instability that is unrelated to patient nonadherence to a medical regimen (Mancini, 2017; Mehra et al., 2016).

Patients are excluded from heart transplantation if they meet any absolute contraindications. These include a systemic illness with a life expectancy of less than 2 years, irreversible pulmonary hypertension (>3 Wood units), severe symptomatic cerebrovascular disease, current substance abuse, multisystem disease, and the inability to comply with drug therapy (Mancini, 2017). A number of relative contraindications for transplant must also be considered. These include currently being treated for cancer. These patients are at risk for their condition to be worsened from the required immunotherapy to prevent graft rejection. Similarly, patients with an active infection cannot receive a heart transplant. The immunosuppressive therapy can increase the severity of the infection.

Age has been considered a relative contraindication for heart transplant. Patients over age 60 to 65 have been excluded in the past. However, physiologic versus chronological age is now being considered and the current listed contraindication is age greater than 70. Heart transplants are now being performed on patients older than 70 if certain added criteria are met (Mancini, 2017). Patients with diabetes mellitus and poor glycemic control (HbA$_{1c}$ >7.5%) or with significant end-organ damage are typically not considered candidates for heart transplant. Other relative exclusion criteria for heart transplant include advanced liver disease, renal dysfunction (serum creatinine >2 mg/dL or

glomerular filtration rate <30 mL/min), advanced peripheral vascular disease, morbid obesity (body mass index >35 kg/m^2), active peptic ulcer disease, cholelithiasis, and diverticulosis. These latter criteria are related to the effects of immunosuppressants such as cyclosporine and calcineurin inhibitors (Mancini, 2017). These agents are discussed later in this chapter.

In addition to the indications and contraindications for heart transplantation, a psychosocial evaluation is paramount to help determine a patient's ability to cope with the waiting time for an organ, the procedure and recovery, and long-term adherence to immunosuppressive therapy. Included in the psychosocial evaluation is determining the extent of alcohol, tobacco, or recreational drug use (Mancini, 2017; Roehm, Vest, & Weiner, 2018).

While absolute and relative exclusion criteria are delineated in the literature, institutional contraindications may also be noted. Therefore, the critical care nurse should be cognizant of those contraindications as well.

Heart Transplantation Procedure

There are two approaches to performing a heart transplant—orthotopic and heterotopic. The orthotopic approach is most commonly performed. With the orthotopic approach, the recipient's heart is replaced with a donor heart. With the heterotopic approach, the recipient's heart is left in place and the donor heart is "piggybacked" to the right side of the recipient's heart. The latter approach is rarely used.

Donor hearts are typically placed either with the more common bicaval approach or the biatrial approach. In the bicaval approach, the donor's right atrium remains intact and the recipient's and donor's left atrium are connected together. This approach allows the sinus node and tricuspid valve to stay intact, lowering atrial dysrhythmias and tricuspid regurgitation. In the biatrial approach, the Lower and Shumway method, the recipient's atria are anastomosed to the donor's left and right atria. This approach is faster and more efficient in the OR but creates larger atrial cavities with increased incidence of tricuspid and mitral regurgitation and atrial dysrhythmias (Nguyen & Banks, 2017).

Regardless of approach, the patient has a median sternotomy incision and is placed on CPB during the transplant procedure (Vega, Schroder, & Nicoara, 2017). Just prior to release of the aortic cross-clamp, a bolus of methylprednisolone (Solu-Medrol®) is administered (Nguyen & Banks, 2017). Once the transplant procedure is completed, pacing wires are secured. The patient may require inotropic and chronotropic support to be removed from CPB. Once the patient is successfully removed from CPB and the donor heart is functioning, protamine (Neutrahep®) is given to reverse the effects of the heparin used in CPB, and the patient is transferred to the ICU for recovery (Nguyen & Banks, 2017).

Care in the Immediate Postoperative Period

When post cardiac transplantation patients arrive in the ICU, they will normally have a pulmonary artery catheter, intra-arterial line, indwelling urinary catheter, and one or more chest tubes in place. Inotropes, vasopressors, and inhaled nitric oxide will likely have been started while in the OR. Pacing wires will be in place and the patient's heart rate will generally be between 90 to 110 beats per minute. The patient will be intubated and sedated. The sternotomy incision could be closed with a dressing in place or left open if the patient is at a higher risk of bleeding, tamponade, or right heart failure or is hemodynamically unstable (Freeman, Koerner, Clark, & Halabicky, 2016; Vega et al., 2017).

Upon arrival in the ICU, the critical care nurse should assess the surgical site for bleeding, and check chest tube output, urine output, and all hemodynamic parameters, including blood pressure (BP), heart rate (HR) and rhythm via bedside monitor, CVP, PAP, PAOP, CO, cardiac index (CI), and systemic vascular resistance (SVR). Pulse oximetry and mixed venous saturation should also be monitored. The critical care nurse should work with the transplant team and the respiratory therapist to optimize oxygen administration, using inotropes, fluids, pacing wires, and inhaled nitric oxide. The nurse will also be responsible for slowly warming the patient to normothermia to prevent bleeding, acidosis, dysrhythmias, and low CO.

Rapid warming can cause vasodilation and hypotension (Freeman et al., 2016; Vega et al., 2017).

Hypercarbia, acidosis, hypoxia, and high inspiratory pressures should be avoided during ventilator management to promote venous return to the heart. Volume status should be closely observed and overload should be avoided. If the renal status declines, renal replacement therapy may be warranted. Frequent laboratory draws will be performed to watch electrolytes, hemoglobin and hematocrit, white cell count, and coagulation status. Some patients may have MCS in place. Preoperative IABP is generally not removed because of increased risk of bleeding due to heparin administration during CPB (Vega et al., 2017). Posttransplant patients are put on protective precautions during hospitalization to reduce the risk of infection. Vasodilatory shock is common and is usually treated with norepinephrine (Adrenaline®), phenylephrine (Neo-Synephrine®), and vasopressin (ADH). Inotropes such as epinephrine, dopamine (Intropin®), milrinone (Primacor®), and dobutamine (Dobutrex®) are used to treat circulatory shock. Pulmonary hypertension and right heart dysfunction are treated with inhaled vasodilators in addition to other agents. All patients are started on IV insulin to maintain a blood glucose less than 140 mg/dL to prevent sternal site infection and poor wound healing (Freeman et al., 2016).

Sedation and IV pain medications are slowly weaned. Heart transplant patients typically remain on mechanical ventilation for 12 to 48 hours and remain in the ICU for 2 to 3 days. Medications, including inotropes, chronotropes, and inhaled pulmonary vasodilators are decreased slowly as tolerated. The insulin infusion is discontinued as the patient begins to eat orally; basal/bolus subcutaneous insulin is initiated if needed. Pacing modes are changed as tolerated. Once the patient has had a stable heart rhythm and has been off chronotropes, pacing wires are removed. Nursing assessments over the next several days should include surgical site assessment for bleeding, infection, or dehiscence. The critical care nurse should monitor for dysrhythmias and signs of cardiac tamponade, systemic infection, graft failure, bleeding, rejection, and neurologic events. The nurse should also continue to monitor all laboratory values, including levels of antirejection medications (Freeman et al., 2016). Interventions for individual complications are detailed next.

Factors Influencing Patient Recovery

After the transplantation procedure is complete, the heart recipient's postoperative care and course will vary depending on many factors. Recipient comorbidities such as prior coronary ischemic injury, prior MCS, history of pulmonary hypertension, or renal or pulmonary dysfunction will affect patient progress. Heart transplant recipients that had higher preoperative instability (i.e., INTERMACS profiles 1 and 2) had the highest risk of in-hospital mortality (Pham, 2018a). Heart transplant recipients who required TAH, mechanical ventilation, or dialysis prior to transplant had the highest risk of 1-year mortality; a prior CABG also conveyed an increased risk of 1-year mortality (Pham, 2018a). Currently, approximately 50% of heart transplant patients are bridged to transplant with VADs, TAH, or ECMO; those bridged with ECMO had worse survival than those on other forms of MCS (Lund et al., 2017).

Donor and harvest factors may influence postoperative course. For example, mismatch of heart size (e.g., a smaller heart being implanted into a larger recipient), older donor age, left ventricular dysfunction, and longer ischemic time of the donor may result in graft dysfunction (Pham, 2018a; Vela, Sáez, & Simon, 2018). Cold ischemic time is also relevant to the recipient's recovery. Cold ischemic time refers to the amount of time from cross-clamping of the donor's aorta with subsequent excision and immersion of the heart in iced saline at 4°C until removal of the cross-clamp after it has been implanted into the patient (Vela et al., 2018). Currently, the maximum cold ischemic time recommended is 6 hours, preferably less than 4 hours (Nguyen & Banks, 2017; Vela et al., 2018). Younger organs tolerate relatively longer ischemic times and older organs tolerate shorter ischemic times (International Society of Heart and Lung Transplantation [ISHLT], 2017a).

Postoperative Complications

Postoperative complications vary based on time since the operation. Early postoperative complications include hyperacute rejection, RV dysfunction or failure, bleeding, graft dysfunction, infection and sepsis, acute kidney injury (AKI), delirium and encephalopathy, and dysrhythmias. Intermediate complications (>30 days since transplantation) include acute rejection, renal dysfunction, and infection. Long-term complications (>1 year since transplant) include chronic renal insufficiency, infection, chronic rejection, hypertension, diabetes mellitus, cardiac allograft vasculopathy, and malignancy (McCartney, Patel, & Del Rio, 2017; Vega et al., 2017).

The immediate postoperative period can be quite challenging for both patients and nurses. While this time generally progresses without complication, patients may demonstrate high levels of vulnerability and low levels of stability. Clinical issues and implications specific to the recovery from anesthesia and CPB were discussed in detail in Chapter 8. Hemodynamic monitoring and care for the patient on mechanical ventilation, including weaning and extubation, were described in Chapters 9 and 11, respectively. Postoperative complications related to CPB were discussed in detail in Chapter 13. Infection and acute and chronic rejection specific to heart transplantation are discussed later in this chapter. The other postoperative complications specific to heart transplantation are discussed next.

Hyperacute Rejection

Hyperacute rejection is rare. It is caused by a preexisting antibody to an allogenic antigen. It may occur within minutes to hours after a transplant and is often fatal. Symptoms are related to rapid graft failure and often manifest as hemodynamic instability. Cardiac function can be supported with inotropes, vasopressors, or MCS. Immediate high-dose immunosuppressants are given, including IV corticosteroids, calcineurin inhibitors (CNIs), and cytolytic induction therapy. Plasmapheresis and IV immunoglobulin (IVIG) can be used to remove and deactivate circulating antibodies. If these treatments do not work, retransplantation can be considered (Vega et al., 2017). Worldwide, the incidence of retransplantation has stayed constant at 2% to 4% (Pham, 2018a).

Bleeding

Postoperative bleeding is a common problem in all cardiac surgery patients. Heart transplant recipients, however, are at greater risk for bleeding than other cardiac surgery patients. Many of these patients have prior sternotomies. For this reason, the new sternotomy wound is often left open, covered with a sterile, occlusive, transparent dressing to permit visualization of accumulating blood and rapid mediastinal exploration, should it be required. In addition, the pericardial sac is larger than normal based on the native heart's enlarged size. Postoperative bleeding may be related to surgery or secondary to a coagulopathy that results from CPB (Birati & Rame, 2014b). Other causes of postoperative bleeding may include hypothermia, administration of heparin for CPB, preexisting hepatic dysfunction from heart failure, and associated low CO. While protamine sulfate is often given in the OR to reverse the heparin effects, an additional dose may be required in the immediate postoperative period.

The ICU nurse should observe the patient for signs of bleeding, including tachycardia, increased chest tube drainage, low CO, low CVP, falling hemoglobin and hematocrit levels, and increasing oxygen requirements. Results of coagulation profiles and platelet count should be evaluated as well. Hypotension and decreasing pulmonary artery and central venous pressures are late signs of bleeding. If the patient is to be transfused with blood or blood products, cytomegalovirus (CMV)–negative patients must receive CMV-negative products (Freeman et al., 2016; Vega et al., 2017).

Strategies employed for bleeding are the same as those used in other cardiac surgery patients. These interventions include eradicating the underlying cause of bleeding, aggressive transfusion of blood products (e.g., fresh frozen plasma, cryoprecipitate) as indicated; use of plasminogen inhibitors (e.g., transexamic acid, aminocaproic acid [Amicar®], aprotinin [Trasylol®]) and factor VII; administration of additional protamine sulfate; and reexploration based on the amount of chest tube output and the patient's coagulation status. Institutional guidelines and protocols regarding appropriate chest tube output after cardiac transplantation vary. If the output is too high, reexploration of the site could be warranted. Gentle milking of chest tubes may be required to dislodge clots and maintain the patency of the chest tubes, if permitted based on institutional policy. Of note, stripping of chest tubes can create large amounts of negative pressure, which can hasten bleeding.

Cardiac Tamponade

Cardiac tamponade may develop either gradually or suddenly in patients who have undergone heart transplantation. It results from fluid accumulating in the pericardial sac, which causes compression of the atria, restriction of venous return to the heart and ventricular filling, and a decrease or cessation of preload and a potential precipitous decline in CO (Yu et al., 2014). Early tamponade may also result from persistent mediastinal bleeding not being evacuated by chest tubes due to clot formation. Cardiac tamponade may also develop following removal of pacing wires or from routine endomyocardial biopsies used to evaluate rejection in the allograft.

The diagnosis of cardiac tamponade may be difficult in heart transplant recipients because hypotension, low CO, elevated CVP, and tachycardia are common scenarios in the immediate postoperative period for all heart transplant recipients. A transesophageal echocardiogram (TEE) can help with diagnosis (Vega et al., 2017). When caring for these patients, the ICU nurse should maintain patency of chest tubes, monitor vital signs and hemodynamic profiles, and observe for signs and symptoms, including those listed in **BOX 19.3**.

If cardiac tamponade develops, initial management should include volume resuscitation to optimize filling pressures (being careful not to overload the right ventricle) and initiation and titration of inotropes if blood pressure is not responsive to fluid resuscitation. Definitive

---

BOX 19.3 Signs and Symptoms of Cardiac Tamponade

- Sudden decrease or cessation of chest tube drainage
- Labile blood pressure
- Tachycardia
- Widened mediastinum on chest x-ray
- Muffled heart tones
- Decreased cardiac output and central venous pressure
- Similar left and right pulmonary artery pressure
- Dyspnea
- Chest pain
- Narrowing pulse pressure
- Paradoxical pulse
- Fatigue
- Malaise
- Dysrhythmias, including tachycardia
- Decreased voltage on ECG
- Cardiac arrest
- Decreased urinary output

ECG, electrocardiogram
Data from Freeman et al, 2016; Kaplow & Iyere, 2017; Yarlagadda, 2017.

treatment entails surgical intervention or emergent bedside sternotomy (Vega et al., 2017). The required equipment and nursing care for the latter procedure were discussed in Chapter 13.

Hypovolemia

Posttransplant hypovolemia has the same etiology in heart transplant recipients as it does in other cardiac surgery patients who have undergone CPB. Cardiopulmonary bypass causes increased capillary permeability, with resultant third spacing of fluid. Intraoperative use of diuretics and initial high post-CPB urinary output further contribute to the postoperative heart transplant patient's hypovolemic state. Hypovolemia, in turn, results in a decrease in preload and cardiac function (Birati & Rame, 2014b).

The ICU nurse must observe heart transplant recipients for hypotension, decreased pulmonary artery pressure and central venous pressure, decreased urinary output, and decreased CO and

CI. Treatment of hypovolemia focuses on volume repletion without volume overload, which can cause right heart failure. This goal may be accomplished through administration of either a crystalloid or a colloid, depending on facility protocol. As discussed in Chapter 17, the debate over the efficacy of crystalloid versus colloid therapy continues. The ICU nurse must carefully monitor the patient's vital signs, urinary output, and hemodynamic profile both during and following volume resuscitation. Development of fluid overload can cause dilation of the right ventricle and pulmonary edema, which can be life threatening (Birati & Rame, 2014b). Fluid resuscitation was discussed in detail in Chapter 17.

Right Ventricular Failure

Right ventricular dysfunction is a major cause of morbidity and mortality in the post heart transplant period. It is the most common reason a patient is unable to wean from CPB following heart transplant and is predominantly due to high mean PAPs (Nguyen & Banks, 2017). Risk factors that contribute to the development of RV failure following a heart transplant can be related to the donor, recipient, or insufficient perfusion of the right ventricle during the procedure. Procedure-related factors are an air embolism in the right coronary artery, hypotension, inadequate myocardial preservation during cardioplegia, and trauma to the organ during harvesting and the transplant procedure. Donor factors include increased cold ischemic time, a reperfusion injury, a thin right ventricular wall, or a donor–recipient size mismatch. Recipient-related factors include high PVR or preexisting pulmonary hypertension. The donor heart may not be accustomed to an elevated PVR, so the implanted right ventricle dilates and fails. The interventricular septal left shift from RV dilation eventually impairs LV filling, causing reduced CO and hypotension (Nguyen & Banks, 2017; Vega et al., 2017; Moore-Gibbs & Bither, 2015).

Right HF is characterized by low CO, elevated CVP, and a normal PAOP (Nguyen & Banks, 2017; Vega et al., 2017). Diagnosis is made by TEE, which generally shows dilation of the tricuspid annulus and resulting tricuspid regurgitation. Treatment of right HF depends on the severity of the condition. The goal of therapy is to support RV function while preventing further elevation in PVR. Right ventricular dysfunction prophylaxis is generally started in the OR even if RV dysfunction is not present (Vega et al., 2017). Interventions include administering fluids while avoiding fluid overload (a maximum CVP of 10 mmHg should be achieved); increasing contractility with inotropes such as dobutamine, epinephrine, milrinone, dopamine, or a combination of these; avoiding hypercarbia, acidosis, and hypoxia; adding vasodilatory agents as needed (discussed below); correcting electrolyte abnormalities; and augmenting low BP with vasopressors (Birati & Rame, 2014b; Nguyen & Banks, 2017; Vega et al., 2017). Patients who do not respond to the above mentioned treatments can be treated with MCS. The ISHLT recommends IABP placement over ECMO or VADs because it is the least invasive (Birati & Rame, 2014b).

Pulmonary Hypertension

Inhaled vasodilators can also be used to lower PVR. Nitric oxide (NO) is frequently used to selectively dilate the pulmonary vasculature without decreasing systemic blood pressure; its administration has been shown to decrease the incidence of RV dysfunction in patients with pulmonary hypertension (Nguyen & Banks, 2017; Vega et al., 2017). Other agents that dilate the pulmonary vasculature (e.g., nitroglycerin [Tridil®], sodium nitroprusside [Nipride®], prostaglandin E-1 [PGE1], and prostacyclin [PGH2]) may cause hypotension and therefore are used less often in post heart transplant patients.

Patients are generally weaned from NO on the first postoperative day or later, depending on the overall clinical picture and their degree of hemodynamic stability. Weaning does not start until the sternal wound is closed. Nitric oxide has a very short half-life, and patients are weaned from it very slowly (over hours) based on BP, PAP, and vasopressor requirements. Abrupt discontinuation of NO causes rebound pulmonary hypertension and acute RV dysfunction. While weaning NO, the critical care nurse must monitor

hemodynamics. The PAP can elevate during weaning. If the CO or urinary output decreases or the CVP increases, the patient may not be tolerating the decrease in NO. If this occurs, the pacing rate or inotrope rate can be changed or the providers could consider diuresis. Acidosis, hypercarbia, and hypoxemia increase PVR. Therefore, patients are hyperventilated to achieve a pH in the range of 7.45 to 7.49 and a $PaCO_2$ in the range of 30 to 35 mmHg. Hypoxemia must be avoided (Freeman et al., 2016; Vega et al., 2017).

Chronotropy (Rate) Issues

Bradycardia may occur in the immediate postoperative period. This complication affects as many as 40% to 50% of orthotopic heart transplant patients, typically taking the form of sinoatrial (SA) node dysfunction. Sinus node dysfunction may occur due to ischemia during hypothermic preservation, intraoperative trauma to the SA node, perinodal atrial tissue, SA artery trauma, rejection, or effects of some pretransplant drugs such as amiodarone (Eisen & Kusmirek, 2017; Wellman, Herrmann, Hagl, & Juchem, 2017). If the latter is the case, the postoperative patient may manifest rhythms originating from the atrioventricular (AV) node. The incidence of sinus node dysfunctions is much lower in bicaval, rather than biatrial, anastomoses, because more sympathetic and parasympathetic fibers are transected during the bicaval technique stimulating regeneration in both branches (Eisen & Kusmirek, 2017).

Bradycardia immediately following surgery has little prognostic significance, but it may affect morbidity secondary to an associated decrease in CO. Sinus node dysfunction may last for up to several weeks following transplant. In the immediate postoperative period, bradycardia should be managed with a temporary pacemaker. Atropine sulfate is not effective in heart transplant patients due to sympathetic and parasympathetic denervation. Bradycardia may be treated with theophylline (Theo-Dur®), terbutaline (Brethine®), or albuterol to keep the heart rate at 80 to 100 beats/min (Birati & Rame, 2014b; Eisen & Kusmirek, 2017). Isoproterenol (Isuprel®) can be given in an emergent situation when pacing wires are not present and should be used cautiously because of associated high myocardial oxygen demand, which has been known to cause acute ischemia. Implantation of a permanent pacemaker may be considered if bradycardia does not resolve within 2 weeks. A dual-chamber pacemaker or an atrial pacemaker in the donor's right atrium is preferred (Eisen & Kusmirek, 2017). In one study of 1,179 heart transplant patients, almost 12% required a permanent pacemaker for bradycardia (Wellman et al., 2017). Management of bradycardia was discussed in detail in Chapter 15.

Tachycardia, which decreases ventricular filling time, and hence the risk of RV dilation, is achieved with an atrial pacer set to the AAI (atria paced, atria sensed, inhibited) mode and a rate of 100 to 120 beats/min via epicardial pacing wires. The AAI mode is selected because transplanted hearts generally have intact conduction systems (unlike in valve surgery patients, who are susceptible to temporary heart blocks). Utilization of the heart's intrinsic conduction system promotes ventricular synchrony, which stabilizes the septum in a manner that facilitates LV and RV function. Tachycardia is also achieved pharmacologically with isoproterenol (which also dilates pulmonary vasculature), dobutamine, and dopamine. Specific tachyarrhythmias following cardiac surgery, including heart transplant, were discussed in detail in Chapter 15. Temporary pacing wires are generally removed when patients have been off chronotropes and their heart rate has been stable for 48 hours (Freeman et al., 2016).

Contractility (Inotropy) Issues

Patients often need support with inotropes following heart transplantation. Therapy may be required for a few days. Weaning from these meds can take place when hemodynamic stability has been attained. Inotropes such as dopamine, dobutamine, epinephrine, and milrinone are used to support RV and LV function (Vega et al., 2017). Milrinone is frequently given at a dose of 0.125 to 0.375 mcg/kg/min and has the added benefit of promoting pulmonary vascular dilation. If these pharmacologic interventions (which were described in detail in Chapter 12) are not

successful in preventing or ameliorating right HF, insertion of an IABP (see Chapter 10) or RVAD may be necessary.

Hypotension

As in other cardiac surgery populations, blood pressure variability is common in patients who have received heart transplants. Hypotension decreases coronary artery perfusion, which is undesirable in all cardiac surgery patients and may contribute to right HF in the heart transplant patient. Treatment is directed at the underlying mechanism.

Vasodilation may be exacerbated by medications such as milrinone. Decreasing the dose of vasodilator medications, if feasible, may mitigate hypotension. Vasopressors such as norepinephrine (Levophed®) and vasopressin are often required to maintain a MAP greater than 65 mmHg. The combination of dobutamine and vasopressin or norepinephrine can be used in patients with hypotension and low CO (Nguyen & Banks, 2017).

Rhythm Disturbance and Electrocardiograph Changes

Development of cardiac dysrhythmias is common following heart transplantation, with AF, atrial flutter (AFL), and supraventricular tachycardia being the most common. For patients who undergo transplants, the likelihood of such abnormalities in heart rhythm is higher in the immediate postoperative period. Such dysrhythmias may result from surgical trauma to the SA and AV nodes, ischemia, suture lines, rejection, and cardiac allograft vasculopathy (Eisen & Kusmirek, 2017; Vega et al., 2017).

Atrial Dysrhythmias. The incidence of AF in heart transplant patients ranges from 10% to 24%; the incidence of AFL is reported at 12% to 15% (Eisen & Kusmirek, 2017). Atrial fibrillation usually occurs within the first 1 to 2 months, while AFL is often a late dysrhythmia (Eisen & Kusmirek, 2017). It has been suggested that AF is attributable to surgical isolation of the pulmonary vein and denervation of the heart. In 5% to 10% of patients, AF develops later; in this instance it is typically associated with loss of function of the transplanted heart and an overall higher mortality rate (Eisen & Kusmirek, 2017; Wellmann et al., 2017). Rivinius and colleagues (2016) found that pretransplant amiodarone use lowered the incidence of AF after transplant and did not increase mortality rates. The ICU nurse should be watchful for AFL as persistent paroxysmal AFL is a strong marker for rejection (Moore-Gibbs & Bither, 2015).

Treatment of atrial dysrhythmias entails controlling ventricular response rate. Immunosuppression is indicated if the cause is thought to be rejection. Atrial flutter may be managed with overdrive pacing; success of greater than 90% has been reported (Eisen & Kusmirek, 2017). Radiofrequency ablation has also been used to treat AFL in heart transplant patients (Eisen & Kusmirek, 2017). Amiodarone should be initiated cautiously in the patient taking calcineurin inhibitors for rejection (Freeman et al., 2016). Patients with chronic AF should be anticoagulated long term similarly to non–heart transplant patients (Eisen & Kusmirak, 2017).

Supraventricular Tachycardia. Types of supraventricular dysrhythmias that have been reported in orthotopic transplant patients include AV reentrant tachycardia, Wolff-Parkinson-White syndrome, and nonparoxysmal atrial tachycardia. Supraventricular tachycardia has been treated successfully with radiofrequency ablation (Eisen & Kusmirek, 2017).

Ventricular Dysrhythmias. Premature ventricular contractions may occur in as many as 100% of orthotopic heart transplant patients early in the postoperative period (Eisen & Kusmirek, 2017). Paroxysmal ventricular tachycardia (VT) decreases in incidence after the initial postoperative period. There may be a correlation between VT, rejection, and transplant vasculopathy. Nonparoxysmal ventricular dysrhythmias are rare in the postoperative heart transplant patient. Development is usually related to severe cardiac allograft vasculopathy or allograft rejection (Eisen & Kusmirek, 2017; Vega et al., 2017). There are reports that implantable cardioverter defibrillators have effectively stopped ventricular

arrhythmias in transplanted patients with severe coronary artery disease (CAD), history of cardiac arrest, or severe left ventricular dysfunction (Eisen & Kusmirak, 2017).

Conduction Delays. Right bundle branch block (RBBB) is a common electrocardiogram (ECG) finding posttransplant, occurring in up to 70% of patients. Development of an RBBB that was not present on the ECG of the donor may be associated with prolonged donor ischemic time and several rejection episodes. Etiologic factors may include RV hypertrophy from elevated PAPs or right bundle damage during endomyocardial biopsy procedures (Eisen & Kusmirek, 2017).

Atrioventricular node function remains intact following a heart transplant. As a consequence, high-degree AV block is rare in posttransplant patients, especially in the early postoperative period. Less than 20% of the permanent pacemakers implanted in heart transplant patients are for AV block. Late development carries an increased mortality rate (Eisen & Kusmirek, 2017).

Neurologic Complications

Twenty percent of all deaths in post cardiac transplant patients are due to neurologic complications (McCartney et al., 2017). In the perioperative period, delirium and encephalopathy are the most common neurologic complications. They occur in 9% of cases (McCartney et al., 2017). Etiologic factors include history of prior stroke, AF, endocarditis-related septic emboli, cardiac catheterization, and perioperative hemodynamic instability.

Other neurologic complications that can occur include stroke, posterior reversible encephalopathy syndrome (PRES), infection, and peripheral neuropathy. Up to 13% of heart transplant patients have a stroke, with ischemic strokes being twice as common as hemorrhagic strokes. Posterior reversible encephalopathy syndrome can occur with the use of CNIs. The approximate 1% of heart transplant patients that experience PRES demonstrate encephalopathy, seizures, headache, and visual disturbances. Reducing the dose of CNIs can ameliorate the symptoms. Seizures can also occur because of focal ischemic injury, anoxic encephalopathy, or metabolic imbalances. Use of long-term antiseizure medications is usually not required. Encephalopathy that occurs in the immediate postoperative period is multifactorial in etiology.

The rate of polyneuropathies is approximately 70% in post cardiac transplant patients. Many of these patients have preexisting neuropathies from diabetes and chronic kidney disease. Long ICU stays and prolonged mechanical ventilation can increase neuromuscular disease. Depression and pain are the most common long-term neurologic complications and are seen in 15% to 37% of post cardiac transplant patients (McCartney et al., 2017). The critical care nurse should be vigilant to watch for signs of these conditions. Neurologic complications were discussed in more detail in Chapter 16.

Allograft Dysfunction or Graft Failure

Graft failure is the most common cause of death in the first 30 days after a heart transplant (McCartney et al., 2017). Graft failure can occur anytime after a transplant; the timing of the failure is key to its diagnosis. Graft failure is divided into early and late graft failure and is characterized by dysfunction of one or both ventricles where the circulatory needs of the patient are not met. Graft failure is manifested as symptoms of acute ventricular dysfunction such as hypotension and decreased CO despite adequate filling pressures.

Early Graft Failure. Early graft failure (EGF) is within the first 30 days of transplant and is generally more severe than late graft failure. While the incidence of EGF varies depending on report, it had a 35.7% mortality rate in cardiac transplants between January 2009 and June 2016 (ISHLT, 2017b). Etiologic factors may be related to the transplant process, patient, or donor. Hormonal effects of brain death in the donor may contribute to graft failure. Massive amounts of catecholamines are released and may lead to systemic hypertension and possibly direct myocardial injury. Age of the donor, cause of donor death, degree of cardiac dysfunction on the part of the donor, and level of inotropic support required prior to procurement

may be other causes. Higher levels of support may lead to myocardial depression. During organ procurement, ischemic time greater than 4 hours may contribute to graft dysfunction. Mismatches between donor and recipient in relation to weight and gender (especially female donor to a male recipient) have also been implicated in the development of graft failure. Effects of hypothermic preservation may be another cause of graft failure. Although hypothermia remains the preferred method for preservation, there is thought that there may be injury to the microcirculation of the heart, which may result in decreased contractility upon reperfusion. Injury during implantation or reperfusion may also cause graft failure (McCartney et al., 2017). Patient factors have also been identified. These include age; need for inotropic, mechanical, or ventilator support; presence of pulmonary hypertension; diabetes; or being overweight. Most forms of early graft dysfunction are reversible, resulting in normal donor heart function if the heart is properly supported during its recovery phase.

Early graft failure can be divided into primary or secondary based on etiology. Primary graft dysfunction (PGD) occurs within 24 hours of surgery and has no obvious cause such as pulmonary hypertension, bleeding, hyperacute rejection, or sepsis. It is generally thought to be related to ischemia from the organ recovery and reimplantation process, reperfusion injury immediately after reimplantation, and preexisting problems with the donor heart. The incidence of PGD following heart transplant is variable but ranges between 2% and 36% with a mortality rate of 10% to 14% (McCartney et al., 2017; Vega et al., 2017). Donor-related risk factors for PGD include female donor to male recipient, donor age, cause of death, presence of CAD or left ventricular hypertrophy (LVH) in the donor age, and the use of catecholamines at the time of death. Recipient-related risk factors include age, increased PVR, and use of either inotropes or MCS at the time of transplantation. Ischemic time, size mismatch, prolonged CPB time, and high transfusion requirement are also important (McCartney et al., 2017).

Ischemia and Reperfusion Injury During Surgery. Primary graft dysfunction may be caused by ischemic time greater than 4 hours, a reperfusion injury, or both. This condition may be only a temporary complication and resolve after 12 to 24 hours after heart transplant. Despite the short duration, the heart does sustain ischemic injury when such dysfunction occurs (Pham, 2018b).

Suboptimal Donor Heart. As the number of heart transplant candidates far exceeds the number of donor hearts available, some transplant programs have been accepting "suboptimal" donors. These are hearts that are from donors older than 55 years of age, hearts with mild LVH or CAD, or hearts that have been treated with higher doses of inotropic agents or vasopressors (Pham, 2018b).

The condition of the donor's heart is one of the factors that can impact early outcomes of the recipient. For example, the presence of LVH in the donor heart can result in less optimal outcomes when compared to a heart without LVH. If the donor had elevated troponin levels, indicating myocardial damage, there is an increased risk of the recipient developing HF early in the postoperative course. Age of the heart itself is reported not to affect long-term survival of the recipient; however, there is an increased chance of CAD being present in hearts over age 40 (Eisen, 2017a).

Treatment of PGD. Inotropes such as milrinone, epinephrine, dopamine, and norepinephrine are used to treat LV and RV function. Inhaled NO or phosphodiesterase inhibitors can be used to treat RV dysfunction. Low-dose nitroglycerin or nitroprusside can be given to decrease RV afterload and increase CO. The PVR should be decreased to reduce afterload. If medical treatment does not improve hemodynamics, MCS with IABP, ECMO, or a VAD should be initiated (Freeman et al., 2016; Pham, 2018b). Intra-aortic balloon pump therapy was discussed in detail in Chapter 10.

Secondary graft failure occurs as a result of the operation or a preexisting condition of the recipient. Common causes include high volumes or pressure loads on the right ventricle, extensive intraoperative bleeding necessitating massive blood transfusions, pulmonary hypertension, and hyperacute rejection. Each of these etiologies was discussed earlier in the chapter.

Late Graft Failure. Late graft failure occurs weeks to years after transplant and is commonly attributed to rejection or development of allograft CAD. Symptoms of rejection include new atrial or ventricular dysrhythmias, elevated jugular venous pressure, new ventricular gallop sounds on auscultation, volume overload, dyspnea on exertion, orthopnea, fatigue, and syncope or near-syncope (Pham, 2018b). Endomyocardial biopsy is generally used to make a diagnosis. Cardiac allograft vasculopathy is an accelerated form of CAD that develops months to years after transplant. Rejection and cardiac allograft vasculopathy are discussed in greater detail later in this chapter.

Acute Kidney Injury

Renal dysfunction, namely acute kidney injury, can occur in the early posttransplant period and lead to further devastating complications such as fluid overload and right heart failure. Renal dysfunction can be caused by prolonged hypotensive episodes causing ischemic reperfusion injuries in the kidneys and medications such as high-dose diuretics and calcineurin inhibitors.

Preexisting renal insufficiency from prolonged low CO states and advanced HF can predispose the patient to posttransplant AKI. Patients who have been receiving high-dose diuretic therapy pretransplant may manifest relative oliguria if the diuretic therapy is stopped abruptly. Combining this diuretic use with abnormal renal perfusion during CPB places the patient at greater risk for renal impairment posttransplant. Diuretics may be used to maintain adequate urinary output in these patients.

Antirejection medications, specifically CNIs, are known nephrotoxic agents that will require monitoring of both renal function (creatinine) and medication levels. Calcineurin inhibitor toxicity is one of the main causes of AKI in heart transplant patients. This is felt to be due to vasoconstriction of the afferent and efferent arterioles causing a decrease in renal blood flow and glomerular filtration rate (GFR) (Bennett, 2015).

In a 2016 study, Fortrie, Manintveid, Caliskan, Bekkers, and Betjes found that 76% of heart transplant patients experienced AKI and 5%

needed renal replacement therapy (RRT). They also found that the 1-year mortality increased from approximately 5% in patients with no AKI to approximately 15% in those with the most severe AKI. Among those who received induction therapy for immunosuppression, their risk of AKI was lower than those who did not receive induction therapy. Romeo and colleagues (2018) reported an AKI in 72% of their patients with 24% requiring RRT and hospital mortality increasing from 0% in those without AKI to 46% in those with the most severe AKI. A higher body mass index, diabetes mellitus, postoperative RV failure, a baseline GFR less than 60 mL/min, and an increased PVR have been found to increase the incidence of AKI (Fortrie et al., 2016; Romeo et al., 2018).

The main determinant of adequate renal function early posttransplant is adequate cardiac performance. As such, optimizing hemodynamics in the immediate postoperative period is essential. When early renal dysfunction is reversed, there typically is no long-term effect following transplant. If renal function is inadequate and refractory to other measures, hemodialysis or continuous RRT may be initiated. These therapies are typically well tolerated in patients with strong cardiac performance.

In the immediate posttransplant period and following CPB, the patient's urinary output will be increased. Once these effects have worn off, it is important that urinary output be maintained at a rate of at least 0.5 mL/kg/hr. The ICU nurse must maintain adequate renal perfusion with fluids, vasoactive agents, or combinations of these to maintain a mean arterial pressure in the range of 60 to 80 mmHg. Monitoring of hourly urinary output and all renal function tests should be performed by the ICU nurse as well.

Postoperative Hypertension

Differences in the physiology between the recipient's original heart and the transplanted heart are related primarily to the fact that the transplanted heart is denervated (afferent and efferent). This means that the nerve supply has been severed and results in the absence of autonomic nervous system innervation of the donor heart. This mechanism is not restored during the transplant process. Efferent denervation has implications for heart rate; afferent denervation has implications for blood pressure. As a result of afferent denervation, there will be impairment of the renin-angiotensin aldosterone system and impairment of normal vasoregulatory responses to changes in cardiac filling pressures. Both of these can result in hypertension. Postoperative hypertension is generally treated with hydralazine (Apresoline®), amlodipine (Norvasc®), or nitroprusside (Nipride®) (Freeman et al., 2016). Prevention and prompt detection and management of hypertension following heart transplantation are essential to prevent surgical site dehiscence.

Psychosocial Conditions

In addition to all of the physiologic stressors associated with heart transplantation, a variety of psychosocial conditions may surface in the postoperative period. Patients are typically and predictably euphoric and relieved that they were recipients of a long-awaited organ. However, depression, anxiety, confusion, aggression, mood swings, and delirium may develop in a few postoperative days and are often related to high doses of steroids. It is common for the patient to inquire about the donor and to experience difficulty coping with the knowledge that a death was associated with the organ procurement. Patients may manifest violent outbursts, attempt to climb out of bed, inappropriately yell at staff, or have hallucinations. Maintaining patient safety during this time is essential. The etiology and specific management of these neurocognitive disorders were discussed in detail in Chapter 16. Maintaining a calm, reassuring environment and demonstrating a high level of caring practices are essential for optimal psychological patient outcomes.

▶ Progression of Care

Transfer to a progressive care unit occurs after the patient is extubated, hemodynamically stable, and no longer receiving any vasoactive medications. The expectation throughout the hospitalization period and beyond is that patients will participate actively and fully in their own recovery.

Pain Management

Transplant patients' requirements for pain medications vary. Back, shoulder, and chest discomfort are common. While the patient is intubated, a continuous infusion of either morphine or sublimaze (Fentanyl®) is typically administered. The narcotic should be titrated so that the patient is easily arousable to verbal stimuli and able to follow simple commands. Once the patient has been extubated, use of acetaminophen (Tylenol®) and oral narcotics (e.g., oxycodone [OxyContin®]) is preferred. Nonsteroidal anti-inflammatory drugs are avoided given the compounded risk of nephrotoxicity when these medications are utilized in conjunction with CNIs to prevent rejection (Bennett, 2015).

Nutrition

Nutritional implications exist for the heart transplant recipient. Adequate nutrition is essential to prevent infection, augment wound healing, carry metabolic demand, and mediate an immune response (Posada-Moreno et al., 2012). Nutritional counseling is provided as patient education.

Recommendations regarding food intake following heart transplant have been published. Patients should be instructed not to consume raw food for the first 6 months following transplant. Casseroles should be cooked at home and eaten immediately after cooking or kept in the refrigerator covered and eaten within 24 hours. Sauces should be kept separate. Patients should consume a diet low in sodium and potassium (Posada-Moreno et al., 2012).

Approximately 10% to 25% of cardiac surgery patients are malnourished (Evans, Hosseinian, Mohabir, Kurtis, & Mechanick, 2015). If the patient had preoperative cachexia, improvements in nutritional status have implications for early and late postoperative morbidity and mortality. Patients should avoid excessive weight gain after undergoing heart transplantation. This is essential to help avoid development of hypertension,

diabetes, or hyperlipidemia. Patients who are obese or underweight 1 year after transplant are at higher risk for rejection than those patients of normal weight or overweight (Posada-Moreno et al., 2012).

Hyperlipidemia (HLD) is common following a heart transplant. Etiologic factors include poor diet, decreased physical activity, immunosuppressant therapy with cyclosporine (Sandimmune®) or steroids, antihypertensive medications, male gender, age, obesity, and diabetes. To prevent HLD, it is recommended to maintain daily total cholesterol intake of less than 300 mg, limit fat intake to less than 30% of total caloric intake, limit saturated fat to less than 10% of total calories, and increase mono- and polyunsaturated fats; the latter should be kept to 7% of total calories (Posada-Moreno et al., 2012).

A clear liquid diet is initiated at the time of extubation and advanced as tolerated. Because many heart transplant recipients are malnourished preoperatively with little nutritional reserve, caloric intake is followed closely and enteral feeding is initiated readily for patients who are not meeting caloric requirements.

Adequate intake of calcium and vitamin D is essential for patients with osteoporosis and for all patients taking chronic steroids. Magnesium depletion has been documented in patients who have undergone heart transplantation. This may be related to diuretic therapy. Similarly, folate and vitamin B6 deficiencies are common, especially in older patients and those with renal insufficiency. Intake of 5 mg of folic acid is recommended daily. L-arginine supplementation results in increased nitric oxide. This improves endothelial function and exercise tolerance following transplant. Each of these dietary interventions may augment quality of life when combined with other therapies (Posada-Moreno et al., 2012).

Data suggest that enteral nutrition is safe following cardiac surgery, even in patients with hemodynamic compromise (Evans et al., 2015). All transplant patients should be followed by a registered dietitian. When providing nutritional education, factors such ethnicity, culture, and social issues need to be considered.

The nurse should be aware of food–drug interactions and herb-drug interactions. A well-known interaction is that of grapefruit juice, which is a potent CYP3A4 inhibitor (Posada-Moreno et al., 2012). Patients should be instructed to avoid nutritional and herbal supplements except as directed by their transplant team. Herbal supplements are increasing in popularity in the United States (Saper, 2018). Because herbal supplements are not regulated by the FDA, a great deal is not known about these products. However, over time, knowledge has been gained about these agents regarding interactions and side effects that can impact recovery of the heart transplant patient. For example, St. John's wort can reduce the effectiveness of warfarin, cyclosporine, and tacrolimus (Prograf®). Garlic decreases concentrations of tacrolimus. Gingko, garlic, chamomile, and saw palmetto can increase the bleeding risk of warfarin while ginseng, green tea, kava kava, milk thistle, and Echinacea can reduce the risk. Both chamomile and Echinacea can increase the effects of cyclosporine while ginger can decrease it. Other herbs that interact with immunosuppressants and should be avoided include peppermint tea, goldenseal, feverfew, and cat's claw (Asher, Corbett, & Hawke, 2017; Colombo, Lunardon, & Bellia, 2014; Ge, Zhang, & Zuo, 2014).

Activity and Exercise

Coughing, deep breathing, and early ambulation are important in heart transplant recipients, as in all postoperative patients. Physical and occupational therapy services are consulted for all transplant patients, and a program of progressive activity is undertaken as soon as the patient's status permits. This program is implemented during hospitalization and continued upon discharge. Patients are also referred for cardiac rehabilitation. Patients are encouraged to assume gradually increasing responsibility for their self-care needs.

The transplanted heart responds differently to exercise than does a native heart. For instance, the resting heart rate is higher because of the lack of vagal innervation. Heart rate is slower to increase with exercise, and slower to return to baseline following physical exertion. In addition, the maximal heart rate is lower in a transplanted heart.

Data support progressive early mobility following cardiac surgery. The type and duration of therapy remains unclear and there are great variations in implementation that exist. There are concerns about weight bearing and upper arm range of motion in patients with a documented sternotomy. General guidelines include using both arms for exercising and activities, avoiding lifting heavy objects (lifting light objects with both arms and keeping the weight of the object close to the body is recommended), and placing arms close to the body to push up from a lying to a sitting position (Katijjahbe et al., 2018).

Exercise ability decreases after a heart transplant. This is thought to be related to preoperative and postoperative factors. Patients with severe, protracted HF who are awaiting transplantation have exercise intolerance due to skeletal muscle atrophy, fatigue, and deconditioning from chronic hospitalizations.

Following a heart transplant, patients should participate in regular weight-bearing exercise as well as muscle strengthening. These are important to help mitigate falls and fractures and side effects of CNIs and to increase bone density. Participation in cardiac rehabilitation is highly recommended. It can improve strength and exercise tolerance (Freeman et al., 2016). Participation in early cardiac rehabilitation can increase long-term survival and promote medication adherence; it has also been found to decrease the adverse effects of immunosuppression and change the endothelium of skeletal muscle (Rosenbaum et al., 2016). Furthermore, Bachmann and colleagues (2018) found that participation in cardiac rehabilitation reduced the 1-year readmission rates for cardiac transplant recipients.

Immunosuppression

The term *immunosuppression* is used in the organ transplant setting to describe methods by which the transplant recipient's immune system is prevented from "attacking" the newly implanted organ. Given that rejection is mediated almost entirely by T cells, with B cells playing a lesser role, immunosuppressants target T-cell function in a variety of ways (Vega et al., 2017).

Immunosuppression regimens generally consist of two phases—induction and maintenance.

Induction therapy offers strong suppression of the immune system in the immediate postoperative period. Use of induction agents also delays the use of immunosuppressants that are nephrotoxic. This is especially important in patients with impaired renal function. The maintenance regimen is lifelong with intensification of treatment or addition of new agents for episodes of rejection. The goals of immunosuppression are to prevent acute and chronic rejection and mitigate toxicities and complications associated with the agents. The particular strategy employed varies by surgeon preference, facility practice, and patient factors, but is uniformly initiated at the time of transplant. The three general principles of immunosuppression are (1) avoid overimmunosuppression, (2) give the highest intensity of medications in the first 3 to 6 months because risk of rejection is highest during this time period, and (3) use low doses of multiple drugs so toxicities do not overlap (Pham, 2018c). A discussion of the most commonly used immunosuppressant medications by phase of immunosuppression follows.

Induction Therapy

The goal of induction therapy is to provide intense immunosuppression when the risk of acute rejection is the highest (Davis & Hunt, 2014). It is also used in those who are at high risk of rejection: patients undergoing retransplantation; patients who are younger, African American, or highly sensitized; or female patients who are multiparous (Briasoulis et al., 2018; Davis & Hunt, 2014; Vega et al., 2017). It can also be used to delay the start of nephrotoxic immunosuppressants in those with renal dysfunction. While not recommended by the ISHLT, induction therapy is used in approximately 50% of all heart transplant programs (Briasoulis et al., 2018). A meta-analysis of immunosuppressive regimens (induction therapy versus no induction therapy) found that patients who received induction therapy had a similar risk of moderate to severe rejection, death, infection, and cancer compared to those who did not receive induction therapy (Briasoulis et al, 2018). Classes

of immunosuppressants used during the induction phase are the interleukin-2 receptor antagonists, polyclonal antithrombocyte antibodies, and monoclonal antibodies.

Interleukin-2 Receptor Agonist. The one interleukin-2 receptor agonist (IL-2RA) available in the U.S. at present is basiliximab (Simulect®). Basiliximab is a chimeric (a combination of mouse and human cells) monoclonal antibody that is used to suppress the immune system. It works by stopping IL-2 from binding to a surface receptor of activated T cells, rather than all T cells. As such, basiliximab prevents T-cell proliferation, which is responsible for the cellular immune response of rejection. It is generally well tolerated with no significant side effects compared to muromonab-CD3 and antithrombocyte medications (Pham, 2018c).

Polyclonal Antibodies. Polyclonal antibodies, or antithymocyte globulins (ATGs), originate from immunized horses (ATGAM®, lymphocyte immune globulin) or rabbits (Thymoglobulin®) with human lymphocytes. These agents have antibodies that work against a number of T lymphocytes, and various mechanisms are involved in reversing rejection with these agents. Side effects include serum sickness (e.g., fever, chills, tachycardia, hypotension, myalgia, and rash) and typically occur with the first or second infusion. Stopping the infusion and then restarting it at a slower rate is suggested. Patients are usually premedicated with an intravenous glucocorticoid, antihistamine, antipyretic, and H_2 blocker to mitigate or prevent reactions. Some patients develop leukopenia and thrombocytopenia, which respond to dose reduction or discontinuation of the agent. Life-threatening side effects include being at risk for cytomegalovirus and other opportunistic infections and malignancies (Pham, 2018c). The use of ATG instead of IL-2RA was found to decrease the risk of moderate to severe rejection (Briasoulis et al., 2018).

Monoclonal Antibodies. Muromonab-CD3 (OKT3) is a murine (mouse-derived) monoclonal antibody that binds to the CD3 site on T lymphocytes. This transiently activates and eliminates nearly all T cells from peripheral circulation, and renders remaining or subsequent T cells incapable of activation. As a result, T cells cannot perform their immunologic function.

Because OKT3 initially activates T cells through binding of the monoclonal antibody with the CD3 surface protein, side effects are those associated with cytokine release. These side effects may range from common, minor flulike symptoms (e.g., fever, chills, and minor pulmonary or GI symptoms) to life-threatening symptoms (e.g., bronchospasm, tachycardia, bradycardia, encephalopathy, seizures, renal insufficiency, and graft thrombosis) (Pham, 2018c). Due to the side effect profile, OKT3 is no longer used in heart transplantation.

Alemtuzumab (Campath-1H), a rat monoclonal antibody, is used in less than 2% of heart transplants. It targets the CD52 antigen expressed on both T and B cells and can result in severe lymphopenia that lasts for 6 months to 3 years (Pham, 2018c). It is used predominantly in kidney transplants, but preliminary results have shown that it decreases the incidence of early acute cellular rejection and allows lower dosages of maintenance immunosuppression.

Maintenance Therapy

The goal of maintenance therapy is to prevent acute rejection. Most of the regimens used for maintenance therapy are comprised of three agents—corticosteroids (administered with tapered dosing), a CNI (e.g., cyclosporine or tacrolimus), and an antiproliferative or antimetabolite agent (mycophenolate mofetil [CellCept®], sirolimus [Rapamune®], or azathioprine [Imuran®]; the latter agent is used less often) (Pham, 2018c).

Corticosteroids. Corticosteroids (e.g., methylprednisolone [Medrol®], prednisone) are useful in all phases of immunosuppression (induction, maintenance, and management of acute rejection), as these agents suppress nearly all mechanisms of the immune system. They alter cytokine expression and leukocyte activity. By suppressing interleukin-1 by macrophages, decreased

T-cell production of interleukin-2 by activated T cells results; this decreases the cellular immune response. It is not completely clear how they reverse acute rejection (Eisen, 2017b).

Long-term use of glucocorticoids is associated with poor wound healing, hyperglycemia, diabetes mellitus, hyperlipidemia, hypertension, fluid retention, myopathy, osteoporosis, and vulnerability for opportunistic infections (Pham, 2018c; Vega et al., 2017). Other reported side effects include emotional instability, headache, peptic ulcers, esophagitis, pancreatitis, pathologic fractures, loss of muscle mass, hypokalemia, pituitary-adrenal insufficiency, herpes zoster, increased intraocular pressure, glaucoma, cataracts, euphoria, dysphoria, depression, mania, and insomnia (Saag & Furst, 2018).

Calcineurin Inhibitors. The CNI category of antirejection agents includes tacrolimus and cyclosporine (CsA). As the name connotes, CNIs inhibit calcineurin. Calcineurin transcribes IL-2. The end result is diminishing of T-lymphocyte activation and proliferation in response to antigens. Each of the available agents forms complexes with different proteins. The drug–protein complexes bind to and inhibit calcineurin. Calcineurin inhibitors block this pathway, thereby inhibiting clonal expansion of T cells (Pham, 2018c). This type of immunosuppression is highly effective, but significant toxicities—most notably nephrotoxicity—limit their use in the posttransplant setting. Side effects of CNIs include hypertension, hyperlipidemia, diabetes mellitus, increased risk of infection, increased risk of malignancy, electrolyte abnormalities, and increased risk for neurotoxicities (Davis & Hunt, 2014; Hardinger & Magee, 2018).

Calcineurin inhibitors are started immediately after surgery unless the patient has chronic renal problems. The nurse should monitor renal function tests and intake and output. Levels (troughs) are followed daily until stable, and then periodically. Because CNIs are metabolized by the CYP3A4 enzyme system, drug interactions are common and can significantly alter drug levels (Hardinger & Magee, 2018). When administered concomitantly, CYP3A4 inhibitors will increase

CsA levels; CYP3A4 inducers will decrease CsA levels (Hardinger & Magee, 2018).

Tacrolimus is the most widely used CNI after heart transplantation. It shows a lower incidence of rejection although survival rates are similar. Tacrolimus also shows lower rates of hypertension and hyperlipidemia than CsA but increases the risk of diabetes mellitus. The side effects are better tolerated although the rates of nephrotoxicity are about equal (Pham, 2018c). Tacrolimus is available in oral and intravenous formulations. The IV dose is one-third of the total daily oral dose and is given as a continuous infusion over 24 hours. Trough levels of tacrolimus are 10 to 15 ng/mL in the first 6 months and 5 to 10 ng/mL thereafter.

Cyclosporine A is also available in oral and intravenous formulations. When administered intravenously, it should also be administered as one-third of the total daily oral dose as a continuous infusion over 24 hours. Cyclosporine A is titrated according to blood levels. The dose should be based on renal function, side effects, infection, and according to the patient's risk of developing rejection. Goal trough levels of CsA are 200 to 300 ng/mL in the first year and 100 to 200 ng/mL thereafter. Side effects specific to CsA include CAD, elevated uric acid levels, dyslipidemia, neurotoxicity, and liver toxicity. Gingival hyperplasia and hirsutism have also been reported with CsA (Pham, 2018c).

Antiproliferative or Antimetabolite Agents

Mycophenolate Mofetil. Mycophenolate mofetil (MMF) is an antiproliferative agent that inhibits purine synthesis, which is necessary for the production of deoxyribonucleic acid (DNA). It inhibits proliferation of T and B cells (Pham, 2018c). It is available in oral and intravenous formulations; the dose is the same for both. Mycophenolate mofetil is used concomitantly with CNIs, corticosteroids, or both. Side effects are largely GI in nature (nausea/vomiting, diarrhea), although leukopenia may occur as well. A connection between MMF and progressive multifocal leukoencephalopathy has been suggested (Pham, 2018c). There is also an increased risk of the patient developing

CMV. Because it causes less bone marrow suppression, is not nephrotoxic, and has been associated with less rejection and improved survival, MMF is the most commonly used antiproliferative agent (Vega et al., 2017). Titration of MMF is based on leukopenia and GI intolerance; drug monitoring is not normally done (Pham, 2018c).

Azathioprine. Azathioprine (AZA) is another antiproliferative agent and has generally been replaced by MMF (Vega et al., 2017). It inhibits DNA, thereby preventing cellular mitosis and proliferation of activated B and T lymphocytes (Pham, 2018c). Azathioprine is typically administered in combination with a glucocorticoid or CNI. Oral and intravenous formulations are available. Side effects include myelosuppression (especially leukopenia), hepatotoxicity, and pancreatitis. Azathioprine should temporarily be discontinued if the patient's white blood cell count decreases by 50% or is less than 3,000 m^3 (Pham, 2018c). As AZA may be more carcinogenic, patients have been switched to other agents. Regardless of which antiproliferative agent is used, the nurse should monitor complete blood counts to evaluate for the presence of associated myelosuppression.

Proliferation Signal Inhibitor or Mammalian Target of Rapamycin Inhibitor

Sirolimus. Proliferation signal inhibitors (PSIs) or mammalian target of rapamycin (mTOR) inhibitors are a fourth class of immunosuppressants that are used in a maintenance regimen. They act through a mechanism similar to, but distinct from, the mechanism used by CNIs. They bind with a protein to inhibit mTOR, which inhibits IL-2 mediated signal transduction and blocks the response of the T- and B-cell activation by cytokines (Hardinger & Brennan, 2018). As a result, there is a lower level of B and T lymphocytes. They are not recommended as initial maintenance treatment in the first 6 months because of a higher rate of rejection and other side effects but they are used in select patients with renal insufficiency, cardiac allograft vasculopathy, or malignancy (Hardinger & Brennan, 2018; Vega et al.,

2017). When used, PSIs generally replace MMF in the immunosuppression regimen (Davis & Hunt, 2014).

Sirolimus (Rapamune®) is an oral agent. Dosage is based on serum drug levels with a goal trough of 5 to 10 ng/mL. Side effects of sirolimus include hyperlipidemia, impaired wound healing, edema, hypertension, headache, progressive multifocal encephalopathy, pancytopenia, venous thrombotic events, dyspnea, interstitial pneumonitis, alveolar hemorrhage, elevated triglycerides, hyperglycemia, new-onset diabetes, acneiform rash, extremity lymphedema, GI upset, proteinuria, urinary tract infections, oral ulcerations, and infertility (Davis & Hunt, 2014; Kaplan, Qazi, & Wellen, 2014). Pericardial and pleural effusions have been reported and pulmonary toxicity is rare (Pham, 2018c). Sirolimus does not cause nephrotoxicity, but when used with a CNI, it can augment the nephrotoxic effects of CNIs. The dosage of CNIs should be reduced by 25% in this instance (Pham, 2018c). Sirolimus is not generally given with CsA unless it is a rescue therapy. If both medications are prescribed, they need to be taken 4 hours apart to minimize interactions (Hardinger & Brennan, 2018). Nursing monitoring of patients receiving mTOR inhibitors includes assessment of complete blood count data to evaluate for the development of myelosuppression and to monitor sirolimus levels (Pham, 2018c).

Everolimus (AFINITOR®) is an analog of sirolimus used predominantly in kidney and liver transplantation. Its half-life is half that of sirolimus. Studies comparing everolimus with MMF showed a reduced progression of coronary wall thickening at 12 months posttransplant with everolimus but a higher rate of drug discontinuation due to side effects. Everolimus is not recommended in the first 3 months posttransplant. Side effects of everolimus are similar to sirolimus but generally less severe (Pham, 2018c).

Rejection

Rejection occurs when T cells recognize the implanted heart tissue as foreign and mount an immune response targeted at eliminating it. The immune response leads to inflammation, cell damage, and death. If left unchecked, progressive decline in organ function ensues. Rejection is prevented by ongoing administration of immunosuppressive agents. Protocols for immunosuppression are facility specific. The components of standard immunosuppression may include a corticosteroid, a CNI, and a purine inhibitor (Koomalsingh & Kobashigawa, 2018).

Three types of rejection are distinguished: hyperacute, acute, and chronic. Hyperacute rejection is discussed earlier in the chapter. Acute rejection occurs when surface cell antigens of the donor heart are recognized as being "nonself." This type of rejection usually occurs within the first few weeks after transplant but may occur years later. The incidence of acute rejection in the first year posttransplant is 25% and accounts for 8% of all deaths (McCartney et al., 2017). There are two types of acute rejection: acute cellular rejection and antibody-mediated rejection. Cardiac allograft vasculopathy, a likely sign of chronic rejection, typically does not occur within the first year of a transplant (McCartney et al., 2017; Vega et al., 2017). It is discussed later in this chapter.

Acute Cellular Rejection

The incidence of acute cellular rejection (ACR) peaks at 1 month posttransplant and then declines over the next 5 months (Eisen, 2017c). Patients experiencing ACR may be asymptomatic or they may demonstrate symptoms consistent with LV failure (e.g., dyspnea on exertion or at rest, paroxysmal nocturnal dyspnea, orthopnea, palpitations, or syncope). They may also experience GI symptoms or atrial dysrhythmias. Left ventricular dysfunction is confirmed on echocardiogram (Eisen, 2017c).

However, most patients are diagnosed during routine endomyocardial biopsy when the patient is asymptomatic. Diagnosis is confirmed by biopsy, which shows inflammatory infiltrates and possibly necrosis (McCartney et al., 2017). Surveillance is discussed later in this chapter. It is graded according to the ISHLT from 0 (no rejection) to 3R (severe rejection). Risk factors include younger recipient, female recipient and female donor, African American recipient, cyclosporine use, and more HLA mismatches between donor and recipient (McCartney et al., 2017).

Mild rejections (grade 1R) are typically not treated unless the patient is experiencing hemodynamic compromise. Moderate rejections (grade 2R) without hemodynamic compromise are usually treated with a temporary increase in dose of corticosteroids, either orally or intravenously. Severe rejections are either grade 2R rejections with hemodynamic compromise, asymptomatic grade 3R rejection, or rejection that does not respond to corticosteroids. Cytolytic therapy (e.g., ATG) is started in addition to the maintenance regimen of CNIs and MMF or AZA if therapeutic blood levels of these medications have been attained (Eisen, 2017c; Vega et al., 2017). This regimen generally reverses 80% to 95% of rejection episodes (Eisen, 2017b).

All symptomatic patients should be hospitalized and treated with IV corticosteroids at a minimum. Corticosteroids will not resolve hemodynamic compromise (Davis & Hunt, 2014). If hemodynamic compromise is present, the patient should be admitted to an ICU and treated for both ACR and antibody-mediated rejection while waiting for biopsy results. Hemodynamic compromise is defined as increased PAP or PAOP, mixed venous oxygen saturation less than 50%, CO less than 4 L/min or CI less than 2 L/min/m², or heart failure symptoms such as profound dyspnea or fatigue (McCartney et al., 2017). Cardiac function should be supported with inotropes or MCS as needed (Davis & Hunt, 2014). After the acute rejection resolves, the maintenance regimen needs to be adjusted for all patients with ACR. Endomyocardial biopsies are obtained at the end of treatment course and again 1 to 2 weeks later for symptomatic patients and 2 to 4 weeks later for asymptomatic patients (Eisen, 2017b; McCartney et al., 2017). Once resolved, the patient returns to the original plan for surveillance biopsies. Posttransplant surveillance is discussed in more detail later in this chapter.

Antibody-Mediated Rejection

Antibody-mediated rejection (AMR) starts when antibodies are developed against the capillary endothelium of the allograft (Vega et al., 2017). The diagnosis of AMR, confirmed by endomyocardial biopsy, is based on immunopathologic features (McCartney et al, 2017). It is less common than ACR with an incidence of 10% to 40% and a worse prognosis (Eisen, 2017c; Vega et al., 2017). It can occur early after transplant (normally seen with graft dysfunction and hemodynamic compromise) or as late as months to years posttransplant (with hemodynamic compromise but less graft dysfunction). Risk factors include female recipient, pretransplant elevated panel reactive antibodies, CMV positivity, prior MCS, allosensitization against anti-HLA, and multiparity (McCartney et al., 2017). Antibody-mediated rejection is treated with plasmapheresis and IVIG to remove antibodies, antilymphocyte antibodies, and high-dose corticosteroids. Rituximab (Rituxan®) can also be used to treat AMR (Eisen, 2017c). Cardiac function should be supported by inotropes, vasopressors, and MCS, if needed. After resolution, the maintenance regimen should be adjusted.

Recurrent or Resistant Rejection

Recurrent or resistant rejection can be treated with photopheresis, which is the separation of leukocytes and their subsequent exposure to ultraviolet light damaging rapidly proliferating leukocytes. This is done twice weekly for 4 weeks. Total lymphoid irradiation and changes in maintenance regimen (by adding methotrexate or changing tacrolimus for cyclosporine) can also be used to treat recurrent or resistant rejection (Eisen, 2017b).

Complications of Immunosuppression
Infectious Disease Following Heart Transplant

Infection is a primary complication following a heart transplant and is a common cause of morbidity and mortality in the first year in this patient population. Heart transplant patients are at increased risk for development of infection for a number of reasons. For example, antirejection medications, especially when used in combination, uniformly increase the risk of infection. Infections posttransplant are divided into three different time periods: the first month posttransplant, 1 to 6 months posttransplant, and more than 6 months since transplant (Fishman, 2017).

In the first month posttransplant, infections are related to either the surgery or hospitalization or are from the donor or recipient. Non-CMV infections are the third most common cause of death (14%) in the first month after transplantation, behind graft failure (40.5%) and multiple organ failure (17.6%) (ISHLT, 2017c). Common nosocomial infections include *Pseudomonas aeruginosa*, *Legionella* species, and other gram-negative bacilli; gram-positive organisms such as the multidrug-resistant organisms vancomycin-resistant enterococci (VRE) and methicillin-resistant *Staphylococcus aureus* (MRSA); azole-resistant *Candida* species; *Aspergillus* species; and *Clostridium difficile*. Common sources of nosocomial infection include invasive lines, catheters, and devices; surgical incisions; and mechanical ventilation equipment. Common viral pathogens include hepatitis B and C. Donor-related pathogens include those with antimicrobial resistance such as azole-resistant *Candida* species, VRE, and MRSA. It can also include human immunodeficiency virus and parasites such as *Trypanosoma cruzi* (Chagas disease) or *Toxoplasma gondii*, which persists in myocardial tissue (Fishman, 2017).

Opportunistic infections are the most common infection from 1 to 6 months posttransplant. These include *Aspergillus fumigatus* (the most common opportunistic pathogen in this time period); *Pneumocystis carinii* pneumonia (PCP); endemic fungi such as histoplasmosis or Cryptococci; viral pathogens such as hepatitis B or C, influenza, or respiratory syncytial virus (RSV); tuberculosis; and *Cryptosporidium* (Fishman, 2017; McCartney et al., 2017). Reactivation of old infections such as Chagas disease or leishmaniasis, cytomegalovirus (CMV), Epstein-Barr virus (EBV), varicella-zoster virus (VZV), and herpes-simplex virus (HSV) also occur during this time. Primary infection by these organisms

is not "cured," but rather is controlled by a competent immune system. Reactivation of infection does not occur in the immunocompetent patient because T and B cells are constantly circulating and immediately respond to any renewed activity of these latent organisms.

More than 6 months after transplant, the most common infections are community acquired due to respiratory viruses such as pneumococcus and *Legionella* species. In the first year after transplant, the most common cause of death was non-CMV infection (31.6%) followed by graft failure (17.8%) (ISHLT, 2017c).

Interventions to prevent development of infection are essential. Prophylactic antibiotic administration based on institutional guidelines is recommended. Strict aseptic technique is required for surgical wound care as well as for management of all invasive lines, catheters, and devices. Once the surgical dressing is removed, usually after 48 hours, cleaning with an antimicrobial solution should be performed until wound healing has taken place. Dry incisions should be left open to air to prevent accumulation of moisture (Moore-Gibbs & Bither, 2015).

Meticulous nursing care is essential to prevent these potentially lethal infections. Preventive measures are crucial in this regard; they include meticulous handwashing, administration of antimicrobial agents (the choices will be facility specific), and discouraging visitation by persons with colds or flu or by persons who recently received a live vaccine. Invasive lines, catheters, and devices should be managed using evidence-based guidelines and removed as early as possible. When feasible, early ambulation should be encouraged. Assessment for and prompt recognition of the presence of signs and symptoms for infection are equally important. These signs may include fever, chills, rigors, mental status changes, elevated white blood cell count, malaise, nausea, and vomiting.

As discussed in Chapter 18, strict glycemic control decreases the risk of deep sternal wound infection. While the patient is intubated and on mechanical ventilation, evidence-based interventions should be implemented to prevent ventilator-associated events (VAEs). Guidelines to prevent VAEs may be found on the American

Association of Critical-Care Nursing's website in the "Recommendations for Practice" section.

Infection Prophylaxis

Several well-established procedures to minimize infectious risks exist. First, the heart donor is screened for HIV, hepatitis B virus (HBV), hepatitis C virus (HCV), CMV, syphilis, EBV, and *T. gondii*. Likewise, the heart recipient is screened before transplant for antibodies to CMV, HIV, HSV, VZV, HBV, HCV, *T. gondii*, endemic fungi, syphilis, and EBV. Presence of antibodies indicates previous infection and confirms the risk for reactivation of these infections in the setting of immunosuppression. The patient also receives a tuberculin skin test (Alexander & Fishman, 2017). Prophylactic medications are used to prevent reactivation of a latent infection when appropriate.

All patients on high-dose steroids or antilymphocyte treatment should receive antibiotics and antiviral therapy, including clotrimazole lozenges (Mycelex Trouch®) to prevent oral candidiasis, acyclovir (Zovirax®) to prevent herpes virus infection, and trimethoprim-sulfamethoxazole (TMP-SMX) to prevent PCP; ganciclovir (Cytovene®) is given in select cases to prevent CMV (Eisen, 2017b; Vega et al., 2017).

Additional antifungal prophylaxis is facility based. *Candida* and *Aspergillus* are the primary fungal organisms seen in heart transplant recipients. Drug interactions with azole drugs and CNIs and mTORs need to be considered when deciding on appropriate preventive measures. Data further suggest that neither ketoconazole (Nizoral®) nor clotrimazole (Mycelex® Troche) decreased the incidence of invasive fungal infections. Patients who should be considered for antifungal prophylaxis include those with kidney or liver dysfunction, large packed red blood cell requirements, prolonged ICU stay, need for additional surgery following transplant, known preoperative colonization with fungus, prior broad-spectrum antibiotic use, or prolonged use of total parenteral nutrition (Alexander & Fishman, 2017).

Cytomegalovirus is the most common opportunistic organism following solid organ transplant. It may be acquired from the donor, blood products, or reactivated in the recipient and generally occurs 1 to 4 months after transplantation. More than 50% of patients who receive a solid organ transplant develop CMV within the first 90 days following transplant (Jani, 2017). Acyclovir, ganciclovir, or valacyclovir (Valtrex®) may be used for prevention (Alexander & Fishman, 2017). Patients with a history of HSV or VZV infection should receive antiviral therapy for 3 to 6 months following transplant and during high-dose antirejection therapy (Alexander & Fishman, 2017).

Prior to transplant, potential recipients are encouraged to be vaccinated against HBV and, if aged 50 to 59, zoster (Alexander & Fishman, 2017). Hepatitis B can be reactivated following heart transplantation due to antirejection medications. Following transplant, vaccine administration is recommended with the dead vaccine for influenza and pneumococcus (Kittleson & Kobashigawa, 2014). The live attenuated intranasal vaccine is contraindicated.

Although these regimens are highly effective in preventing infectious complications, infection remains a significant cause of mortality through the 1-year mark following transplant.

Malignancies

Malignancy is the most common cause of death 5 to 10 years posttransplant (Lund et al., 2017) and the incidence increases over time (Pham, 2017a). By 10 years posttransplant, 28% of heart transplant recipients will have a malignancy, with skin (18%) and lymphoma (1.8%) carcinomas being the most common (Lund et al. 2017). The use of sirolimus and everolimus shows less progression to malignancy (Kittleson & Kobashigawa, 2014).

Chronic Kidney Disease

Calcineurin inhibitors, such as tacrolimus and cyclosporine, contribute to long-term renal dysfunction (i.e., chronic kidney disease). Chronic kidney disease (CKD) is seen in up to 50% of heart transplant patients 5 years posttransplant, with 6% of patients requiring dialysis and approximately 4% requiring renal transplant 10 years posttransplant (Lund et al., 2017; McCartney et al., 2017).

Risk factors for CKD include decreased pretransplant GFR, pretransplant hypertension or diabetes mellitus, increased age, female gender, or postoperative AKI (McCartney et al., 2017).

Cardiac Allograft Vasculopathy

Cardiac allograft vasculopathy (CAV) refers to allograft CAD in the transplanted heart. After first-year posttransplantation, it is one of the three most common causes of death (McCartney et al., 2017). Cardiac allograft vasculopathy in transplant recipients is distinguished from CAD in other populations in that it results in diffuse, longitudinal, and concentric luminal narrowing rather than discrete lesions. Therefore, it is often not amenable to percutaneous or surgical intervention. The prevalence of CAV in survivors at 1, 5, and 10 years posttransplantation is 8%, 29%, and 47%, respectively (Gustafsson, 2018).

Some of the etiologic factors associated with CAV include older age of the donor, donor history of hypertension, male donor, Caucasian donor, tobacco use or diabetes mellitus in the donor, younger age of the recipient, greater number of HLA mismatches, history of acute rejection, and the recipient's pretransplant history of ischemic heart disease (Eisen, 2017d; Gustafsson, 2018).

Cardiac allograft vasculopathy develops slowly. Its diagnosis may be difficult based on symptomatology. Because of afferent and efferent denervation, patients rarely develop angina. As such, silent myocardial infarction, progressive HF, and sudden cardiac death may be how the patient presents with CAV. The most common symptoms are weakness, palpitations, dyspnea, and GI symptoms (Gustafsson, 2018; McCartney et al., 2017).

Patients may have changes found on echocardiogram or changes in allograft function found on echocardiogram or right cardiac catheterization. Other invasive options are available. Coronary angiography will reveal vessel narrowing and filling of the coronary arteries but lacks sensitivity for early-stage CAV and severely underestimates its presence (Gustafsson, 2018). Intravascular ultrasound (IVUS) can be used when angiography findings do not explain the left ventricular dysfunction and can confirm CAV. Ultrasound will detect thickening of the intimal layer of coronary arteries (Gustafsson, 2018).

Noninvasive diagnostic studies are not sensitive enough to be performed in lieu of coronary angiography. Select low-risk patients may be followed with noninvasive methods. If abnormalities are noted, coronary angiography can then be performed. Elevations in biomarkers, such as C-reactive protein, predict a high likelihood of CAV (Eisen, 2017d).

Current recommendations for CAV screening include annual coronary angiography in the first 5 years if the GFR is greater than 30 mL/min. If the GFR is less than 30 mL/min, annual dobutamine stress testing is recommended. More than 5 years posttransplantation, those at low risk should receive annual dobutamine stress testing. Those with evidence of CAV should undergo annual coronary angiography (Gustafsson, 2018).

Prevention of CAV is essential because of poor outcomes associated with this complication. Preventive strategies that are reported include administration of statins, which should be started 1 to 2 weeks posttransplant (McCartney et al., 2017). Patients who are transplant recipients have a high incidence of hyperlipidemia. Statin administration decreases the risk of CAV and improves mortality rates. One concern about this therapy is the associated development of myopathy. This is especially true when statins are administered with cyclosporine or tacrolimus. Both of these antirejection medications inhibit the CYP3A4 enzyme system, which metabolizes most of the statin medications. One statin, pravastatin (Pravachol®), is not metabolized by the CYP3A4 enzyme so the risk of myopathy is less with this statin (Eisen, 2017e).

Administration of the mTOR inhibitors has been shown to decrease the incidence of CAV. Sirolimus decreases cell production. Its use in the prevention of CAV, however, may be concerning because of reports of poor wound healing with this agent. Some reports recommend the use of sirolimus in patients with documented vasculopathy (Eisen, 2017e). Patients who used everolimus had a smaller increase in the maximal intimal thickness than azathioprine and a reduction in rejection but higher rates of side effects and mortality (Eisen, 2017e).

Because oxidative stress has been implicated in the development of CAV, it is logical that antioxidants be considered to help prevent this condition. More data are needed. Administration of antioxidants (vitamins C and E), when given with pravastatin, has been shown to decrease the progression of atherosclerosis. This effect is thought to be due to decreased oxidative stress effects with antioxidants (Eisen, 2017e).

In some initial studies, administration of diltiazem (Cardizem®), if started shortly after a heart transplant, has been shown to prevent development of CAV. The data are not definitive to support diltiazem's contribution regarding CAV prevention and recent studies have not found a reduction in CAV (Eisen, 2017e). However, it is suggested that it may be considered in patients early after transplant if hypertension is present. The need for a prudent lifestyle and preventive measures are emphasized to include smoking cessation, control of hypertension, and cholesterol reduction (with diet and medications) (Eisen, 2017e). Other medications that can slow the progression of CAV include ACE inhibitors and ganciclovir. Angiotensin converting enzyme inhibitors improve the microvascular endothelial dysfunction in allografts, and the use of ganciclovir for CMV prophylaxis has been shown to slow the progression of CAV (Birati & Rame, 2014b).

At present, the only definitive treatment for CAV is retransplantation. Ethical issues surround this treatment option given the limited number of organs available for transplant. Some question why a person should get a second heart while so many are awaiting transplantation of a first (Eisen, 2017e; Kittleson & Kobashigawa, 2014). Other treatment options that are described in the literature include altering the immunosuppression regimen by either increasing the dosage of the agents or changing them and revascularization (percutaneous or surgical). Increasing the dose of immunosuppressants is not recommended because of the increased risk of infection and malignancy. Percutaneous coronary intervention in symptomatic patients with abnormal stress tests has been used as a palliative procedure in patients with single-vessel disease. An immediate success of 92% to 94% has been found with a restenosis rate

of 20% to 55% at 6 to 12 months (Eisen, 2017e). There are limited data to suggest that angioplasty with stenting can lead to a decreased incidence of restenosis when compared to angioplasty alone and the efficacy of drug-eluting stents with CAV needs to be evaluated (Eisen, 2017e). Coronary artery bypass grafting has been performed on a small number of patients. The efficacy data are inconsistent and CABG is not currently recommended (Eisen, 2017e; Fujita et al., 2014).

Posttransplant Surveillance

Patients who undergo heart transplantation receive lifetime follow-up to monitor for rejection, drug toxicity, infection, malignancy, and other complications of therapy. The frequency of the monitoring is based on the amount of time since transplantation and the patient's postoperative course. In general, patients receive follow-up every week for the first month after transplant; biweekly for the second month; monthly for the next few months; then bimonthly for the next 6 months. Frequency of follow-up is increased if problems develop (Freeman et al., 2016).

An ECG, biomarkers, cardiac imaging, coronary angiography, IVUS, and endomyocardial biopsies are performed at regular intervals to monitor for development of rejection (Eisen, 2017c; Freeman et al., 2016). Complications of myocardial biopsy include pneumothorax, cardiac perforation, and tricuspid valve injury. Levels of immunosuppressive agents are monitored in addition to complications of these agents. Assessment of bone density while the patient continues on bisphosphonate therapy continues every 1 to 2 years. Bisphosphonate therapy is required following a heart transplant because of the increased rate of bone loss and risk for fractures (Zhao, Wang, & Hu, 2015).

▸ Outcomes After Heart Transplant

According to the ISHLT, the total number of adult heart transplants through June 30, 2016, was 120,991

(Lund et al., 2017). The 1-year survival rate following heart transplant is reported to be as high as 82% and the overall 5-year survival rate is 69% (McCartney et al., 2017). The median survival rate is 10.7 years in adults (Lund et al, 2017). *The Registry of the International Society for Heart and Lung Transplantation's 34th Official Adult Heart Transplantation Report* provided detailed data on outcomes following transplant. These data are summarized in **TABLE 19.2**.

The leading causes of death are graft failure, infection, malignancy, and multiple organ failure. Graft failure is seen more often in the first 30 days while infection is more common in the first year. Long-term leading causes of death include malignancy, CAV, and renal failure (Lund et al., 2017).

Other Long-Term Complications

Hypertension

Up to 91% of patients report hypertension within 5 years of a heart transplant (McCartney et al., 2017). It is thought to be due to CNIs. The treatment of hypertension is the same as it is for non–heart transplant patients. Interventions include lifestyle modification (e.g., sodium restriction, weight loss, exercise). Patient and family education should begin as early as feasible in the postoperative period. Medication selection depends on patient response. Calcium channel blockers, ACE inhibitors, or ARBs may be used. The latter two classes of agents may be preferred in patients with diabetes. Calcium channel blockers can increase edema and the levels of CNIs. Beta blockers are avoided as they can cause fatigue in heart transplant patients. Modification of risk factors may also include management of diabetes and elevated lipids; change to the immunosuppressive therapy may be indicated as well (Kittleson & Kobashigawa, 2014).

Diabetes Mellitus, Hyperlipidemia, Osteoporosis, Gout

Hyperglycemia is due to chronic steroid use and use of tacrolimus. A diagnosis of diabetes mellitus increases posttransplant to 23% to 36% of

TABLE 19.2 Cumulative Morbidity Rates in Survivors of Adult Heart Transplant Recipients, January 1, 1994, to June 30, 2015

	Within 1 Year (%)	Within 5 Years (%)	Within 10 Years (%)
Renal Dysfunction			
All	25.7	51.1	68.4
Abnormal creatinine (<2.5 mg/dL)	17.2	32.7	39.2
Creatinine (>2.5 mg/dL)	6.3	13.8	18.7
Long-term dialysis	1.9	3.2	6.7
Renal transplant	0.4	1.4	3.8
Diabetes	22.2	35.5	---
Coronary artery vasculopathy	7.8	29.3	47.4

Data from Lund et al., 2017.

patients in the first 2 years (Lund et al., 2017; McCartney et al., 2017). Early steroid withdrawal can reverse a new diagnosis of diabetes mellitus. Diabetes can increase the risk of CAV, renal dysfunction, stroke, and infection and should be managed with diet modifications and medications. Metformin should be avoided (Kittleson & Kobashigawa, 2014).

Hyperlipidemia is common, occurring in up to 88% of heart transplant patients 5 years posttransplant (Lund et al, 2016). Pravastatin is the statin of choice as it is not metabolized by cytochrome 3A4 (Kittleson & Kobashigawa, 2014). Osteoporosis, exacerbated by chronic steroid use, can cause vertebral compression fractures. Weight-bearing exercise is recommended. A bone density screening should be performed annually and the patient should take calcium and vitamin D supplements and bisphosphonates (Kittleson & Kobashigawa, 2014). Gout is often seen posttransplant due to CNI and diuretic use and renal insufficiency. Colchicine (Colcrys®) can be used for gout flares but can cause myelosuppression when used with CNIs. Allopurinol (Zyloprim®) can be used for maintenance therapy unless azathioprine is used; the combination of allopurinol and azathioprine can also cause myelosuppression (Kittleson & Kobashigawa, 2014).

Psychosocial Conditions

Long-term psychological disorders are also prevalent. One study found that within 3 years of transplant, almost 40% of heart transplant recipients developed a mood or anxiety disorder. Another found that the risk for major depression after a heart transplant was 41%. Depressed patients were five times more likely to develop rejection (Conway et al., 2014). Psychosocial issues are discussed in detail in Chapter 24.

▶ Patient Teaching

Patients are discharged when pacing wires have been removed and there is no evidence of rejection. A follow-up appointment is scheduled with the cardiac surgeon several weeks postdischarge. After cardiac rehabilitation is complete, a visiting nurse should be scheduled to ensure that patients are adherent to medications and dressing changes and all questions are answered.

As part of patient teaching, the nurse must review the anticipated schedule of return visits. Clearance to return to work or school or to resume driving will depend on each individual's progress. Physical restrictions include no lifting, pulling, or pushing of any item weighing more than 10 pounds for the first 6 to 8 weeks posttransplant. This is followed by orders not to lift, pull, or push anything weighing more than 25 pounds for at least 12 weeks. Heart recipients should not drive for 6 weeks. Scuba diving, extreme mountain climbing, and extreme contact sports are prohibited for life. Patients should also be provided with a MedicAlert® bracelet.

The complexity of transplant care and the consequences of noncompliance make effective patient teaching critically important. Adherence to mandated care regimens is more likely if patients understand why these practices are important. For this reason, several educational strategies are used to relay information and confirm understanding. Methods of teaching include provision of printed information, verbal instruction from multidisciplinary team members, opportunities to practice skills, demonstration, and return demonstration. Patients and their families are also provided with contact information so they can call with questions.

A number of resources and opportunities for collaboration among disciplines are available for patients following heart transplantation. These include home health nurses, assistance with cardiac rehabilitation, psychological support, nutritional planning, and support groups. The latter is important for both the patient and caregiver.

Infection Avoidance

Because infection poses one of the greatest threats to the transplant patient, avoidance and recognition of infection constitute a major focus of teaching. Common signs of infection are reviewed and patients are instructed to call if they develop any of these signs. Response to infection will be blunted in the immunosuppressed patient, so signs of infection may be nonspecific (e.g., malaise, "don't feel right"). Patients are advised to avoid people who have received live vaccines and to check with their transplant provider before receiving any immunization. Other routine practices include proper handwashing; avoiding contact with people who are ill; observing standard food hygiene procedures; and avoiding stagnant water, gardening, and digging. Patients frequently assume that the risk of gardening can be avoided if their hands are protected with gloves; in reality, the risk with gardening relates to inhalation of spores mobilized by manipulation of dirt. Dental follow-up is recommended; prophylactic antibiotics should be taken prior to any dental work. Finally, patients are encouraged to avoid any unnecessary medical procedures in the first 6 months after transplant.

Sexual Activity

Issues related to sexuality are also included in discharge teaching. Specific instructions are provided, as well as opportunity to discuss concerns. Sexual activity may be resumed as soon as the patient feels ready. For 6 weeks, patients should avoid putting weight on their arms and chest. Sexual activity may be aerobic and should be approached as such, with appropriate warm-up (e.g., foreplay) and cool-down (e.g., cuddling) periods being employed.

Patients should be given the opportunity to discuss other sexuality-related issues, such as anxiety, lack of desire, and body image concerns, and should be reassured that these concerns are not unusual. They should be invited to speak openly about their concerns and ask questions as they arise.

Family planning and pregnancy should be discussed prior to transplant. The reason for transplant is important; if the patient had a peripartum cardiomyopathy, it could happen again. Pregnancy should be avoided in the first year and conception that first year is important as fertility is not affected by immunosuppressants. Pregnancy should be discouraged if graft dysfunction and severe CAV will prevent a successful outcome. Prior to pregnancy, current medications should be reviewed to reduce the risk to the fetus. Mycophenolate mofetil and mTOR inhibitors should be avoided as they can cause birth defects. Breastfeeding is discouraged because cyclosporine and tacrolimus can be passed to the infant (Foley, 2017).

Other Instructions

Other instructions included in discharge teaching include recommendations regarding pet care, travel, and procedure for contacting the donor family. Transplant recipients should not change cat litter due to the risk of toxoplasmosis. Travel is not prohibited; destination-specific immunizations should be cleared by the transplant team. Using sunscreen and wearing hats and protective clothing are encouraged due to the risk of photosensitivity and increased risk of skin cancer associated with immunosuppressive medications (Coghill et al., 2016). Skin cancers are a significant cause of morbidity and mortality in organ transplant patients (Lund et al., 2017). Heart transplant recipients should continue routine cancer screenings, including mammography, colonoscopy, Papanicolaou tests, and dermatologic visits.

Medications

Transplant patients are prescribed multiple medications that must be taken exactly as prescribed. The consequences of noncompliance (whether intentional or inadvertent) may be devastating. Every effort is made to ensure that the patient understands the dosing and administration regimen for all medications to be taken. Printed information should be provided to patients listing each medication prescribed along with its mechanism of action, side effects, interactions, dosing schedule, and procedures to be followed for missed doses. Due to the risk of interactions or compounded toxicities, patients are instructed not to take any over-the-counter medication without clearance from the transplant provider. Exceptions to this rule include acetaminophen, acetylsalicylic acid, docusate sodium (Colace®), senna, loperamide (Imodium®), and bismuth subsalicylate (Kaopectate®).

New prescriptions from nontransplant care providers should also be cleared by the transplant team. Patients are instructed to avoid all nonsteroidal anti-inflammatory drugs. Herbal teas, medications, and other nutritional supplements should also be cleared with the transplant team.

▶ Summary

The ICU nurse plays a pivotal role in optimizing outcomes of patients and families during HF exacerbations and the wait for a heart transplant. High levels of critical thinking are required to care for the patient on inotropic or mechanical support. Evaluating the patient's candidacy for transplant and supporting the patient and family as they await availability of a suitable donor heart require high levels of clinical inquiry and caring practices. The ICU nurse also has a role as a facilitator of learning as the patient and family learn about management strategies for HF and about the transplant process.

Posttransplant patients have a high degree of vulnerability in the immediate postoperative period. The ICU nurse must monitor for, promptly recognize, and treat the significant complications that can affect short-, intermediate-, and long-term survival following heart transplantation.

🔍 CASE STUDY

P. J., a 46-year-old male patient with a 5-year history of HF, has been diagnosed with end-stage HF. He originally had viral myocarditis that resulted in a dilated cardiomyopathy. He has slowly deteriorated even though he has had medical intervention of a biventricular pacemaker and home-delivered inotropic medication. He had been on the transplant list for a heart for 3 months when a donor was identified.

Critical Thinking Questions

1. What should the nursing assessment include upon admission from the operating room to the ICU?
2. How should the nurse anticipate treating vasodilatory shock?
3. How should the nurse anticipate treating postoperative pulmonary hypertension?

Answers to Critical Thinking Questions

1. The ICU nurse should assess the surgical site for bleeding, and check chest tube output, urine output, and all hemodynamic parameters, including BP, HR and rhythm, CVP, PAP, PAOP, CO, CI, and SVR. Pulse oximetry and mixed venous saturation should also be monitored. The nurse will also be responsible for slowly warming the patient to prevent bleeding, acidosis, dysrhythmias, and low CO. Hypercarbia, acidosis, hypoxia, and high inspiratory pressures should be avoided during ventilator management to promote venous return to the heart. Volume status should be closely observed and overload should be avoided. Frequent laboratory draws will be performed to watch electrolytes, hemoglobin and hematocrit, white cell count, and coagulation status.
2. Vasodilatory shock is usually treated with norepinephrine, phenylephrine, and vasopressin.
3. Pulmonary hypertension and right heart dysfunction are treated with inhaled vasodilators and other agents.

Self-Assessment Questions

1. Which heart failure patient may be a candidate for heart transplantation? A patient:
   A. with irreversible pulmonary hypertension.
   B. who has a predicted 1-year survival rate of at least 35%.
   C. who has a maximum oxygen consumption of less than 12 mL/kg/min who is receiving beta blockers.
   D. with severe symptomatic cerebrovascular disease.

2. Which patient will not be considered for a heart transplantation? A patient with:
   A. bilirubin 2.0 mg/dL.
   B. creatinine clearance less than 50 mL/min.
   C. diabetes with an HbA_{1c} 8.0%.
   D. body mass index 28 kg/m^2.

3. Which patient is a candidate for a heart transplant? A patient with a history of:
   A. peptic ulcer disease.
   B. cirrhosis.
   C. end-stage renal disease.
   D. mild depression.

4. Which statement is true regarding extracorporeal membrane oxygenation (ECMO)?
   A. It can provide support to the patient awaiting heart transplant for months.
   B. It uses a centrifugal pump to propel blood from the left ventricle to the systemic circulation.
   C. A sternotomy is required for direct access and cannulation of the heart and great vessels.
   D. Blood is withdrawn via a central vein to a gas exchanger so that the heart and lungs are bypassed.

5. Following ventricular assist device placement, the nurse should anticipate administration of:
   A. anticoagulants.
   B. broad-spectrum antibiotics.
   C. judicious fluid administration.
   D. inotropic support.

6. A patient with which arterial blood gas result is most likely to experience increased pulmonary vascular resistance?

	pH	pCO$_2$	pO$_2$	HCO$_3$
A.	7.49	30	73	19
B.	7.30	38	79	18
C.	7.51	31	65	25
D.	7.29	50	58	28

7. Which should the nurse include in teaching patients being discharged home with a left ventricular assist device?
   A. Wipe dust from a computer screen before use.
   B. Rinse the ventricular filter with water weekly.
   C. Avoid extreme temperatures when tub bathing.
   D. Obtain a backup generator.

8. Which should the nurse anticipate if the postoperative heart transplant patient is rewarmed too rapidly?
   A. Hypotension
   B. Alkalosis
   C. Peripheral vasoconstriction
   D. Increased cardiac output

9. Which of the following is an early sign of bleeding in a postoperative heart transplant patient?
   A. Pulmonary artery pressures of 13/9 mmHg
   B. Blood pressure of 80/40 mmHg
   C. Cardiac output of 4 L/min
   D. Heart rate of 130 beats/min

10. Which is indicative of cardiac tamponade following heart transplantation?
    A. Heightened R wave
    B. Widening pulse pressure
    C. CVP 12 mmHg
    D. Cardiac output 4.2 L/min

Answers to Self-Assessment Questions

1. **C. who has a maximum oxygen consumption of less than 12 mL/kg/min who is receiving beta blockers**
   Rationale: Presence of irreversible pulmonary hypertension or severe symptomatic cerebrovascular disease is an absolute contraindication for heart transplantation. Life expectancy less than 2 years is another absolute contraindication for heart transplantation.

2. **C. diabetes with an HgbA$_{1c}$ 8.0%**
   Rationale: Patients with diabetes with poor glycemic control (HgbA$_{1c}$) will not be considered for heart transplantation. Other patients include those with advanced liver disease, creatinine clearance less than 30 mL/min, and those with a BMI greater than 35 kg/m^2.

3. **D. mild depression**
   Rationale: Patients must be able to cope with the waiting time for an organ. Peptic ulcer disease, cirrhosis, and end-stage renal disease are relative contraindications for heart transplantation.

4. **D. Blood is withdrawn via a central vein to a gas exchanger so that the heart and lungs are bypassed.**
   Rationale: Extracorporeal membrane oxygenation allows for heart-lung bypass. It can provide support for days to weeks. It uses standard CPB equipment that has been modified. Cannulation is via percutaneous vessels.

5. **A. anticoagulants**
   Rationale: Anticoagulation is needed to prevent pump thrombosis and thrombotic events. Other infection prevention strategies are required, but antibiotic therapy is not required. Neither judicious fluid administration nor inotropic support is indicated.

6. **D. 7.29 / 50 / 58 / 28**
   Rationale: Presence of acidosis, hypercarbia, and hypoxemia increase pulmonary vascular resistance.

7. **D. Obtain a backup generator.**
   Rationale: Backup equipment must be kept nearby in case of a power failure. The computer screen should not be touched. The ventricular filter should be cleaned and inspected daily. Patients should not participate in any activities that involve water immersion.

8. **A. hypotension**
   Rationale: Hypotension may occur from vasodilation if the patient is warmed too rapidly. Other sequelae include acidosis, peripheral vasodilation, and decreased cardiac output.

9. **D. heart rate of 130 beats/min**
   Rationale: Tachycardia is an early sign of bleeding. A decrease in PAP, hypotension, and low cardiac output are late signs of bleeding.

10. **C. CVP 12 mmHg**
    Rationale: An increase in CVP is an indication of presence of cardiac tamponade. Other indications include low voltage QRS complexes, narrowing pulse pressure, and decreased cardiac output.

CLINICAL INQUIRY BOX

Question: What are the early postoperative pulmonary complications in heart transplant recipients?

Reference: Firat, A. C., Kömürcü, Ö., Zeyneloglu, P., Türker, M., Sezgin, A., & Pinat, A. (2015). Early postoperative pulmonary complications following heart transplantation. *Critical Care, 19*(Suppl 1), S270. Retrieved from https://ccforum.biomedcentral.com/articles/10.1186/cc14350

Objective: To determine early postoperative pulmonary complications in patients who undergo heart transplantation.

Method: A retrospective chart review.

Results: Twenty-five patients (34.7%) developed early postoperative complications following heart transplantation. The most frequently reported complications were pleural effusion (26.4%), atelectasis (8.3%), ARDS (6.9%), and pulmonary edema (4.2%). The length of time on mechanical ventilation was 44.2 ± 59.2 hours. The ICU length of stay was 10.1 ± 5.8 hours. Hospital length of stay was similar for both groups. There was no difference in mortality between the two groups.

Conclusion: Respiratory complications are relatively common in heart transplant patients in this study. Complications were self-limiting and did not impact mortality rates.

References

Alexander, B. D., & Fishman, A. A. (2017). *Prophylaxis of infection in solid organ transplantation*. Retrieved from http://uptodate.com/contents/prophylaxis-of-infection-in-solid-organ-transplantation

Al Musa, T., Chue, C. D., & Lim, H. S. (2017). Mechanical circulatory support for decompensated heart failure. *Current Heart Failure Reports, 14*, 365–375.

Arabia, F. A., Cantor, R. S., Koehl, D. A., Kasirajan, V., Gregoric, I., Moriguchi, J. D., . . . Kirklin, J. K. (2018). Interagency registry for mechanically assisted circulatory report on the total artificial heart. *The Journal of Heart and Lung Transplantation*. doi:10.1016/j.healun.2018.04.004

Asher, G. N., Corbett, A. H., & Hawke, R. L. (2017). Common herbal dietary supplement-drug interactions. *American Family Physician, 96*(2), 101–107.

Bachmann, J. M., Shah, A. S., Duncan, M. S., Greevy Jr, R. A., Graves, A. J., Ni, S., . . . Freiberg, M. S. (2018). Cardiac rehabilitation and readmissions after heart transplantation. *The Journal of Heart and Lung Transplantation, 37*(4), 467–476.

Benjamin, E. J., Virani, S. S., Callaway, C. W., Chamberlain, A. M., Chang, S. . . . Mutner, P. (2018). Heart disease and stroke statistics—2018 update. *Circulation, 137*, e67–e492.

Bennett, W. M. (2015). *Cyclosporine and tacrolimus nephrotoxicity*. Retrieved from http://www.uptodate.com/contents/cyclosporine-and-tacrolimus-nephrotoxicity

Birati, E. Y., & Rame, J. E. (2014a). Left ventricular assist device management and complications. *Critical Care Clinics, 30*(3), 607–627.

Birati, E. Y., & Rame, J. E. (2014b). Post-heart transplant complications. *Critical Care Clinics, 30*(3), 629–637.

Briasoulis, A., Inampudi, C., Pala, M., Asleh, R., Alvarez, P., & Bhama, J. (2018). Induction immunosuppressive therapy in cardiac transplantation: A systematic review and meta-analysis. *Heart Failure Reviews*. https://doi-org.proxy.library.emory.edu/10.1007/s10741-018-9691-2

Centers for Medicare and Medicaid Services. (2016). *VAD destination therapy facilities*. Retrieved from https://www.cms.gov/Medicare/Medicare-General-Information/MedicareApprovedfacilitie/VAD-Destination-Therapy-Facilities.html

Chaudhry, S., & Stewart, G. C. (2016). Advanced heart failure prevalence, natural history and prognosis. *Heart Failure Clinics, 12*, 323–333.

Chmielinski, A., & Koons, B. (2017). Nursing care for the patient with a left ventricular assist device. *Nursing, 45*(5), 34–41.

Coghill, A. E., Johnson, L. G., Berg, D., Resler, A. J., Leca, N., & Madeleine, M. M. (2016). Immunosuppressive medications and squamous cell skin carcinoma: Nested case-control study within the skin cancer after organ transplant (SCOT) cohort. *American Journal of Transplantation, 16*(2), 565–573.

Colombo, D., Lunardon, L., & Bellia, G. (2014). Cyclosporine and herbal supplement interactions. *Journal of Toxicology, 2014*. Retrieved from http://www.hindawi.com/journals/jt/2014/145325/

Colvin, M., Smith, J. M., Hadley, N., Skeans, M. A., Carrico, R., & Kasiske, B. L. (2018). OPTN/SRTR 2016 annual data report: Heart. *American Journal of Transplantation, 18*(S1), 291–362.

Conway, A., Schadewaldt, V., Clark, R., Ski, C., Thompson, D. R., Kynoch, K., . . . Doering, L. (2014). The effectiveness of non-pharmacological interventions in improving psychological outcomes for heart transplant recipients: A systematic review. *Cardiovascular Nursing, 13*(2), 108–115.

Davis, M. K., & Hunt, S. A. (2014). State of the art: Cardiac transplantation. *Trends in Cardiovascular Medicine, 24*, 341–349.

Desai, S. R., & Hwang, N. C. (2018). Advances in left ventricular assist devices and mechanical circulatory support. *Science Direct, 32*, 1193–1213.

Eisen, H. J. (2017a). *Heart transplantation (beyond the basics)*. Retrieved from http://www.uptodate.com/contents/heart-transplantation-beyond-the-basics

Eisen, H. J. (2017b). *Acute cardiac allograft rejection: Treatment*. Retrieved from http://www.uptodate.com/contents/acute-cardiac-allograft-rejection-treatment

Eisen, H. J. (2017c). *Acute cardiac allograft rejection: Diagnosis*. Retrieved from http://www.uptodate.com/contents/acute-cardiac-allograft-rejection-diagnosis

Eisen, H. J. (2017d). *Pathogenesis of and risk factors for cardiac allograft vasculopathy*. Retrieved from http://www.uptodate

.com/contents/pathogenesis-of-and-risk-factors-for-cardiac-allograft-vasculopathy

Eisen, H. J. (2017e). *Prevention and treatment of cardiac allograft vasculopathy.* Retrieved from http://www.uptodate.com/contents/prevention-and-treatment-of-cardiac-allograft-vasculopathy

Eisen, H. J., & Kusmirek, L. S. (2017). *Arrhythmias following cardiac transplantation.* Retrieved from http://www.uptodate.com/contents/arrhythmias-following-cardiac-transplantation

Ergle, K., Parto, P., & Krim, S. R. (2016). Percutaneous ventricular assist devices: A novel approach in the management of patients with acute cardiogenic shock. *The Ochsner Journal, 16*, 243–249.

Evans, A. S., Hosseinian, L., Mohabir, T., Kurtis, S., & Mechanick, J. I. (2015). Nutrition and the cardiac surgery intensive care unit patient—an update. *Journal of Cardiothoracic and Vascular Anesthesia, 29*(4), 1044–1050.

Fishman, J. A. (2017). *Infection in the solid organ transplant recipient.* Retrieved from http://www.uptodate.com/contents/infection-in-the-solid-organ-transplant-recipient

Foley, M. R. (2017). *Pregnancy after cardiac transplantation.* Retrieved from http://www.uptodate.com/contents/pregnancy-after-cardiac-transplantation

Fortrie, G., Manintveid, O. C., Caliskan, K., Bekkers, J. A., & Betjes, M. G. H. (2016). Acute kidney injury as a complication of cardiac transplantation: Incidence, risk factors, and impact on 1-year mortality and renal function. *Transplantation, 100*(8), 1740–1749.

Freeman, R., Koerner, E., Clark, C., & Halabicky, K. (2016). Cardiac transplant postoperative management and care. *Critical Care Nursing Quarterly, 39*(3), 214–226.

Fujita, T., Kobayashi, J., Hata, H., Murata, Y., Suguchi, O., Yanese, M., . . . Nakatani, T. (2014). Off-pump coronary artery bypass grafting for a left main lesion due to cardiac allograft vasculopathy in Japan: First report of a case. *Surgery Today, 44*(10), 1949–1952.

Ge, B., Zhang, Z., & Zuo, Z. (2014). Updates on the clinical evidenced herb-warfarin interactions. *Evidence-Based Complementary and Alternative Medicine, 2014*, 1–18.

Go, A., Mozaffarian, D., Roger, V., Benjamin, E., Berry, J., Borden, W., . . . Turner, M. B. (2013). Heart disease and stroke statistics—2013 update. *Circulation, 127*, e6–e245.

Gustafsson, F. (2018). *Clinical manifestations, diagnosis, and prognosis of cardiac allograft vasculopathy.* Retrieved from http://www.uptodate.com/contents/clinical-manifestations-diagnosis-and-prognosis-of-cardiac-allograft-vasculopathy

Habal, M. V., & Garan, A. R. (2017). Long-term management of end-stage heart failure. *Best Practice and Research Clinical Anaesthesiology, 31*, 153–166.

Hardinger, K., & Brennan, D. C. (2018). *Pharmacology of mammalian (mechanistic) target of rapamycin (mTOR) inhibitors.* Retrieved from https://www.uptodate.com/contents/pharmacology-of-mammalian-mechanistic-target-of-rapamycin-mtor-inhibitors

Hardinger, K., & Magee, C. C. (2018). *Pharmacology of cyclosporine and tacrolimus.* Retrieved from https://www.uptodate.com/contents/pharmacology-of-cyclosporine-and-tacrolimus

Hayward, C., & Jansz, P. (2015). Mechanical circulatory support for the failing heart—progress, pitfalls and promises. *Heart, Lung and Circulation, 24*, 527–531.

International Society of Heart and Lung Transplantation. (2017a). [Graph illustration of risk factors for one-year survival, ischemic time and donor age]. Heart transplant: Adult recipients from the International Thoracic Organ Transplant (TTX) registry data slides. Retrieved from https://ishltregistries.org/registries/slides.asp

International Society of Heart and Lung Transplantation. (2017b). [Graph illustration of adult heart transplants: relative incidence of leading causes of death]. Heart transplant: Adult recipients from the International Thoracic Organ Transplant (TTX) registry data slides. Retrieved from https://ishltregistries.org/registries/slides.asp

International Society of Heart and Lung Transplantation. (2017c). [Graph illustration of adult heart transplants: cause of death]. Heart transplant: Adult recipients from the International Thoracic Organ Transplant (TTX) registry data slides. Retrieved from https://ishltregistries.org/registries/slides.asp

Jani, A. A. (2017). *Infections after solid organ transplant.* Retrieved from http://emedicine.medscape.com/article/430550-overview

Kaplan, B., Qazi, Y., & Wellen, J. R. (2014). Strategies for the management of adverse events associated with mTOR inhibitors. *Transplantation Reviews, 28*(3), 126–133.

Kaplow, R., & Iyere, K. (2017). When cardiac tamponade puts the pressure on. *Nursing, 47*(2), 24–30.

Katijjahbe, M. A., Granger, C. L., Denehy, L., Royse, A., Royse, C., Bates, R., . . . El-Ansary, D. (2018). Standard restrictive sternal precautions and modified sternal precautions had similar effects in people after cardiac surgery via median sternotomy ('SMART' Trial): A randomised trial. *Journal of Physiotherapy, 64*(2), 97–106.

Khoshbin, E., & Dark, J. H. (2017). Heart transplantation. *Surgery, 35*(7), 360–364.

Kirklin, J. K., Pagani, F. D., Kormos, R. L., Stevenson, L. W., Blue, E. D., Myers, S. L., . . . Naftel, D. C. (2017). Eighth annual INTERMACS report: Special focus on framing the impact of adverse events. *The Journal of Heart and Lung Transplantation, 31*(2), 117–126.

Kittleson, M. M., & Kobashigawa, J. A. (2014). Long-term care of the heart transplant patient. *Current Opinions in Organ Transplantation, 19*(5), 515–524.

Koomalsingh, K., & Kobashigawa, J. A. (2018). The future of cardiac transplantation. *The Annals of Cardiothoracic Surgery, 7*(1), 135–142.

Kwak, J., Majewski, M., & LeVan, P. T. (2018). Heart transplantation in the era of mechanical circulatory support. *The Journal of Cardiothoracic and Vascular Anesthesia, 32*, 19–31.

Lima, B., Bansla, A., Abraham, J., Rich, J. D., Lee, S. S., Soleimani, B., . . . Joseph, S. M. (2018). Controversies and challenges of ventricular assist device therapy. *The American Journal of Cardiology, 121,* 1219–1224.

Lund, L. H., Edwards, L. B., Dipchand, A. I., Goldfarb, S., Kucheryavaya, A. Y., Levvey, B. J., . . . Stehlik, J. (2016). The registry of the International Society for Heart and Lung Transplantation: Thirty-third official adult heart transplant report—2016; Focus theme: Primary diagnostic indications for transplant. *The Journal of Heart and Lung Transplantation, 35*(10), 1158–1169.

Lund, L. H., Khush, K. K., Cherikh, W. S., Goldfarb, S., Kucheryavaya, A. Y., Levvey, B. J., . . . Stehlik, J. (2017). The registry of the International Society for Heart and Lung Transplantation: Thirty-fourth official adult heart transplant report—2017; Focus theme: Allograft ischemic time. *The Journal of Heart and Lung Transplantation, 36*(10), 1037–1046.

Mancini, D. (2017). *Indications and contraindications for cardiac transplantation in adults.* Retrieved from http://www.uptodate.com/contents/indications-and-contraindications-for-cardiac-transplantation.

Martonik, H. (2017). Caring for patients with a left ventricular assist device. *American Nurse Today, 12*(5). Retrieved from https://www.americannursetoday.com/caring-patients-left-ventricular-assist-device/

McCartney, S. L., Patel, C., & Del Rio, J. M. (2017). Long-term outcomes and management of the heart transplant recipient. *Best Practice and Research Clinical Anaesthesiology, 31,* 237–248.

Mehra, M. R., Canter, C. E., Hannan, M. M., Semigran, M. J., Uber, P. A., Baran, D. A. . . . Zuckermann, A. (2016). The 2016 Internal Society for Heart Lung Transplantation listing criteria for heart transplant: A 10-year update. *The Journal of Heart and Lung Transplantation, 35*(1), 1–23.

Miller, L. W., & Rogers, J. G. (2018). Evolution of left ventricular assist device therapy for advanced heart failure: A review. *JAMA Cardiology,* e1–e9. doi:10.1001/jamacardio.2018.0522xx

Moore-Gibbs, A., & Bither, C. (2015). Cardiac transplantation: Considerations for the intensive care unit nurse. *Critical Care Nursing Clinics of North America, 27,* 565–575.

Nguyen, L., & Banks, D. A. (2017). Anesthetic management of the patient undergoing heart transplant. *Best Practice & Research Anaesthesiology, 31,* 189–200.

Organ Procurement and Transplant Network (OPTN). (2017). *Proposal to modify the adult heart allocation system. OPTN/UNOS Briefing Paper; OPTN/UNOS Thoracic Organ Transplantation Committee; Department of Health and Human Services.* Retrieved from https://optn.transplant.hrsa.gov/media/2028/thoracic_policynotice_201612.pdf

Paul, S., & Hice, A. (2014). Role of the acute care nurse in managing patients with heart failure using evidence-based care. *Critical Care Nursing Quarterly, 37*(4), 357–376.

Pham, M. X. (2018a). *Prognosis after cardiac transplantation.* Retrieved from http://www.uptodate.com/contents/prognosis-after-cardiac-transplantation

Pham, M. X. (2018b). *Graft dysfunction after orthotopic cardiac transplantation.* Retrieved from http://www.uptodate.com/contents/prognosis-after-cardiac-transplantation

Pham, M. X. (2018c). *Induction and maintenance of immunosuppressive therapy in cardiac transplantation.* Retrieved from http://www.uptodate.com/contents/induction-and-maintenance-of-immunosuppressive-therapy-in-cardiac-transplantation

Posada-Moreno, P., Ortuño-Soriano, I., Zaragoza-García, I., Rodríguez-Martinez, D., Pacheco-del-Cerro, J., Martínez-Rincón, C., . . . Villarino-Marín, L. (2012). Nutritional intervention in heart transplant recipients—dietary recommendations. In S. Moffatt-Bruce (Ed.), *Cardiac transplantation.* Retrieved from http://www.intechopen.com/books/cardiac-transplantation/nutritional-intervention-in-people-with-heart-transplant-dietary-recommendations

Rivinius, R., Helmschrott, M., Ruhparwar, A., Schmack, B., Erbel, C., Gleissner, C. A., . . . Doesch, A. O. (2016). Long-term use of amiodarone before heart transplantation significantly reduces early post-transplant atrial fibrillation and is not association with increased mortality after heart transplantation. *Drug Design, Development and Therapy, 10,* 677–686.

Roehm, B., Vest, A. R., & Weiner, D. E. (2018). Left ventricular assist devices, kidney disease, and dialysis. *American Journal of Kidney Disease, 71*(2), 257–266.

Romeo, F. J., Varela, C. F., Norberto, V., Rodolfo, P., Gustavo, G., Ricardo, P., . . . Belziti, C. A. (2018). Acute kidney injury following cardiac transplantation: Foe or common innocent bystander? *Transplantation Proceedings.* doi.org/10.1016/j.transproceed.2018.03.106

Rosenbaum, A. M., Kremers, W. K., Schirger, J. A., Thomas, R. J., Squires, R. W., Allison, T. G., . . . Edwards, B. S. (2016). Association between early cardiac rehabilitation and long-term survival in cardiac transplant recipients. *Mayo Clinic Proceedings, 91,* 149–156.

Saag, K. G., & Furst, D. E. (2018). *Major side effects of systemic glucocorticoids.* Retrieved from http://www.uptodate.com/contents/major-side-effects-of-corticosteroids

Saper, R. B. (2018). *Overview of herbal medicine and dietary supplements.* Retrieved from http://www.uptodate.com/contents/overview-of-herbal-medicine-and-dietary-supplements

Schaheen, B. W., Thiele, R. H., & Isbell, J. M. (2015). Extracorporeal life support for adult cardiopulmonary failure. *Best Practice and Research Clinical Anaesthesiology, 29,* 229–239.

Smith, E. M., & Franzwa, J. (2015). Chronic outpatient management of patients with a left ventricular assist device. *Journal of Thoracic Disease, 7*(12), 2112–2124.

Subramaniam, K. (2015). Mechanical circulatory support. *Best Practice and Research Clinical Anaesthesiology, 29,* 203–227.

SynCardia Systems, LLC. (2018). *What is the total artificial heart?* Retrieved from https://syncardia.com/clinicians/home

Takayama, H., Takeda, K., Doshi, D., & Jorde, U. (2014). Short-term continuous-flow ventricular assist devices. *Current Opinion in Cardiology, 29*(3), 266–274.

Toega, H., Ruel, M., & Haddad, H. (2015). Anticoagulation strategies for left ventricular assist devices. *Current Opinion in Cardiology, 30*(2), 192–196.

Torregrossa, G., Anyanwu, A., Zucchetta, F., & Gerosa, G. (2014). SynCardia: The total artificial heart. *Annals of Cardiothoracic Surgery, 3*(6), 612–620.

Vega, E., Schroder, J., & Nicoara, A. (2017). Postoperative management of heart transplantation patients. *Best Practice and Research Clinical Anaesthesiology, 31*, 201–213.

Vela, M. M., Sáez, D. G., & Simon, A. R. (2018). Current approaches in retrieval and heart preservation. *Annals of Cardiothoracic Surgery, 7*(1), 67–74.

Wellmann, P., Herrmann, F. E. M., Hagl, C., & Juchem, G. (2017). A single center study of 1,179 heart transplant patients—factors affecting pacemaker implantation. *Pacing and Clinical Electrophysiology, 40*, 247–254.

Yancey, C. W., Jessup, M., Bozkurt, B., Butler, J., Casey, D. E., Colvin, M. M., . . . Wilkoff, B. L. (2017). ACC/AHA/HFSA focused update of the 2013 ACCF/AHA guideline for the management of heart failure. *Circulation, 136*, e137–e161.

Yancey, C. W., Jessup, M., Bozkurt, B., Butler, J., Casey, D. E., Drazner, M. H., . . . Wilkoff, B. L. (2013). 2013 ACCF/AHA guideline for the management of heart failure. *Circulation, 128*, e240–e327.

Yarlagadda, C. (2017). *Cardiac tamponade clinical presentation.* Retrieved from http://emedicine.medscape.com/article/152083-clinical

Yoshioka, D., Takayama, H., Colombo, P. C., Yuzefpolskaya, M., Garan, A. R., Topkara, V. K., . . . Takeda, K. (2017). Changes in end-organ function in patients with prolonged continuous-flow left ventricular assist device support. *Cardiothoracic Anesthesiology, 103*, 717–724.

Yu, Z., Kittleson, M., Patel, J., Liou, F., Yabuno, J., Piponniau, L., . . . Kobashigawa, J. (2014). Moderate pericardial effusions after heart transplant: Do they require proactive intervention? Abstract C1590. *Transplantation, 98.* Retrieved from https://journals.lww.com/transplantjournal/Fulltext/2014/07151/Moderate_Pericardial_Effusions_After_Heart.1417.aspx

Zhao, J., Wang, C., & Hu, Z. (2015). Efficacy and safety of bisphosphonates for osteoporosis or osteopenia in cardiac transplant patients: Meta-analysis. *Transplantation Proceedings, 47*(10), 2957–2964.

Web Resources

Cardiac surgery: http://www.youtube.com/watch?v=qVYiGdQKP4s

Deciding whether to have transplant surgery: http://www.youtube.com/watch?v=Q0qQX6Ps79c

ECMO: http://www.youtube.com/watch?v=Psci-wZKN_s

ECMO cannulation technique: https://www.youtube.com/watch?v=ntBiTpwnKK4

Heart-lung transplantation: http://www.youtube.com/watch?v=zuG3mJQ3p40

Life on the transplant list: http://www.youtube.com/watch?v=xS7v4M-VmGw

Orthotopic heart transplant: http://www.youtube.com/watch?v=N7etGEtdCCk

Ventricular assist device: http://www.youtube.com/watch?v=DLV6kIfvSDA

UNOS guidelines for Transplant: Https://optn.transplant.hrsa.gov

CHAPTER 20

Post-ICU Care and Other Complications

Courtenay W. Brown

▶ Introduction

Cardiac surgery consists of operations to repair or correct cardiac or thoracic abnormalities. The most common surgical procedures include coronary artery bypass grafting (CABG), valve replacements or repairs, congenital or acquired defects, and repair or replacement of the aortic root. Less common are removal of intracardiac tumors and heart transplantation. Over the past 20 years, the cardiac surgery patient has become more acute, with sicker patients being operated upon. The number of elective cases has decreased from 75% to approximately 40%, while urgent cases have increased from 25% to 50%. Despite this increase in acuity, the expected mortality rate for the cardiac surgery population has remained constant, at approximately 2% (Ginwalla, Faraday & Whitman, 2014). This decline in mortality and morbidity has occurred, even though there have been increases in patient age, comorbid conditions, and procedural complexity. Most of the substantial achievements in outcomes can be attributed to advances in the intraoperative phase, critical care management, and postoperative management of the cardiac surgical patient. The prevention and management of post–intensive care unit (post-ICU) complications requires a thorough understanding of high-risk patients and the ability to proactively identify therapeutic strategies and interventions. For cardiac surgery patients who develop complications, early diagnosis, prevention, and treatment have become integral parts of the care plan. This chapter is designed to review the post-ICU phase, and the physiologic disturbances and complications that can occur once the patient has transitioned to the intermediate or stepdown unit.

▶ Cardiac Complications

The goal of recovery from cardiac surgery is to assess and optimize cardiac function. Appropriate management requires knowledge of the surgery type, comorbidities, risk factors, and early recognition of clinical changes. Cardiac dysfunction in patients after surgery can result from a number of different factors and can be demanding to manage.

Original contributions from Kristine J. Peterson

Many of the factors associated with cardiac compromise in the post-ICU clinical area can be attributed to the patient's cardiac history, surgical type, length of stay in the ICU, length of time on mechanical ventilation, ICU medication management, and the development of any other postoperative complications as outlined in Chapter 13. Discharge from the ICU historically has occurred 1 to 3 days after cardiothoracic surgery. By reducing the amount of time spent in the ICU, patients' outcomes should improve. The criteria for ICU discharge can vary depending on the type of surgery and preoperative risk factors. Cardiogenic shock, age greater than 80 years, dialysis-dependent renal failure, and surgery performed emergently are some factors that can delay a transfer from the ICU. Some institutions utilize predictive models, acuity tools, and fast tracking protocols to assist with clinical decision making if patients are stable enough to transfer out of the ICU.

The primary objective of post-ICU management of the cardiac surgery patient is to maintain adequate cardiac output and hemodynamic stability while assisting the patient to the ultimate goal of discharge. Post-ICU management requires the patient to be on continuous telemetry, frequent vital sign monitoring, and continued vigilance for any signs of complications that may arise. Transfer from the ICU means that the patient's clinical progression is in the right direction; however, the nature of cardiac surgery still places the patient at risk for cardiac complications to arise.

Dysrhythmias

The trauma of cardiac surgery predisposes patients to atrial and ventricular dysrhythmias. These dysrhythmias contribute to prolonged hospital stays, higher costs, increased risk of stroke, and increased morbidity and mortality. The high frequency of postoperative dysrhythmias and the potential for serious adverse events make it vital to identify and treat them appropriately and quickly. **BOX 20.1** outlines the risk factors that have been most commonly attributed to the development of dysrhythmias. During the post-ICU phase, cardiac surgery patients are placed on continuous telemetry to aid in the recognition

---

BOX 20.1 Risk Factors for Postoperative Dysrrhythmias

Advanced age
Obesity
Sleep apnea
Previous history of arrhythmias
Previous cardiac surgery
Low-intensity physical activity the year prior to surgery
Electrolyte disturbances (hypokalemia and hypomagnesemia)
Hypothermia
Preexisting preoperative comorbidities (e.g., COPD, diabetes, CHF, MI, cardiomegaly, mitral valvular disease, severe right coronary artery stenosis)
Myocardial irritation
Atrial distension
Proarrhythmic drug usage (e.g., sotalol, quinidine)
Longer duration of CPB and aortic clamp times
Bicaval venous cannulation
Sympathetic hyperactivity
Inadequate myocardial protection during CPB
Mechanical irritation from an indwelling CVC

CHF, congestive heart failure; COPD, chronic obstructive pulmonary disease; CPB, cardiopulmonary bypass; CVC, central venous catheter; MI, myocardial infarction.
Data from Lee, 2017; Stephens & Whitman, 2015; Ginwalla, Faraday & Whitman, 2014; Silvery, 2017.

---

of rhythm changes. Rhythm deviations and electrocardiogram (ECG) changes may occur suddenly and cause significant clinical deterioration. To improve hemodymamic stability and optimization of heart rate and rhythm, medications, cardioversion/defibrillation, or pacing may be warranted to correct or reverse any dysrhythmias. Dysrhythmia management includes correction of transient and modifiable predisposing factors, as well as specific therapy for the dysrhythmia. The urgency for and type of treatment are determined by the clinical manifestations of the dysrhythmia. Self-terminating dysrhythmias, in the setting of a transient stressor and without overt cardiac disease, often are not medically treated. However, the development of hemodynamically significant dysrhythmias in patients under critical stress conditions such as systemic infections or pulmonary issues needs a therapy for restoring the patient to a stable clinical status (Peretto, Durante, Limite, & Cianflone, 2014). Postoperative dysrhythmias were discussed in detail in Chapter 15.

Bradycardia

Sinus bradycardia, junctional rhythm, and atrioventricular (AV) conduction disturbances comprise the majority of bradycardias after cardiac surgery. Bradycardias are particularly common after valve surgery and are most likely an outcome of direct surgical injury and local edema. Bradycardias can also be potentiated by anti-tachyarrhythmia prophylaxis (Stephens & Whitman, 2015). The slow heart rate of the bradycardias may cause hemodynamic compromise and a decrease in cardiac output. High-grade conduction blockade (i.e., new bifascicular or trifascicular block and complete heart block) is the most serious of these as it is frequently associated with significant hemodynamic instability and reflects an intraoperative injury to the conduction system that may be permanent (Ginwalla et al., 2014; Silvestry, 2017). Atrioventricular conduction problems may not be immediately apparent but can develop several days after surgery. Therefore, AV conduction problems may appear after the patient has transferred from the ICU. Atrioventricular conduction problems such as third-degree AV block is a critical problem in the postoperative patient since the ventricular escape rate may be only 30 to 40 beats per minute.

It is standard practice to attach temporary epicardial pacing wires to the right ventricle to allow pacing to occur externally if needed; most often atrial wires are also placed. In low-risk patients, ventricular wires may be sufficient. If temporary pacing is desired or required, atrial pacing is preferred. If conduction through the AV node is preserved, pacing the atrium alone is the favored mode because stroke volume is increased when the electrical impulse is generated above the AV node. In the event of an atrioventricular conduction block, atrioventricular sequential pacing is the next choice. Ventricular pacing should largely be used as a rescue mode in the event of cardiac standstill or failure of atrial leads to capture. Likewise, pacing too rapidly can adversely affect cardiac performance by decreasing filling time, exacerbating ischemia, or inducing heart block (Silvestry, 2017; Stephens & Whitman, 2015; Yazdchi & Rawn, 2017). It is vital the nurse ensures that the pacer is working properly and can sense appropriately to avoid pacer dysfunction causing lethal dysrhythmias. A daily check of the patient's underlying rhythm, the minimum current that the pacemaker is able to sense (sensitivity), the pacing capture threshold, and the battery life of the pacer should be performed.

Once the patient has transitioned to the post-ICU phase, the pacing wires will be capped to prevent disruption or pulling of the wires as the patient recovers. Capping of the epicardial pacing wires may occur prior to transfer from the ICU, and can be achieved with a capping device or method. Most epicardial pacing wires will be removed 1 to 2 days prior to discharge. The coagulation status of the patient should be assessed prior to wire removal and heparin if administered should be discontinued in a sufficient time frame prior to wire removal. The wires are removed with gentle continuous pressure while the patient is continuously monitored on telemetry. After the wires are removed, the nurse must monitor the patient frequently for any signs and symptoms of bleeding or cardiac tamponade. Current guidelines recommend measuring vital signs frequently during the first 4 hours after temporary pacing wire removal. The emphasis on nursing assessment should be on new or worsening bleeding, hypotension, and dyspnea which may signal impending cardiac tamponade (Hoit, 2017). If serious bleeding or tamponade occurs as a result of wire removal, an emergent resternotomy may be needed. Emergent resternotomy was discussed in Chapter 13.

If the patient has a bradycardic event and the pacing wires have been removed, symptomatic bradycardia can be treated acutely with atropine. A backup method utilizing a transcutaneous pacemaker via cutaneous external pacing pads applied to the skin is indicated for the patient with poor signs of perfusion who cannot be paced. This external method can also be employed for conduction blockade disturbances while waiting for placement of a permanent pacer.

Atrial Fibrillation

Postoperative atrial fibrillation (POAF) is the most frequent atrial dysrhythmia encountered after cardiac surgery, with incidence rates varying between 15% and 60% depending on the type of procedure and the criteria for diagnosis. POAF has been reported in up to 15% to 40% of patients after isolated CABG surgery, in 37% to 50% after valvular surgery, and in approximately 60% after combined procedures. The incidence increases with increasing age. POAF is associated with increased rates of stroke, renal dysfunction, infection, increased lengths of stay, and mortality. Patients with POAF are also predisposed to a significantly higher postoperative risk of thromboembolism, bleeding from anticoagulation, hemodynamic compromise, and side effects of antiarrhythmic drug therapy (Habbab & Chu, 2016; Lee, 2017; Phan et al., 2015; Silvestry, 2017).

POAF causes a loss of atrial contraction, which can disturb normal atrioventricular synchrony and result in a 15% to 25% reduction in cardiac output. POAF may reduce diastolic filling and cardiac output and increase myocardial oxygen consumption thus resulting in hypotension and myocardial ischemia (Peretto et al., 2014). It is usually self-limited, as 15% to 30% convert within 2 hours and up to 80% in 24 hours. The mean duration of POAF was found to last 11 to 12 hours, with more than 90% converting to sinus rhythm 6 to 8 weeks following surgery (Lee, 2017). The evidence also suggests that performing CABG surgery without the use of the bypass machine (off-pump) may be associated with a lower incidence of postoperative atrial dysrhythmias (Habbab & Chu, 2016; Stephens & Whitman, 2015). There are numerous risk factors that contribute to the development of this atrial dysrhythmia; however, none of the risk factors has adequate predictive accuracy to identify the individual patient at risk for POAF. As a result, several risk models have been developed that use multiple factors to stratify patients into low-, medium-, and high-risk categories. The risk factors and other components of atrial fibrillation were covered in Chapters 13 and 15.

The incidence of POAF can be reduced by approximately 50% by the initiation of prophylactic treatment with beta blockers, amiodarone, or sotalol. Use of beta blockers for the prevention of POAF is supported by the highest level of evidence. For that reason, beta blockers should be started or resumed as soon as they can be safely tolerated following cardiac surgery. The greatest benefits are seen when beta blockers are initiated prior to or immediately after surgery and are independent of the agent or dose. Beta blockers appear to provide more effective prophylaxis when they are dosed with high frequency and titrated to produce an effect on heart rate and blood pressure. Prophylactic administration of oral beta blockers reduces the incidence of POAF by as much as 40% (Lee, 2017; Stephens & Whitman, 2015). Research has also been conducted on an ultra-short-acting beta blocker, landiolol hydrochloride, for the prevention of atrial fibrillation (AF). Postoperative AF (POAF) was reduced with the treatment of landiolol hydrochloride and no hypotension or bradycardia developed as a side effect, indicating the safety of the administration of this drug for prophylaxis (Liu, Bian, Zhang, Jian, & Liu, 2014). Further studies need to be conducted on the dosage and efficacy of landiolol hydrochloride before it can be widely accepted into practice.

Additionally, preoperative loading of amiodarone is more effective than postoperative loading; however, both methods reduce the incidence of POAF. In meta-analyses of multiple trials, amiodarone had a significant impact on reducing postoperative stroke incidence and was the only effective converter of atrial fibrillation to sinus rhythm. Several different studies of the administration of amiodarone preoperatively have been conducted. It has been given orally 1 to 7 days before surgery, intravenously immediately following surgery, or intravenously for 24 hours followed by oral therapy for 4 days. The outcomes show that more research is needed to determine the optimum dosing time frame (Peretto et al., 2014). Daily magnesium started preoperatively and continued for 4 days postoperatively has also been shown to reduce the incidence of POAF after CABG (Ginwalla et al., 2014; Habbab & Chu, 2016; Lee, 2017; Yazdchi & Rawn, 2017). Recent studies have also examined the role of vitamin C in the prevention of POAF. Oxidative stress plays a role in ischemia-reperfusion injury, which occurs in open heart surgery. Oxidative stress is also involved in the pathogenesis of AF. Vitamin C is a water-soluble antioxidant that may protect against oxidative stress. Some studies showed that cardiac surgery decreased vitamin C levels consistent with increased oxidative stress. Preliminary findings show that prophylactic administration of vitamin C shortened the duration of hospital and ICU stays of cardiac surgery patients. However, further research is needed to determine the optimal dosage protocol and to identify the patient cohorts who would benefit the most (Hemilä & Suonsyrjä, 2017). Some nonantiarrhythmic drugs have the potential to protect against the development of POAF due to their antioxidant or anti-inflammatory properties. Angiotensin-converting enzyme (ACE) inhibitors and statin drugs seem to lower the incidence of POAF, but the evidence remains inconclusive (Lee, 2017; Peretto et al., 2014).

When POAF does occur, it often happens within the first few days of surgery. The dysrhythmia will commonly develop on the second or third day postop with the etiology for this time frame being unknown. In a multicenter study of 4,657 patients, the majority of first episodes of POAF occurred by day 2, while the majority of recurrent episodes occurred by day 3 (Lee, 2017; Stephens & Whitman, 2015). The likelihood of POAF occurring after transferring from the ICU is high. Thus it is useful to educate and notify patients preoperatively about the possibility of the dysrhythmia. Because the probability is high for this postoperative complication to occur, the intermediate or stepdown cardiac surgical unit nurses must meticulously assess for this alteration. POAF can be confirmed based on the results of a 12-lead electrocardiogram (ECG), and typically presents with an abrupt change in rhythm with loss of P waves on a surface ECG or with continuous telemetry monitoring. This requires close monitoring of the continuous ECG rhythm from the telemetry machine to alert the nurse to any acute changes. It is also imperative for the nurse to assess cardiac function and to ascertain how the patient feels if POAF occurs. For many patients,

the ventricular rate response to AF is usually 110 to 150 beats per minute, and this rate is generally tolerated without any physiologic alterations. With the onset of tachycardia or a rate higher than 150, patients may begin to become symptomatic. Patients may become anxious, short of breath, diaphoretic, and warm in response to this increase in rate. At the onset of POAF, the nurse's role is to assess for any symptoms, obtain a blood pressure and mean arterial pressure, ensure line patency, and inform the health care team of the rhythm change. The ultimate goal for treatment is to slow heart rate, to restore and maintain normal heart rhythm, and to prevent blood clots that may lead to a stroke. Underlying comorbidities, such as older age, previous cerebrovascular disease, presence of carotid bruit, peripheral vascular disease, and CPB time, play an integral role in the development of in-hospital stroke in adjunction to the dysrhythmia itself (Peretto et al., 2014).

The treatment of POAF requires a comprehensive management of antithrombotic therapy to prevent thromboembolic events, and antiarrhythmic treatment including both rate and rhythm control strategies. Patients with POAF are at an increased risk of thromboembolic events. The risk is increased in patients with POAF of more than 48 hours' duration and is greater in patients with certain high-risk features such as hypertension, heart failure, rheumatic mitral valve disease, and previous thromboembolism (Lee, 2017; Peretto et al., 2014). The role of short- and long-term anticoagulation in patients with POAF is not clear. There is uncertainty regarding the reduction of the incidence of stroke on anticoagulants. Furthermore, the bleeding risk is increased with anticoagulation during the postoperative period. Many patients with POAF following cardiac surgery spontaneously revert to and maintain sinus rhythm, potentially negating the need for anticoagulants. However, when anticoagulation is started, the patient should be carefully and closely monitored. This monitoring will be performed with the health care team and should include following the 2008 American College of Clinical Pharmacy (ACCP) guidelines on antithrombotic therapy. The guidelines suggest oral anticoagulation for patients with POAF after cardiac surgery lasting more than 48 hours if bleeding risk is acceptable. The recommended target international normalized ratio (INR) is 2.5 (range 2.0–3.0). The guidelines also suggest that oral anticoagulation should be continued for 4 weeks, particularly in patients with risk factors for thromboembolism (Lee, 2017; Peretto et al., 2014). Patients with a prior history of AF or who remain in permanent POAF after surgery should be anticoagulated with warfarin based upon their long-term embolic risk. The evidence also suggests that the routine use of heparin as a bridge to therapeutic anticoagulation levels is not necessary. Rate control strategy with anticoagulation represents a reasonable first approach to hemodynamically stable patients due to the transient nature of the dysrhythmia. This approach is associated with early discharge and has been demonstrated to be safe (Peretto et al., 2014).

Additionally, antiarrhythmic therapy is utilized as a treatment for POAF. In patients with POAF, there is a higher threshold for long-term antiarrhythmic therapy. The therapeutic options for POAF include rate control and electrical or pharmacologic cardioversion. Electrical cardioversion is indicated for symptomatic patients, and is unnecessary for well-tolerated POAF due to the self-limited course (Lee, 2017; Peretto et al., 2014). Pharmacologic cardioversion can be achieved with class IA, IC, or III antiarrhythmic drugs, either orally or by intravenous infusion. Chapter 15 discussed the pharmacologic treatments and therapies for POAF in greater detail.

The post-ICU management of anticoagulant and antiarrhythmic therapy for POAF includes monitoring for any adverse events and educating patients. With anticoagulant usage, the nurse will need to monitor INR levels, educate the patient on the importance of dietary restrictions and bleeding complications, and monitor for any changes in vital signs or assessment parameters. Additionally, antiarrythmic therapy with intravenous amiodarone requires the nurse to be watchful for vital sign changes on drug initiation, adverse side effects, and other complications. Amiodarone, a class III antiarrhythmic agent, is commonly used in patients with unstable atrial dysrhythmias. The preferred method of amiodarone infusion is through a central line; however, the appearance of atrial fibrillation may initially occur once the patient has been transferred to the intermediate unit. Oftentimes, the central venous catheter has already been removed prior to transfer. Thus the route of administration on the intermediate unit may be through a peripheral intravenous catheter (PIVC). Infusing amiodarone through a PIVC can increase the incidence and severity of phlebitis occurring. Phlebitis is identified as warmth, tenderness, erythema, or palpable venous cord (Ray-Barruel, Polit, Murfield, & Rickard, 2014). Other commonly used descriptors include pain, swelling, induration, and purulent drainage. Phlebitis can be categorized as mechanical or chemical. Phlebitis caused by amiodarone infusion through a PIVC is considered to be chemical. Chemical phlebitis is caused by the drug or fluid being infused through the cannula. Factors such as pH and osmolality of the substances have a significant effect on the incidence of phlebitis (Norton et al., 2013). Moreover, it is the reason why nurses need to assess the PIVC site frequently during amiodarone infusion. If phlebitis does occur, the nurse needs to be able to properly rate the severity of symptoms. A systematic review of the literature reveals a plethora of phlebitis scales that can be utilized to assess phlebitis. Additionally, no uniformity exists as to how many signs must be present to qualify as phlebitis and/or warrant PIVC removal. Many tools consider the presence of two or more symptoms as phlebitis with other scales requiring only one sign. A lack of consensus on phlebitis measures has likely contributed to disparities in reported phlebitis incidence and thus requires further study (Ray-Barruel et al., 2014). The most widely used phlebitis scales are the Infusion Nurses Society (INS) phlebitis scale and the Visual Infusion Phlebitis Scale. For this discussion, the INS phlebitis scale will be illustrated as an example of an assessment tool that can be utilized to look for signs and symptoms of phlebitis. **BOXES 20.2** and **20.3** outline the nursing interventions and assessments that need to occur to reduce the incidence and increase recognition of intravenous peripheral amiodarone infusion phlebitis.

BOX 20.2 Interventions to Reduce the Incidence of Phlebitis During Intravenous Peripheral Amiodarone Infusion

1. Use a small-bore PIVC (22 gauge or smaller), as preferred.
2. Place PIVC in a large vein, antecubital or above.
3. Avoid placing the PIVC in the hand.
4. Use an inline (0.22-micron filter) when administering amiodarone via a central or PIVC to minimize the risk of phlebitis.
5. Change IV tubing and inline filter every 24 hours.
6. Assess the PIVC site in which the amiodarone is infusing every 4 hours. If any signs/ symptoms of redness, swelling, or pain, discontinue the PIVC site and resume the infusion via a new catheter/catheter site location on the unaffected arm.
7. Determine and document the degree of the phlebitis utilizing a phlebitis rating scale.

PIVC, peripheral intravenous catheter
Data from Norton, Ottoboni, Varday, et al., 2013; Spiering, 2014.

BOX 20.3 Phlebitis Rating Scale

0 = No clinical symptoms
0+ = Pain at site, but no clinical symptoms
1+ = Erythema at access site with or without pain
2+ = Pain at access site with erythema and/or edema
3+ = Pain at access site with erythema and/or edema, streak formation, or palpable venous cord
4+ = Pain at site with erythema and/or edema, or palpable venous cord over 1 inch in length, purulent drainage

Ray-Barruel, Polit, Murfield, & Rickard, 2014.
Phlebitis Scale: Infusion Nurses Society Standards of Practice, 2006.

Ventricular Dysrhythmia

The hemodynamic instability of patients with ventricular dysrhythmias is variable and depends upon a number of factors, such as the rate of the dysrhythmia and left ventricular systolic and diastolic function. Nonsustained ventricular tachycardia (NSVT) is common following cardiac surgery and typically a reflection of perioperative ischemia/reperfusion injury, electrolyte abnormalities (hypokalemia and hypomagnesemia), or an increase in exogenous or endogenous sympathetic stimulation. NSVT is defined as 3 or more ventricular beats occurring at a rate of more than 100 per minute lasting less than 30 sec or without hemodynamic compromise (Silvestry, 2017; Yazdchi & Rawn, 2017). Occasional episodes of NSVT do not require treatment. If episodes of NSVT persist, particularly in association with vital sign changes or hemodynamic instability, then more aggressive treatment may be required. Additionally, premature ventricular contractions (PVCs) are impulses that arise in an ectopic ventricular focus. PVCs are common after open heart surgery; and are usually not a problem in and of themselves, but may serve as an indicator of other issues. Patients with isolated and uncomplicated PVCs postoperatively do not exhibit an increased risk of malignant ventricular dysrhythmias. On the other hand, frequent PVCs (>30/hr) may have an impact on short-term outcome by reducing ventricular function (Peretto et al., 2014). Dysrhythmias were discussed in further detail in Chapter 15.

The intermediate care unit nurse must monitor for signs and symptoms of cardiac compromise related to the development of ventricular dysrhythmias. NSVT and PVCs are usually readily identifiable by continuous telemetry monitoring and the assessment for them should be incorporated into the routine care for the cardiac surgical patient. If an episode of NSVT or run of PVCs occurs, the intermediate care nurse should assess for any changes in heart rate, blood pressure, and if the patient has any symptoms as a result of the dysrhythmia. Additional assessments include ruling out electrolyte imbalances and hypoxia as a potential cause. If the patient is symptomatic or the NSVT becomes sustained, the nurse should anticipate the administration of further medications, electrical cardioversion, implantable cardioverter defibrillator (ICD) by the electrophysiologist, or transfer to a higher level of care.

Mechanical Complications

Mechanical complications can occur during the post-ICU phase. They are usually detected by echocardiography or invasive hemodynamic assessment, and are usually treated with surgery. Examples of mechanical complications include spasm or occlusion of a coronary artery graft, hematoma, and cardiac tamponade (Silvestry, 2017). The predominant mechanical complication during the post-ICU phase is cardiac tamponade.

Cardiac Tamponade

Cardiac tamponade is common in patients after open heart surgery due to postoperative bleeding or postcardiotomy syndrome. Cardiac tamponade results from an accumulation of pericardial fluid under pressure, leading to impaired cardiac filling and hemodynamic instability. Most often with cardiac surgery, cardiac tamponade can occur from an anastomotic leak or improper drainage of mediastinal chest tubes from clot formation (Floerchinger et al., 2013; Hoit, 2017). Cardiac tamponade was thoroughly discussed in Chapter 13.

Once patients transfer out of the cardiovascular intensive care unit (CVICU), they are still at risk for developing cardiac tamponade. The anastomosis from surgery may leak, chest tube clot formation may occur, and tamponade can happen after pacing wires are removed. The nurse in the post-ICU setting needs to remain attentive to the symptoms of cardiac tamponade and be able to assist if emergent resternotomy is warranted.

Prosthetic Valve Endocarditis

Surgical replacement of a diseased heart valve with a prosthetic valve or transcatheter implantation of a prosthetic valve can provide great clinical benefits. However, such procedures can exchange the deleterious effects of native disease for prosthesis-related complications (Gaasch & Zoghbi, 2017). Prosthestic valve endocarditis (PVE) is a potential risk for any patient who has had cardiac surgery. PVE can arise early or late after surgery. The timing of the infection reflects different pathogenic mechanisms that, in turn, influence the microbiology, pathology, and clinical manifestations of the infection. In early infection, microorganisms can come in contact with the valve prosthesis by contamination intraoperatively or via hematogenous spread during the initial days and weeks after surgery (Karchmer, 2017). The mechanisms of endocarditis involve the disposition of fibrin and platelets at the site of endothelial damage or at the location of the sutures and/or at the valve sewing ring. The organisms can adhere to these structures and initiate infection. Infective endocarditis following surgical valve replacement occurs in 1% to 6% of patients and is associated with high morbidity and mortality, with the greatest risk during the initial 3 months after surgery. The infection generally occurs with equal frequency at the aortic and mitral sites and on mechanical and bioprosthetic devices during the first postoperative year (Karchmer, 2017).

The diagnosis of PVE is based on positive blood cultures. At least three sets of blood cultures should be obtained from separate venipuncture sites prior to initiation of antibiotic therapy (Karchmer, 2017). Additionally, transesophageal echocardiography (TEE) is considered the procedure of choice and is essential for both the diagnosis and management of PVE. The TEE is able to detect leakage around the valve and the presence of vegetations.

Patient education should include instruction regarding the risk of infective endocarditis, the importance of optimal dental hygiene and regular dental care, the need for endocarditis prophylaxis at the time of dental procedures, and the importance of seeking appropriate medical attention if symptoms of infection arise.

Postpericardiotomy Syndrome

Patients can present with postpericardiotomy syndrome (PPS) several days postoperatively. Clinical symptoms may occur as late as several weeks to months after surgery and may be associated with significant morbidity. It is believed that PPS results from a heightened immune system response to injury following cardiac surgery (Alraies et al., 2014). The incidence of PPS varies between

9% and 50% depending on the populations studied (Lehto, Gunn, Karjalainen, Airaksinen, & Kiviniemi, 2015). Postpericardiotomy syndrome can oocur anywhere from a few days to a few weeks after cardiac surgery. It is diagnosed by the presence of at least two of the following clinical features: fever in the absence of infections source, pleuritic chest pain, pericardial friction rub, pleural effusion, and a persistent pericardial effusion 1+ weeks after surgery (Alraies et al., 2014). The severity of PPS can present as acute or recurrent pericarditis, pericardial effusion with or without tamponade, or constrictive pericarditis with hemodynamic instability requiring surgery. Postpericardiotomy syndrome is often characterized by a new pericardial effusion and fever. Treatment with colchicine in combination with nonsteroidal anti-inflammatory drugs (NSAIDs) may be useful in treating PPS. For severe cases oral steroids may be needed. Treatment that is not alleviated with medications include procedural interventions, including pericardiocentesis or pericardial widow for tamponade, or pericardiectomy for constrictive pericarditis in the postoperative period (Alraies et al., 2014).

Sudden Cardiac Arrest and Sudden Cardiac Death

Sudden cardiac arrest (SCA) and sudden cardiac death (SCD) refer to the sudden cessation of cardiac activity with hemodynamic collapse, typically due to sustained ventricular tachycardia or ventricular fibrillation. Sudden cardiac arrest is also known as aborted SCD if an intervention such as defibrillation or spontaneous reversion restores circulation. If the patient dies, the event is known as SCD (Podrid, 2017). For cardiac surgery patients in the post-ICU setting, mostly all cardiac arrest or SCD events are observed secondary to the monitoring capabilities of the continuous telemetry devices. In cardiac surgery patients, SCA and SCD may occur as a terminal event in patients with a deteriorating clinical course in the ICU despite aggressive therapy, or may occur unexpectedly during the postoperative phase in hemodynamically stable patients. It is estimated that of the 400,000 patients who undergo cardiac surgery in the United States annually, 0.7% to 8% will experience a cardiac arrest after cardiac surgery (Dunning et al., 2017). In the post-ICU setting, SCA or SCD can be related to mechanical complications such as tamponade, graft malfunction, valve obstruction, or nonmechanical complications such as dysrhythmias, ischemia, and pulmonary embolism. It is paramount that nurses in the post-ICU setting pay attention to the vital signs (blood pressure and heart rate) and ECG interpretations. The continuous telemetry monitor must be attached to the patient and functional to be able to detect changes in ECG rhythm. Cardiac surgical patients present a unique opportunity for high survival thanks to optimal monitoring and close recognition of SCA from predictable cases and patient populations. Additionally, highly trained health care providers who work in an environment with specialized interventions such as defibrillation and emergent resternotomy help to improve the outcomes of patients with cardiac arrest (Ley, 2015). Ultimately patients who suffer SCA or SCD in the hospitalized setting have the best chance of successful resuscitation; however, the event must be managed quickly and appropriately.

In the post-ICU setting if a patient is experiencing SCA the nurse's primary responsibility is to initiate cardiopulmonary resuscitation (CPR), including immediate external cardiac compressions at a rate of 100/min and a depth of 2 inches as promoted by the American Heart Association (AHA) guidelines. After sternotomy, there is an additional risk of displacement of the sternum with external compressions. Also, if the patient has sternal wires, cardiac tissues or bypass grafts can be damaged or lacerated by the wires or bone edges from the sternotomy. However, this does not negate the need for compressions to occur. The actual incidence of events related to compressions for cardiac surgical patients is unknown (Ley, 2015). The goal standard of therapy for SCA is defibrillation. Immediate defibrillation of shockable rhythms is of vital importance to survival and, once available, takes priority over all other therapies (Ley, 2015). CPR should be immediately resumed for 2 minutes following defibrillation shocks, even if the rhythm appears to have changed, before stopping to study the ECG tracing. Potentially reversible causes of cardiac arrest include hypovolemia, hypoxia, myocardial ischemia, metabolic abnormalities, overdoses, tension pneumothorax, and pulmonary embolism. These causes need to be ruled out or treated if they are suspected to have caused the SCA. For asystole or severe bradycardia, pacing wires should be utilized when available prior to initiating chest compressions (Yazdchi & Rawn, 2015).

Ventricular fibrillation (VF) is the most common cause of SCA, particularly during the postoperative period. Pulseless ventricular tachycardia is also a dangerous phenomenon. In the event of either of these dysrhythmias, prompt defibrillation is key to increase the chance of successful resuscitation. The most important factors contributing to survival following SCA are prompt defibrillation and immediate, high-quality, and uninterrupted chest compression. Additionally, use of epinephrine should be limited and not follow standard algorithms in the resuscitation of cardiac surgery patients because of the potential for hypertension leading to suture line disruption and hemorrhage (Yazdchi & Rawn, 2015). In some instances, cardiac massage or internal defibrillation may be warranted to restore heart function.

In Chapter 13, advanced cardiac life support (ACLS) guidelines coupled with emergent resternotomy practices were discussed in detail for cardiac surgical patients. Emergent resternotomy may be required for 0.8% to 2.7% of all patients undergoing cardiac surgery (Dunning et al., 2017). Emergent resternotomy outside of the ICU is associated with poor survival, although patients occasionally survive. While emergent resternotomy may be less effective outside of the ICU, defibrillation, pacing strategies, and epinephrine recommendations remain appropriate and are preferred if the patient has undergone cardiac surgery. Although the rates of survival may be suboptimal, the Society for Thoracic Surgeons (STS) expert consensus suggests that emergency resternotomy should be an integral part of the cardiac arrest protocol until postoperative day 10. It is the belief of the taskforce that significant adhesions would be unlikely to be present until at least 10 days postoperatively. Additionally, the consensus suggests that local protocols for emergency resternotomy outside of the ICU should be drawn up and rehearsed (Dunning et al., 2017). If emergent resternotomy is performed in the post-ICU setting, staff who are well trained and experienced is optimal.

Effective teamwork is a critical component of effective CPR and resuscitation. Additionally, team leaders need to be identified and closed-loop communication should be utilized. The post-ICU nurse should have knowledge of the patient's medical problems, operative details, and postoperative course to help guide the resuscitation strategies. After successful resuscitation from SCA, the patient should be moved to the ICU for additional monitoring and nursing care.

▶ Pulmonary Complications

Performing cardiac surgery requires either a midline sternotomy or a thoracotomy to gain access to the heart and the surrounding structures. Temporary compromise of respiratory function can occur due to the disruption of the thoracic cage and alterations in diaphragmatic movement in the chest wall. Issues with ventilation and gas exchange are not uncommon after cardiac surgery. Cardiac surgery is associated with a marked reduction in pulmonary function that peaks 24 hours after surgery and gradually improves over the next several weeks (Ginwalla et al., 2014). However, some patients who have undergone cardiac surgery can experience a spectrum of pulmonary complications during the postoperative phase. Patients' comorbidities and risk factors can play a role in the development of pulmonary complications. Patients undergoing cardiac surgery for structural or congenital heart disease who have pulmonary hypertension are at a higher risk for morbidity following cardiac surgery. Additionally, the lungs can become atelectatic during bypass surgery and edema can occur due to fluid shifts and the inflammatory response caused by the bypass circuit (Yazdchi & Rawn, 2017). Impaired pulmonary function after cardiac surgery can result from prolonged ventilations, complications during the intraoperative period, difficultly weaning, or extubation failure. Many of the complications have been treated or managed during the ICU phase; however, post-ICU pulmonary complications can still occur. Cardiac surgery patients are most at risk for atelectasis, pneumothorax, pleural effusions, pneumonia, pulmonary embolism, and pulmonary hypertension during the post-ICU phase. Some therapies such as deep breathing exercises, incentive spirometry, and early mobilization after surgery are risk reduction strategies that can decrease the incidence of pulmonary complications (Smetana, 2017). Patient education regarding lung expansion and other interventions should begin prior to surgery for the best results. Chapter 13 discussed several pulmonary complications in detail; other complications that more commonly occur during the post-ICU phase will be examined in this chapter.

Pleural Effusions

A postoperative pleural effusion, which is a collection of fluid in the pleural space, is common after cardiac surgery. Most effusions develop as a consequence of the surgical procedure and follow a benign course. Pleural effusions of a generally benign nature occur after cardiac transplantation, coronary artery bypass grafting, and less often with mitral and aortic valve replacement surgery. These effusions can arise in the early (≤30 days) or late (>30 days) postoperative period (Heffner, 2017). Postoperative effusions can be caused by hemothorax, pneumonia, pleural infections, mediastinitis, PPS, central line erosion in the pleural space, chylothorax, and fluid overload (Heffner, 2017; Yadzchi & Rawn, 2017). Most postoperative effusions occur on the left side, and encompass an area smaller than two intercostal spaces. They are small to moderate in size, present within 1 to 2 days after surgery, and are not associated with respiratory symptoms. Many of the small effusions resolve over time and may require diuretic therapy. Early effusions may also be seen before the usual onset of PPS, which can develop during the second or third postoperative week. Defining characteristics of PPS include fever, leukocytosis, pericardial rub, elevated erythrocyte sedimentation rate and C-reactive protein, and pulmonary infiltrates (Heffner, 2017). Nonsteroidal anti-inflammatory agents and colchicines can be used to treat PPCS (Yazdchi & Rawn, 2017). Larger or symptomatic pulmonary effusions, particularly in patients with impaired lung function, will result in dyspnea, chest pain or heaviness, and hypoxia, and can be treated with a thoracentesis and analysis of the pleural fluid. It is rare for large effusions to require decortication for repair.

Nursing management in the post-ICU phase for pleural effusions should focus on assessing the breath sounds, respiratory effort, pulse oximetry, and pain levels of the patient. Additionally, the nurse should monitor for any lab value changes, elevations in body temperature, or any other signs that PPCS is occurring. If thoracostomy drainage or chest tubes are required, smaller diameter tubes or blakes are often better tolerated than traditional chest tubes (Yazdchi & Rawn, 2017). It is the nurse's responsibility to assess the color, consistency, amount of drainage, and dressing site. Any abnormalities or increases in the amount of drainage need to be communicated to the health care team.

Pulmonary Hypertension

Pulmonary hypertension (PH) may develop as a result of long-standing valvular heart disease or other causes and is considered chronic PH. Chronic or preexisting PH is commonly caused by left-sided heart failure, aortic stenosis, mitral valve disease, and pulmonary disease (Yazdchi & Rawn, 2017). Over time, the pulmonary artery pressure approaches the systemic blood pressure and patients are at increased risk when cardiac surgery is performed. Pulmonary hypertension is defined as an elevated mean arterial pressure at or above 25 mmHg at rest. It has several etiologies and can be a progressive and fatal disease if left untreated (Rubin & Hopkins, 2017). Patients with PH are at high risk of cardiovascular collapse and death when undergoing anesthesia, mechanical ventilation, and major surgery. With severe PH, the risk of postoperative right ventricular failure and death following surgery is greatly increased; therefore, severe PH in the preoperative phase may be a surgical contraindication. Patients undergoing cardiac surgery for structural or congenital heart disease frequently have PH, which can complicate the postoperative management.

Acute postoperative PH can also develop and must be managed aggressively to avoid right ventricular failure. Acute postoperative PH can be caused by perioperative ischemia or infarction, or by acute increases in peripheral vascular resistance (PVR). Acute increases in PVR are commonly caused by left ventricular dysfunction, mitral valve insufficiency or stenosis, volume overload, pulmonary edema, hypoxia, or acidosis (Yazdchi & Rawn, 2017). Symptoms and signs of PH initially are exertional dyspnea and fatigue. Over time, patients may develop symptoms of severe PH with overt right ventricular failure, which can include exertional chest pain, syncope, ascites, anorexia and/or abdominal pain in the right upper quadrant due to passive hepatic congestion, and peripheral edema (Rubin & Hopkins, 2017). The nursing management of postoperative pulmonary hypertension may include the IV administration of diuretics, milrinone, inhaled nitric oxide, inhaled prostacyclin, and oral sildenafil. By reducing the PVR, the function of the right ventricle should improve, which can result in increased cardiac output and oxygenation (Hopkins & Rubin, 2017). Some of the treatment agents can also reduce systemic vascular resistance (SVR), which can cause systemic hypotension. The balance of managing PH and systemic hypotension can be challenging, often requiring a combination of agents (Yazdchi & Rawn, 2017).

During the post-ICU phase of care, nursing care is centered on the assessment and management of fluid balance, oxygenation, blood pressure, and heart rate. Also, administration of PH-specific medications is paramount.

▶ Hematologic Complications

One of the principle challenges of cardiac surgery is to achieve sufficient anticoagulation while the patient is on the bypass machine, and to prevent excessive bleeding postoperatively. Patients who undergo off-pump CABG experience significantly less bleeding and blood transfusion requirements. Excessive postoperative bleeding can lead to additional complications, including blood transfusions and transfusion-related complications, which can cause an increase in morbidity and mortality.

Postoperative Bleeding

As discussed in Chapter 13, quantitative assessment of postoperative bleeding is critical to document the extent of hemorrhage and the associated patient response while rectifying the situation. Postoperative bleeding is common, with severe bleeding occurring in 3% to 5% of patients who have undergone cardiopulmonary bypass (CPB). Severe bleeding is defined as requiring transfusion of more than 10 units of packed red blood cells. Such extensive bleeding can be caused by the following factors: incomplete surgical hemostasis, residual heparin effect after CPB, clotting factor depletion, hypothermia, postoperative hypotension, hemodilution, and platelet abnormalities (Silvestry, 2017). Chest tube drainage has also commonly been used to define excessive or severe bleeding. A recent expert panel has proposed a more universal definition of perioperative bleeding in adult cardiac surgery. This definition identifies five classes of bleeding ranging from insignificant (class 0) to massive (class 4). The definition is based on several variables such as delayed sternal closure, chest tube output over 12 hours, blood products transfused, and need for surgical reexploration. This classification appears to predict the risk of mortality; however, its application in the clinical setting remains undetermined (Stephens & Whitman, 2015).

Recent guidelines have highlighted the risks associated with blood transfusion and advocate for restrictive transfusion protocols. The Society for Thoracic Surgery (STS) guidelines recommend transfusion for patients who have bled more than 30% of their blood volume or who are bleeding uncontrollably. In stable postoperative patients, it is recommended that transfusion only be considered if the hemoglobin falls below 7 g/dL or hematocrit below 21% (Yazdchi & Rawn, 2017).

During the post-ICU phase, the potential for postoperative bleeding still exists. Cardiac surgery patients are at risk for cardiac tamponade, anastomotic leak, and are still vulnerable to postoperative anemia. The nurse needs to follow the blood volume lab values, hemoglobin, and hematocrit to be able to ascertain if a descent occurs. In the event that the blood values have a precipitous decline, a blood transfusion may be warranted to maintain clinical stability.

▶ Transfusion-Related Complications

Cardiac surgery is a common procedure that requires large numbers of red blood cells (RBCs). It is estimated that approximately 20% of the total blood supply is consumed by patients undergoing cardiac surgery. Blood transfusions are necessary for the correction of anemia and bleeding disorders, even though they can be associated with higher morbidity and mortality. Blood transfusion is the most commonly performed hospital procedure, with more than 19 million transfusions administered in the United States during 2013 (Henneman et al., 2017). During cardiac surgery due to hemostatic abnormalities, intraoperative and postoperative bleeding are commonly seen, which can result in postoperative anemia (Bilgin & Van de Watering, 2013). Although a blood transfusion is typically a safe procedure, the potential for transfusion-associated adverse events (TAAEs) does exist. A common misperception is that the most frequently encountered TAAE is a hemolytic reaction in a patient who receives incompatible blood. However, the incidence of other adverse events and complications that may cause a transfusion-related fatality is higher. Transfusions can be associated with an increased risk of pneumonia, bacteremia, sternal wound infection, and *Clostridium difficile* after cardiac surgery (Stephens & Whitman, 2015). A number of complications that can occur as a result of a transfusion and cause TAAEs are transfusion-associated circulatory overload (TACO) and posttransfusion purpura. Additionally, transfusion-related acute lung injury (TRALI) can also occur posttransfusion and was discussed in detail in Chapter 13.

Transfusion-Associated Circulatory Overload

Transfusion-associated circulatory overload refers to pulmonary edema after the transfusion of blood products. It is a form of circulatory volume overload that can occur with transfusion of any blood component (e.g., RBCs, platelets, fresh frozen plasma [FFP] or other plasma product, cryoprecipitate). The risk factors for developing TACO are outlined in **BOX 20.4**. TACO is a potentially life-threatening complication of hemotherapy, accounting for up to 24% of transfusion-associated patient fatalities. In addition to increased mortality, TACO is associated with increased morbidity, increased length of stay, and increased hospital costs (Henneman et al., 2017). Transfusion-associated circulatory overload should be considered in any patient who has respiratory distress or hypertension during or within 6 hours of completing a transfusion, especially in individuals with underlying cardiac disease and who have a positive fluid balance.

BOX 20.4 Risk Factors for the Development of TACO

Age (<3 years, >60 years)
Female sex
Underlying cardiac, renal, or pulmonary conditions (HF, COPD)
Small stature
Low body weight
Hypoalbuminemia
Faster rate of infusion
Vasopressors (recent)
Positive fluid balance
History or hemodialysis
Number of units transfused

COPD, chronic obstructive pulmonary disease; HF, heart failure; TACO, transfusion-associated circulatory overload.
Data from Silvergleid, A. J., Kleinman, S. & Tirnauer, J. S., 2017; Henneman et al., 2017.

The clinical manifestations of a patient with TACO are similar to respiratory distress. The patient may experience dyspnea or orthopnea and the severity is variable, from mild dyspnea to acute respiratory decompensation. Patients may have a cough, crackles and/or wheezing on auscultation, tachycardia, elevated blood pressure, decreased oxygen saturation, tachypnea, increased jugular venous distention (JVD), and S3 heart sound on auscultation. Headache is common and seizures have been reported in some cases. Symptoms typically occur after a significant portion of the blood products or multiple units have been infused, up to approximately 6 hours following the completion of an infusion (Silvergleid, Kleinman, & Tirnauer, 2017). Clinical findings typically present during the transfusion or between 2 and 6 hours afterward; however, cases have been reported as late as 24 hours posttransfusion (Henneman et al., 2017). Transfusion-associated circulatory overload is not known to cause fever, hives, or angioedema, so patients with these symptoms should be evaluated for other TAAEs.

Chest radiography (CXR) may be helpful in determining the diagnosis of TACO. It should be obtained to confirm pulmonary edema and rule out any other causes of respiratory distress (e.g., pneumothorax). The typical finding on CXR of TACO includes pulmonary edema and in some cases cardiomegaly. Echocardiography is not routinely done to diagnose TACO. If TACO is suspected, treatment should not be delayed while waiting on the CXR results. An exception is when it is unclear whether the patient is experiencing TACO versus TRALI, since the administration of diuretics, which is critical to the management of TACO, may be harmful in a patient with TRALI (Silvergleid et al., 2017). The differences in TRALI and TACO are outlined in **TABLE 20.1**.

Nurses are the key providers responsible for the recognition that TACO may be occurring. They must be knowledgeable and aware of the signs and symptoms and respond appropriately. TAAEs, including TACO, TRALI, and hemolytic reactions due to mismatched blood types, may present similarly in a clinical setting. As a result, all potential transfusion-associated adverse events must be managed initially in the same manner,

TABLE 20.1 TACO versus TRALI

Symptoms	TRALI	TACO
Onset of symptoms	Less than 6 hours	Mainly less than 6 hours
Respiratory symptoms	Dyspnea	Dyspnea
Fluid balance	Positive or negative	Positive
Chest x-ray	Bilateral infiltrates	Bilateral infiltrates with signs of fluid overload
Echocardiography	Normal EF	Decreased EF
B-type natriuretic peptide	Low or normal	Elevated

EF, ejection fraction; TACO, transfusion-associated circulatory overload; TRALI, transfusion-related acute lung injury.
Data from Silvergleid, A. J., Kleinman, S. & Tirnauer, J. S., 2017.

which consists of immediately stopping the infusion and notifying the provider and blood bank. The nurse must do further assessments by auscultating the lungs, checking for signs of JVD, and checking the vital signs. Nurses in the post-ICU unit are oftentimes aware of the potential complications due to transfusions, and have protocols and procedures in place to check on the patients frequently. Ideally, the nurse should assess for any risks for TACO prior to beginning the transfusion and monitor, assess, and document vital signs and patient presentation. Additionally, avoidance of multiple unit transfusions and the administration of split units to high-risk patients should minimize and mitigate the risk of TACO occurring. In the event that TACO is confirmed, the nurse should anticipate the administration of diuretics, supplemental oxygen, and elevating the head of the bed to position the patient upright to assist with any respiratory compliance.

▶ Venous Thromboembolism (Deep Vein Thrombosis and Pulmonary Embolism)

Venous thromboembolism (VTE), encompassing both deep vein thrombosis (DVT) and pulmonary embolism (PE), is the third leading cause of cardiovascular death. The incidence and the significance of VTE in cardiac surgery patients have not been well defined or thoroughly studied (Mufti, Baskett, Arora, & Légaré, 2015). The incidences of DVT and PE following cardiac surgery appear to be lower than those for other major surgical procedures due to the fact that heparin is utilized during the operation. Additionally, impaired platelet function post-CPB, increased use of antiplatelet agents and anticoagulants, and early ambulation may reduce the incidence of clot formation. The reported incidence of PE ranges from 0.5% to 3.5%, accounting for only 0.3% to 1.7% of perioperative deaths (Yazdchi & Rawn, 2017). Cardiac patients have multiple VTE risk factors such as immobility, prolonged preoperative hospitalization, obesity, and prothrombotic conditions such as heparin-induced thrombocytopenia (HIT) and other complicating factors. However, it is not clear that routine thromboprophylaxis is indicated in the cardiac surgical population. The practice of VTE prophylaxis after cardiac surgery is controversial. According to the European Association for Cardiothoracic Surgery (EACTS) guidelines, prophylactic anticoagulation for VTE should be commenced from the first postoperative day. However, an increased risk of bleeding and cardiac tamponade resulting from pharmacologic thromboprophylaxis remains a major concern for patients who have undergone

cardiac surgery. The American College of Chest Physicians clinical practice guidelines have also stressed that patients after cardiac surgery are at high risk of major bleeding complications with only moderate risk for VTE and suggest that pharmacologic VTE prophylaxis is only needed for those with prolonged hospitalization post-surgery (Ho, Bham, & Pavey, 2015). These recommendations were based on consensus among experts and weak evidence. More recent evidence suggests that a prothrombotic state (any agent or condition that leads to thrombosis) is common after cardiac surgery from postoperative day 1, reaches a peak prothrombotic state between days 3 and 5 after surgery, and can last up to 30 days postoperatively. Therefore, patients after cardiac surgery are not necessarily protected from VTE from day 1 postoperatively, despite their tendency for bleeding during the immediate postoperative period. The topic remains contentious on whether the benefits of VTE prophylaxis would outweigh its possible harm in patients after cardiac surgery.

Pulmonary embolism is a form of VTE that can be common postoperatively and sometimes fatal. The presentation can be variable and sometimes nonspecific, making the diagnosis challenging. PE refers to obstruction of the pulmonary artery or one of its branches by material (e.g., thrombus, air, tumor, or fat). The overall incidence is approximately 112 cases per 100,000 and is slightly more common in males than females (Thompson & Kabrhel, 2017). The clinical symptoms of PE may be sudden hemodynamic collapse due to a large embolus, or the gradual development of dyspnea and chest pain due to smaller emboli. Typically, the patient suffers respiratory distress with increased work of breathing, anxiety, chest pain, cough, sense of impending doom, and decreased oxygen saturations. The patient may also experience some leg swelling and warmth particularly if a DVT is present and has broken off and caused the embolus. The pathogenesis of PE is similar to that of DVT. Most emboli arise from lower extremity proximal veins; however, they can also originate in the upper extremity veins, right heart, inferior venal cava, and pelvic veins (Thompson & Kabrhel, 2017). Initial resuscitative efforts for patients with suspected PE should focus on oxygenation and stabilization. The therapeutic treatment of choice is systemic anticoagulation and the risk and benefits of bleeding are weighed objectively by the provider.

Deep vein thrombosis can occur in superficial or deep veins of the lower and upper extremities. The thrombi can form in the proximal or distal veins. Patients may experience warmth, tenderness, and swelling of the affected extremity. Doppler ultrasonography is the diagnostic tool utilized to confirm DVT. Anticoagulation is the mainstay of therapy for patients with acute lower extremity DVT. Intravenous unfractionated heparin is initially utilized with a transition to warfarin for at least 3 months. Patients with recurrent DVTs or PEs, despite anticoagulation, may be candidates for the placement of an inferior vena caval filter (Lipp & Hull, 2017).

During the post-ICU phase of care, the nurse must ensure that the patient has some form of VTE prophylaxis. Due to the controversy for the administration of pharmacologic prophylaxis, many institutions utilize mechanical prophylaxis such as alternating leg pressure devices (ALPs) or sequential compression devices to prevent the stasis of blood and to maintain adequate blood flow. For patients in whom mechanical prophylaxis is contraindicated, pharmacologic prophylaxis with LMWH (e.g., enoxaparin [Lovenox®]) may be utilized. Nursing actions include assessing the patient for any respiratory alterations, assessing for signs of DVT development, and educating and encouraging the patient to ambulate as tolerated.

▸ Gastrointestinal Complications

Gastrointestinal (GI) complications occur in approximately 1% to 4% of patients undergoing cardiac surgery. They are often insidious in onset, difficult to detect, and severe in their consequences. Additionally, the presentation may differ from the complication in a noncardiac surgery patient. One likely cause of these GI complications

is hypoperfusion during surgery or the early postoperative phase. **BOX 20.5** lists a number of risk factors that place patients at risk for the development of GI complications (Schwartz, Lindsey, Khabiri, & Stawicki, 2013). The most common complication is upper GI bleeding, usually from duodenal or gastric ulceration. The incidence of GI bleeding and stress ulcer formation can be reduced with the administration of H2 inhibitors, proton pump inhibitors, and sucralfate. All patients undergoing cardiac surgery should receive stress ulcer prophylaxis. Additionally, postoperative ileus is a GI complication following cardiac surgery (Yazdchi & Rawn, 2017).

BOX 20.5 Risk Factors for Postoperative Gastrointestinal Complications

Older age
Decreased LVEF (<40%)
Postoperative low cardiac output
DM
Renal failure
PVD
Valvular surgery or combined CABG/valve operation
Prolonged mechanical ventilation
Emergent surgery
Prolong CPB time
Need for IABP
Vasopressors during or after surgery
Need for reexploration following surgery (resternotomy)
Preexisting gastric ulcer disease
Stroke
Postoperative sepsis/infections, complications (including sternal wound infections)
Open surgery versus minimally invasive
Intraoperative and postoperative bleeding
Opioid usage

CABG, coronary artery bypass graft; CPB, cardiopulmonary bypass; DM, diabetes mellitus; IABP, intra-aortic balloon pump; LVEF, left ventricular ejection fraction; PVD, peripheral vascular disease.
Data from Schwartz, Lindsey, Khabiri & Stawicki, 2013: Kalff, Wehner & Litkouhi, 2017)

Postoperative Intestinal Ileus

Failure of the intestinal contents to progress normally through the GI tract is not uncommon following major surgery. To some extent, intestinal ileus is present in all patients following cardiac surgery; however, when prolonged it will increase the length of stay and may lead to other complications. The incidence of ileus in cardiothoracic patients is between 1% and 2%. It can manifest itself in a number of forms, from isolated gastric distension to prolonged bowel dysfunction. The development of a new ileus with severe abdominal pain may indicate a more clinically significant problem such as mesenteric ischemia or pancreatitis (Schwatz et al., 2013; Yazdchi & Rawn, 2017). Symptoms of a postoperative ileus (POI) may include nausea, vomiting, inability to tolerate enteral food and fluids, constipation, and abdominal distention. After surgery, motility returns to the small intestine within 24 hours, followed by the return of gastric motility within 24 to 48 hours, and motility to the colon returns at 48 to 72 hours (Katrancha & George, 2014; McCutcheson, 2013). In a small number of patients, the ileus persists past the fourth postoperative day, requiring the use of suppositories, enemas, and promotility agents such as metoclopramide (Reglan®). Additionally, the avoidance of narcotics and the possible placement of a nasogastric suction tube may be warranted.

The nursing management of GI complications in the post-ICU or intermediate care unit includes the nurse carefully assessing for bowel sounds, diet tolerance, passage of flatus, complaints of nausea/vomiting or abdominal pain, and observation of the color of stool if the patient has a bowel movement. In the event the nurse suspects a POI, in addition to bowel sounds, the nurse should assess for distention. An abdominal radiograph or plain abdominal films are often the diagnostic evaluation ordered to determine if an ileus exists. The plain abdominal radiographs may show dilated loops of bowel but should demonstrate air in the colon and rectum without a transitions zone to suggest bowel obstruction (Kalff et al., 2017).

▶ Hospital-Acquired Infections

Of cardiac surgery patients, 10% to 20% develop a nosocomial infection (Yazdchi & Rawn, 2017). A hospital-acquired infection can be due to iatrogenic therapy and interventions done while the patient is hospitalized. Infections can occur related to the surgical site, invasive central venous catheter, intubation, and the use of an indwelling catheter. Catheter-associated urinary tract infections (CAUTIs), sternal wound infections, and hospital-acquired pneumonia related to intubation are complications that can be seen during the post-ICU phase of care. Hospital-acquired pneumonia was discussed in detail in Chapter 13.

Catheter-Associated Urinary Tract Infections

Urinary tract infections (UTIs) associated with urinary catheters are the leading cause of secondary health care–associated bacteremia. Approximately 20% of hospital-acquired bacteremias arise from the urinary tract, and the mortality associated with this condition is about 10% (Fekete, Calderwood, & Bloom, 2017). Catheter-associated urinary tract infection can be defined as either symptomatic bacteriuria or asymptomatic bacteriuria, with the distinguishing difference being the presence of symptoms, including fever, costovertebral angle tenderness, altered mental status, hypotension, or evidence of a systemic inflammatory response syndrome. A CAUTI may be extralumial or intraluminal. Extraluminal infection occurs via entry of bacteria into the bladder along the biofilm that forms around the catheter in the urethra. Intraluminal infection occurs due to urinary stasis because of drainage failure or due to contamination of the urine collection bag with subsequent ascending infection. Extraluminal CAUTIs are more common, occurring 66% versus 34% in one study (Fekete et al., 2017). Patients who have cardiac surgery have an indwelling catheter inserted perioperatively to keep up with the urinary output intra- and postoperatively. The indwelling catheters are necessary for the interdisciplinary team to manage the fluid status and functionality of the kidneys postoperatively. The risk factors for cardiac surgery patients developing a CAUTI are outlined in **BOX 20.6**.

Symptoms of CAUTI include fever, flank or suprapubic discomfort, costovertebral angle tenderness, leukocytosis, hypotension, and catheter obstruction. Nonspecific findings include new-onset delirium or other systemic manifestations that suggest an infection. Patients who develop a CAUTI soon after removal of a catheter may be more likely to have the typical urinary symptoms of dysuria, frequency, and urgency. Diagnosis is generally made based on symptoms and by obtaining a urine culture. The treatment approach of CAUTI includes antimicrobial therapy and catheter management. Antimicrobial selection should be based upon the culture results when available. Depending on the clinical response, the infecting organism, and the agent used for treatment, 7 to 14 days of therapy is generally appropriate. If the organism is susceptible and the patient is well enough to take oral medication with adequate absorption, oral therapy can be used for some or all of the treatment course (Fekete et al., 2017).

A component of the post-ICU care of the cardiac surgery patient is ensuring the early removal of the indwelling catheter. Many institutions have adopted the standard of removing the indwelling catheter 48 hours or by postoperative day 2, unless specific indications for continued catheter presence are warranted. Additionally, some institutions have nurse-driven protocols, which help the nurse to autonomously decide if the urinary catheter can be removed. If the urinary catheter is still indicated and in place when the patient is transferred out of the ICU, the nurse should advocate for the catheter removal as soon as possible to prevent the development of a CAUTI. If the indications are not met for removal, the nurse should implement the CAUTI bundle interventions to help decrease and prevent the development of a CAUTI. Components of the bundle include keeping the catheter bag below the bladder, securing the catheter to the leg with a securement device, emptying the catheter bag frequently to ensure that it doesn't get too full, and not contaminating the catheter outlet valve during urine collection bag emptying. Additional information on insertion guidelines, indications for use, and other CAUTI prevention and bundle strategies can be found at www.cdc.gov and www.ahrq.gov.

BOX 20.6 Risk Factors for Cardiac Surgery Patients Developing CAUTI

Older age
Female gender
DM
Cardiogenic shock
Urgent or emergent operation
PRBC units transfused
Presence of DSWI
Increased ICU LOS
Bacterial colonization of the drainage bag
Errors in catheter care (nonsterile insertion
    technique, break in the closed drainage
    system)
Duration of catherization

CAUTI, catheter-associated urinary tract infection; DM, diabetes mellitus; DSWI, deep sternal wound infection; ICU, intensive care unit; LOS, length of stay; PRBC, packed red blood cells.
Data from Gillen, Isbell, Michaels, Lau & Sawyer, 2015; Fekete, Calderwood & Bloom, 2017

Sternal Complications and Mediastinitis

Postoperative wound complications and infections in cardiac surgery are complex and multifactorial. Preoperative interventions such as clipping chest hair, utilizing chlorhexidine gluconate (CHG) wipes, administering adequate prophylactic antibiotics prior to skin incision, ensuring good intraoperative hemostasis, and adequately closing with sutures and topical adhesive (Dermabond©) versus staples can reduce the incidence of wound complications in cardiac surgery (Yazdchi & Rawn, 2017). Moreover, early detection and treatment of sternal wound breakdown or sternal instability may prevent subsequent complications such as infection or nonunion. Sternal wound complications can be limited to the superficial tissues or extend deeply through all the layers of closure. Soft tissue dehiscence refers to the separation of the superficial tissues such as the skin, subcutaneous fat, and muscle layers. The sternum is stable to palpate and the soft tissue dehiscence is considered a minor complication. Sternal dehiscence refers to the separation of the edges of the sternum from one another and can be caused by wire fracture loosening or pulling through the sternal edge. Patients may complain of painful chest motion and clicking. This is considered a surgical emergency, since patients with sternal dehiscence have an increased risk of ventricular rupture due to sharp wires or bone fragments rubbing against the heart. When sternal dehiscence occurs during the postoperative phase, the patient is taken back to the operating room for reexploration (Orgill, 2017). Deep sternal wound infection (DSWI), also known as mediastinitis, is a postoperative sternal wound complication that can also occur. The incidence of postoperative mediastinitis ranges from 0.4% to 5%, with the incidence in most centers being between 1% and 2% (Sexton, 2017). Coronary artery bypass grafting and other surgical procedures involving the median sternotomy carry the risk of sternal wound complications that can lead to increased morbidity, reduced quality of life, prolonged or repeated hospitalizations, increased health care costs, and, for serious cases, mortality rates of 15% to 40% (Adams et al., 2016). Furthermore, sternal wound complications and infections occur late, 1 to 2 weeks past surgery and sometimes after discharge (Ginwalla et al., 2014). There are numerous risk factors that can lead to the development of postoperative mediastinitis (**BOX 20.7**). Postoperative mediastinitis can occur from preoperative, intraoperative, and postoperative contamination and disruption. Preoperative skin colonization with potentially pathogenic or highly resistant organisms, interruption of the blood supply to the sternum during surgery, tissue trauma due to electrocautery, intraoperative wound contamination, and postoperative wound disruption due to coughing can contribute to the development of mediastinitis (Sexton, 2017). The majority of patients with

---

BOX 20.7 Risk Factors for Postoperative Mediastinitis

COPD
Renal dysfunction
DM or perioperative hyperglycemia
Blood transfusions
Immunosuppression
Malnutrition and low serum albumin
Osteopenia
Obesity
Peripheral artery disease
Tobacco use
Preoperative chest deformities (pectus excavatum, barrel chest)
Prior cardiac surgery/resternotomy
Macromastia (enlarged breasts)
Presence of multiple drains and thoracostomy tubes (portals for entry of bacteria)
Mobilization of the internal mammary arteries
Prolonged surgical procedure (>5 hours)
Prolonged postoperative intensive care
Return to the OR within 4 days postoperatively (e.g., to control bleeding)

COPD, chronic obstructive pulmonary disease; DM, diabetes mellitus; OR, operating room.
Data from Ginwalla, Faraday & Whitman, 2014; Sexton, 2017; Orgill, 2017

---

postoperative mediastinitis have monomicrobial infections that can be caused by virtually any organism. The most common organisms causing mediastinitis are methicillin-susceptible *Staphylococcus aureus* (MSSA) (45%), methicillin-resistant *S. aureus* (MRSA) (16%), gram-negative bacilli (17%), coagulase-negative staphylococci (13%), and streptococci (5%). Postoperative mediastinitis due to MSSA appears to occur more often in the setting of preoperative nasal MSSA colonization, whereas MRSA appears to happen more often due to nosocomial transmission between patients (Sexton, 2017). Signs and symptoms of mediastinitis include fever, tachycardia, chest pain, sternal instability, redness, and purulent drainage from the mediastinum. The chest pain is typically out of proportion to what should be experienced so many days out from surgery in the post-ICU setting. Patients may also experience some edema and crepitus of the chest wall. Laboratory and diagnostic findings may also show leukocytosis, mediastinal widening, or air on radiologic tests. Computed tomography (CT) is better than plain radiography films in diagnosis with the two hallmark features of mediastinitis being localized mediastinal fluid and pneumomediastinum. Additionally, bacteremia or systemic infection is common and occurs in 57% of patients with postoperative mediastinitis (Sexton, 2017). Bacteremia with positive blood cultures may be the first sign of mediastinitis and should be evaluated carefully in patients following cardiac surgery. In recent years, there has been an increased focus on the prevention of hospital-acquired conditions, including mediastinitis. Restrictions on the reimbursement of medical expenses, particularly in the last years, have magnified the importance of preventing postsurgical complications. In October 2008, the Centers for Medicare Services (CMS) in the United States implemented a policy that eliminated reimbursement for mediastinitis following coronary artery bypass surgery (Gorlitzer et al., 2013; Sexton, 2017).

The treatment of mediastinitis requires a combination of surgical debridement and antimicrobial therapy. Due to the variability of the presentation and clinical course, there are no consensus guidelines for the surgical treatment of mediastinitis. Effective therapy requires immediate and aggressive wound debridement with placement of vascularized tissue, muscle, and even omentum, in the anterior mediastinal space (Ginwalla et al., 2014).

The debridement of nonviable tissue is essential and indicated in the presence of necrotic tissue or purulent drainage. The endpoint of sternal debridement is the clinical appearance of well-vascularized healthy bone. After debridement, the sternum can be rewired or plated if adequate bone stock is present and infection is absent. Flap closure is reserved for patients who have an inadequate amount of bone after debridement or if the infectious process is not under control. After debridement, the sternum can be closed immediately or following an interval of open wound management. For those patients who are not candidates for immediate primary sternal or flap

closure, the open sternum can be managed with conventional moist gauze dressings or alternatively using negative-pressure wound therapy, also known as vacuum-assisted closure (VAC) therapy, while awaiting delayed closure. VAC therapy stabilizes the chest wall, removes excess fluid, and facilitates wound healing. Although VAC therapy is associated with decreased times to delayed closure and a reduction in patient mortality, a small number of deaths have been reported in association with this therapy, primarily due to cardiac rupture (Ginwalla et al., 2014; Orgill, 2017). The nurse must be sure to provide a barrier dressing between the gauze or foam and the heart to minimize the delivery of excessive negative pressure directly to the heart muscle. The exploration, debridement, and closure of the sternal wound should be performed in the operating room as a collaborative effort between the cardiac and plastic surgery services.

Additionally, appropriate and prolonged antibiotics are required. The selection of antimicrobial therapy should be based on deep sternal drainage, blood, and mediastinal wound cultures obtained at the time of mediastinal exploration or when the mediastinitis is suspected. Deeper postoperative mediastinitis can require intravenous antibiotics for 6 weeks.

During the post-ICU phase of care, the nurse should focus on assessing the sternal wound frequently for any alterations or signs and symptoms of infection. This includes proper cleaning of the sternal wound. Some organizations utilize CHG wipes daily to assist with decreasing the incidence of colonization of the sternal wound before and after cardiac surgery. Effective glycemic control is also needed in the post-ICU phase. Research has shown that successful glucose control for at least 3 days postoperatively is associated with a significantly lower sternal wound infection rate (Yazdchi & Rawn, 2017). The typical incubation time for postoperative mediastinitis is within 14 days of surgery; however, the onset may be delayed for months. It is imperative that the post-ICU nurse educate patients and families about the signs and symptoms of postoperative mediastinitis and what to do if it occurs. Teaching should center on the normal progression and appearance of wound healing and the recognition of infection. Additionally, patients should be taught how to properly protect the sternum prior to discharge using sternal precaution techniques. Sternal precautions include weight restrictions, not pushing up when rising from sitting to standing, and performing only pain-free bilateral arm movements (Adams et al., 2016). For patients with macromastia (enlarged breasts), a support bra or sternal stabilizing device may be utilized to prevent postoperative mediastinitis.

▶ Neurologic Complications

Neurologic complications have been a major concern throughout the history of cardiac surgery. Technological advances and techniques have led to minimally invasive and endovascular therapies to repair vascular, valvular, and myocardial alterations. Despite these advances in therapy, neurologic complications such as stroke, delirium, and cognitive decline still frequently occur. The incidence of postoperative neurologic sequelae after CABG surgery is approximately 2% to 6%, with the frequency increasing among older patients (Silvestry, 2017). Neurologic complications can range from stroke, to transient ischemic attacks (TIAs), to encephalopathy, seizures, delirium, and postoperative cognitive dysfunction. Delirium, postoperative cognitive dysfunction, and seizures are complications that can occur during the post-ICU phase of care. Chapters 13 and 16 explored the complications related to stroke and other neurologic dysfunctions.

Delirium

Postoperative delirium is a common neurologic complication following cardiac surgery. Delirium is defined as an acute confusional state characterized by an alteration of consciousness with reduced ability to focus, sustain, or shift attention. It can develop over a short period of time and tends to fluctuate throughout the course of the day. Delirium occurs in 3% to 32% of cardiac surgery patients, particularly those with preexisting organic mental disorders such as stroke, dementia, prior alcohol consumption, advanced age, or intracranial cerebral artery disease (O'Neal & Shaw, 2016). The incidence of delirium increases if the patient is intubated or is of advanced age. There are 3 subtypes of delirium that can occur anytime during the postoperative period: hypoactive, hyperactive, and mixed. Patients with hyperactive delirium may be agitated, combative, and have loud behavior; hypoactive patients are withdrawn and display quiet behavior. The most common type of delirium is hypoactive; it is often misdiagnosed or undetected by health care professions.

Delirium is associated with many negative consequences, such as an increase in the length of stay, increased risk to fall, prolonged mechanical ventilation, reduced cognitive and functional recovery, and an increase in morbidity and mortality. Delirium is a complex phenomenon that is multifactorial in nature, which makes the exact etiology and pathophysiology hard to detect. Several precipitating and predisposing risk factors contribute to the development of delirium. Precipitating risk factors are triggers that cause delirium, and predisposing risk factors are baseline conditions that increase the risk of delirium. These are summarized in **TABLE 20.2**.

There are many proposed pathophysiologic mechanisms for delirium, including neurotransmitter dysfunction, inflammatory response with an increase of inflammatory markers such as chemokines and interleukin-6, blood-brain barrier disruption, and decreased cholinergic activity. It has also been theorized that the release of stress hormones (cortisol) during the intraoperative period for cardiac surgery is a contributing factor (Francis, 2017). There are many risk factors for the development of delirium that commonly occur in cardiac surgery patients, including fever, sepsis, pressor requirements, and the use of medications such as benzodiazepines, opiates, and anticholinergics. Mechanically ventilated patients appear to be at especially high risk for developing delirium during and after their ICU stay. Given the range of risk factors, symptoms, and subtypes, the diagnosis and recognition of delirium may

TABLE 20.2 Risk Factors Contributing to the Development of Delirium After Cardiac Surgery

Predisposing Risk Factors	Precipitating Risk Factors
Age over 65 years Male Dementia/cognitive impairment History of stroke History of alcohol or substance abuse Diabetes mellitus Atrial fibrillation Depression Functional impairment Malnutrition Sensory impairment (visual and hearing) Severe illness Fracture of trauma Urgent need for operation	Medications administered during the perioperative period (fentanyl and propofol) Duration of surgery Hypoxia Prolonged intubation Hematocrit levels of lower than 30% Surgery type Red blood cell transfusion Elevation of inflammatory markers (chemokines and interleukin-6) and plasma cortisol levels Infection/fever, pneumonia, central venous catheter infection, sepsis, or CAUTI Cardiogenic shock Dehydration Use of indwelling catheter and fecal retention Metabolic/electrolyte imbalances LCOS Sedation/narcotics: opioids, benzodiazepines, corticosteroids, anticholinergics, diuretics, and general anesthetics Polypharmacy and the treatment with multiple drugs Decreased mobility Disruption of the sleep–wake cycle No visitors Use of physical restraints Pain/anxiety

CAUTI, catheter-associated urinary tract infection; LCOS, low cardiac output syndrome.

Data from Francis, 2017; Jannati, Bagheri, Sohrabi, Cherati & Mazdarani, 2014; O'Neal & Shaw, 2016; Norkienė, Ringaitienė, Kuzminskaitė & Šipylaitė, 2013

be difficult and underrecognized by health care professionals (Francis, 2017; Mangusan, Hooper, Denslow, & Travis, 2015; O'Neal & Shaw, 2016).

The recognition of delirium can be ascertained by utilizing various screening tools. During the post-ICU phase, the Confusion Assessment Method (CAM), Nursing Delirium Screening Tool (NUDESC), Delirium Observation Screening Scale (DOSS), and NEECHAM Confusion Scale can be utilized in the general unit setting to screen and asses for delirium (Poikajärvi, Salanterä, Katajisto, & Junttila, 2017). CAM is the most commonly used validated instrument by clinicians to detect delirium. The CAM and CAM-ICU have gained widespread recognition in everyday

clinical practice and was developed to assist in the detection of delirium by non-psychiatrists. The CAM has a sensitivity of approximately 94% to 100%, and has a specificity of approximately 90% to 95% (McDonagh et al., 2014; Smulter, Lingehall, Gustafson, Olofsson, & Engström, 2015). The optimum goal is to recognize the risk factors, screen appropriately, and prevent patients from developing delirium. With early recognition and implementing nonpharmacologic and pharmacologic interventions, the incidence and occurrence of delirium can be reduced. Some nonpharmacologic interventions include family presence, normalizing the sleep–wake cycle, early mobilization, music therapy, reorientation, utilizing visual and hearing aids, validation therapy, physical and occupational therapy, and restraint reduction (Francis, 2017; O'Neal & Shaw, 2016). When non-pharmacologic interventions are ineffective, pharmacologic therapy may be needed. Haloperidol is the traditional agent for the pharmacologic treatment of delirium; second-generation antipsychotics (quetiapine, risperidone, ziprasidone, and olanzapine) have been used as an alternative treatment. The newer atypical antipsychotic agents have fewer side effects and appear to have similar efficacy to haloperidol (Francis, 2017). Other agents such as lorazepam may also be administered separate or concomitantly to achieve desired effects. In the ICU setting, dexmedetomidine is often utilized as a pharmacologic therapy. Dexmedetomidine is a selective alpha-2 adrenergic receptor agonist that has sedative, analgesic, and opioid-sparing effects. Generally, patients receiving dexmedetomidine are able to cooperate with nursing as they are easily awakened. It has been shown to be as effective as propofol or midazolam for light sedation during prolonged mechanical ventilation with possible advantages of shorter time to extubation and a possible decrease in delirium when compared to propofol (McLauglin & Marik, 2016).

During the post-ICU phase, the nurse should assess the patient for the onset of delirium every shift using a validated tool (NEECHAM, NUDESC, or CAM), and should include nursing interventions to prevent delirium development. If delirium is screened and diagnosed, the focus should be on preventing the patient from self-harm and implementing nonpharmacologic and pharmacologic strategies if necessary until the episode resolves. The patient should be provided a quiet environment and, if appropriate, given his or her eyeglasses and hearing aids. Catheters should be removed as soon as possible. Nursing efforts should be made to restore the patient's normal sleep cycle. For hyperactive patients, a sitter may be necessary to closely watch the patient. If acute agitation is assessed, haloperidol may be required. Haloperidol has the potential to prolong the QT interval and should be used with care in patients who are receiving antiarrhythmics or other drugs that may potentiate this problem. If necessary, properly applied physical restraints with appropriate documentation of the need for their use may be required. The Society of Critical Care Medicine (SCCM) has also published recommendations for practice related to the ABCDEF bundle. The newly-published pain agitation/sedation, delirium, immobility, and sleep disturbances guidelines are available online. The websites can be found in the Web Resources section at the end of this chapter.

Postoperative Cognitive Dysfunction

Postoperative cognitive dysfunction (POCD) is linked to delirium and is frequently mistaken to be delirium. POCD and delirium are two primary forms of postoperative central nervous system dysfunction. POCD is a subtle disorder of thought processes, which may influence isolated domains of cognition such as verbal memory, visual memory, language comprehension, executive function, and the speed of processing information. It is to be distinguished from postoperative delirium, which tends to be transient and a fluctuating disturbance that occurs shortly after surgery (Morimoto, 2016). Postoperative cognitive dysfunction has been associated with longer hospital stays and increased mortality. Hypoperfusion, emboli, hyperthermia, edema, and inflammation related to the use of cardiopulmonary bypass have been associated with the mechanisms of POCD. The incidence of POCD is higher in patients undergoing cardiac surgery. The high incidence of POCD in cardiac surgery patients has been attributed to microembolic events during the use of CPB. The microembolic events may cause focal cerebral infarcts leading to postoperative cognitive impairment. Additionally, there does not appear to be a reduced incidence of cognitive dysfunction with on-pump CABG surgery versus off-pump CABG (Morimoto, 2017). Postoperative cognitive dysfunction can be subclassified into short-term and long-term. Short-term POCD is usually transitory and is defined as cognitive decline lasting up to 6 weeks postoperatively. This occurs in 20% to 50% of patients undergoing cardiac surgery. However, POCD can be long-term, which is defined as a subtle deterioration in cognitive function 6 months after surgery. This occurs in 10% to 30% of cardiac patients (Tan & Amoako, 2013). The pathophysiology of POCD is multifactorial and it can be associated with a wide range of surgical, anesthetic, and patient factors. Some risk factors and causes include age, history of alcohol abuse, use of anticholinergic medications, postoperative hypoxia, baseline cognition, and preoperative cognitive dysfunction. Additionally, there has been interest in the role of intraoperative monitoring in POCD. It has been hypothesized that POCD may be related to cerebral hypoperfusion. Devices such as cerebral oximetry may be used to maintain regional cerebral oxygen saturation (rSO_2) within predefined limits, as cognitive decline after cardiac surgery may be associated with decreases in cerebral oxygen desaturations (McDonagh et al., 2014; Tan & Amoako, 2013). Likewise, cardiac surgeons commonly use hypothermia during surgery to reduce metabolism, minimize damage to vital organs, and for its neuroprotective properties. Patients need to return to normothermia following surgery; however, neurons may be injured during the rewarming process. Prolonged mild hypothermia and slow rewarming may prevent the development of cognitive dysfunction after cardiac surgery (Wang et al., 2014).

POCD following cardiac surgery has been a controversial topic. The main reason for the controversy is that it is difficult to quantify and diagnose. Different studies have used various test score thresholds and methods to define the disorder. Likewise, POCD is not a clinical diagnosis, it is not listed in the fifth edition of the *Diagnostic and Statistical Manual of Mental Disorders*, and patients cannot be described as having the disorder unless they undergo a formal preoperative cognitive testing battery (McDonagh et al., 2014). Nevertheless, it is a phenomenon and complication seen in patients who have cardiac surgery. POCD has been associated with reduced quality of life and increased 1-year mortality, which strongly indicates that it is an important problem that affects some patients (McDonagh et al., 2014).

Prudent postoperative management in the post-ICU phase should include encouraging a good diet, early mobility, and neurologic assessments.

As there is no evidence POCD can be treated successfully, emphasis should be on prevention and implementing coping strategies. It is important to recognize potential risk factors and to educate patients and families of the occurrence of POCD. Additionally, nursing should offer reassurance about the recovery of POCD in the preceding months. Coping strategies should be discussed, including using lists and calendars to assist with everyday tasks. Nursing's ultimate goal is to provide supportive care and to educate the patients and their families.

Seizures

Postoperative seizures are a relatively uncommon complication of cardiac surgery. The incidence of seizures after cardiac surgery varies between 0.5% and 7.6% Seizures may be caused by a number of factors such as thromboembolic ischemic stroke, cerebral air embolism, medication toxicity related to antibiotics, or other perioperative drugs such as tranexamic acid (TXA) (Manji, Grocott, Manji, Menkis, & Jacobsohn, 2015). Other risk factors and causes are outlined in **BOX 20.8**. Electroencephalogram (EEG) should be considered in patients who are unresponsive 18 to 24 hours after

---

BOX 20.8 Risk Factors for Seizures Following Cardiac Surgery

Preoperative cardiac arrest
Procedures involving the thoracic aorta
Hypoxemia
Metabolic disturbances (hyponatremia, hypoglycemia)
Drug toxicity (lidocaine, procainamide)
Structural brain injury (stroke)
Administration of TXA
APACHE II scores >20
Previous cardiac surgery
Open chamber procedure
CPB time >150 min
Preoperative neurologic disease

APACHE, Acute Physiology and Chronic Health Evaluation; CPB, cardiopulmonary bypass; TXA, tranexamic acid.
Data from Manji, Grocott, Manji, Menki, et al., 2015; McGarvey, Cheung & Stecker, 2017

surgery to detect possible nonconvulsive seizure activity (McGarvey, Cheung, & Stecker, 2017).

Nursing care for a patient experiencing recurrent seizures during the post-ICU phase should center on safety management (e.g., padding the side rails) and the administration of anticonvulsants as ordered.

▸ Other Complications in Post-ICU Care

As a result of hospitalization and extensive cardiac surgery, many patients are still at risk for additional complications during the post-ICU phase of care. Patients may have had a prolonged ICU stay and developed additional complications that continue to need to be addressed as the patient transitions to a lower level of care. This section of the chapter explores additional complications that occur after cardiac surgery.

Chest Tube–Related Complications

Postoperative drainage of surgical sites is a standard component of many operations and is employed routinely after cardiac surgery. After open heart surgery, patients have chest tubes inserted to drain excess fluids, air, and blood. The placement of the tube is needed to drain fluid or create additional negative-pressure suctioning for lung reexpansion, or both. Placement of a least one mediastinal tube is traditional; however, patients may also have a second pleural tube (Kruse, Wahl, Guthrie, & Sendelbach, 2017). Patent chest tubes are necessary to alert nurses to internal bleeding, anastomotic leaks, and air leaks. Any occlusion or blockage of the chest tubes can lead to life-threatening complications, including cardiac tamponade, tension pneumothorax, and sepsis (Huggins & Carr, 2017). Additional complications that can occur with chest tubes include subcutaneous emphysema, tube malposition, and a blocked tube. Reexploratory surgery may be warranted if occluded chest tubes lead to the development of empyema, or a hemothorax that is large enough to cause loss of lung volume. The

incidence of chest tube complications ranges from 1% to 6% and is related to the diameter of the tube, with small-bore tubes having fewer complications. However, the incidence of blockage is higher with small-bore tubes (Huggins & Carr, 2017). The quality and status of postoperative hemostasis and the occurrence of bleeding from surgical sites are often assessed by the volume and character of drainage output. Chest tube drainage is traditionally accomplished via large-bore CTs, which must be properly situated and managed. However, many surgeons use the small-bore more pliable silastic or blake tubes for chest tube drainage. Many surgeons consider the potential for clogging when they choose the diameter size and number of chest tubes placed after surgery. In cardiac surgical patients, chest tubes are susceptible to clotting and thrombus formation after surgery, and the occlusion of chest tubes by thrombus can lead to serious complications such as acute tamponade, hemothorax, and pleural effusion (Karimov et al., 2013). Additionally, chest tube complications can lead to hemodynamic instability, which can prolong the length of stay and adversely influence patient outcomes.

Traditional management of chest tubes for patients after open heart surgery includes use of up to -20 cm H_2O of wall suction to help remove potentially large amounts of drainage and, in patients with pleural tubes, to allow air to leave the chest (Kruse et al., 2017). However, no known research supports managing chest tubes in patients after cardiac surgery by using -10 to -20 cm H_2O wall suctioning from immediately after surgery until the tubes are removed. Numerous studies have focused on the duration of the placement of chest tubes and not on the use of suctioning and postoperative outcomes. In a systematic review, the findings showed that few researchers had examined the best methods for managing drainage via mediastinal chest tubes and found no differences in chest tube output or incidence of tamponade for different levels of suctioning and manipulation techniques of the tube (Kruse et al., 2017). Likewise, the management of chest tubes has traditionally included improvised mechanical methods such as milking or stripping and tapping to remove clots to ensure patency of the chest tubes. The issue with this practice is that milking, fan-folding, stripping, and tapping are not standardized and are thus difficult to compare. Additionally, the evidence shows the practice of milking does not significantly improve fluid drainage and may inadvertently cause dangerously high negative intrapleural pressure of -400 cm H_2O. What is known from the literature is that the management of chest tubes varies and the evidence is unclear on which form of manipulation is more effective, if manipulation and suction is best, or if manipulation alone is harmful. Many of these questions remain controversial, and oftentimes institutions are doing what the surgeon may have learned to be effective during medical training.

In the post-ICU phase of care, the nurse must continue to assess the patient for any signs of an air leak, occlusion, subcutaneous emphysema, and tamponade. This requires the intermediate care nurse to check the chest tube drainage system suction settings, air leak detector, and quality and amount of drainage frequently. If the institution permits, milking or stripping of the tube can be performed, although this is controversial. Tamponade should be suspected for chest tube outputs over 400 mL/hr for 1 hour, over 300 mL/hr for 2 to 3 hours, and 200 mL/hr for 4 hours (Yazdchi & Rawn, 2017). If a suspected air leak, the nurse needs to visualize the air leak detector for vigorous bubbling or fluctuation in the chest tube drainage system. The patient's lungs, work of breathing, use of accessory muscles, and pulse oximetry should also be assessed as indicators of any respiratory compromise. Another nursing intervention that may be performed during the post-ICU phase is the conversion of a silastic blake chest tube to a bulb suction. The nurse must be sure not to introduce any air into the system when converting to bulb suction. Additionally, the bulb must be compressed to create adequate suction. Output goals and the color/consistency of the drainage must also be met prior to chest tube removal. Once the chest tube output has diminished and the patient is hemodynamically stable, it can be removed. Many chest tube removal procedures include placing petroleum gauze on the chest tube sites under a dry sterile dressing. However, the use of petroleum gauze has never been shown to decrease the risk of post–pull pneumothorax. There is the theoretical risk that the petroleum gauze may cause delayed wound healing at the chest tube site (Huggins & Carr, 2017). The chest tube can be removed at end inspiration; others advocate for end expiration. A small study comparing these two techniques did not show a difference in post–pull pneumothorax. Whichever technique is used, the patient should be educated on and rehearse several times prior to the actual tube removal. Once the tube is removed a dressing with or without petroleum gauze is applied. One of the major complications of chest tube removal is pneumothorax formation; therefore, a chest radiograph should be performed to evaluate for the occurrence of a pneumothorax (Huggins & Carr, 2017).

Sleep

Altered sleep patterns are a common problem among cardiac patients and are one of the most frequently reported symptoms by patients in the postoperative period of cardiac surgery. The sleep pattern of patients is changed during the recovery period and is characterized by shorter periods, frequent awakenings, and a perception of poor sleep quality. As a result of the broken sleep pattern, patients may experience fatigue, irritability, and daytime sleepiness. Due to the decreased amount and quality of sleep, some patients may be unable to perform in physical or rehabilitative therapy, which can prolong the recovery phase and increase the length of stay. Decreased or dysfunctional sleep patterns can be caused by a number of factors such as age, gender, previous sleep issues or disorders, the environment, and pain. The disruption in sleep may also be multifactorial in nature with contributing reasons being pain, nausea, lights and noise in the environment, and the patient being away from home. Conventional pharmacologic therapy can be utilized to assist with improving the quality of sleep. Sleep aids such as zolpidem tartrate (Ambien®) and temazepam (Restoril®) can be administered during the post-ICU phase. However, there have been several studies examining nonpharmacologic strategies on how to improve sleep after cardiac surgery in the postoperative phase. Studies suggest that a combination of interventions used to actively reduce anxiety and pain, as well as controlling environmental factors, is efficacious in decreasing the incidence of sleep disorders (Machoda, Souza, Poveda, & Costa, 2017). A study performed in 2015 utilized progressive muscle relaxation therapy on 100 subjects and found that sleep quality was significantly better in the intervention group versus the control group, which participated in regular physical exercise and care (Ranjbaran, Dehdari, Sadeghniiat-Haghighi, & Majdabadi, 2015). Additional studies examined guided imagery using music and headphones, and a sleeping mask and earplugs, and the use of white noise to impact the quality of sleep in postoperative patients. It was found that patients undergoing cardiac surgery listened to white noise to help environmental stimuli and led to relaxation, which contributed to falling asleep faster and maintaining sleep. It was posited that white noise decreased the difference between baseline noise and peaks of noise, decreasing the reflex response on individuals in the face of intense stimuli (Casida et al., 2013; Hu, Jiang, Hegadoren, & Zhang, 2015; Machoda et al., 2017).

During the post-ICU phase, the nurse should assess the amount and quality of sleep a patient is getting and how it is impacting the healing process. Nurses should value sleep as an integral part of their practice to ensure the recovery of patients, thus decreasing complications, costs, and the length of stay. If a patient reports poor quality or amount of sleep, the nurse needs to advocate for adding a short-term pharmacologic sleep aid and/or the institution of other interventions to help with sleep hygiene. These interventions may include the patient's family bringing in familiar objects (e.g., pillow, blanket) from home, performing cultural practices such as tea before bedtime, or helping make the hospital environment more conducive to sleep by dimming the lights and reducing noise from monitors and alarms.

Pain

Pain after cardiac surgery may occur for some patients. Pain may originate from the sternotomy, chest tube sites, and harvest graft sites. Additionally, stiffness and pain or tightness in the back or upper shoulders is common. Adequate pain control is necessary to improve pulmonary function, decrease delirium, increase patient satisfaction, and facilitate the healing process. It is imperative for the nurse to assess the type, quality, and location of pain prior to the administration of an analgesic agent. In the post-ICU phase of care, numeric pain scales or behavioral scales are used for patients to rate their pain. For pain control, systemic opioids are the mainstay of analgesia in the early postoperative phase. Commonly used opioids include fentanyl, morphine, hydromorphone, and meperidine. Once patients are able to take oral medications, they are typically changed to oral narcotics for pain management. There are some data supporting the use of ketorolac in patients with normal renal function, but a high degree of caution should be used with all NSAIDs due to adverse effects on platelet and kidney function, and their tendency to induce gastric ulcer formation (Stephens & Whitman, 2015).

Nonpharmacologic interventions such as music therapy, repositioning, guided imagery, and hot/cold packs may improve pain control in lieu of medications. During the post-ICU phase, the nurse needs to ensure adequate pain control and to discuss the expectation of pain and goal of pain control. Nurses need to educate patients on how to splint or brace when coughing, and to not wait until pain becomes unbearable to take medications. Ultimately, the nurse should serve as the patient advocate and communicate with the care team if adequate pain control is not achieved. Nurse-driven protocols can help to facilitate pain assessment and rapid treatment of postoperative pain.

Post–Intensive Care Syndrome

Critical care medicine has advanced rapidly and has resulted in a growing population of survivors of critical illness. Many survivors experience impairment in cognition, mental health, and physical function, known as post–intensive care syndrome (PICS). Of the 5 million patients who receive critical care in the United States each year, 50% to 70% will acquire PICS. Post-intensive care syndrome is a grouping of post–critical care complications that includes persistent cognitive dysfunction, acquired weakness, and intrusive memories akin to post-traumatic stress disorder (PTSD) (Meyers, Smith, Allen, & Kaplan, 2016). Post-intensive care syndrome may occur in as few as 2 days after a patient receives critical care, and can also affect the patient's family members (PICS-F). It is a complicated and multifaceted diagnosis that has variable risk factors. The patient's previous comorbidities, severity of illness, and other factors play a role in the development of PICS. Several risk factors that contribute to the development of PICS include preexisting neuromuscular disorders, dementia, psychiatric illness, delirium, sepsis, and acute respiratory distress syndrome. The signs and symptoms of PICS improve over the first 6 to 12 months following discharge from the ICU; however, about 50% of patients do not return to work after 1 year, and 30% never return to work, increasing the burden on family members (Mikekelsen, Netzer, & Iwashyna, 2017).

The American Association of Critical-Care Nurses has created a bundle that is targeted at addressing the key elements that may cause PICS. The ABCDEF bundle incorporates elements to specifically address the components of PICS. Additionally, the bundle embraces the family as essential partners in the patient's recovery.

Advances in postdischarge care and post-ICU clinics have occurred in the United Kingdom. Post-ICU programs that offer ICU survivors and their relatives a chance to see the ICU, meet the ICU staff, and discuss their experiences are key to helping with PICS. This program has proven to be a valued service. Additionally, post-ICU programs can be a source of important feedback from patients to ICU professionals, offering opportunities for improved treatment and care protocols (Meyers et al., 2016; Mikekelsen et al., 2017; Svenningsen, Langhorn, Agard, & Dreyer, 2015).

Understanding the causes, progression, symptoms, and possible treatments is vital to improving critical care for survivors and their families. All health care providers should be collaborating to ensure the development of a multidisciplinary treatment plan inclusive of the family to help prevent or reduce the incidence of PICS.

▶ Summary

The post-ICU phase after cardiac surgery is a dynamic time, characterized by organ system lability and fluctuations in the patient's progression to healing. To achieve the goal of stability and safe discharge, the intermediate care nurse must be clinically aware and able to assess for complications and changes. While there is some degree of complications that are predictable, the preexisting comorbidities and the procedural complexity have increased the acuity of cardiac surgery patients. The higher acuity of the cardiac surgery patient causes the predictable nature of complications to be more varied. Likewise, increased length of postoperative ICU stay and hospital stay after cardiac surgery are associated with an increased likelihood of in-hospital mortality (Mazzeffi, Zivot, Buchman, & Halkos, 2014).

The implementation of clinical pathways, protocols, or checklists can assist nurses in consistently providing a set standard of care to ensure safe patient outcomes. The delivery of care to cardiac surgical patients can be complex and tenuous. Nurses and other health care providers must constantly assimilate large amounts of information on a daily basis to provide safe and effective care. Reliance on individual performance can drastically vary. Clinical pathways and protocols help to standardize care, reduce the incidence of medical errors, and infuse evidence-based practices into the care delivered by the health care team. The best approach to the development of protocols and clinical pathways is including all members of the health care team and in some instances previous cardiac surgical patients. The utilization of the clinical pathways and protocols can assist in the delivery of care in the post-ICU setting.

The intermediate care or post-ICU nurse plays an integral part in identifying, treating, and preventing post-ICU alterations. Increased vigilance, astute assessment skills, and implementing evidence-based practice interventions support the nurse with helping the patient and families to an optimum state of health and ultimately to a safe discharge.

$\wp$ *CASE STUDY*

T. G., a 77-year-old male admitted with chest pain and severe CAD, undergoes a quad-vessel CABG. The patient was unable to be weaned quickly off the ventilator due to a history of smoking and mild COPD. After 3 days in the CVICU, the patient's urinary catheter is removed and he is transferred to the stepdown unit. The admitting nurse assesses the patient to have 2L NC with oxygenation saturation 96%, sinus rhythm on the telemetry monitor, BP 136/72, and two chest tubes to 20 cm H_2O wall suction. The patient's midline incision is open to air and appears to be healing appropriately. The nurse would like to ambulate the patient and get him walking; however, the patient appears withdrawn and somnolent. The patient's wife arrives to the room and states the patient's disposition is not the norm for him. As the wife is trying to get the patient to participate in his daily care, the patient begins to complain that he is not feeling well. The patient appears to have some difficulty in breathing, and his oxygenation saturation is 90% on 2LNC. The patient's blood pressure is obtained and it is 96/62, HR is 142 and irregular. The patient states that his heart feels like it is racing. The nurse obtains an order for a 12-lead ECG.

Critical Thinking Questions

1. What postoperative complication is the patient experiencing?
2. What interventions or therapies does the nurse anticipate being a part of the clinical pathway or the patient's plan of care since he is post-op day 3?
3. What other complications is the patient at risk for?
4. What topics should the nurse anticipate teaching the patient and family about postoperatively?

Answers to Critical Thinking Questions

1. The patient could be experiencing several complications, and definitive diagnostic tests would need to be completed to isolate or diagnose the specific complication. Based on the patient description of symptoms, the change in heart rate and regularity, and the clinical picture, point to the most common postoperative dysrhythmia of atrial fibrillation with rapid ventricular rate (RVR). The 12-lead ECG would help to clinically diagnose if the dysrhythmia is present. An antiarrhythmic drug will be administered to assist with the management of the POAF. Typically, amiodarone is bolused first and then an infusion is started. Additionally, the patient may be experiencing the early stages of hypoactive delirium, since the wife reported that he is not typically somnolent, lethargic, and withdrawn. The nurse would need to screen the patient for delirium and assess the medical record for any recent changes in medications and/or lab values. It would also be helpful to assess if the patient utilizes hearing or visual aids, and to have the wife provide them as soon as possible.
2. The nurse should anticipate the following interventions during the post-ICU phase for the patient's plan of care:
   a. Ambulation
   b. Incentive spirometry usage
   c. Incision care and assessment (CHG wipes)
   d. Chest tube management (drainage, dressing, output documentation, assessing for air leak and other complications such as crepitus)
   e. Intake and output documentation
   f. Harvest/graft site assessment
   g. Pain control
   h. Medication teaching
   i. Central/peripheral line maintenance
   j. Systems assessment (neurologic assessment to monitor for s/s of CVA; GI assessment for bowel sounds, etc.)
   k. Mechanical or pharmacologic VTE prophylaxis

(continues)

⌕ CASE STUDY (continued)

3. The patient is at risk for several other complications such as delirium, postoperative ileus, deep vein thrombosis, pulmonary embolus, bleeding, pneumothorax, sudden cardiac arrest, and stroke.
4. The patient and family will need to be taught a number of topics during the post-ICU phase. The topics include:
   - Incision and harvest/graft site care and management
   - Signs and symptoms of infection
   - Medication side effects
   - Activity level and restrictions
   - Sternal precautions
   - Diet/alcohol consumption
   - Smoking cessation
   - Constipation
   - Emotional changes
   - Cardiac rehabilitation as ordered
   - When to call the doctor or report to the emergency department

Self-Assessment Questions

1. Reducing hospital-acquired infections in patients after cardiac surgery should include which of the following interventions?
   A. Routine central venous catheter dressing changes performed every 72 hours to minimize the risk of central line–associated bloodstream infections
   B. Administration of sliding scale insulin at regular intervals to control blood glucose levels during the postoperative phase of care
   C. Administration of prophylactic intravenous antibiotics for the duration of the inpatient stay to reduce occurrence of *Clostridium difficile*
   D. Removal of the urinary catheter as soon as possible once the patient is clinically stable

2. A patient admitted to the post-ICU area after 2 weeks in the CVICU is at an increased risk for post–intensive care syndrome (PICS) if there is a previous history of which condition?
   A. Dementia
   B. Rheumatoid arthritis
   C. Depression
   D. Rheumatic heart disease

3. Three days following a CABG ×4 the patient dumps 490 mL into his chest tube sanguineous drainage collection system over 2 hours. The most likely cause of this increased output is:
   A. heparin-induced thrombocytopenia.
   B. bleeding at the anastomosis site.
   C. protamine reversal syndrome.
   D. adhesions on the pacing wires.

4. Which signs and symptoms of transfusion-associated circulatory overload (TACO) are not seen on assessment of a patient with this condition?
   A. Decreased oxygenation saturation
   B. Increased respiratory effort (tachypnea)
   C. Increased jugular venous distention (JVD)
   D. S4 heart sounds on auscultation

5. Which cardiac surgical procedure puts a patient at greater risk for developing postoperative seizures?
   A. Mitral valve repair
   B. Thoracic aortic arch aneurysm repair
   C. CABG ×3
   D. Implantation of left ventricular assist device

6. When teaching a patient about how to care for his or her sternotomy incision, which information should not be taught to patients and families for postincision care?
   A. Holding a pillow to the chest when coughing
   B. Minimal scrubbing with mild soap and water on the incision site
   C. Utilizing the arms to bear weight when rising or with position changes
   D. Checking the incision daily for signs of redness, discharge, or swelling

7. In the post-ICU setting, the nurse is caring for an adult congenital heart disease (ACHD) patient who has undergone a mitral valve replacement (MVR) 3 days ago. The mediastinal and pleural chest tubes have been converted to bulb suction, and the patient is ambulating in the halls. The nurse rounds on the patient an hour later and notices a large output of sanguinous blood in the bulbs, and the patient is hypotensive. A stat complete blood count (CBC) is ordered. The nurse anticipates administering a blood transfusion for which of the following results?
   A. Hemoglobin 8.2 and hematocrit 22
   B. Hemoglobin 7.4 and hematocrit 24
   C. Hemoglobin 6.9 and hematocrit 20
   D. Hemoglobin 7.1 and hematocrit 21

8. Which is the best strategy to utilize to reduce the incidence of phlebitis in a patient receiving the intravenous antiarrhythmic medication amiodarone for postoperative atrial fibrillation?
   A. Infusing amiodarone through an inline 0.22-micron filter for peripheral intravenous catheters
   B. Infusing amiodarone through a 24-gauge or larger peripheral intravenous catheter
   C. Infusing amiodarone through a 20-gauge peripheral intravenous catheter in the hand
   D. Infusing amiodarone through a 22-gauge peripheral intravenous catheter and rotating the site daily

9. A nurse is caring for a patient 4 days postoperative from CABG ×3 with AVR. The sternal incision appears red and the patient reports tenderness and pain. Upon further assessment, the nurse notices that the patient has edema and yellow drainage at the site. What interventions does the nurse anticipate occurring?
   A. Evacuation of the drainage at bedside using needle aspiration
   B. Wound and blood cultures to be obtained for the source of bacteremia and colonization
   C. Chlorohexidine gluconate (CHG) wipes every 2 hours to neutralize the bacterial growth
   D. Localized debridement of the site and administration of antibiotic solution

10. What is the goal standard of therapy for a patient who is experiencing SCA to facilitate resuscitation and return of spontaneous circulation (ROSC)?
    A. Administration of 1 mg epinephrine every 3 to 5 minutes
    B. Chest compression 120 compressions/minute
    C. Cardioversion with 250 Joules or hospital standard
    D. Defibrillation with 120 Joules or hospital standard

Answers to Self-Assessment Questions

1. **D. removal of the urinary catheter as soon as possible once the patient is clinically stable**
   Rationale: Removal of the indwelling urinary catheter as soon as possible reduces the risk of CAUTI. Urinary tract infections are the most common hospital-acquired infection, and the incidence is directly related to the duration of the indwelling catheter in the bladder.

2. A. **dementia**
   Rationale: Dementia is a risk factor that can contribute to the development of post–intensive care syndrome (PICS).

3. B. **bleeding at the anastomosis site**
   Rationale: Bleeding at the anastomosis site will produce high volumes of sanguinous output in the chest tube drainage collection device within a relatively small amount of time.

4. D. **S4 heart sounds on auscultation**
   Rationale: S4 heart sounds on auscultation will not be heard in a patient with signs and symptoms of TACO. Patients with TACO typically present with respiratory symptoms such as tachypnea, decreased oxygen saturation, increased work of breathing, increased JVD, and S3 heart sounds on auscultation.

5. B. **thoracic aortic arch aneurysm repair**
   Rationale: Thoracic aortic arch aneurysm repair surgery places a patient at greater risk for the development of a postoperative seizure.

6. D. **checking the incision daily for signs of redness, discharge, or swelling**
   Rationale: Utilizing the arms to bear weight when rising or with position changes is not appropriate techniques related to sternal precautions and patients should be taught to restrict the amount of pressure or weight bearing with the upper extremities.

7. C. **hemoglobin 6.9 and hematocrit 20**
   Rationale: The STS guidelines recommend transfusion for stable postoperative patients be considered only if hemoglobin falls below 7 g/dL and hematocrit below 21%.

8. A. **infusing amiodarone through an inline 0.22-micron filter for peripheral intravenous catheters**
   Rationale: Infusing amiodarone through an inline 0.22-micron filter for peripheral intravenous catheter decreased the incidence of phlebitis in patients receiving amiodarone through a peripheral IV.

9. B. **Wound cultures to be obtained for source of bacteremia and colonization**
   Rationale: Wound cultures need to be drawn to identify the type of bacteria. Oftentimes broad-spectrum antibiotics may initially be ordered until the type of bacteria is identified with either the blood or wound cultures, then a more specific antibiotic can be administered.

10. D. **defibrillation with 120 Joules or hospital standard**
    Rationale: Defibrillation is the intervention that increases a patient's chance of ROSC after SCA.

CLINICAL INQUIRY BOX

Question: Are nursing interventions able to improve a patient's sleep quality after open heart surgery?

Reference: Greve, H., & Pedersen, P. U. (2016). Improving sleep after open heart surgery-effectiveness of nursing interventions. *Journal of Nursing Education and Practice*, 6(3), 15–25.

Objective: To see if systematic training and education in sleep anamneses and sleep hygiene enhances nurses' awareness on sleep problems, and as a result makes nurses able to propose appropriate interventions during hospitalization after open heart surgery.

Method: The study design is a controlled intervention study. Patients in the control group received usual care. Patients in the intervention group received nursing care focused on improving sleep by use of sleep-anamneses and sleep hygienic principles. Patients' sleep quality was measured via self-report preoperatively, and 1 and 2 months postoperatively by use of PSQI-questionnaire and sleep diaries.

Results: There was no significant effect on the intervention, though there were several signs that had some effect 2 months after discharge. The total sleep time, sleep efficiency, sleep medication, and sleep quality were affected 2 months after discharge.

Conclusion: Systematic education and training of nurses in sleep and sleep hygiene practices has some effect on patients' self-reported sleep quality 2 months after open heart surgery.

References

Adams, J., Lotshaw, A., Exum, E., Campbell, M., Spranger, C. B., Deveridge, J., . . . Schussler, J. M. (2016). An alternative approach to prescribing sternal precautions after median sternotomy, "keep your move in the tube." *Baylor University Medical Proceedings, 29*(1), 97–100.

Alraies, M. C., Aljoroudi, W., Shabrang, C., Yarmohammadi, H., Klein, A., & Tamarappoo, B. K. (2014). Clinical features associated with adverse events in patients with post-pericardiotomy syndrome following cardiac surgery. *American Journal of Cardiology, 114*(9), 1426–1430.

Bilgin, Y. M., & Van de Watering, L. M. (2013). Complications after cardiac surgery due to allogenic blood transfusions. *Journal of Clinical & Experimental Cardiology, 7*, 5. doi:10.4172/2155-9880.S7-005

Casida, J. M., Yaremchuk, K. L., Shpakoff, L., Marrocco, A., Babicz, G., & Yarandi, H. (2013). The effects of guided imagery on sleep and inflammatory response in cardiac surgery: A pilot randomized controlled trial. *Journal of Cardiovascular Surgery, 54*(2), 269–279.

Devlin et al., (2018). Clinical practice guidelines for the prevention and management of pain, agitation/sedation, delirium, immobility, and sleep disruption in adult patients in the ICU. *Critical Care Medicine, 46*(9), e825–e873. doi:10.1097/CCM.0000000000003299 Available at https://www.ncbi.nlm.nih.gov/pubmed/30113379

Dunning, J., Levine, A., Ley., J., Strang, T., Lizotte, D. E., Lamarche, Y. . . . Bakaeen, F. G. (2017). The Society of Thoracic Surgeons expert consensus for the resuscitation of patients who arrest after cardiac surgery. *Annals of Thoracic Surgery, 103*(3), 1005–1020.

Fekete, T., Calderwood, S. B., & Bloom, A. (2017). *Catheter-associated urinary tract infections.* Retrieved from www.uptodate.com/contents/catheter-associated-urinary-tract-infection-in-adults

Floerchinger, B., Camboni, D., Schopka, S., Kolat, P., Hilker, M., & Schmid, C. (2013). Delayed cardiac tamponade after open heart surgery—is supplemental CT imaging reasonable? *Journal of Cardiothoracic Surgery, 8*, 158. doi:10.1186/1749-8090-8-158

Francis, J. (2017). *Delirium and acute confusional states: Prevention, treatment and prognosis.* Retrieved from http://www.uptodate.com/contents/delirium-and-acute-confusional-states-prevention-treatment

Gaasch, W. H., & Zoghbi, W. A. (2017). *Overview of the management of patients with prosthetic heart valves.* Retrieved from https://www.uptodate.com/contents/overview-of-the-managment-of-patients-with-prosthetic-heart-valves

Gillen, J. R., Isbell, J. M., Michaels, A. D., Lau, C. L., & Sawyer, R. G. (2015). Risk factors for urinary tract infections in cardiac surgical patients. *Surgical Infections, 16*(5), 504–508.

Ginwalla, R., Faraday, N., & Whitman, G. (2014). Postoperative management of the cardiac surgical patient. In D. Yuh, L. Vricella, S. Yang, & J. R. Doty (Eds.), *Textbook of cardiothoracic surgery.* New York, NY: McGraw-Hill Education.

Gorlitzer, M., Wagner, F., Pfeiffer, S., Folkmann, S., Meinhart, J., Fischlein, T., . . . Grabenwoeger, M. (2013). Prevention of sternal wound complications after sternotomy: Results of a large prospective randomized multicentre trial. *Interactive CardioVascular and Thoracic Surgery, 17*, 515–522. doi:10.1093/icvts/ivt240

Habbab, L. M., & Chu, V. F. (2016). Intrapericardial amiodarone for the prevention of postoperative atrial fibrillation. *Journal of Cardiac Surgery, 31*, 253–258.

Heffner, J. E. (2017). *Pleural effusions following cardiac surgery.* Retrieved from http://www.uptodate.com/contents/pleural-effusions-following-cardiac-surgery

Hemilä, H., & Suonsyrjä, T. (2017). Vitamin C for preventing atrial fibrillation in high risk patients: A systematic review and meta-analysis. *BMC Cardiovascular Disorders, 17*, 180. doi:10.1186/s12872-017-0478-5

Henneman, E. A., Andrzejewski, C., Gawlinski, A., McAfee, K., Panaccione, T., & Dziel, K. (2017). Transfusion-associated circulatory overload: Evidence-based strategies to prevent, identify, and manage a serious adverse event. *Critical Care Nurse, 37*(5), 58–66.

Ho, K. M., Bham, E., & Pavey, W. (2015). Incidence of venous thromboembolism and benefits and risks of thromboprophylaxis after cardiac surgery: A systematic review and meta-analysis. *Journal of the American Heart Association, 4*, e002652. doi:10.1161/JAHA.115.002652

Hoit, B. (2017). *Cardiac tamponade.* Retrieved from https://www.uptodate.com/contents/cardiac-tamponade/print?search=cardiac%20tamponade

Hopkins, W., & Rubin, L. J. (2017). *Treatment of pulmonary hypertension in adults.* Retrieved from https://www.uptodate.com/contents/treatment-of-pulmonary-hypertension-in-adults

Hu, R. F., Jiang, X. Y., Hegadoren, K. M., & Zhang, Z. H. (2015). Effects of earplugs an eye masks combined with relating music on sleep, melatonin and cortisol levels in ICU patients: A randomized controlled trial. *Critical Care, 19*, 1–9. Retrieved from https://www.ncbi.nlm.nih.gov/pmc/articles/PMC4391192/pdf/13054_2015_Article_855.pdf

Huggins, J. T., & Carr, S. (2017). *Placement and management of thoracostomy tubes.* Retrieved from https://www.uptodate.com/contents/placement-and-management-of-thoracostomy-tubes

Jannati, Y., Bagheri-Nesami, M., Sohrabi, M., Yazdani-Cherati, Y., & Mazdarani, S. (2014). Factors associated with post-surgical delirium in patients undergoing open heart surgery. *Oman Medical Journal, 29*(5), 340–345.

Kalff, J. C., Wehner, S., & Litkouhi, B. (2017). *Postoperative ileus.* Retrieved from https://www.uptodate.com/contents/postoperative-ileus

Karchmer, A. W. (2017). *Epidemiology, clinical manifestations, and diagnosis of prosthetic valve endocarditis.* Retrieved from https://www.uptodate.com/contents/epidemiology-clinical-manifestations-and-diagnosis-of-prosthetic-valve-endocarditis

Karimov, J. H., Gillinov, A. M., Schenck, L., Cook, M., Kosty Sweeney, D. K., Boyle, E. M., . . . Fukamachi, K. (2013). Incidence of chest tube clogging after cardiac surgery: A single-centre prospective observational study. *European Journal of Cardio-Thoracic Surgery, 44,* 1029–1036. doi:10.1093/ejcts/ezt140

Katrancha, E. D., & George, N. M. (2014). Postoperative ileus. *MEDSURG Nursing, 23*(6), 387–391.

Kruse, T., Wahl, S., Guthrie, P. F., & Sendelbach, S. (2017). Place atrium to water seal (paws): Assessing wall suction versus no suction for chest tubes after open heart surgery. *Critical Care Nurse, 37*(4), 17–28.

Lee, R. (2017). *Atrial fibrillation and flutter after cardiac surgery.* Retrieved from https://www.uptodate.com/contents/atrial-fibrillation-and-flutter-after-cardiac-surgery

Lehto, J., Gunn, J., Karjalainen, P., Airaksinen, J., & Kiviniemi, T. (2015), Incidence and risk factors of postpericardiotomy syndrome requiring medical attention: The Finland postpericardiotomy syndrome study. *The Journal of Thoracic and Cardiovascular Surgery, 15,* 51–53.

Ley, S. J. (2015). Standards for resuscitation after cardiac surgery. *Critical Care Nurse, 35*(2), 30–37.

Lipp, G. Y., & Hull, R. D. (2017). *Overview of the treatment of lower extremity deep vein thrombosis (DVT).* Retrieved from https://www.uptodate.com/contents/overview-of-the-treatment-of-lower-extremity-deep-vein-thrombosis

Liu, S., Bian, C., Zhang, Y., Jian, Y., & Liu, W. (2014). Landiolol hydrochloride for prevention of atrial fibrillation after cardiac surgery: A meta-analysis. *Pace, 37,* 691–696.

Machoda, F. S., Souza, R. C., Poveda, V. B., & Costa, A. L. (2017). Non-pharmacological interventions to promote the sleep of patients after cardiac surgery: A systematic review. *Revista Latino-Americana de Enfermagem, 25,* e2926. doi:10.1590/1518-8345.1917.2926

Mangusan, R. F., Hooper, V., Denslow, S. A., & Travis, L. (2015). Outcomes associated with postoperative delirium after cardiac surgery. *American Journal of Critical Care, 24*(2), 156–162.

Manji, R. A., Grocott, H. P., Manji, J. S., Menkis, A. H., & Jacobsohn, E. (2015). Recurrent seizures following cardiac surgery: Risk factors and outcomes in a historical cohort study. *Journal of Cardiothoracic and Vascular Anesthesia, 29*(5), 1206–1211.

Mathew, S. E., Beavers, C. J., & McNeely, E. (2016). The national practice patterns of venous thromboembolism prophylaxis post-cardiothoracic surgery. *Journal of Pharmacy Practice, 30*(4), 394–399.

Mazzeffi, M., Zivot, J., Buchman, T., & Halkos, M. (2014). In-hospital mortality after cardiac surgery: Patient characteristics, timing, and association with postoperative length of intensive care unit and hospital stay. *Annals of Thoracic Surgery, 97,* 1220–1226.

McCutcheson, T. (2013). The ileus and oddities after colorectal surgery. *Gastroenterology Nursing, 36*(5), 368–375.

McDonagh, D. L., Berger, M., Mathew, J. P., Graffagnino, C., Milano, C. A., & Newman, M. F. (2014). Neurological complications of cardiac surgery. *Lancet Neurology, 13,* 490–502.

McGarvey, M. L., Cheung, A. T., & Stecker, M. M. (2017). *Neurological complication of cardiac surgery.* Retrieved from http://www.uptodate.com/contents/neurological-complications-of-cardiac-surgery

McLaughlin, M., & Marik, P. E. (2016). Dexmedetomidine and delirium in the ICU. *Annals of Translational Medicine, 4*(11), 224. doi:10.21037/atm.2016.05.44

Meyers, E. A., Smith, D. A., Allen, S. R., & Kaplan, L. J. (2016). Post-ICU syndrome: Rescuing the undiagnosed. *Journal of the American Academy of Physicians Assistants, 29*(4), 34–37.

Mikekelsen, M. E., Netzer, G., & Iwashyna, T. (2017). *Post-intensive care syndrome.* Retrieved from https://www.uptodate.com/contents/post-intensive-care-syndrome-pics

Morimoto, Y. (2016). Postoperative cognitive dysfunction after cardiac surgery. *Anaesthesia Pain & Intensive Care, 20*(1), S146–S149. Retrieved from http://www.apicareonline.com/postoperative-cognitive-dysfunction-after-cardiac-surgery

Mufti, H. N., Baskett, R. J., Arora, R. C., & Légaré, J. (2015). The perception of evidence for ventous thromboembolism prophylaxis current practices after cardiac surgery: A Canadian cross-sectional survey. *Thrombosis, 2015.* doi:10.1155/2015/795645

Norkienė, I., Ringaitienė, D., Kuzminskaitė, V., & Šipylaitė, J. (2013). Incidence and risk factors of early delirium after cardiac surgery. *BioMed Research International,* Article ID 323491, 1–5. doi:10.1155/2013/323491

Norton, L., Ottoboni, L. K., Varady, A., Yang-Lu, C. Y., Becker, N., Cotter, T., . . . Wang, P. (2013). Phlebitis in amiodarone administration: Incidence, contributing factors, and clinical implications. *American Journal of Critical Care, 22*(6), 498–505.

O'Neal, J. B., & Shaw, A. D. (2016). Predicting, preventing, and identifying delirium after cardiac surgery. *Perioperative Medicine, 5*(7), 1–8. doi:10.1186/s13741-016-0032-5

Orgill, D. P. (2017). Surgical management of sternal wound complications. Retrieved from http://www.uptodate.com/contents/surgical-managment-of-sternal-wound-complications

Peretto, G., Durante, A., Limite, L., & Cianflone, D. (2014). Postoperative arrhythmias after cardiac surgery: Incidence, risk factors and therapeutic management. *Cardiology Research and Practice, 2014,* 615987. doi:10.1155/2014/615987

Phan, K., Ha, H., Phan, S., Medi, C., Thomas, S. P., & Yan, T. D. (2015). New-onset atrial fibrillation following coronary bypass surgery predicts long-term mortality: A systematic review and meta-analysis. *European Journal of Cardiothoracic Surgery, 48*(6), 817–824.

Podrid, P. J. (2017). *Overview of sudden cardiac arrest and sudden cardiac death.* Retrieved from http://wwww.uptodate.com/contents/overview-of-sudden-cardiac-arrest-and-sudden-cardiac-death

Poikajärvi, S., Salanterä, S., Katajisto, J., & Junttila, K. (2017). Validation of Finnish Neecham confusion scale and nursing delirium screening scale using confusion assessment method algorithm as a comparison scale. *BMC Nursing, 16*(7), 1–10. doi:10.1186/s12912-016-0199-6

Ranjbaran, S., Dehdari, T., Sadeghniiat-Haghighi, K., & Majdabadi, M. M. (2015). Poor sleep quality in patients after coronary artery bypass graft surgery: An intervention study using the PRECEDE-PROCEED model. *Journal of Tehran University Heart Center, 10*(1), 1–8. Retrieved from https://www.ncbi.nlm.nih.gov/pubmed/26157457

Ray-Barruel, G., Polit, D. F., Murfield, J. E. & Rickard, C. M. (2014). Infusion phlebitis assessment measures: A systematic review. *Journal of Evaluation in Clinical Practice, 20*(2), 191–202.

Rubin, L., & Hopkins, W. (2017). *Clinical features and diagnosis of pulmonary hypertension in adults.* Retrieved from http://www.uptodate.com/contents/classification-and-diagnosis-of-pulmonary-hypertension

Rubin, L. J., & Hopkins, W. (2017). *Classification and prognosis of pulmonary hypertension in adults.* Retrieved from http://www.uptodate.com/contents/classification-and-prognosis-of-pulmonary-hypertension

Schwartz, J., Lindsey, D. E., Khabiri, H., & Stawicki, S. P. (2013). Gastrointestinal complications in cardiothoracic surgery: A synopsis. In M. J. Firstenberg (Ed.), *Principles and practice of cardiothoracic surgery* (pp. 355–371). Retrieved from https://cdn.intechopen.com/pdfs-wm/45021.pdf. doi:10.5772/54348

Sexton, D. J. (2017). *Postoperative mediastinitis after cardiac surgery.* Retrieved from http://www.uptodate.com/contents/postoperative-mediastinitis-after-cardiac-surgery

Silvergleid, A. J., Kleinman, J., & Tirnauer, J. S. (2017). *Transfusion-associated circulatory overload.* Retrieved from http://www.uptodate.com/contents/transfusion-associated-circulatory-overload-taco

Silvestry, F. (2017). *Postoperative complications among patients undergoing cardiac surgery.* Retrieved from http://www.uptodate.com/contents/postoperative-complications-among-patients-undergoing-cardiac-surgery

Smetana, G. W. (2017). *Strategies to reduce postoperative complications in adults.* Retrieved from http://www.uptodate.com/contents/strategies-to-reduce-postoperative-pulmonary-complications

Smulter, N., Lingehall, H. C., Gustafson, Y., Olofsson, B., & Engström, K. (2015). Validation of the confusion assessment method in detecting postoperative delirium in cardiac surgery patient. *American Journal of Critical Care, 24*(6), 481–487.

Spiering, M. (2014). Peripheral amiodarone-related phlebitis: An institutional nursing guideline to reduce patient harm. *Infusion Nurses Society, 37*, 453–460.

Stephens, R. S., & Whitman, G. J. (2015). Postoperative critical care or the adult cardiac surgical patient: Part 1: Routine postoperative care. *Critical Care Medicine, 43*(7), 1477–1497.

Svenningsen, H., Langhorn, L., Agard, A. S., & Dreyer, P. (2015). Post-ICU symptoms, consequences, and follow-up: An integrative review. *British Association of Critical Care Nurses, 22*(4), 212–220.

Tan, A. M., & Amoaka, D. (2013). Postoperative cognitive dysfunction after cardiac surgery. *Continuuing Education in Anaesthesia. Critical Care & Pain, 13*(6), 213–223. Retrieved from https://academic.oup.com/bjaed/article-abstract/13/6/218/247009

Thompson, B. T., & Kabrhel, C. (2017). *Overview of acute pulmonary embolism in adults.* Retrieved from https//www.uptodate.com/contents/overview-of-acute-pulmonary-embolism-in-adults

Wang, W., Wang, Y., Wu, H., Lei, L., Xu, S., Shen, X., . . . Wang, F. (2014). Postoperative cognitive dysfunction: Current developments in mechanism and prevention. *Medical Science Monitor, 20*, 1908–1912. doi:10.12659/MSM.892485

Yazdchi, F., & Rawn J. D. (2017). Postoperative care of cardiac surgery patients. In L. H. Cohn & D. H. Adams (Eds.), *Cardiac surgery in the adult* (5th ed.). New York, NY: McGraw-Hill. Retrieved from http://accesssurgery.mhmedical.com.proxy.library.emory.edu/content.aspx?bookid=2157&sectionid=164290048

Web Resources

American Association of Critical-Care Nurses. www.aacn.org.

Recommendations for practice for the management of delirium
CAUTI implementation and bundles: www.ahrq.gov
CAUTI implementation and bundles: www.ihi.org
CAUTI information: www.cdc.gov/infectioncontrol/guidelines/cauti/index.html
Delirium and Post-Intensive Care Syndrome (PICS)/ABCDEF bundle: www.aacn.org
Delirium recognition and management: www.icudelirium.org

CHAPTER 21

Implications of Obesity of the Cardiac Surgery Patient

Dalton Skipper

▶ Introduction

Approximately 39.8% of adults in the United States are obese. Comorbidities associated with obesity result in annual medical costs that are $1,429 higher for people who are obese as compared to those of normal weight. Estimates of the annual costs of medical care in the United States will be approximately $147 to $210 billion. Compounding these costs is obesity-associated job absenteeism, which is estimated at $4.3 billion (State of Obesity, 2004–2018).

Obesity does not affect all racial groups equally. The group with the highest age-adjusted rate of obesity is non-Hispanic blacks (47.8%). This is followed by Hispanics (42.5%), non-Hispanic whites (32.6%), and non-Hispanic Asians (10.8%). Further, the highest rate of obesity occurs in adults 40 to 59 years of age (42.8%). This is compared to adults 20 to 39 years of age (35.7%) and those age 60 and older (41%) (Hales, Carroll, Fryar, & Ogden, 2017).

Obesity is defined based on body mass index (BMI). A person's BMI can be determined using a calculator that is available free of charge online on any of several websites. It is based on the ratio of weight (in kilograms) and height (in centimeters). Many of the online BMI calculators allow users to enter their weight in pounds and height in inches. The World Health Organization (WHO) classifies obesity based on BMI. A person is classified as overweight with a BMI of 25 to 29.9 kg/m^2; obesity is defined as a BMI greater than 30 kg/m^2. Obese class I corresponds with a BMI of 30 to 34.99 kg/m^2, class II is a BMI of 35 to 39.99 kg/m^2, and class III is a BMI of 40 kg/m^2 or higher (WHO, n.d.). Waist circumference is another way to classify presence of obesity. This method has not yet been uniformly adapted into clinical practice.

A number of comorbidities are associated with obesity. These include type II diabetes, several forms of cancer diseases, and almost all forms of cardiovascular disease, asthma, gallbladder disease, osteoarthritis, and chronic back pain (Böhmer & Wappler, 2017). Additionally, obese patients may experience obstructive sleep apnea and are more at risk for complications related to anesthetic drugs and difficulties during intubation (Demirel, Bolat, & Altun, 2017). As the number of persons with obesity increases, so too will the number requiring cardiac surgery. Nurses caring for these patients require an understanding

Original contribution from Roberta Kaplow

of the physiologic changes that are associated with obesity and must modify their care to meet the individual needs of this patient population. This chapter describes the physiologic changes that occur as a result of obesity and issues surrounding the patient with obesity who is undergoing cardiac surgery. Implications of care during the preoperative, intraoperative, and postoperative phases are also described.

▶ Physiologic Changes Associated with Obesity

A number of physiologic changes occur in patients with obesity. The changes are typically due to an increase in body mass or adiposity. Changes in the cardiovascular, respiratory, gastrointestinal (GI), and renal systems are addressed in the sections that follow.

Cardiovascular Changes

Both cardiovascular and hemodynamic changes occur as a result of increased body mass. There is an increase in cardiac output (CO) to meet the increase in metabolic demands. Dilation of the left ventricle occurs due to the increase in venous return; this results in left ventricular hypertrophy (LVH). Obese patients have higher resting cardiac filling pressures that result in cardiac remodeling, ventricular dysfunction, and subsequent heart failure (HF) (Alpert, Lavie, Agrawal, Aggarwal, & Kumar, 2014). Other cardiovascular changes include increases in stroke volume, myocardial workload, myocardial oxygen demand, and decreased vascular resistance. Hypertension and cardiomegaly result from increases in CO and stroke volume, leading to cardiac remodeling, thus increasing mortality. Compared to their normal-weight counterparts, data suggest an overall increased risk of death associated with cardiovascular disease in those who are obese (Borrell & Samuel, 2014).

Respiratory Changes

There are changes in the respiratory system related to obesity. Obesity causes an increase in carbon dioxide (CO_2) production and oxygen consumption. There is a decrease in chest wall compliance due to the extra weight around the ribs, below the diaphragm, and in the abdominal area. Decreased chest wall compliance results in reduced total lung capacity related to body habitus and increases in oxygen demand and pulmonary blood volume (Steier, Lunt, Hart, Polkey, & Moxham, 2014). The expiratory reserve volume (the maximum amount of air that can be exhaled from the lungs following a normal exhalation) and functional residual capacity (FRC, the amount of air left in the lungs at the end of exhalation) are also dramatically reduced (Steier et al., 2014). Patients with obesity often have lower tidal volume with an associated increase in respiratory rate. Decreases in lung volumes and chest wall movement may result in increased work of breathing and oxygen consumption. Restrictive lung disease may develop in patients with obesity from increases in intra-abdominal pressure and decreased compliance of the chest wall (Backman et al., 2016; Steier et al., 2014). Additional abdominal pressure may come from patient positioning as with the supine position (Backman et al., 2016). Mild hypoxia may exist due to ventilation-perfusion mismatch from basilar atelectasis from immobility. Upon ambulation or repositioning, ventilation-perfusion mismatch is improved (Backman et al., 2016). Intrapulmonary shunting is mild to moderately increased (1%–16%) in the obese population (Rivas et al., 2015).

Patients with obesity may also develop obstructive sleep apnea (OSA). It results in chronically low oxygen levels, elevated CO_2 levels, and pulmonary and systemic vasoconstriction. These put the obese patient at increased risk for intrapulmonary shunting and ischemia (cardiac and cerebral), even in patients as young as 15 years (Mandviwala, Khalid, & Deswal, 2016; Mitchell et al., 2015). Obstructive sleep apnea may complicate opioid-based pain management due to the alteration in both pain processing and sensitivity to opioid effect (Chung, Abdullah, & Liao, 2016). Considerations should be made for those with respiratory concern, including continuous peripheral capillary oxygen saturation (SpO_2) monitoring and capnography (Gupta et al., 2018).

Gastrointestinal Changes

Obesity is associated with a number of GI changes. For example, incidence of gastroesophageal reflux is higher because of increased intra-abdominal pressure. Obese patients have larger fasting gastric volumes than those of nonobese patients (Acosta et al., 2015). Nonneoplastic disorders are more prevalent in obese patients, such as Barrett's esophagus, along with neoplastic diseases (Feakins, 2016). Data suggest that GI microbiota is altered in obesity, affecting metabolism and absorption (Graham, Mullen, & Whelan, 2015). High-fat, low-fiber diets often consumed by the obese are understood to be the cause of GI cancers and microbiota changes (Feakins, 2016; Graham et al., 2015).

Renal Changes

Presence of obesity puts the patient at greater risk for developing hypertension and diabetes; both of these are implicated in the development of end-stage renal disease. Obesity also has effects on hemodynamics in the kidney; patients with fewer nephrons are more likely to develop these hemodynamic effects. Etiology factors of obesity-related kidney disease include hyperfiltration and increased wall tension on the glomerular capillaries (Hall et al., 2014).

▶ Drug Pharmacokinetics and Pharmacodynamics

The pharmacokinetics and pharmacodynamics of drugs are altered in patients with obesity. The distribution and elimination of drugs will be affected as a result of obesity-related decreased total body water and increased CO, volume of distribution, adiposity, and renal and hepatic blood flow. It has been suggested that patients be dosed for medications based on ideal body weight (Knibbe et al., 2015). Since obesity can impact the clearance of drugs, pharmacokinetic parameters are a concern to determine therapeutic maintenance dosages of medications such as antibiotics and blood thinners (Knibbe et al., 2015).

▶ The Preoperative Phase of Cardiac Surgery

As described in Chapter 4, the nurse plays a pivotal role in performing a preoperative evaluation prior to cardiac surgery. During this time, a comprehensive history and physical may reveal pivotal information that can impact the patient's intraoperative and postoperative trajectory. The nurse should inquire about and assess for symptoms of OSA, obese hypoventilation syndrome (OHS), and obesity-associated comorbidities (e.g., hypertension, angina, diabetes, and impaired renal and hepatic function). Appropriate diagnostic tests should also be obtained (e.g., chest radiograph, electrocardiogram, and labs). Because OSA is often undiagnosed, it is suggested that a tool to screen patients be used. An example of an OSA screen is the STOP-Bang questionnaire. This eight-question screening tool assesses for the presence of snoring, feeling tired, and observed apnea. Neck size, gender, BMI, and age are all considered in determining the probability of presence of OSA (Chung et al., 2016).

Obesity hypoventilation syndrome is characterized by alveolar hypoventilation during sleep and wakefulness and is present when an obese person has a CO_2 level greater than 45 mmHg while awake (Shetty & Parthasarathy, 2015). It is reported to be present in up to 25% of patients with OSA. Obesity hypoventilation syndrome is reported to be more common in patients with severe obesity (BMI >40 kg/m^2) and those with dyspnea on exertion. For patients deemed to be at risk for having OHS, the nurse performing the preoperative evaluation should obtain an order for an arterial blood gas to determine if hypercarbia is present. If a patient is found to have CO_2 retention, referral for sleep studies or to a pulmonologist is recommended prior to the patient having surgery, if possible (Raveendran, Wong, Singh, Wong, & Chung, 2017).

During the preoperative evaluation, baseline vital signs should be obtained. If the patient has poorly controlled hypertension (systolic pressure >160 mmHg or diastolic pressure >100 mmHg), it should be determined if surgery can be delayed so that blood pressure control can be attempted (Hartle et al., 2016).

Evaluation of the patient's management of diabetes should also occur during the preoperative evaluation. Data including degree of glycemic control and blood glucose range will be helpful during the perioperative period. Presence of metabolic syndrome, defined as the coexistence of type 2 diabetes and cardiovascular disease risk factors (e.g., hyperglycemia, dyslipidemia, hypertension, and abdominal obesity), is associated with an increased risk of postoperative complications. Optimization of any of these components prior to surgery is recommended. Baseline data will also help with perioperative management (Böhmer & Wappler, 2017).

▶ Preparation of the Operating Room and Staff

To best prepare the patient with obesity for cardiac surgery, the operating room (OR) staff and anesthesia provider must be aware of the patient's weight, as the surgical table must be able to accommodate it; two tables pushed together may be required. Need for additional padding, linen, and lifting equipment should be anticipated. Additional staff may be required to assist with patient transfer and proper positioning. Appropriately sized monitoring and safety equipment (e.g., blood pressure cuff and sequential compression sleeves) should be procured. Because of the conical shape of the upper arm that may exist in patients with obesity, it may not be possible to place the blood pressure cuff in that location; alternative sites may need to be considered (e.g., lower arm or lower leg). Allotment of additional surgical time should be anticipated. Surgical procedures of obese patients can extend longer than anticipated (Kadry et al., 2014).

Additional equipment may be needed to administer anesthesia to a patient with obesity. Needles with extra length may be required for administration of any epidural anesthesia or nerve blocks as well as ultrasound equipment to determine optimal placement in the epidural or intrathecal space (Elsharkawy, Sonny, & Chin,

2017). Because of the increased amount of adipose tissue in the pharyngeal walls, upper airway collapse may result; difficulty with bag-valve-mask ventilation, intubation, or both may be realized (Turnbull et al., 2017; Whyte & Gibson, 2018).

Morbidly obese patients may pose additional challenges to anesthetists in the perioperative and postoperative settings because of their increased cardiopulmonary complications (Chung, 2016). A BMI greater than 40 kg/m^2 is shown to be associated with increased morbidity and mortality from thromboembolic, infectious, and general surgical complications (Chung et al., 2016). Superobese patients (BMI >50 kg/m^2) have been shown to not be candidates for ambulatory surgery (Chung et al., 2016).

Supine positioning during cardiac surgery may further decrease FRC. Compliance of the chest wall and lungs also decreases when the patient with obesity is in a supine position. This may result in hypoventilation and barotrauma while on mechanical ventilation. Prone positioning is known to be beneficial in the obese patient population by increasing FRC, lung compliance, and oxygenation intraoperatively (Shah, Wong, Wong, & Chung, 2016).

Patients with OSA will have further decreases in lung volume and compliance when they receive anesthesia. This places them at greater risk for the development of atelectasis during the induction of anesthesia. An increase in intrapulmonary shunting can result. During induction, these patients are also at increased risk for aspiration due to the aforementioned GI changes associated with obesity.

▶ Postoperative Care

Patients typically remain intubated for a period of time following cardiac surgery. It is common for lung volumes to remain low and for atelectasis to be present following open heart surgery. This results in increased intrapulmonary shunting and consequent hypoxemia (Parida & Bidkar, 2016). There remains a dilemma as to which mode of ventilation to use (pressure or volume controlled) because of the risk of ventilation-induced injury.

No differences between these two modes of ventilation are reported; however, advanced pressure modes of ventilation have a theoretical advantage over conventional modes (Nouri, Sohrabi, Moradian, & Ghiasi, 2016; Parida & Bidkar, 2016). It is suggested that the goal of mechanical ventilation focus on using peak inspiratory pressures and positive end-expiratory pressure that are adequate to open and keep open collapsed alveoli. Extubation failure is not uncommon in the immediate postoperative period for patients with obesity. This is especially true of patients with chronic obstructive pulmonary disease. Advanced pressure modes assure a target tidal volume delivery at reasonable pressures, helping reduce atelectasis and pulmonary edema postoperatively (Parida & Bidkar, 2016).

The incidence of atelectasis is reported to be more common following cardiopulmonary bypass procedures than in other surgical procedures. Atelectasis correlates well with intrapulmonary shunt (Parida & Bidkar, 2016). Use of noninvasive ventilation methods such as continuous positive airway pressure (CPAP) and bilevel positive airway pressure (BiPAP) is reported to decrease the incidence of atelectasis and intubation in patients with obesity (Band & Marcolini, 2018; Shah et al., 2016). Because of the increased work of breathing that is typically present in postoperative patients with obesity (Steier et al., 2014), the positive pressure associated with BiPAP may be beneficial. Because of the changes in lung volumes and the enhancement of these effects when placed in a supine position, patients with obesity should be in a semi-sitting position unless contraindicated (Steier et al., 2014; Türk, Aydoğdu, & Gürsel, 2018).

During handoff from the OR, the intensive care unit (ICU) nurse should inquire about any difficulties encountered during intubation. If these were present, diligence should be exercised when determining readiness for extubation. Once successfully extubated, strategies should be implemented to prevent postoperative respiratory complications. Since obese patients have a lower total lung capacity and breathe at a lower FRC, obese patients are much more sensitive to the demands of breathing postoperatively (e.g., developing atelectasis and other changes in lung volumes) (Steier et al., 2014).

Patients with obesity, OSA, or both may be more sensitive to respiratory depression associated with the administration of sedatives and opioids (Chung et al., 2016; Tsai & Schumann, 2016). There is a potential for airway obstruction to occur when sedated. Patients should be monitored with pulse oximetry and an end-tidal CO_2 detector (capnography).

Complications of cardiac surgery reported in the literature include increased length of stay (Almashrafi, Elmonstri, & Aylin, 2016; Azarfarin, Ashouri, Totonchi, Bakhshandeh, & Yaghoubi, 2014), increased mortality rates (Azarfarin et al., 2014; Gelijns et al., 2014), sternal wound dehiscence (Orgill, 2018), wound infection (Almashrafi et al., 2016; Gelijns et al., 2014), mediastinitis (Gelijns et al., 2014), readmission to the ICU (Gelijns et al., 2014), acute kidney injury (30% of patients) (O'Neal, Shaw, & Billings, 2016), atrial fibrillation (Melduni et al., 2015), and increased prothrombotic state (Chung et al., 2016; Kindo et al., 2014).

There are conflicting data on the incidence of complications and mortality rates following cardiac surgery when comparing obese patients with those who are not. Some data suggest no difference in the incidence of these complications or mortality rates in patients with obesity, while other data suggest a statistically significant increased incidence of these outcome variables (Ghanta et al., 2017; Hysi et al., 2014). The former has been called the "obesity paradox" (Akin & Nienaber, 2015; Lavie, Carbone, & Agarwal, 2018). Recent data suggest leaner patients have higher mortality rates than those with higher BMIs (Carnethon & Khan, 2017).

▶ Summary

Nurses caring for patients with obesity who underwent cardiac surgery procedures should anticipate the presence of and observe for signs and symptoms of these complications and promptly intervene if they manifest. Early recognition and prompt intervention are essential to optimize patient outcomes.

🔍 CASE STUDY

G. S., a 55-year-old female patient with a history of metabolic syndrome and OSA, was admitted to the ICU immediately following coronary artery bypass grafting. Her intraoperative course was uncomplicated. She is intubated and on mechanical ventilation. She is receiving a continuous infusion of morphine as well as dexmedetomidine to prevent inadvertent extubation and promote comfort.

Critical Thinking Questions

1. How should the ICU nurse position this patient?
2. For which complications should the ICU observe?
3. What changes in respiratory physiology should the ICU nurse anticipate?

Answers to Critical Thinking Questions

1. The patient should be positioned in a semi-sitting position to mitigate intrapulmonary shunting that is associated with a supine position in patients with obesity.
2. The nurse should observe for early signs of wound infection, acute renal failure, and atrial fibrillation. The nurse should also be aware that in the event of premature extubation, the patient may have a difficult reintubation.
3. Respiratory parameters the ICU should anticipate include hypercarbia, increased oxygen consumption, decreased chest wall and lung compliance, decreased chest wall expansion, decreased tidal volume, increased respiratory rate, increased work of breathing, mild hypoxia, increased shunt, and signs and symptoms of OSA.

Self-Assessment Questions

1. Which is a cardiovascular change associated with obesity?
   A. Decreased cardiac output
   B. Decreased metabolic demand
   C. Increased vascular resistance
   D. Increased stroke volume

2. Which is an etiologic factor of hypertension and cardiomegaly associated with obesity?
   A. Increased cardiac output
   B. Decreased stroke volume
   C. Increased myocardial workload
   D. Decreased vascular resistance

3. Which is a respiratory change associated with obesity?
   A. Decreased respiratory rate
   B. Increased pulmonary compliance
   C. Increased oxygen consumption
   D. Decreased pulmonary blood volume

4. Which is an etiologic factor associated with restrictive lung disease associated with obesity?
   A. Increased chest wall compliance
   B. Increased intra-abdominal pressure

   C. Decreased intrapulmonary shunting
   D. Decreased expiratory reserve volume

5. Which is a sequela of obstructive sleep apnea?
   A. Vasodilation of the pulmonary vasculature
   B. Low carbon dioxide levels
   C. Vasodilation of the systemic vasculature
   D. Low oxygen tension

6. Which should the nurse anticipate affecting the pharmacokinetics of drugs administered to patients with obesity?
   A. Increased total body water
   B. Decreased volume of distribution
   C. Increased cardiac output
   D. Decreased renal blood flow

7. Which should be anticipated to occur upon induction of anesthesia in the patient with obesity undergoing cardiac surgery?
   A. Increased chest wall compliance
   B. Decreased functional residual capacity
   C. Increased lung compliance
   D. Decreased aspiration risk

8. Which complication is a patient with obesity likely to experience in the immediate

postoperative period following cardiac surgery?
A. Ventilator-associated barotrauma
B. Wound infection
C. Atelectasis
D. Atrial fibrillation

9. Which occurs as a result of increased cardiac output and left ventricular hypertrophy associated with obesity?
A. Heart failure
B. Ventricular tachycardia
C. Decreased myocardial oxygen demand
D. Ventilation-perfusion (V/Q) mismatch

10. Which is a gastrointestinal change associated with obesity?
A. Increased intra-abdominal pressure
B. Increased gastric motility
C. Decreased gastric emptying
D. Decreased fasting gastric volume

Answers to Self-Assessment Questions

1. D. **increased stroke volume**
Rationale: Stroke volume increases to meet metabolic demands. Cardiac output and metabolic demand also increase in response to obesity.

2. A. **increased cardiac output**
Rationale: Hypertension and cardiomegaly result from the increases in cardiac output and stroke volume, leading to heart remodeling.

3. C. **increased oxygen consumption**
Rationale: There is an increase in oxygen consumption due to the increase in metabolic demand. Patients with obesity typically have a lower tidal volume, which is associated with an increased respiratory rate. Obesity also leads to increased carbon dioxide production and increased oxygen consumption. There is also an associated decrease in chest wall compliance due to the extra weight around the patient's ribs. The decrease in chest wall compliance results in increased pulmonary vascular volume.

4. B. **increased intra-abdominal pressure**
Rationale: Restrictive lung disease may develop in patients with obesity from increases in intra-abdominal pressure. There is also an associated decrease in compliance of the chest wall and increased intrapulmonary shunting in patients with obesity.

5. D. **low oxygen tension**
Rationale: Obesity can lead to obstructive sleep apnea, which can result in chronically low oxygen tension. It also causes vasoconstriction of the pulmonary vasculature and increased carbon dioxide levels.

6. C. **increased cardiac output**
Rationale: Distribution and elimination of drugs are affected as a result of obesity-related increased cardiac output.

7. B. **decreased functional residual capacity**
Rationale: Supine positioning during cardiac surgery may further decrease functional residual capacity. There is an increased risk of aspiration, and a decrease in chest wall and lung compliance when the patient is in the supine position.

8. C. **atelectasis**
Rationale: Lung volumes may remain low following cardiac surgery, which can result in atelectasis. Ventilator-associated barotrauma is not a complication associated with cardiac surgery in the immediate postoperative time. Wound infection and atrial fibrillation are known complications of cardiac surgery but there are conflicting data regarding obese versus nonobese patients.

9. A. **heart failure**
Rationale: Dilation of the left ventricle occurs due to increases in cardiac output and increased venous return; these lead to ventricular hypertrophy. Obese patients have higher resting cardiac filling pressures that result in cardiac remodeling, ventricular dysfunction, and subsequent heart failure.

10. A. **increased intra-abdominal pressure**
Rationale: Obesity results in an increase in intra-abdominal pressure, increased fasting gastric volume, and increased gastric emptying.

CLINICAL INQUIRY BOX

Question: What is the effect of obesity on cost following cardiac surgery?

Reference: Ghanta, R. K., La Por, D. J., Zhang, Q., Devarkonda, V., Isbell, J. M., Yarboro, L. T., . . . Ailawadi, G. (2017). Obesity increases risk-adjusted morbidity, mortality, and cost following cardiac surgery. *Journal of the American Heart Association.* doi:10.1161/JAHA.116.003831

Objective: To determine if there is an increase in cost as a result of obesity following cardiac surgery.

Method: Medical record review of 13,637 consecutive patients who underwent coronary artery bypass grafting, valve surgery, or a combination of these procedures comprise the Society of Thoracic Surgery database.

Results: Morbidly obese patients experienced approximately 60% higher mortality than their normal weight counterparts, greater than 2-fold increase in renal failure, and 6.5-fold increase in deep sternal wound infection. Higher body mass index was significantly associated with mortality and major morbidity. Total hospital costs increased with body mass index (17.2% higher costs in this patient population).

Conclusion: Higher body mass index is associated with increased mortality, significant morbidity, and increased costs of hospital care.

References

Acosta, A., Camilleri, M., Shin, A., Vazquez-Roque, M., Iturrino, J., Lanza, I. R., . . . Zinsmeister, A. R. (2015). Association of *UCP-3*-rs-1626521 with obesity and stomach functions in humans. *Obesity (Silver Spring), 23*(4), 898–906.

Akin, I., & Nienaber, C. A. (2015). "Obesity paradox" in coronary artery disease. *World Journal of Cardiology, 7*(10), 603.

Almashrafi, A., Elmontsri, M., & Aylin, P. (2016). Systematic review of factors influencing length of stay in ICU after adult cardiac surgery. *BMC Health Services Research, 16*(1), 318.

Alpert, M. A., Lavie, C. J., Agrawal, H., Aggarwal, K. B., & Kumar, S. A. (2014). Obesity and heart failure: Epidemiology, pathophysiology, clinical manifestations, and management. *Translational Research, 164*(4), 345–356.

Azarfarin, R., Ashouri, N., Totonchi, Z., Bakhshandeh, H., & Yaghoubi, A. (2014). Factors influencing prolonged ICU stay after open heart surgery. *Research in Cardiovascular Medicine, 3*(4), e20159.

Backman, H., Eriksson, B., Hedman, L., Stridsman, C., Jansson, S. A., Sovijärvi, A., . . . Lundbäck, B. (2016). Restrictive spirometric pattern in the general adult population: Methods of defining the condition and consequences on prevalence. *Respiratory Medicine, 120*, 116–123.

Band, M., & Marcolini, E. (2018). Airway and ventilation management. In *Neurocritical care for the advanced practice clinician* (pp. 387–406). New York, NY: Springer.

Böhmer, A. B., & Wappler, F. (2017). Preoperative evaluation and preparation of the morbidly obese patient. *Current Opinion in Anesthesiology, 30*(1), 126–132.

Borrell, L. N., & Samuel, L. (2014). Body mass index categories and mortality risk in US adults: The effect of overweight and obesity on advancing death. *American Journal of Public Health, 104*(3), 512–519.

Carnethon, M. R., & Khan, S. S. (2017). An apparent obesity paradox in cardiac surgery. *Circulation, 135*(9), 864–866.

Chung, F., Abdullah, H., & Liao, P. (2016). STOP BANG questionnaire. *Chest, 149*(4), 631–638.

Demirel, I., Bolat, E., & Altun, A. Y. (2017). Obesity and anesthesia management. *Current Topics in Anesthesiology.* Retrieved from https://www.intechopen.com/books/current-topics-in-anesthesiology/obesity-and-anesthesia-management

Elsharkawy, H., Sonny, A., & Chin K. J. (2017). Localization of epidural space: A review of available technologies. *Journal of Anaesthesiology Clinical Pharmacology, 33*(1), 16–27.

Feakins, R. M. (2016). Obesity and metabolic syndrome: Pathological effects on the gastrointestinal tract. *Histopathology, 68*(5), 630–640.

Gelijns, A. C., Moskowitz, A. J., Acker, M. A., Argenziano, M., Geller, N. L., Puskas, J. D., . . . Miller, M. A. (2014). Management practices and major infections after cardiac surgery. *Journal of the American College of Cardiology, 64*(4), 372–381.

Ghanta, R. K., LaPar, D. J., Zhang, Q., Devarkonda, V., Isbell, J. M., Yarboro, L. T., . . . Ailawadi, G. (2017). Obesity increases risk-adjusted morbidity, mortality, and cost following cardiac surgery. *Journal of the American Heart Association, 6*(3), e003831.

Graham, C., Mullen, A., & Whelan, K. (2015). Obesity and the gastrointestinal microbiota: A review of associations and mechanisms. *Nutrition Reviews, 73*(6), 376–385.

Gupta, K., Prasad, A., Nagappa, M., Wong, J., Abrahamyan, L., & Chung, F. F. (2018). Risk factors for opioid-induced respiratory depression and failure to rescue: A review. *Current Opinion in Anesthesiology, 31*(1), 110–119.

Hales, C. M., Carroll, M. D., Fryar, C. D., & Ogden, C. L. *Prevalence of obesity among adults and youth: United*

States, 2015–2016. Retrieved from https://www.cdc.gov/nchs/data/databriefs/db288.pdf

Hall, M. E., do Carmo, J. M., da Silva, A. A., Juncos, L. A., Wang, Z., & Hall, J. E. (2014). Obesity, hypertension, and chronic kidney disease. *International Journal of Nephrology and Renovascular Disease*, *7*, 75.

Hartle, A., McCormack, T., Carlisle, J., Anderson, S., Pichel, A., Beckett, N., . . . Heagerty, A. (2016). The measurement of adult blood pressure and management of hypertension before elective surgery. *Anaesthesia, 71*(3), 326–337.

Hysi, I., Picon, C., Guesnier, L., Gautier, L., Renaut, C., Geronimi, H., . . . Fabre, O. (2014). Results of elective cardiac surgery in patients with severe obesity (body mass index >35 kg/m²). *Archives of Cardiovascular Disease, 107*(1), 540–545.

Kadry, B., Press, C. D., Alosh, H., Opper, I. M., Orsini, J., Popov, I. A., . . . Macario, A. (2014). Obesity increases operating room times in patients undergoing primary hip arthroplasty: A retrospective cohort analysis. *Peer J, 2*, e530.

Kindo, M., Minh, T. H., Gereli, S., Meyer, N., Schaeffer, M., Perrier, S., . . . Mazzucotelli, P. (2014). The prothrombotic paradox of severe obesity after cardiac surgery under cardiopulmonary bypass. *Thrombosis Research 134*(2), 346–353.

Knibbe, C. A., Brill, M. J., van Rongen, A., Diepstraten, J., van der Graaf, P. H., & Danhof, M. (2015). Drug disposition in obesity: Toward evidence-based dosing. *Annual Review of Pharmacology and Toxicology, 55*, 149–167.

Lavie, C. J., Carbone, S., & Agarwal, M. A. (2018). An obesity paradox with myocardial infarction in the elderly. *Nutrition, 46*, 122–123.

Mandviwala, T., Khalid, U., & Deswal, A. (2016). Obesity and cardiovascular disease: A risk factor or a risk marker? *Current Atherosclerosis Reports, 18*(5), 21.

Melduni, R. M., Schaff, H. V., Bailey, K. R., Cha, S. S., Ammash, N. M., Seward, J. B., & Gersh, B. J. (2015). Implications of new-onset atrial fibrillation after cardiac surgery on long-term prognosis: A community-based study. *American Heart Journal, 170*(4), 659–668.

Mitchell, A. B., Cole, J. W., McArdle, P. F., Cheng, Y. C., Ryan, K. A., Sparks, M. J., . . . Kittner, S. J. (2015). Obesity increases risk of ischemic stroke in young adults. *Stroke, 46*(6), 1690–1692.

Nouri, J. M., Sohrabi, B., Moradian, S. T., & Ghiasi, S. M. S. (2017). Effect of adaptive support ventilation weaning mode in conventional or standard methods on respiratory and hemodynamic performance indices: A randomized clinical trial. *Trauma Monthly, 22*(5), e37663.

O'Neal, J. B., Shaw, A. D., & Billings, F. T. (2016). Acute kidney injury following cardiac surgery: Current understanding and future directions. *Critical Care, 20*(1), 187.

Orgill, D. P. (2018). *Surgical management of sternal wound complications*. Retrieved from https://www.uptodate.com/contents/surgical-management-of-sternal-wound-complications

Parida, S., & Bidkar, P. U. (2016). Advanced pressure control modes of ventilation in cardiac surgery: Scanty evidence or unexplored terrain? *Indian Journal of Critical Care Medicine, 20*(3), 169.

Raveendran, R., Wong, J., Singh, M., Wong, D. T., & Chung, F. (2017). Obesity hypoventilation syndrome, sleep apnea, overlap syndrome: Perioperative management to prevent complications. *Current Opinion in Anesthesiology, 30*(6), 146–155.

Rivas, E., Arismendi, E., Agustí, A., Sanchez, M., Delgado, S., Gistau, C., . . . Rodriguez-Roisin, R. (2015). Ventilation/perfusion distribution abnormalities in morbidly obese subjects before and after bariatric surgery. *Chest, 147*(4), 1127–1134.

Shah, U., Wong, J., Wong, D. T., & Chung, F. (2016). Preoxygenation and intraoperative ventilation strategies in obese patients: A comprehensive review. *Current Opinion in Anesthesiology, 29*(1), 109–118.

Shetty, S., & Parthasarathy, S. (2015). Obesity hypoventilation syndrome. *Current Pulmonology Reports, 4*(1), 42–55.

State of Obesity. (2004–2018). *The healthcare costs of obesity*. Retrieved from https://state of obesity.org/healthcare-costs-obesity

Steier, J., Lunt, A., Hart, N., Polkey, M. I., & Moxham, J. (2014). Observational study of the effect of obesity on lung volumes. *Thorax, 69*(8), 752–759.

Tsai, A., & Schumann, R. (2016). Morbid obesity and perioperative complications. *Current Opinion in Anesthesiology, 29*(1), 103–108.

Türk, M., Aydoğdu, M., & Gürsel, G. (2018). Effects of modes, obesity, and body position on non-invasive positive pressure ventilation success in the intensive care unit: A randomized controlled study. *Turkish Thoracic Journal, 19*(1), 28.

Turnbull, C. D., Wang, S. H., Manuel, A. R., Keenan, B. T., McIntyre, A. G., Schwab, R. J., . . . Stradling, J. R. (2017). Relationships between MRI fat distribution and sleep apnea and obesity hypoventilation syndrome in very obese patients. *Sleep and Breathing*. doi:10.1007/s11325-017-1599

Whyte, A., & Gibson, D. (2018). Imaging of adult obstructive sleep apnoea. *European Journal of Radiology, 102*, 176–187.

World Health Organization. (n.d.) *Obesity*. Retrieved from https://www.who.int/topics/obesity/en/

Web Resources

Centers for Disease Control and Prevention: *Overweight and Obesity*; contains several obesity facts, including obesity statistics by state: http://www.cdc.gov/obesity/data/adult.html

National Heart, Lung, and Blood Institute: *Calculate Your Body Mass Index* (BMI calculator); uses standard and metric for entries: http://www.nhlbi.nih.gov/health/educational/lose_wt/BMI/bmicalc.htm

CHAPTER 22

Cardiogenetics

Joyce King

▶ Introduction

Typically, intensive care unit (ICU) nurses do not consider genetics an important part of their requisite knowledge base to care for critically ill patients. Many nursing programs do not include genetics in the curriculum and continuing education opportunities in the field of genetics, specifically, cardiogenetics is limited. Although nurses are diligent in reviewing the family history with patients and their families, the usefulness of this information has not fully been utilized in nursing practice. This chapter is intended to give the ICU nurse a broad, generalized overview of genetic/genomic considerations that may be integral to their patient management. Management strategies are briefly discussed. An exhaustive review of management of conditions with a cardiogenetics basis exceeds the scope of this chapter.

▶ History

Genetics has been a cornerstone of the science of medicine for many years; however, it has only been within the past 20 years that genetics has taken a more central role in patient management.

Where did genetics begin? Gregor Mendel, an Austrian monk who observed changes in his pea plants has been named the father of modern genetics. Gregor Mendel found that when a yellow pea and a green pea were bred together, the offspring pea was always yellow. However, in the next generation of plants, green peas reappeared at a ratio of 1:3. Thus, the terms *dominant* and *recessive* inheritance were coined. Although this information was remarkable, Mendel's work did not become famous until the 20th century. Another important genetic discovery occurred in 1871 when Dr. Miescher discovered "nuclein." Through various experiments, Dr. Miescher found that he could isolate components of the cytoplasm that only contained phosphorus and nitrogen and not sulfur. "Nuclein" was later named deoxyribonucleic acid (DNA), which is now known to be the carrier of inheritance (Axelson-Fisk, 2015). More famously, in the mid-20th century, James Watson and Francis Crick discovered the double helix structure of DNA. Through these discoveries, the groundwork was laid to begin understanding how genetic instructions are encoded into the cells of all living organisms.

In 1990, the U.S. government together with international partners initiated the Human Genome Project. The project had dual goals: to determine

Original contributions by Tracey Andrews and Sonya R. Hardi

the sequence of chemical base pairs that makes up human DNA and to identify/map all of the genes found in humans from both a physical and functional standpoint. The project was declared complete in 2003. Twenty universities and research centers within the United States, United Kingdom, France, Germany, Japan, and China were used for genetic sequencing. Although the initial plan was to study all DNA, this was not done. About 8% of the human genome was not sequenced secondary to DNA complexity within heterochromatic areas (Harmon, 2010). Around the same time that the Human Genome Project was in the planning phase, forensic science was beginning the use of DNA profiling to assist with criminal investigations, paternity testing, and immigration disputes (Newton, 2008).

Genetics plays a role in many diseases including cancer, diabetes, and heart disease. Cardiogenetics is the specialized focus on genetics related to the cardiovascular system within humans. This field focuses on any condition that can have cardiovascular impact, including conduction disorders, structural abnormalities, and syndromes. Identifying the underlying genetic cause of heart disease can guide therapy. This chapter focuses on the most commonly seen disorders within the cardiac surgery practice area, specifically in cardiothoracic surgery ICUs.

▶ Genetics Terminology

In order to be able to discuss genetics, the reader should be familiar with basic genetic terms. The intent of this chapter it is not to provide exhaustive genetic information; rather, it is to encourage further study into genetic information that is pertinent to the nurse's own practice. **TABLE 22.1** provides commonly used genetic terms that should be reviewed prior to proceeding with this chapter.

▶ Family History

Pedigrees (also known as genograms) are diagrams of a family history. Family pedigrees provide a wealth of information about possible genetic links to diseases. Given that nurses are the frontline health care provider, the nurse generally is the provider that completes the patient's pedigree. Pedigree construction is relatively easy to complete and can be done as the nurse asks family history. At least three generations of both paternal and maternal family histories should be included. Some clinicians focus only on practice-specific pedigrees; this should be discouraged. Many times, syndromes that would not normally contribute to disease processes can be key to uncovering important genetic causal factors in disease diagnosis, severity, and prognosis. An example of this is Duchene muscular dystrophy (DMD), which is an X-linked genetic disorder where the mother passes on a genetic mutation to her son. It is highlighted by profound muscular weakness that progresses to death. Because of the X-link inheritance pattern, only males can be diagnosed with DMD; however, females can be carriers and can also have manifestations of this gene mutation. With regard to cardiogenetics, females with the DMD gene mutation can have dilated cardiomyopathy (DCM). Therefore, gathering as much information as possible is extremely important. Another example: A nurse is taking a family history. The patient reveals that her brother died in a single-vehicle accident at the age of 23. During further discussion, the nurse notes that several of the patient's family members have required internal cardioverter-defibrillator (ICD) implantations or have died from "heart attacks." How does the young man fit into this? There is a high suspicion for a possible arrhythmogenic basis for this young man's death. Even if disorders of family members uncovered during this interview process do not seem to be important to the overall cause of a patient's condition, making note of those disorders may actually provide invaluable insight into the patient's condition.

The 2009 Heart Failure Society of America (HFSA) guideline recommends a careful family history for three or more generations for all patients with cardiomyopathy (Hershberger et al., 2009). The initial discussion with the patient should include family history and pedigree analysis for unexplained heart failure before age 60 or sudden cardiac death in the absence of ischemic disease. Referral to a center with expertise in genetic cardiomyopathies should be considered, because these

TABLE 22.1 Common Genetic Nomenclature

Term	Definition
Allele	One of the alternative versions of a gene at a given location.
Autosomal	Refers to any of the chromosomes other than sex-determining chromosomes.
Autosomal dominant	Inheritance pattern whereby there is a 50% chance of having a mutated gene passed onto offspring.
Autosomal recessive	Inheritance pattern where offspring must receive a copy of a mutated gene from both parents in order to inherit the disease.
Chromosome	Organized packet of DNA found in the nucleus of cells. In the human, each cell contains 23 pairs of chromosomes.
Consultant	The individual who presents for genetic counseling; not necessarily the proband.
Gene	Functional and physical heredity unit passed from parent to offspring. Genes provide the code for the synthesis of proteins and are located on chromosomes.
Genotype	An individual's collection of genes.
Heterozygous	An individual who has inherited two different alleles, usually one is normal one is abnormal.
Heritability	Degree at which information contained within genes can be transmitted from parent to offspring.
Heterogeneity	Medical condition that may have one or more etiologies.
Homozygous	Where an individual inherits the same alleles for a particular gene from both parents.
Locus	The site or location of a specific gene on a chromosome.
Mitochondrial inheritance	Mitochondria also have DNA that is inherited and can be mutated. This inheritance pattern is passed on by mothers because during fertilization, only the nucleus of the sperm enters the egg and none of the sperm mitochondria.
Pedigree	A diagram showing genetic relationships and medical history of a family using standardized symbols and terminology.
Penetrance	How often, within a population, a gene is expressed when it is present.

(continues)

TABLE 22.1 Common Genetic Nomenclature	*(continued)*
Phenotype	Observable characteristics of gene expression; clinical presentation.
Polymorphism	Polymorphism is extremely common; it is a kind of variation related to biodiversity, genetic variation, and adaptation. Examples include human blood groups and Rh factor
Proband	Affected individual through whom a family with a genetic disorder is determined.
X-linked	Genes on the X chromosome are said to be X-linked. Mutations of these genes can be inherited as recessive or dominant. Most X-linked disorders are passed on by mothers to their sons.

Data from United States Library of Medicine: Genetics Home Reference, 2014.

centers can provide comprehensive genetic counseling and testing. This is especially true when dealing with syndrome-related disease. Finally, these centers often maintain a comprehensive database that assists in research and treatment advances.

When completing family histories, there are cardiogenetic red flags to watch for during the interview process, including:

- "Heart attack" in a person younger than 50 years old (could be cardiomyopathy, aortic dissection, or arrhythmias)
- Two or more closely related family members on the same side of the family with the same or related condition (e.g., heart disease, arrhythmia, stroke)
- Unexplained sudden death (could be indicative of myocardial infarction [MI], cardiomyopathy, arrhythmia, aortic dissection)
- An individual who has been diagnosed with a specific type of hereditary disease (e.g., hypertrophic cardiomyopathy [HCM], Marfan syndrome)
- Coronary heart disease (CHD) at an early age (males younger than 55; women younger than 65)
- Two or more family members with congenital heart defects/disease
- Family history of symptoms and procedures suspicious for hereditary arrhythmia syndrome: syncope, seizures, multiple family members with pacemaker/implantable cardioverter defibrillator, sudden death, or sudden infant death syndrome

▶ Clinical Screening

Screening is an important consideration when dealing with cardiomyopathies. Genetic testing has moved to the forefront of clinical practice. Several disease-specific testing panels for cardiomyopathies are commercially available (McDonald et al., 2017). Dilated cardiomyopathy, HCM, arrhythmogenic right ventricular cardiomyopathy (ARVC), and other cardiomyopathies often are present in asymptomatic people. Progressive disease may occur within a relatively short period of time in those asymptomatic people; however, they may already have begun to have electrocardiographic or echocardiographic findings consistent with cardiomyopathy. As such, clinical screening protocols have been developed.

The 2009 HFSA genetic evaluation of cardiomyopathy guideline recommends the following screening for first-degree relatives of patients with DCM. This screening should include history (with special focus on heart failure symptoms, arrhythmias, presyncope, and syncope), physical examination (special attention to cardiac/skeletal muscle systems), electrocardiogram (ECG), echocardiogram, and serum CK-MM. Even though initial screening may not reveal any problems, asymptomatic patients should be re-screened at 3- to 5-year intervals beginning in childhood or at any time symptoms begin to appear. Repeat clinical screening at 1 year is suggested in first-degree relatives with any abnormal clinical screening tests (Hershberger et al., 2009).

▶ Genetic Counseling/Testing

Genetic and family counseling is recommended for all patients with cardiac-related genetic disorders. According to McDonald and colleagues (2017), genetic counsellors are fundamental to the health care of patients and their families that have inherited diseases. Because of the complexity of genetic testing/counseling, referral to specialized genetic cardiomyopathy/aortopathy centers should take place. All patients who are offered genetic testing should receive genetic counseling, including the explanation of genetic disease and risk, test sensitivities, heritability, and possible test outcomes, including the possibility of inconclusive or false-positive/-negative results. Genetic testing should be considered for the one most clearly affected person in a family to facilitate family screening and management.

Counseling and explanation of the Genetic Information Nondiscrimination Act, a U.S. Act of Congress, was passed in 2008 to prevent the use of genetic information in health insurance and employment for all U.S. citizens, except for those employed by the U.S. Armed Forces. Screening the most affected person in the family increases the likelihood of detecting a relevant mutation. This premise is held with all conditions involving cardiogenetics as well. For those patients with DCM and prominent conduction system disease, a family history of premature unexpected sudden death, or any combination of these, the European Heart Rhythm Association recommended through their consensus statement that comprehensive or targeted (LMNA and SCN5A) gene testing be performed (Ackerman et al. 2011).

▶ Cardiac Generalizations

It is not new news that heart disease "runs in families." Recent research indicates that genetic causes of heart failure is associated with many syndromes, including hypertrophic, arrhythmogenic, and dilated cardiomyopathies. Understanding the underlying genetic cause of a disorder can help to guide therapy.

Most inherited cardiovascular diseases (CVDs) have an autosomal dominant pattern indicating a 50% chance of a person passing a disorder on to their offspring. Characteristically, a "traditional" inheritance pattern is seen with genetic disorders. This, however, is not true in CVD genetics. A lack of a traditional inheritance pattern often makes prognosis difficult. This does not mean that diagnosis will be difficult, as long as the health care provider pays close attention to the family history and doesn't overlook an individual who typically does not have a high cardiovascular risk (e.g., young women, non-obese patients).

As defined in the genetics terminology table, penetrance refers to the frequency with which a heritable trait or condition coded by a gene is manifested in individuals carrying the identified gene. Specifically, in medical genetics, penetrance refers to the proportion of people with a genetic mutation who exhibit clinical symptoms. Consider the following example. If a disorder is passed through an autosomal dominant mode of inheritance, this means that there is a 50% chance of passing on the disorder. Some genes have different penetrance levels; these levels are measured in percentages. If the autosomal dominant gene mutation has 95% penetrance, then 95% of those who inherited the gene mutation will develop the disease. In many genetic disorders, this is a relatively clear-cut view of penetrance. Unfortunately, cardiovascular genetics does not fit that pattern. Incomplete penetrance is often seen. This means that people who carry the genetic mutation do not always develop the disorder. The basis for this variation has been found to be multifactorial where the environment, diet, gender, socioeconomic status, and other factors may contribute to this incomplete penetrance. It is important to note, that individuals who have the gene mutation but do not express it can still transmit this gene to their children who may express the gene and develop the disease.

▶ Cardiomyopathies

Cardiomyopathies are diseases of the heart muscle that result in structural and functional abnormalities that result in failure of myocardial performance. This can be a mechanical dysfunction leading to congestive heart failure, or can result in life-threatening arrhythmias.

There are two categories of cardiomyopathies: primary and secondary. Primary cardiomyopathy means that the heart is the main organ affected; secondary cardiomyopathies are a component of a systemic or multi organ disorder. The American Heart Association classification subdivided cardiomyopathies into genetic, mixed, and acquired forms (Arbustini et al., 2014). The most commonly known cardiomyopathies include DCM, HCM, left ventricular non-compaction cardiomyopathy (LVNCC), ARVC, and restrictive cardiomyopathy (RCM). Hypertrophic cardiomyopathy, LVNCC, and ARVC are classified as genetic cardiomyopathies. Other common genetic cardiomyopathies include the 5'-AMP-activated protein kinase subunit gamma-2 (PRKAG2) gene, Danon glycogen storage diseases, conduction defects, mitochondrial myopathies, and ion channel disorders. Dilated cardiomyopathy and RCM are classified as mixed cardiomyopathies. Acquired cardiomyopathies include myocarditis, Takotsubo, peripartum, and tachycardia-induced cardiomyopathies. Cardiomyopathies are clinically heterogeneous diseases where factors such as gender, age of onset, risk for heart failure, and likelihood of sudden death are different among the different subtypes. For example a patient with DCN may have a mildly enlarged and mildly dysfunctional left ventricle yet develop a life-threatening ventricular arrhythmia while another patient with an extremely enlarged and dysfunctional left ventricle may be at low risk for developing an arrhythmia. The MOGE(S) classification system, published in 2013, not only includes phenotypic characterization of cardiomyopathies, but also incorporates knowledge regarding genetic mutations, acquired causes of cardiomyopathies (i.e., intramyocardial inflammation, viral infections), and other conditions that may induce a cardiomyopathy (i.e. storage diseases, toxicity). The system is based on the following five attributes in the description of cardiomyopathies.

1. Morphofunctional characteristics: provides the clinical diagnosis (e.g., M_D = dilated cardiomyopathy)

2. Organ involvement: Indicates if heart and/or extracardiac involvement is present (e.g., O_{H+K} = heart and kidney involvement)

3. Genetic/familial inheritance: Nature of genetic transmission (e.g., G_{AD} = autosomal dominant)

4. *Etiology*: Description of a specific cause (e.g., E_{G-MYH7})

5. (*S*)tage: Describes the functional status according to the New York Heart Association (NYHA) functional class (I to IV) (e.g., S_{C-II} = Stage C/NYHA Functional Status II) (Arbustini, 2014)

Dilated Cardiomyopathy

Dilated cardiomyopathy is characterized by ventricular dilation and progressive contractile dysfunction usually associated with ventricular hypertrophy. Frequently, despite a thorough evaluation, the specific etiology cannot be determined. Increasingly familial or genetic forms are being identified although DCM can result from a variety of acquired causes including myocarditis, alcohol and other toxins, peripartum cardiomyopathy, iron overload from multiple transfusions, and superphysiologic stress (e.g., hyperthyroidism, excess catecholamines). Dilated cardiomyopathy is one of the main causative factors for congestive heart failure (CHF) as well as a common diagnosis in patients referred for cardiac transplantation. Dilated cardiomyopathy can occur at any age, although it most often occurs between the ages of 20 and 50, is diagnosed more frequently in the African-American population, and has a higher prevalence in men than in women. The genetic type of DCM is called familial cardiomyopathy. Some studies indicate that 30% to 35% of what was initially diagnosed as idiopathic DCM may be familial DCM. Thus far, more than 40 genes have been shown to be associated with DCM. (Das et al., 2015)

Most familial DCM is transmitted in an autosomal dominant inheritance pattern although X-linked, autosomal recessive, and mitochondrial inheritance patterns also occur. Mestroni and colleagues (1999) demonstrated the spectrum of familial DCM in a study that evaluated 350 patients with DCM and 281 of their relatives from 60 families. This study identified subtypes of DCM. These subtypes include autosomal dominant DCM with normal skeletal muscle examination/histology, autosomal recessive DCM (16%) with younger age of onset and rapid progression to death or transplant, X-linked (10%) in males with severe progressive heart failure associated with mutations of the dystrophin gene, a form of autosomal dominant DCM (7.7%) associated with subclinical skeletal muscle disease with variable levels of serum CK-MM and with dystrophic changes on skeletal muscle biopsy, familial DCM associated with conduction disorders (2.6%), and unclassified forms (7.7%) (Ackerman et al., 2011).

DCM Genes

Thirty percent of familial DCM cases are caused by abnormalities involving sarcomere protein. Sarcomere genes play a role in muscular development and function. The most common mutations have been identified in the beta myosin heavy chain (MYH7), alpha myosin heavy chain (MYH6), cardiac troponin T (TNNT2), titin (TTN), alpha-tropomyosin (TPM1), and cardiac troponin C (TNNC1) genes. Different mutations in these genes can also cause HCM, which is discussed later in this chapter. Other genes beyond sarcomeric involvement are also documented. The most common mutations have been found in laminin-alpha 4 (LAMA4), vinculin (VCL), ABCC9, delta-sarcoglycan (SGCD), and the presenilins (PSEN1 and PSEN 2). LMNA mutations occur in 4% to 8% of DCM cases and are associated with conduction system defects and confer a more ominous prognosis, including sudden cardiac death. LMNA cardiomyopathy usually occurs with heart block (first degree that progresses to second then third degree), supraventricular arrhythmias (atrial fibrillation/flutter), and sick sinus syndrome, with progressively worsening ventricular arrhythmias including ventricular tachycardia and fibrillation. Dilated cardiomyopathy can occur at any point in the development of conduction system disease. Most patients with this mutation will require pacemaker insertion. SCN5A is a gene that codes for sodium channels

therefore mutations in this gene lead to conduction disorders and ventricular dysfunction. Sinoatrial node dysfunction and atrial arrhythmias are also common. In a report from Olson and colleagues (2005), 27% of patients with SCN5A mutations had early features of DCM (mean age of diagnosis: 20), 38% had DCM (mean age of diagnosis: 48), and 43% had atrial fibrillation (AF) (mean age of diagnosis: 28).

X-linked DCM transmission is also documented. Familial DCM that is transmitted as an X-linked trait most often results from mutations in Xp21, the dystrophin gene, a cytoskeletal protein that provides structural support to the myocyte. Most dystrophin mutations produce either Duchenne or Becker muscular dystrophy, both of which are associated with cardiac involvement. Another X-linked DCM gene is tafazzin, a gene that is associated with Barth syndrome. This syndrome is characterized by DCM, weakness in skeletal muscles, and neutropenia. Autosomal recessive transmission is rare but still occurs. Mutations in the ALMS1 gene on chromosome 2p13 produces the most common autosomal recessive disorder with cardiac involvement, Alström syndrome. Alström syndrome is characterized by multiple organ dysfunction, including DCM (Bozkurt et al., 2016).

Evaluation of DCM

It is recommended that in patients with idiopathic DCM a 3-generational family history should be obtained to assist in the diagnosis of familial DCM. It is also recommended that first-degree relatives of patients with familial DCM be evaluated with serial echocardiographic screening. After identification of a DCM-causative mutation, family members should also receive mutation-specific genetic testing. Genetic testing should be done in conjunction with genetic counseling.

Treatment of DCM

Medical therapy is recommended based on the cardiac phenotype outlined in general guidelines provided by heart failure experts and not by finding a specific genetic mutation. Exclusion to this would be in the event of DCM with associated conduction disorders. Patients who have idiopathic DCM or those with known desmin or LMNA mutations should be considered for prophylactic pacemaker insertion. Early treatment with angiotensin-converting enzyme (ACE) inhibitors has been shown to slow progression of LV enlargement in patients who have not shown evidence of decreased LV function; the greatest efficacy has only been shown with those patients with LV ejection fraction (LVEF) of less than 35% to 40%. Some experts have recommended initiation of ACE inhibitor or beta blocker therapy with early signs of familial DCM; however, this approach has not been adopted in major society guidelines.

Hypertrophic Cardiomyopathy

Hypertrophic cardiomyopathy is a common genetic cardiac disorder with an incidence of 1 in 500 individuals. It is characterized by myocardial hypertrophy, decreased left ventricular compliance and in some cases ventricular outflow obstruction. Hypertrophic cardiomyopathy is a major cause of sudden cardiac death (SCD) in young people (i.e., younger than 30 years) and is the most common cause of SCD in young athletes, accounting for 36% of deaths. The incidence of HCM-related SCD in adults is 0.5% to 1%. Approximately 50% of HCM-related deaths occur during or just after the individual has done some type of physical activity. Sudden cardiac death is often the first and only indication of the presence of HCM. Ninety percent of HCM-related deaths in athletes occur in males. This is potentially due to the increased frequency of participation at a higher intensity sports with male athlete; however, a true understanding of this gender bias has not been fully elucidated (Ackerman et al., 2011).

Genetic Basis of HCM

As is seen with DCM, there are different types of HCM with extensive genetic heterogeneity. Hypertrophic cardiomyopathy is usually inherited through an autosomal dominant inheritance pattern with variable penetrance. More than 400 different known mutations in nine different genes have been identified (Mitchell, 2015). Sarcomere protein gene mutations cause most forms of HCM, with 80% of cases being associated with MYH7, MYBPC3, TNNT2, and TNNI3 mutations. As was discussed with DCM, sarcomere genes involve muscle formation and function. The genetic mutations associated with HCM result in force generation malfunctions. The two most common genes responsible for approximately half of patients with familial HCM are mutations MYH7 and MYBPC3 (which code for myosin binding protein C). De novo MYH7 mutations have also been noted in patients who have HCM but have no family history of the disease. This type of mutation causes early onset of HCM and is often associated with early decompensation requiring cardiac transplantation. MYBPC3 is considered a milder form of sarcomere protein gene mutation and results in later onset of HCM, usually around the age of 50–60 years. TNNT2 mutation (gene codes for cardiac troponin I) is associated with a high incidence of SCD. An insertion/deletion polymorphism of the gene responsible for encoding ACE is also associated with HCM. The deletion/deletion (D/D) genotype of ACE is associated with more marked LV hypertrophy and may be associated with higher rates of SCD (Marian et al, 2017).

Genetic Testing in HCM

It is recommended that patients who have been diagnosed with HCM should undergo genetic testing. Currently available techniques will identify causal variants in approximately 30% to 50% of probands with HCM (Marian et al., 2017). Genetic testing should be accompanied by genetic counseling by both a genetic counselor as well as a cardiologist who specializes in cardiogenetics. Specifically, discussion of HCM pathophysiology, symptoms, prohibition of sports participation, SCD, testing of family members, and possible need for invasive intervention should be included.

HCM Screening and Diagnosis

Hypertrophic cardiomyopathy screening has become prevalent in young athletes. Health care providers have been taught that 80% of diagnoses are accomplished through the history and physical examination. In the case of HCM, however, physical exam and medical history are ineffective, since only 3% of cases are identified in this manner. The clinical diagnosis of HCM is based on the presence of left ventricular hypertrophy with an end-diastolic ventricular septal thickness in adults ≥13 mm. Seventy percent of asymptomatic HCM is diagnosed by using the ECG, although this test cannot distinguish between the different types of hypertrophic abnormalities. Upon recognition of LVH in ECG readings, most clinicians will do further studies, such as cardiac magnetic resonance imaging to investigate the specific cause of LVH (Marian et al., 2017).

Treatment

Because of HCM pathophysiology, dehydration must be avoided at all costs. Because of the tachycardia and dehydration associated with sports, young patients with HCM are counseled to avoid participating in competitive sports or intensive exercise although most patients may participate in low-intensity sports such as golf.

Pharmacologic therapy is the cornerstone of treating symptomatic patients. Beta blockade agents are used to reduce myocardial oxygen demand as well as to maintain a lower heart rate. For those who do not tolerate beta blockade therapy, calcium channel blockers are an acceptable alternative as long as the patient has preserved LV function. For those patients who continue to have symptoms despite optimization of medical management, there are more invasive management alternatives.

Alcohol septal ablation (ASA) is a minimally invasive procedure performed by interventional cardiologists. This procedure is for patients with left ventricular outflow tract obstruction who do not respond to pharmacotherapy and meet certain criteria such as have suitable coronary artery anatomy, are greater than 60 years of age, and have unacceptable surgical risks due to comorbidities (Spirito, Rossi, & Maron, 2017). The success rate is approximately 80% with a low (1% to 2%) procedural mortality rate (Sorajja, 2017).

The procedure is performed by introducing a catheter-based injection of absolute alcohol into the septal perforator to induce a controlled infarction of the hypertrophied septum. This helps abolish the dynamic outflow obstruction. Gradient reduction has been shown to correlate with significant clinical improvement in patient symptoms as well as assist with LV remodeling. The most common complication of ASA has been conduction issues, where up to 10% of patients undergoing this procedure have had complete heart block refractory to medication, thereby requiring permanent pacemaker insertion. Myocardial infarction is a less common complication but has been seen in up to 3.5% of patients undergoing ASA. Another consideration of ASA is that this procedure induces myocardial tissue necrosis, thereby leaving a scar. This scar can result in an arrhythmogenic substrate that predisposes some patients to lethal re-entrant ventricular tachycardia. An increasing number of patients undergoing ASA redevelop hypertrophic septal tissue that requires myectomy (Quintana, Bajona, Arguis, & Prat-González, 2017).

Surgical myectomy is a surgical procedure for HCM when other treatments have failed. This procedure is considered the gold standard of care for symptomatic obstructive HCM. Since the procedure has a greater than 90% success rate and low operative risk when performed by an experienced surgeon in a center that has a high volume of these types of cases (Sorajja, 2017). In this procedure, a rectangular, 3 to 4 cm myectomy trough is created by a cardiac surgeon from just below the aortic valve to the site of mitral–septal contact and intraventricular obstruction. As a result, the redundant tissue causing LV outflow tract obstruction is surgically removed. This allows for improved hemodynamics and LV remodeling.

Complications of myectomy include the usual post-cardiac surgery complications, including infection, atrial arrhythmias, and bleeding. Specifically, because the atrioventricular conduction system can be affected, high-degree conduction blocks may occur necessitating permanent pacemaker insertion. Less than 2% of cases of HCM require cardiac transplantation.

▶ Familial Hypercholesterolemia

Familial hypercholesterolemia (FH) is characterized by elevated serum low-density lipoprotein (LDL) cholesterol levels, which result in excess cholesterol in tissues. This leads to an acceleration of atherosclerosis and increased risk for premature CHD. Because of the markedly elevated LDL levels, deposition of LDL-derived cholesterol, called xanthomas, can also be found in tendons and the skin.

Genetics

More than 90% of mutations in patients with FH occur in the LDLR gene, the gene that codes for the LDL receptor. LDLR mutation databases currently list more than 800 different mutations. Another form of FH involves mutations of apolipoprotein B (apoB) and proprotein convertase subtilisin/kexin type 9 (PCSK9), mutations that cause less than 10% of cases. Mutations in apoB tend to have incomplete penetrance, thereby resulting in a milder form of FH than that seen in LDLR mutations. PCSK9 mutations are associated with a particularly severe clinical phenotype although patients do seem to respond to statin therapy (Bourbon et al, 2017).

The most common inheritance pattern for FH is autosomal dominant. Autosomal recessive FH is extremely rare and involves the LDLRAP1 mutation. Patients with this type of mutation often have a milder form of FH. Autosomal recessive FH is more commonly seen in patients with a family history of consanguinity.

Two types of autosomal dominant FH exist: homozygous and heterozygous. Heterozygous FH is the milder type with plasma cholesterol levels between 300 mg/dL and 400 mg/dL while homozygous FH is more severe with plasma cholesterol levels between 600 mg/dL and 1,200 mg/dL Inheritance of heterozygous type FH occurs in approximately 1 in 500 persons while homozygous inheritance only occurs in 1 in one million individuals. Both types are associated with premature development of CAD.

The LDL receptor gene is located on the short arm of chromosome 19. There are more than 1,000 different mutations that have been identified that have been grouped into five different classes. Class 1 includes null alleles, which results in the production of a defective protein. Class 2, the most common mutation, results in a protein that cannot move from the endoplasmic reticulum to the Golgi apparatus. Class 3 mutations result in a receptor that is unable to correctly bind the LDL. Class 4, the rarest mutation, where the protein cannot get to where it is supposed to go on the cell surface to internalize LDL through the process of endocytosis. Class 5 gives rise to receptors that cannot recycle properly. Patients with heterozygous FH that have one normal allele and one mutant allele and are able to take up LDL at approximately half the normal rate. Those with homozygous FH have two mutant alleles, which result in total or near-total inability to bind and take up LDL (Repas & Tanner, 2014).

Screening

Approximately 85% of patients with FH have not been diagnosed and are not on appropriate lipid-lowering therapy (Repas & Tanner, 2014). Familial hypercholesterolemia begins at the age of 3 in patients with a family history. Cholesterol levels should be checked frequently. Cardiac catheterization to ascertain the presence of early CHD is done at earlier ages than in the general population. Patients with homozygous FH will often have cardiac catheterizations in early childhood.

Management

Statin therapy is initiated at an early age (usually around age 15–18) in those with heterozygous FH and most patients will likely need increasing doses as they age. Lomitapide (Juxtapid®) is a new medication that has been specifically designed for treating FH. Patients with homozygous FH are under constant surveillance and frequent cardiac catheterizations are common.

Percutaneous coronary intervention and coronary artery bypass grafting are often required, even in children. Medications to combat hypercholesterolemia are ineffective in patients with homozygous FH; frank discussion regarding stringent heart-healthy lifestyle is paramount in this patient population.

Because of the higher incidence of development of ischemic cardiomyopathy, heart failure is common in patients with homozygous FH. Cardiac transplantation is typically not explored in this population because of the high likelihood for CAD development in the transplanted organ. Moreover, tacrolimus, an anti-rejection medication, has a propensity to cause early development of CAD. In some cases, heart transplantation can be explored if concomitant liver transplant is also performed. With liver transplantation, the goal is that the new organ will assist in LDL uptake improvement, thereby decreasing the risk for early CAD development (Repas & Tanner, 2014).

▶ Aortopathies

Aortopathy refers to any disease or malfunction of the aorta. There are five main aortopathic conditions that have clinical relevance: Marfan syndrome (MFS), Loeys–Dietz syndrome (LDS), Ehlers–Danlos syndrome (EDS Types I/II, IV, and VI), idiopathic thoracic aneurysm/dissection, and coarctation of the aorta. Note that three of the five are syndromes, which indicates that multiple body systems are affected by the disease process. Marfan syndrome, LDS, EDS, and coarctation of

the aorta all have genetic components. This chapter focuses on the first three syndromes without discussion of coarctation of the aorta because of its usual repair in pediatric settings.

Marfan Syndrome (MFS)

Marfan syndrome is an inherited connective tissue disease that is associated with decreased life expectancy. The gene responsible for MFS was not discovered until 1991 when Dr. Francesco Ramirez discovered the occurrence of misfolding of the protein fibrillin-1 (FBN1). There are no currently documented gender, geographical, or ethnic biases associated with MFS. Fifteen to thirty percent of MFS cases occur secondary to a de novo genetic mutation—not inheritance from a parent. Therefore, sole reliance on pedigree/family history can cause missed MFS diagnosis in some patients. The most recent Ghent criteria for the diagnosis of MSF is listed in **TABLE 22.2**. The Ghent clinical criteria was developed to facilitate the accurate recognition of MFS as well as to improve patient management and counseling.

MFS Genetics

MFS results from a defect in an extracellular glycoprotein called fibrillin-1. Glycoproteins are essential components of elastic fiber formation in connective tissue. The gene that codes for fibrillin-1 (FBN1) is

TABLE 22.2 Revised Ghent Criteria for the Diagnosis of Marfan Syndrome	
In the absence of family history:	▪ Aortic root dilatation Z score ≥ 2 and ectopia lentis (Z score it equivalent to the number of standard deviations the actual aortic root diameter differs from the mean of a group of health controls) ▪ Aortic root dilatation Z score 2 or greater and an FBN1 mutation ▪ Aortic root dilatation Z score 2 or greater and systemic score 7 or more points (see **TABLE 22.3**) ▪ Ectopic lentis and FBN1 mutation with known aortic root dilatation
In the presence of family history:	▪ Ectopia lentis and family history of MFS (as defined above) ▪ A systemic score 7 or more points and family history of MFS (as defined above) ▪ Aortic root dilatation Z score 2 or greater above 20 years old, 3 or greater below 20 years, plus family history of Marfan syndrome (as defined above)

Data from Loeys, B., (2010).

TABLE 22.3 Scoring of Features According to the Revised Ghent Nosology

Scoring of systemic features:

- Wrist and thumb sign – 3 (wrist or thumb sign – 1)
- Pectus carinatum deformity – 2 (pectus excavatum or chest asymmetry – 1)
- Hind foot deformity – 2 (plain pes planus – 1)
- Pneumothorax – 2
- Dural ectasia – 2
- Protrusio acetabuli – 2
- Reduced US/LS and increased arm/height and no severe scolosis – 1
- Scoliosis or thoracolumbar kyphosis – 1
- Reduced elbow extension – 1
- Facial features (3/5) – 1 (dolichocephaly, enophthalmos, downslanting palpebral fissures, malar hypoplasia, retrognathia)
- Skin striae – 1
- Myopia .3 diopters – 1
- Mitral valve prolapse (all types) – 1

Maximum total: 20 points; score 7 or greater indicates systemic involvement; US/LS – upper segment/lower segment ratio.

Data from Radke & Baumgartner, 2014.

located on Chromosome 15. More than 600 distinct mutations of the FBN1 gene have been identified in individuals with MFS. Fibrillin-1 is a major component of microfibrils that form a scaffold for the formation of elastin, a component of all connective tissue. There are thought to be two forms of fibrillin. Fibrillin-1 has a direct role in connective tissue formation and maintenance. Fibrillin-1 also has a direct relationship with transforming growth factor beta (TGF-β). Misregulated TGF-β has injurious effects on vascular smooth muscle development and the integrity of the extracellular matrix. Marfan syndrome has notable excess TGF-β in the lungs, aorta, and heart valves. Fibrillin-2 (encoded on chromosome 5) plays a major role in joint and musculoskeletal formation. Fibrillin-2 malfunctions are seen in Beals syndrome, also known as congenital contractural arachnodactyly. Marfan syndrome has an autosomal dominant inheritance pattern (Mitchell, 2015; Radke & Baumgartner 2014).

MFS Key Cardiac Characteristics

Cardiovascular compromise is common in MFS. Many patients will have sluggish peripheral

circulation, resulting in cold feet, hands, or both. Mitral valve prolapse is seen in approximately 28% to 45% of patients with MFS. Aortic valve formation and function have also been noted to be problematic in MFS. Many patients will have aortic valvular prolapse, resulting in aortic insufficiency. The most worrisome cardiovascular concern in MFS is the high propensity of aortic aneurysms and dissections. The most vulnerable parts of the aorta for MFS patients are the aortic root and ascending aorta. Descending thoracic aorta aneurysms are also common. Less commonly, aneurysms of the iliac and renal arteries are noted (less than 1% of cases). Other systems that also are involved in MFS include skeletal (kyphosis, scoliosis, pectus excavatum), the eye (dislocation of the lens), and the skin (striae). Pulmonary complications of MFS including obstructive sleep apnea, and deformity of the thoracic cage with restrictive lung disease may also be present (Pyeritz, 2016; Radke & Baumgartner, 2014).

MFS Screening/Testing

Since MFS is a multi-system disease, multiple modalities and methods have to be used for the diagnosis and follow-up. Cardiac and aortic complications are of major concern, therefore transthoracic echocardiography is the primary imaging tool in the diagnosis of MFS. Magnetic resonance imaging, another key technique in the diagnosis and management of MFS, allows detailed assessment of the aortic root and the heart when echocardiography may not be possible due to chest deformities.

Genetic testing is not mandatory according to the revised nosology (disease classification) as most often the diagnosis can be made of phenotype alone. A recent study showed genetic testing altered the final diagnosis in only 11% of patients. It is recommended that genetic testing be done in phenotype positive patients to validate the clinical diagnosis, exclude alternative diagnoses, and to facilitate diagnosis in the patients' offspring. In patients who the phenotype is not clear cut, genetic testing is controversial. A suggested approach is that have patients have clinical features that involve at least two or three organ systems, genetic testing for FBN1 mutation is reasonable (Radke & Baumgartner, 2014).

MFS Management

Management includes both medical and surgical recommendations. It is currently recommend that all MFS patients, regardless of aortic size, receive β-blocker therapy. Other antihypertensive drugs should be utilized if β-blockers are not tolerated.

Current recommendation advises prophylactic surgery (valve-sparing root repair) when aortic root diameter is greater than 50 mm or with a family history of aortic dissection 46 to 50 mm (Pyeritz, 2016). Annual follow-up with transthoracic echocardiograms is needed in all patients to monitor progression of aortic dilatation. More frequent evaluation may be indicated with rapid progression. Follow-up of other systems such as annual ophthalmological evaluation is also essential. All patients with MFS should also receive counseling regarding lifestyle restrictions (e.g. avoid isometric exercises, exercising to exhaustion, contact sports) to prevent risks for aortic dissection (Pyeritz, 2016).

Loeys-Dietz Syndrome (LDS)

Loeys-Dietz syndrome is a genetic disorder that also affects the body's connective tissue and is associated with aortopathies. Loeys-Dietz syndrome is inherited in an autosomal dominant pattern and is caused by mutations in one of five genes: LDS-1 transforming growth factor beta-receptor 1 (TGFβR1), LDS-2 transforming growth factor beta-receptor2 (TGFβR2), LDS-3 mothers against decapentaplegic homolog (SMAD-3), LDS-4 transforming growth factor beta-2 ligand (TGFβ2), and LDS-5 transforming growth factor beta-e ligand (TGFβ3). As was noted in MFS, these receptors play a major role in vascular stability. Included in the most common characteristics of LDS is aortic aneurysm (MacCarrick et al., 2014).

Clinical Presentation

Since connective tissue is found throughout the body, other than aortic aneurysms, the syndrome has many other clinical manifestations such as arterial tortuosity, congenital heart defects, craniofacial defects, skin changes, and osteoporosis to name a few. Rapid progression of aortic aneurysms is a distinct feature of LDS. This is especially notable in patients with LDS 1 or 2. These patients are known to have aortic rupture at young ages and at a smaller dimension than those with other aortopathies. Aortic dissection has been reported in patients as young as 3 months to 3 years. Mean age of death of patients with LDS has been reported as 26.1 years, with aortic dissection and cerebral hemorrhage as the major causes of death.

Bicuspid aortic valves (BAV), atrial septal defects, or patent ductus arteriosus are frequently seen in LDS 1 or 2. Mitral valve prolapse can be seen in all types of LDS, with mild to severe mitral valve disease being reported. Twenty-four percent of patients with LDS 3 have been noted to have chronic AF and LVH. Left ventricular hypertrophy associated with LDS has been reported as mostly concentric in the absence of aortic stenosis or hypertension and ranges from mild to moderate. LDS 1 has associated decreased systolic function, heart failure, and arrhythmias.

Arterial tortuosity can occur throughout the body but is seen more frequently in neck vessels. Type B (descending thoracic aorta) dissections have been reported in minimally or non-dilated aortas (3.7–4.2 cm) in LDS 1, 2, and 3. There have also been reports of rapid expansion of aneurysms within dissections within a few days. Aneurysms and dissections of other major arteries have also been reported (MacCarrick et al., 2014).

LDS Genetic Testing/Screening

Because of its relatively new status as a diagnosis, recommendations for genetic testing are still being developed. Aortopathy panels readily include the five associated LDS genes, which increases the likelihood of appropriate diagnosis (MacCarrick et al., 2014).

LDS Management

Patients with LDS should have echocardiograms at least every 6 months Because of the aggressive and rapidly progressive aortic aneurysms associated with LDS, valve-sparing aortic root replacement is advised. In MFS, aortic root dimensions of 5 cm or greater are deemed the appropriate measurement necessitating surgery. However, experts advise LDS patients to undergo surgery when aortic root dimensions reach 4 cm. Valve-sparing surgery is more widely done to avoid the need for anticoagulation, given these patients often have a higher incidence of bleeding problems. Postoperative echocardiograms should be done at 3- to 6-month intervals for 1 year after surgery and every 6 months thereafter because of the report of coronary button aneurysms developing after valve-sparing aortic root replacement. Patients with known aortic dissections should be monitored every 2 to 3 months with surveillance computed tomography (CT) scans. Because of the higher incidence of arterial tortuosity, especially in the neck, ultrasound-guided catheter placement needed for post-surgical management should be performed. Angiotensin receptor blocker (ARB) therapy has shown to be effective in aortic stabilization as well as hypertension management (MacCarrick et al., 2014).

Ehlers-Danlos Syndromes (EDS)

EDS are a group of inherited disorders caused by abnormalities in the production and structure of collagen. The inheritance pattern of EDS varies by type with some types being inherited in an autosomal dominant pattern and other types in an autosomal recessive pattern. Many patients with EDS will have crossover symptoms that appear in multiple syndromes; therefore, diagnosis is often missed or misdiagnosis occurs.

According to the EDS Society, there are currently 13 types of EDS. Type 4 is associated with cardiac implications and is caused by COL3A1 gene mutation. This type is the most clinically worrisome because it affects vascular collagen/connective tissue. Twenty-five percent of patients with Type 4 EDS develop significant health problems, including heart failure, by the age of 20. More than 80% develop life-threatening complications by age 40. The COL3A1 genetic mutation causes the vascular connective tissue to be extremely fragile resulting in spontaneous blood vessel and organ rupture (Rombaut et al., 2011).

Clinical Presentation

Vascular problems seen in EDS are often as severe, if not more severe, than those seen in MFS. All blood vessels, not just the aorta, are fragile and have a tendency toward aneurysm. Arterial rupture has been seen with Type 4 EDS. Mitral valve prolapse is also seen in Type 4 EDS and is often associated with endocarditis. Finally, these patients often have platelet aggregation failure and have a tendency to bleed (Byers et al., 2017). Other clinical features associated with different types of EDS include fragile, hyperextensible skin vulnerable to trauma, hypermobile joints, and poor wound healing (Mitchell, 2015)

EDS Screening/Testing

Ehlers-Danlos syndrome is often a diagnosis of exclusion because of its associated crossover and often vague symptoms. Genetic testing and counseling should only be performed by those associated with a strong background in this type of disorder.

EDS Management

Ehlers-Danlos syndrome has no cure. Palliative treatment is the primary cornerstone of management with the maintenance of blood pressure in the normal or low normal range and prevention of surges in blood pressure. The goal is to minimize the risk for arterial dissection or rupture. Even if genetic testing does not provide definitive diagnosis of Type 4 EDS, close monitoring of these patients' cardiovascular systems should be done. Those patients with valvular malfunction or aortic aneurysm may require surgery with surgery generally occurring after the aneurysm or rupture (Byers et al., 2017). Unlike those with MFS, prognosis does not necessarily improve with aortic replacement. These patients may still have spontaneous rupture of other organs. These patients also have been seen to have a high incidence of bleeding and profound hematoma development after arterial and venous catheter placement. As a result, these patients require careful line insertion by qualified personnel.

▶ Bicuspid Aortic Valve Disease

Normal aortic valves are tricuspid. Bicuspid aortic valve disease is the most common congenital cardiac abnormality that affects an estimated 0.5% to 2% of adults (Masri et al., 2016). Bicuspid aortic valve disease is almost three times more common in males than females. Some data suggest that African Americans are more likely to develop severe aortic stenosis than Caucasian patients (Patel et al., 2014). Earlier data suggest just the opposite (Chandra et al., 2012).

Pathogenesis

Embryologically, the definitive fetal cardiac structure is developed by 8 weeks gestation. The semilunar valves form the division between the truncus arteriosus and create two separate channels that form the aortic and pulmonary trunks. The channels are created by the fusion of two truncal ridges across the lumen. Small swellings appear on the inferior margins of each truncal ridge, forming the basis for adult valve leaflets. A third channel is created in each channel occurring opposite the first, which will form the third leaflet. In the normal aortic valve, the left and right leaflets of the adult valve are formed from the respective swellings, while the posterior leaflet is formed from an off branch of the aortic trunk. The exact pathophysiology of the formation of BAV is not fully understood. It is thought to have a genetic component, especially given the association of BAV with other congenital abnormalities such as coarctation of the aorta. Three types of BAV are described in the literature:

1. *Type 1*: Two commissures (area where two valve leaflets have abnormally come together) of the BAV are located in an anteroposterior direction giving left and right cusps
2. *Type 2*: Commissures located on the right and left sides of the annulus leading to anterior posterior cusps
3. *Type 3*: Fusion of the left and non-coronary cusps (most rare: seen in fewer than 1%)

A raphe, or seam that forms the junction between two fused valve leaflets, is present on the right and anterior cusps, respectively. This makes the valve appear tricuspid on echocardiography. The site of cusp fusion can have prognostic effects of BAV. Type 1 BAV has been associated with a higher incidence of aortic stenosis; Type 2 valves tend to have complications at younger ages, with most having aortic regurgitation (Masri et al., 2016).

Coronary anatomy may also be abnormal with BAV. With normal anatomy, the posterior descending artery (PDA) supplies the inferior wall of the left ventricle and inferior part of the septum. The coronary artery that supplies the PDA determines coronary dominance. Approximately 70% of people have right coronary artery dominant circulation, meaning that the PDA originates from the right coronary artery. Twenty percent have codominance, meaning both the right coronary artery and circumflex artery feed the PDA. Ten percent are left coronary dominant, meaning that the circumflex alone supplies the PDA

(Pelter, Al-Zaiti, & Carey, 2011). Most patients with BAV disease have a left dominant coronary circulation. This left coronary vessel can arise from the pulmonary artery. The left main coronary artery (LMCA) can also be up to 50% shorter than in normal patients and occurs in up to 90% of BAV cases. This is an extremely important consideration in any aortic valve surgery. The most common non-valvular abnormality associated with BAV is thoracic aortic dilatation. This is thought to be due to alteration in aortic flow but is also due to cellular structural abnormalities including decreased fibrillin, which causes smooth muscle cell detachment and cellular death. A recent systematic review of 13 studies showed that the most serious complication associated with BAV (i.e., aortic dissection) was rare of an incidence rate of 0.4% over a follow-up period of 2–16 years (Masri et al., 2016). Coarctation of the aorta is also seen in 20% to 85% of cases. Coarctation-mediated hypertension associated with BAV increases the risk for aortic dissection. Aortic coarctation associated with BAV occurs more frequently in men than women (4:1). Other conditions associated with BAV include labile hypertension, mitral regurgitation, and patent ductus arteriosus.

BAV Genetics

Heritability of BAV is well established with loci on chromosomes 18, 5, and 13 being implicated. The most recognized genetic link to the pathology of BAV is mutations in *NOTCH1*. Notch is a key signaling pathway in the cardiac valve development during embryogenesis. *NOTCH1 gene* mutations are associated with left ventricular outflow abnormalities including BAV (Kostina et al., 2016).

Screening

Although the 2% incidence of BAV may be higher than currently reported, there have been no guidelines suggesting BAV screening in the general population. Rather, screening for BAV in patients with first-degree relatives known to have BAV has been recommended by the American College of Cardiology (ACC) and AHA. Screening includes echocardiography to screen for evidence of BAV

and aortic root dilatation in addition, Doppler evaluation for aortic coarctation is also recommended. If the aortic root and/or ascending aorta cannot be assessed completely by echocardiography, magnetic resonance angiography or CT angiography is indicated.

BAV Diagnosis

Type 1 BAV is the most common type. In these patients, presentation is typically from ages 40 to 60 years. In this population, aortic stenosis is the most common diagnosis. However, mixed aortic stenosis and aortic insufficiency is not uncommon. In Type 2 BAV, presentation usually is seen between the ages of 20 and 30. These patients tend to present with mild to severe aortic regurgitation and ascending aortic aneurysms. Physical examination will usually be limited to auscultation with most patients having a systolic ejection murmur associated with aortic stenosis that is best heard at the apex. An ECG will usually be normal; however, if there is moderate to severe aortic stenosis, associative LVH may be noted. The mainstay of BAV diagnosis is echocardiography (both transthoracic and transesophageal). With adequate images, there is a 92% sensitivity and a 96% specificity for definitive BAV diagnosis. Parasternal short axis views allow for the best and direct visualization of aortic valve cusps. In this view, the normal triangular opening shape is lost. The commonly described "fish mouth"–like appearance can be noted. This appearance is similar to that of the mitral valve. This "fish mouth" appearance is especially pronounced in systole. In diastole, the raphe can appear similar to a commissure of the third cusp, which can result in inaccurate diagnosis of a tricuspid aortic valve rather than BAV. If echocardiography cannot fully quantify the extent of any aortopathy; cardiac magnetic resonance imaging or CT is indicated.

BAV Treatment

The only curative treatment for BAV is surgical replacement of the aortic valve. Medical therapy is used to alleviate symptoms and to slow the progression of aortic valve disease and aortopathies. The

ACC/AHA joint guidelines suggest beta blockers as a first-line therapy in patients with BAV (Allen et al., 2016). Angiotensin receptor blocker therapy may have a role, but there is a lack of supporting evidence of their efficacy. Surgical management is dependent on the patient. Valvular replacement is usually not deemed as practical, because patients outgrow the prosthetic valve. The 2010 ACCF/AHA/ATTS/ACR/ASA/SCA/SCAI/SIR/STS/SCM guidelines recommend operative intervention to repair or replace the aortic root or the ascending aorta in asymptomatic patients if the diameter of the aortic root or ascending aorta is 5.5 cm or greater. If additional risk factors are present (i.e., family history of aortic dissection) or if the patient is at low surgical risk, operative intervention may be considered if the diameter is 5.0 cm or greater (Hiratzka et al., 2010). An estimated 15 years of freedom from complications was 86% in patients with an aortic diameter less than 4 cm, dropping down to 81% in those with 4 to 4.4 cm, and 43% in patients with an ascending aortic diameter 4.5 cm or greater. New techniques of repair, such as transcatheter aortic valve implantation, have been reported.

▶ **Pharmacogenomics**

As has been demonstrated in this chapter, cardiogenetics can play a huge role in disease development. Similarly, ICU nurses may be faced with challenges related to pharmacogenomics or pharmagogenetics, which is the study of how inherited variations in DNA affect the way people respond to medications. Specifically, pharmacogenomics refers to the study of genetic/genomic differences in *multiple* genes' influence on variability in drug response (e.g., efficacy, toxicity) while pharmacogenetics refers to the study of how genetic differences in a *single* gene influences variability in drug response. Components of both pharmacogenomics and pharmacogenetics include drug targets and transporters, drug-metabolizing enzymes, pharmacodynamics, and pharmacokinetics. All of these factors play roles in the variability seen in drug efficacy and toxicity.

Other factors that contribute to drug distribution and action variability include age, gender, ethnicity/race, concomitant drug administration, concomitant diseases, psychosocial factors, and socioeconomic factors. When considering the clinical relevance of this emerging field, two questions should come to mind: (1) Can we predict who will derive an optimal response? and (2) Can we predict who will have toxicity? These questions have been the cornerstone of pharmacogenomics research, and evidence supports the idea that patient genotype determines the optimal drug therapy approach; however, pathogen genotype can also determine optimal drug approach.

Drug Metabolism Pharmacogenetics

Drug metabolism considerations are considered pharmacogenetics rather than genomics because of their monogenic nature. This means that a single gene is the focus of the metabolic difference. Drug metabolism mutations have a phenotype-to-genotype approach, meaning that the characteristics presented in the clinical setting are considered prior to exploring genetic mutations/cause. Drug metabolism can occur in several organs although the liver frequently has the greatest metabolic capacity and is the major site for drug metabolism. Chemical modifications to drugs occur so they can eventually be eliminated. These chemical reactions usually increase water solubility to promote elimination. In the case of genetic mutations, these chemical reactions may be slowed down, accelerated, or altered in some manner. In the liver, the drug-metabolizing enzyme cytochrome P450 is well known. This enzyme has subunits that often have genetic mutations that cause significant clinical consequences.

Warfarin

The widely known drug warfarin (Coumadin®) has a narrow range between efficacy and toxicity. Warfarin metabolism and subsequent inactivation are mediated by a family of CYP450 isoenzymes (e.g., CYP2C1, CYP1A2). There are several known variants of the CYP2C isoenzyme: CYP2C9*1 is associated with normal enzyme activity and the normal metabolizer phenotype while CYP2C9*2 and

CYP2C9*3 variants are associated with reduced or nearly abolished function, respectively. With mutation of CYP2C9, there is up to three times higher risk of serious or life-threatening bleeding episodes in patients requiring warfarin therapy. Greater than 90% of deleterious CYP2C9 mutations are found in Caucasians. Clinical sensitivity for other racial and ethnic groups are still being investigated.

Vitamin K, the antidote for warfarin, regulates clotting in humans. Vitamin K epoxide reductase enzyme (VKOR) is the target for warfarin and is coded for by the VKORC1 gene. Patients who carry 1639G, a variant in the promoter region of the VKORC1 gene have increased sensitivity to warfarin and require lower doses. The CYP2C9 (*2 and *3) variants together with the VKORC1 promoter mutations are estimated to account for 40% to 63% of therapeutic warfarin dosing variability. Genetic testing is available; caution should be used when ordering. Mutations other than those previously described will not be detected. Mutations in other genes and non-genetic factors that may affect drug metabolism (e.g., drug–drug interactions) are not detected. Genetic variant detection does not replace the need for therapeutic drug monitoring or other appropriate clinical monitoring (Dean, 2016).

CYP2C19 Mutations

CYP2C19 protein regulation is controlled by the CYP2C19 gene (a member of the cytochrome P450 gene family). This protein, like CYP2C9, produces an enzyme that controls drug metabolism for several antidepressants (e.g., tricyclics, selective serotonin reuptake inhibitors), anti-epileptics (diazepam [Valium®], phenytoin [Dilantin®], phenobarbital [Luminal®]), proton pump inhibitors (omeprazole [Prilosec®], lansoprazole [Prevacid®], pantoprazole [Protonix®]), clopidogrel (Plavix®), beta blockers (propranolol, Inderal®), non-steroidal anti-inflammatory drugs (indomethacin [Indocin®]), and warfarin. Three to five percent of Caucasians and 15% to 20% of Asians with CYP2C19 mutations are deemed "poor metabolizers" with no CYP2C19 function. In the case of clopidogrel, this could lead to considerable risk, including MI, stroke, and death. As a result, in 2010, the U.S. Food and Drug Administration put a black box warning on clopidogrel for health care providers and patients to be aware that CYP2C19 poor metabolizers, representing up to 14% of patients, are at high risk for treatment failure and that genetic testing for a CYP2C19 mutation is available. A Roche AmpliChip® CYP450 test is used to identify CYP2C19 and CYP2D6 mutations. Pharmacies have begun routine testing for this mutation when new clopidogrel prescriptions are received. There are other CYP mutations, such as CYP2D2, which may affect drug metabolism, including commonly used analgesic agents used in the ICU.

▶ Cardiogenetic Nursing Considerations

ICU nurses employed at academic, or tertiary centers, will most likely provide care for patients with a genetic foundation for their disease process. For that reason, these nurses should familiarize themselves with common cardiogenetic disorders that may be routinely seen in their patients. For those nurses who practice in smaller community hospitals, this does not mean that they will be excluded from seeing patients with cardiogenetic disorders. Given that many patients present without prior symptoms, whenever a nurse performs patient assessment, the "red flags" of genetic risk should be kept in mind.

Careful review of pathophysiology is paramount. For example, when caring for a patient who has undergone surgical myectomy for HCM, the nurse must be aware that the left ventricle will require time to recover from the HCM-associated stiffness and high pressure gradient. As such, the patient will most likely be volume dependent for several hours in the postoperative phase. Therefore, early diuresis with diuretics should be avoided. Further, given postoperative patients have autodiuresis, extra volume may be required to maintain adequate filling pressures. Tachycardia should be avoided. This can usually be controlled by volume resuscitation; pharmacological intervention may also be required. Conversely, patients who undergo cardiac surgery who have DCM will require early diuresis because of their higher risk for CHF.

Patients with familial aortopathic disease will also have connective tissue problems. Many patients with Marfan syndrome have spontaneous pneumothoraces; close observation after chest tube removal is mandatory. Increased intrathoracic pressure created with vomiting can increase the risk for pneumothoraces; early use of anti-emetics should be employed.

▶ Summary

Understanding the importance of history taking of the patient with a focus on family health is crucial to the identification of a genetic predisposition to cardiovascular disorders associated with hereditary.

🔍 CASE STUDY

A 20-year-old college tennis player presents to her primary care physician for clearance to continue participating in collegiate sports. Upon examination, a grade 1/6 systolic ejection murmur is auscultated. The patient is long-legged, and has long arms, fingers, and toes in relation to her trunk size. Her arm span is wider than her height. Her weight is appropriate for her height. Her joints hyperextend. Stretch marks are present on her hips and lower back area; she denies significant weight loss. Her heart rate was 48 (regular), which she states is her normal slow rate. Her physical exam is otherwise unremarkable; no respiratory or neurological issues were identified. She is in no distress and reports no discomfort. Her family history is negative for cardiac disease. Her primary care physician suspects Marfan syndrome.

Critical Thinking Questions

1. What factors led the physician to suspect the presence of Marfan syndrome?
2. Why is the patient at risk for the development of a pneumothorax?
3. What cardiac issues is the patient at risk to develop?

Answers to Critical Thinking Questions

1. The physician based the suspicion of Marfan syndrome on the review of systems. Despite not having respiratory distress or neurologic findings, which are typically associated with Marfan syndrome, the patient's extremities were elongated, there was a presence of stretch marks in the lower back and hips despite no significant weight loss being reported. Her joints are able to be hyperextended. All of these are symptoms associated with Marfan syndrome.
2. With Marfan syndrome, the alveoli are less elastic than normal. In addition, increased intrathoracic pressure created with vomiting can increase the risk for development of a pneumothorax.
3. The patient is at risk for mitral regurgitation, aortic regurgitation, aortic aneurysm, tricuspid regurgitation, and pulmonic regurgitation. Mitral valve issues are reported more commonly in females. The mitral valve leaflets are of abnormal size, composition, and stretch. The leaflets are then too large for the opening between the left atrium and ventricle. This results in the leaflets bellowing backwards during systole, which leads to mitral valve prolapse (Thacoor, 2017).

Self-Assessment Questions

1. Pedigrees (also known as genograms) are schematic renderings of family history and should include _____ generation(s) of both paternal and maternal family history.
   A. one
   B. two
   C. three
   D. four

2. With regard to cardiogenetics, females with the Duchene muscular dystrophy gene mutation should be evaluated for which disorder?
   A. Hypertrophic cardiomyopathy
   B. Arrhythmogenic right ventricular cardiomyopathy
   C. Dilated cardiomyopathy
   D. Left ventricular non-compaction cardiomyopathy

3. The 2009 HFSA genetic evaluation of cardio-myopathy guideline recommends screening for first-degree relatives of patients with DCM. If a first-degree relative has an abnormal clinical screening test, they should be reevaluated within which time period?
   A. 3 months
   B. 6 months
   C. 9 months
   D. 12 months

4. Most inherited cardiovascular diseases have a(n) _____ pattern.
   A. autosomal dominant
   B. autosomal recessive
   C. Y-linked inheritance
   D. X-linked inheritance

5. The "G" of the MOGE(S) classification stands for:
   A. glycogen storage diseases.
   B. level of generation.
   C. gradient pressures.
   D. nature of genetic transmission.

6. Which is the most common cause of sudden cardiac death in young athletes?
   A. Hypertrophic cardiomyopathy
   B. Arrhythmogenic right ventricular cardiomyopathy
   C. Dilated cardiomyopathy
   D. Left ventricular non-compaction cardiomyopathy

7. Which is associated with Loeys-Dietz Syndrome?
   A. Venous tortuosity
   B. Skin changes
   C. Endocarditis
   D. Ventricular dysrhythmias

8. Diagnosis of Marfan syndrome may be misleading if relying totally on pedigree/family history because some patients have:
   A. a de novo genetic mutation.
   B. poor penetrance levels.
   C. an autosomal dominant gene mutation.
   D. glycogen storage diseases.

9. A patient is diagnosed with Loeys-Dietz syndrome. The nurse should anticipate management to include administration of:
   A. metoprolol (Lopressor®).
   B. phenylephrine (Neo-Synephrine®).
   C. valsartan (Diovan®).
   D. digitoxin (Digoxin®).

10. A distinct feature of Loeys-Dietz syndrome is:
    A. severe muscle weakness.
    B. outflow obstruction.
    C. keloid formation.
    D. aortic aneurysm.

Answers to Self-Assessment Questions

1. C. **Three**
   Rationale: At least three generations on both the paternal and maternal family histories should be included in a genogram.

2. C. **Dilated cardiomyopathy**
   Rationale: Females with Duchene muscular dystrophy gene mutation can have dilated cardiomyopathy. It is related to diastolic dysfunction and fibrosis, which can progress to dilated cardiomyopathy.

3. D. **12 months**
   Rationale: The guideline recommends repeat clinical screening at one year in any first-degree relatives with any abnormal screening tests.

4. A. **Autosomal dominant**
   Rationale: Most inherited cardiovascular diseases have an autosomal dominant pattern. This means that only one parent needs to have the gene.

5. D. **Nature of genetic transmission**
   Rationale: The G step refers to genetic/familial inheritance or the nature of genetic transmission.

6. A. **Hypertrophic cardiomyopathy**
   Rationale: Hypertrophic cardiomyopathy is a major cause of death in those younger than 30 years of age and accounts for 36% of deaths in young athletes.

7. B. **Skin changes**
   Rationale: Loeys-Dietz syndrome is a genetic disorder that affects connective tissue. Since connective tissue is found throughout the body, skin changes are among the clinical manifestations of the condition.

8. A. **a de novo genetic mutation**
Rationale: Up to 30% of patients with Marfan syndrome are due to a de novo genetic mutation.

9. C. **valsartan (Diovan®).**
Rationale: Angiotensin receptor blockers, such as valsartan, have been shown to be effective in aortic stabilization and hypertension management.

10. D. **aortic aneurysm**.
Rationale: Included in the most common characteristics of Loeys-Dietz syndrome is aortic aneurysm.

CLINICAL INQUIRY BOX

Question: Is there a relationship between vitamin D deficiency and coronary artery ectasia?

Reference: Demir, M., Demir, C., & Keçeoğlu, S. (2014). The relationship between vitamin D deficiency and coronary artery ectasia. *Postepy W Kardiologii Interwencyjnej, 10*(4), 238–241.

Objective: To compare vitamin D levels of patients with coronary artery ectasia.

Method: Prospective comparative study of vitamin D and parathyroid hormone levels of patients with coronary artery ectasia.

Results: The average vitamin D level was lower and parathyroid hormone level was higher in patients with coronary artery ectasia.

Conclusion: There is a relationship between vitamin D deficiency and the presence of coronary artery ectasia.

References

Ackerman, M., Priori, S., Willems, S., Berul, C., Brugada, C., Brugada, R., . . . Zipes, D. P. (2011). HRSA/EHRA expert consensus statement on the state of genetic testing for the channelopathies and cardiomyopathies. *Heart Rhythm, 8*(8), 1308–1318.

Allen, B. D., Marki, M., Barker, A. J., van Ooij, P., Carr, J. C., Malaisrie, C., . . . Kansal, P. (2016). Influence of beta-blocker therapy on aortic blood flow in patients with bicuspid aortic valve. *International Journal of Cardiovascular Imaging, 32*(4), 621–628.

Arbustini, E., Narula, N., Tavazzi, L., Serio, A., Grasso, M., Favalli, V., . . . Narula, J. (2014). The MOGE(S) classification of cardiomyopathy for clinicians. *Journal of the American College of Cardiology, 64*(3), 304–318.

Axelson-Fisk, M. (2015). Annotation pipelines for next-generation sequencing projects. In M. Axelson-Fisk (Ed). *Comparative gene finding. Models, algorithms and implementation* (pp. 325–368). Gothenburg, Sweden: Springer.

Bourbon, M., Alves, A., & Sibrands, E. (2017). Low-density lipoprotein receptor mutational analysis in diagnosis of familial hypercholesterolemia. *Current Opinion in Lipidology, 28*(2), 120–129.

Bozkurt, B., Colvin, M., Cook J., Cooper, L., Deswal, A., Fonarow, G., . . . Yancy, C. (2016). Current diagnostic and treatment strategies for specific dilated cardiomyopathies. *Circulation, 134*, e579–e646.

Chandra, S., Lang, R. M., Nicolarsen, J., Gayat, E., Spencer, K. T., Mor-Avi, V., . . . Bowman, M. A. (2012). Bicuspid aortic valve: Inter-racial difference in frequency and aortic dimensions. *JACC: Cardiovascular Imaging, 59*(10), 981–989.

Das, S., Biswas, A., Kapoor, M., Seth, S., Bhargava, B., & Rao, B. (2015). Epidemiology of cardiomyopathy—A clinical and genetic study of dilated cardiomyopathy: The EPOCH-D Study. *Journal of the Practice of Cardiovascular Sciences, 1*(1), 30–34.

Dean, L. (2016). Warfarin therapy and the genotypes *CYP2C9* and *VKORC1*. Retrieved from https://www.ncbi.nlm.nih.gov/books/NBK84174/

Hershberger, R., Lindenfeld, J., Mestroni, L., Seidman, C., Taylor, M., & Towbin, J. (2009). Genetic evaluation of cardiomyopathy—A Heart Failure Society of America practice guideline. *Journal of Cardiac Failure, 15*(2), 83–89.

Hiratzka, L. F., Bakris, G. L., Beckman, J. A., Bersin, R. M., Carr, V.F., Casey, D. E. Jr, Eagle, K. A., Hermann, L. K., Isselbacher, E. M., Kazerooni, E. A., Kouchoukos, N.T., Lytle, B. W., Milewicz, D. M., Reich, D. L., Sen, S., Shinn, J.A., Svensson. L.G., & Williams, D. M. (2010). ACCF/AHA/AATS/ACR/ASA/SCA/SCAI/SIR/STS/SVM Guidelines for the diagnosis and management of patients with thoracic aortic disease: a report of the American College of Cardiology Foundation/American Heart Association Task Force on Practice Guidelines, American Association for Thoracic Surgery, American College of Radiology, American Stroke Association, Society of Cardiovascular Anesthesiologists, Society for Cardiovascular Angiography and Interventions, Society of Interventional Radiology, Society of Thoracic

Surgeons, and Society for Vascular Medicine. *Circulation,* 121, e266–e369.

Kostina, A., Uspensky, V., Irtyuga, O., Ignatieva, E., Freylikhman, O., Gavriliuk, A., . . . Malashicheva, A. B. (2016). Notch-dependent EMT is attenuated in patients with aortic aneurysm and bicuspid aortic valve. *Biochimica et Biophysica Acta, 1862*(4), 733–740.

Loeys, B., Dietz, H., Braverman, C., Callewaert, L., De Backer, J., Devereux, R., . . . De Paepe, A. M. (2010). The revised Ghent nosology for the Marfan syndrome. *Journal of Medical Genetics, 47*(7), 476–485.

MacCarrick, G., Black, J., Bowdin, S., El-Hamamsy, I., Frischmeyer-Guerrerio, P., Guerrerio, A., . . . Dietz, H. C., III. (2014). Loeys-Dietz syndrome: A primer for diagnosis and management. *Genetics in Medicine, 16,* 576–587.

Marian, A. J. & Braunwald, E. (2017). Hypertrophic cardiomyopathy: Genetics, pathogenesis, clinical manifestations, diagnosis, and therapy. *Circulation Research, 121*(7), 749–770.

Masri, A., Svensson, L. G., Griffin, B. P., & Desai, M. Y. (2017). Contemporary natural history of bicuspid aortic valve disease: A systematic review. *Heart, 103*(17), 1323–1330.

McDonald, M. A., Ashley, E. A., Fedak P. W., Hawkins, N., Januzzi, J. L., McMurray, J. J., . . . Virani, S. (2017). Mind the gap: Current challenges and future state of heart failure care. *Canadian Journal of Cardiology, 33*(11), 1434–1449.

Mitchell, R. N. (2015). Heart. In V. Kumar, A. Abbas, & J. Aster (Eds.) *Pathologic basis of disease* (10th ed., pp. 399–440). Philadelphia: Elsevier Saunders.

Newton, G. (2008). *Discovering DNA fingerprinting.* Retrieved from http://genome.wellcome.ac.uk/doc_wtd020877.html

Olson, T., Michels, V., Ballew, J., Reyna, S., Karst, M., Herron, K., . . . Anderson, J. L. (2005). Sodium channel mutations and susceptibility to heart failure and atrial fibrillation. *Journal of the American Medical Association, 293*(4), 447–453.

Orho-Melander, M. (2015). Genetics of coronary heart disease: Towards causal mechanisms, novel drug targets and more personalized prevention. *Journal of Internal Medicine, 278*(5), 433–446.

Patel, D. K., Green, K. D., Fudim, M., Harrell, F. E., Wang, T. J., & Robbins, M. A. (2014). Racial differences in the prevalence of severe aortic stenosis. *Journal of the American Heart Association, 3,* e000879. Retrieved from http://jaha.ahajournals.org/content/ahaoa/3/3/e000879 .full.pdf

Pelter, M., Al-Zaiti, S., & Carey, M. (2011). Coronary artery dominance. *American Journal of Critical Care, 20*(5), 401–402.

Pyeritz, R. (2016). Recent progress in understanding the natural and clinical histories of the Marfan syndrome. *Trends in Cardiovascular Medicine, 26,* 423–428.

Quintana, E., Bajona, P., Arguis, M. J., & Prat-González, S. (2017). Septal myectomy after failed septal alcohol ablation. *Annals of Cardiothoracic Surgery, 6*(4), 394–401.

Radke, R., & Baumgartner H. (2014). Diagnosis and treatment of Marfan syndrome: An update. *Heart, 100,* 1382–1391.

Repas, T., & Tanner, J. (2014). Preventing early cardiovascular death in patients with familial hypercholesterolemia. *Journal of the American Osteopath Association, 114*(2), 99–108.

Roberts, W. (1992). Morphologic aspects of cardiac valve dysfunction. *American Heart Journal, 123*(6), 1610–1632.

Rombaut, L., Malfait, F., De Wandele, L., Cools, A., Thijs, Y., De Paepe, A., . . . Calders, P. (2011). Medication, surgery, and physiotherapy among patients with the hypermobility type of Ehlers-Danlos syndrome. *Archives of Physical Medical Rehabilitation, 92*(7), 1106–1112.

Sorajja, P. (2017). Alcohol septal ablation for obstructive hypertrophic cardiomyopathy. *Journal of the American College of Cardiology, 70*(4), 489–494.

Spirito, P., Rossi, J., & Maron, B. (2017). Alcohol septal ablation: In which patients and why? *Annals of Cardiothoracic Surgery, 6*(4), 369–375.

Thacoor, A. (2017). Mitral valve prolapse and Marfan syndrome. *Congenital Heart Disease, 12*(4), 430–434.

Web Resource

Ehlers-Danlos National Foundation: This website has excellent information and support resources for patients with EDS as well as for health care providers: http://ednf.org

CHAPTER 23

Nutritional Issues of the Patient Undergoing Cardiac Surgery

Roberta Kaplow

▶ Introduction

Up to 25% of patients who are to undergo cardiac surgery lack proper nutrition as a result of heart disease. Decreased food intake, lack of physical activity, aging, and alterations in metabolism are suggested etiologies (van Venrooij et al., 2013). Critically ill patients, in general, and postoperative cardiac surgery patients are typically in a catabolic state (Makikado, Lasierra, Pérez-Vela, & Gonzalez, 2014; McClave et al., 2016). The catabolic state is partially attributed to fasting preoperatively (Stoppe et al., 2017).

Inadequate nutrition puts postoperative cardiac surgery patients at risk for a number of infectious and noninfectious complications that can impact patient outcomes (Cangelosi, Rodday, Saunders, & Cohen, 2014; Gonçalves et al., 2016; Snider et al., 2014; Tyler & Guenter, 2017; van Venrooij et al., 2013). These include infection, increased length of hospital and intensive care unit (ICU) stays, costs of care, readmission rates, risk of pressure ulcer development, risk of death, and lower quality of life (Lomivorotov et al., 2013a; Ohkuma et al., 2017; Pathirana et al., 2014; Sanchez, Sanchez, & Dudrick, 2011; Thourani et al., 2011; van Venrooij et al., 2011; van Venrooij et al., 2012).

Undernutrition can be defined by the presence of 10% or more weight loss in the 6 months prior to cardiac surgery and a low free-fat mass index (van Venrooij et al., 2013). Malnutrition is "an acute, subacute, or chronic state of nutrition in which a combination of varying degrees of overnutrition or undernutrition (with or without inflammatory activity) have led to a change in body composition and diminished function" (American Society for Parenteral and Enteral Nutrition, 2018). It is also defined as "any imbalance in nutrition; from overnutrition to under-nutrition" (Pathirana et al., 2014). This chapter will discuss the cardiac surgery patient's need for nutrition, strategies to assess nutritional status, and treatment modalities.

▶ Cardiac Surgery Patients' Need for Nutrition

As a source of stress, surgery results in a hypermetabolic state that requires additional protein and calories. Protein, fat, and glycogen from fat tissue move to the liver and viscera, which can result in protein calorie malnutrition (Fairfield & Askari, 2017).

An adequate nutritional status is essential for recovery from cardiac surgery. Yet, following cardiac surgery, patients' nutritional status may be impacted for several reasons. These include pain, medications, anorexia, and anxiety. Further, the inflammatory response and release of proinflammatory mediators (associated with cardiopulmonary bypass [CPB]) is suggested to produce subtle damage to the gastrointestinal (GI) tract as well as other body organs (Gonçalves et al., 2016; Sanchez et al., 2011; Stoppe et al., 2017). As a result, caloric intake may be inadequate for optimal recovery of patients who undergo open heart surgery (Rahman et al., 2016). The effects of reperfusion injury following cardiac surgery have also been noted to impact nutritional status (Sanchez et al., 2011).

The etiologies of undernutrition in postoperative cardiac surgery patients include decreased intake of food, changes in metabolism, age, poor absorption of nutrients, increase in nutritional requirements, excess loss of nutrients, or decreased physical activity (Pathirana et al., 2014; van Venrooij et al., 2013). Decreased intake of food causes fat, muscle, skin, bone, and viscera loss; this results in weight loss and an increase in the amount of extracellular fluid. It also results in increased vulnerability for infection and pressure ulcers, impaired wound healing, and overgrowth of bacteria in the intestinal tract. Finally, malnutrition results in dysfunction of the immune system by impairing neutrophil, lymphocyte, and macrophage function and activation of the complement system (Fairfield & Askari, 2017).

Data over the past decade support the need for adequate nutritional intake in patients undergoing cardiac surgery (Chermesh et al., 2014). Outcomes such as improved wound healing, maintenance of gut integrity, and energy metabolism are cited as improved with adequate nutrition (Tepaske et al., 2001).

▶ Assessment of Nutrition

Nutrition screening is "a process to identify an individual who may be malnourished or at risk for malnutrition and to determine if a detailed nutrition assessment is indicated. It entails comprehensive medical, nutrition, and medication histories; physical exam, anthropometric measurements (measurement of the human body); and lab data" (Tyler & Guenter, 2017, p. 3).

The challenges associated with conducting a comprehensive assessment of the nutritional status of a patient undergoing cardiac surgery have been documented. Pivotal information, including lab and anthropometric data, complete history, and physical findings (e.g., unintended weight loss, decreased strength or stamina, diminished appetite, changes in digestive patterns) may alert the clinician of the possibility of alterations in nutrition and the potential impact these alterations may have on postoperative recovery from cardiac surgery (Sanchez et al., 2011).

Physical Exam

On conducting a physical exam, it is important to note whether the patient has a history of unintended weight gain or loss. Presence of chronic diseases (e.g., diabetes), infection, recent required hospitalization, and surgical history (especially GI surgery) should be assessed. Determination of whether the patient uses dietary supplements (e.g., protein shakes) should be made. Body mass index (BMI) should be calculated; this can be performed using any BMI calculator available online. The nurse should also assess for the presence of edema and for other symptoms of malnutrition, including loss of subcutaneous fat, hair loss, bleeding or sores in the oral cavity, stomatitis, evidence of heart failure, and loss of muscle mass in the extremities (Fairfield & Askari, 2017).

The American Society of Parenteral and Enteral Nutrition (ASPEN) (2015) delineates seven indications of adult patients being of nutritional risk: (1) unintended weight loss of 10% in the past 6 months or unintended 5% weight loss in the past month, (2) unintended increase or decrease in weight of 10 pounds (4.5 kg) within the past 6 months, (3) BMI less than 18.5 kg/m^2 or greater than 25 kg/m^2, (4) presence of chronic disease, (5) an increase in metabolic activity, (6) changes in diet or diet schedules, and (7) insufficient intake of nutrition for more than 1 week.

Lab Data

Three protein markers are used. While these markers do not directly reflect a patient's nutritional status, they do reflect a patient's severity of illness and can be used to determine therapy when evaluated concomitantly with other parameters.

Serum Albumin

A low serum albumin level ($<$2.2 g/dL) is an indicator of a negative catabolic state. Data on elderly patients who underwent general surgery reveal a correlation between a low serum albumin level and poor patient outcomes. The researchers concluded that, along with weight loss, serum albumin level is a reliable predictor of risk for nutrition decline and a complicated postoperative course (van Stijn et al., 2013). Hypoalbuminemia can occur with stress (including that associated with surgery) and liver or kidney disease (Fairfield & Askari, 2017).

Serum Transferrin

Serum transferrin levels can be used to evaluate a patient's protein status over the previous 2 to 4 weeks. It also reflects a patient's iron status. If a patient's iron level is within range, low serum transferrin levels can be used as an indicator of a patient's protein status (Fairfield & Askari, 2017).

Serum Prealbumin

Serum prealbumin levels decrease rapidly with the onset of malnutrition and increase quickly when there is adequate protein intake. However, serum prealbumin levels can be impacted with the onset of an inflammatory response. Production of prealbumin, in addition to the presence of cytokines associated with inflammation, can also be reduced in the presence of liver or kidney disease. As such, serum prealbumin levels are the least valuable to evaluate nutritional status (Fairfield & Askari, 2017).

Other Labs

A basic metabolic profile, including serum magnesium, phosphorus, and calcium levels, may be useful to evaluate a patient's overall clinical and fluid status. Addition of these electrolytes to the basic metabolic panel should be considered more so in patients with poor oral nutrition intake or in the presence of diarrhea (Fairfield & Askari, 2017).

Nutrition Risk Scoring Systems

Screening a patient's nutritional status is a "process of identifying characteristics known to be associated with malnutrition risk" (Pathirana et al., 2014). This is compared to a nutrition assessment, which reveals if a patient has malnutrition (Pathirana et al., 2014).

A number of scoring systems have been reported that can be used to assess patients' risk of nutritional deficits. Validity of these scoring systems have not been determined in patients who are critically ill. Ideally, a scoring system should be able to predict patients who will develop critical levels of malnutrition rather than just identifying patients who already have malnutrition (Stoppe et al., 2017). Screening tools that are easy to use and quick to complete are important (van Venrooij et al., 2013) to identify patients at risk for undernutrition postoperatively.

Lomivorotov and colleagues (2013b) evaluated five preoperative screening scoring systems in patients who were undergoing CPB surgery. Of the Subjective Global Assessment (SGA), Nutritional Risk Screening 2002 (NRS-2002), Malnutrition Universal Screening Tool (MUST), Mini-Nutritional Assessment (MNA), and Short Nutritional Assessment Questionnaire (SNAQ), the researchers concluded that the MUST and MNA tools best predicted postoperative cardiac surgery complications. The presence of malnutrition using the SNAQ, MUST, NRS-2002, and

MNA correlated with identified postoperative complications. The MUST, NRS-2002, MNA, and SGA determined malnutrition was associated with increased ICU length of stay in patients who underwent cardiac surgery. The SNAQ, MUST, and MNA determined malnutrition was associated with an increased hospital length of stay. The MUST and MNA determined malnutrition was associated with postoperative complications following cardiac surgery (Pathirana et al., 2014).

The Cardiac Surgery-Specific Malnutrition (CSSM) instrument combines data from the MUST with gender (female) and age (ages 65 or older) to patients at risk for undernutrition. The Cardiac Surgery-Specific Undernutrition Screening Tool (CSSUST), which takes into account decreased food intake and inactivity, is reported to be more sensitive than the CSSM in predicting undernutrition in patients undergoing cardiac surgery (van Venrooij et al., 2013). The Johns Hopkins Hospital Nutrition Support Score has been shown to predict patient need for nutritional support following cardiac surgery (Ohkuma et al., 2017).

The Nutrition Risk in Critically Ill (NUTRIC) tool identifies postoperative critically ill patients' nutritional risk. This scoring system identifies postoperative patients who are at high risk to develop malnutrition and who will benefit from aggressive nutritional support (Heyland, Dhaliwal, Wang, & Day, 2013). The NUTRIC score also discriminates between patients who are at a low risk for malnutrition who would not benefit or may be harmed by nutritional support (Stoppe et al., 2017).

Other Assessments

A noninvasive method to measure muscle mass that is described is performance of an ultrasound of the quadriceps muscle. This procedure can be performed to see if there are changes in amount of muscle and fat (Stoppe et al., 2017; Tillquist et al., 2014). The rectus femoris has also been used to evaluate skeletal muscle wasting (Puthucheary et al., 2013). Radiologic studies such as computed tomography and magnetic resonance imaging have also been described to assess for loss of muscle due to a catabolic state, to identify severe muscle loss, and to assess the effectiveness

of interventions being used to treat muscle wasting (Baracos & Kazemi-Bajestani, 2013).

According to expert consensus, for a diagnosis of malnutrition to be made, at least two of the following must be present: (1) inadequate caloric intake, (2) weight loss, (3) muscle mass loss, (4) subcutaneous fat loss, (5) accumulation of fluid (this may hide weight loss), and (6) decreased functional status as evidenced by strength of hand grasps (Fairfield & Askari, 2017).

Gonçalves and colleagues (2016) evaluated the preoperative nutritional status of patients who were undergoing elective cardiac surgery. They used nutritional screening, adductor pollicus (a muscle in the hand that is used to adduct the thumb) muscle thickness measurement (anthropometry), and lab testing (i.e., serum albumin, lymph cytometry, and lipid panel) to monitor patients for up to 10 days postoperatively. They reported a correlation between serum albumin levels and renal complications and anthropometry measurement of the nondominant hand with infectious complications. Over 51% of patients were found to be overweight and approximately 14% were underweight. Over 14% had diminished muscle reserves; the highest incidence was in elderly cardiac surgery patients. The sample also had 12.5% with hypoalbuminemia. Over 62% of patients developed postoperative complications. The highest incidence of complications was reported in patients who underwent myocardial revascularization or mitral valve replacement, but there was no statistically significant difference between patients who did and did not develop complications in these two groups. Similarly, there was no statistically significant difference in patients who were overweight or had hypoalbuminemia.

▶ Challenges to Attaining an Adequate Nutritional Status

Several small studies dating back to the 1970s documented the need for nutritional support in patients undergoing cardiac surgery, some of the associated challenges (Stoppe et al., 2017), and the inadequate intake of protein and calories in this vulnerable patient population (Rahman et al., 2016).

Several challenges for optimizing a patient's nutritional status following cardiac surgery have been identified. One of these includes a decrease in taste sensitivity. Keith, Mokbel, San Emeterio, Song, and Errett (2010) reported alterations in taste sensitivity for sweet, salt, sour, and bitter in patients who underwent coronary artery bypass graft surgery. These taste changes were still present 4 months postoperatively.

LaSierra and colleagues (2015) evaluated patients who underwent cardiac surgery who were hemodynamically unstable and who required mechanical ventilation for more than 24 hours. Of the 37 patients studied, just over 40% reached their caloric intake goal.

Similarly, Berger, Revelly, Cayeux, and Chiolero (2005) studied older (aged ≥70) postoperative on-pump cardiac surgery patients with left ventricular dysfunction. They also concluded that enteral nutrition (EN) is feasible in this patient population despite hemodynamic instability, but caloric needs could not adequately be met.

Older adults are now considered candidates for cardiac surgery given advances in the procedures. These patients may present with decreased nutritional status. Their metabolic reserves may also be altered. These conditions may pose challenges to this group of patients, especially when cardiac surgical procedures are not as clear-cut as planned (Sanchez et al., 2011).

Cardiac cachexia associated with heart failure is often seen in patients with end-stage heart disease. This specific type of protein-calorie malnutrition is associated with severe muscle wasting as well as fat and bone tissue loss and may put patients at risk for complications if they undergo cardiac surgery (Sanchez et al., 2011). The incidence of cachexia in patients with heart failure is 15%; up to 50% of patients with heart failure have malnutrition (Rahman et al., 2015). Collaboration with a nutritionist along with preoperative and postoperative nutritional support are recommended for this vulnerable patient population (Sanchez et al., 2011).

Data from one study reveals differences in caloric intake of patients who underwent open versus closed cardiac surgery. Patients in the former group had a lower intake of calories than their closed cardiac surgery counterparts. The differences in caloric intake decreased as the recovery time progressed. Statistical differences were not reported in this study (Hosain, Akter, Rasheed, Maruf, & Ahmed, 2009).

The timing of initiation of nutritional therapy in patients undergoing cardiac surgery is also challenging. While it may be optimal to perform a nutritional risk assessment preoperatively, most patients are admitted on their day of surgery. As such, a nutritional risk assessment should occur preoperatively so that the patient's nutritional status can be optimized prior to surgery (at least 2 to 7 days preoperatively) (Stoppe et al., 2017).

▶ Patients at Risk

Stoppe and colleagues (2017) identified risk factors that should be considered during the various phases patients experience when undergoing cardiac surgery. During the prehospital phase, patient demographics such as age, functional status, and frailty are identified. Patients with a BMI less than 20, those who have experienced weight loss over the previous 6 months, or those with comorbid conditions that cause an inflammatory response are also at risk. During the preoperative phase, patients with hemodynamic instability, with decreased oral intake, who required ICU admission prior to surgery, who had rescheduled surgery, or who are fasting are at risk. During the intraoperative phase, patients with hemodynamic instability or undergoing CPB are noted to be at risk for nutritional abnormalities and will likely require intense nutritional support postoperatively. Patients with postoperative hemodynamic instability or who have an extended ICU length of stay or postoperative complications are also at risk. Data are inconsistent regarding the relationship between BMI and postoperative surgery mortality (Costa et al., 2015; Thourani et al., 2011; Stamou et al., 2011; Vaduganathan et al., 2012).

▶ Evidence-Based Recommendations

The Guidelines for the Provision and Assessment of Nutrition Support in the Adult Critically Ill Patient: Society of Critical Care Medicine (SCCM) and ASPEN (hereafter, "guidelines") recommend performing a nutrition risk assessment on all patients admitted to the ICU if nutritional intake is deemed to be potentially altered. Six bundle statements are inherent within the guidelines. In addition to performing a nutrition risk assessment, which includes determining energy and protein requirements, initiation of enteral nutrition is recommended within 1 to 2 days of ICU admission with the goal of nutrition therapy to be reached over 1 week; implementation of measures to mitigate aspiration risk (e.g., head of bed elevation at 30 to 45 degrees, considering use of chlorhexidine mouthwash) and augment tolerance to the EN (e.g., administration of a prokinetic agent, continuous feeds); not using gastric residual volumes; and initiation of parenteral nutrition (PN) when EN is not adequate or achievable (McClave et al., 2016).

According to the guidelines, feeding may offset the metabolic effects of the stress response, mitigate oxidative cell injury, and alter immune responses in a positive way (McClave et al., 2016).

Given the few randomized controlled trials that have been conducted on nutritional status of patients undergoing cardiac surgery, the International Multidisciplinary Expert Group on Nutrition in Cardiac Surgery felt unable to provide compelling endorsements for adoption into practice. They did, however, publish six key recommendations:

1. Preoperatively, use a nutritional risk scoring system to identify patients in need of nutrition optimization.
2. Patients undergoing cardiac surgery who are deemed malnourished preoperatively should receive 2 to 7 days of nutritional therapy (Gustafsson et al., 2013).
3. All postoperative cardiac surgery patients should have a daily assessment of nutritional intake on postoperative day 3; all patients should be evaluated for alterations in nutrition. The goal of attaining at least 80% of their required protein and caloric intake with EN or PN should be met as soon as possible.
4. Postoperative cardiac surgery patients who are deemed high risk for alterations in nutrition and have an anticipated extended ICU length of stay should have nutritional support initiated 0 to 24 hours postoperatively.
5. Patients who have nutritional support initiated after a prolonged period of starvation or with malnutrition at baseline should be monitored for refeeding syndrome. These patients should have their nutrition needs advanced more slowly (over 3 to 4 days to attain their goal) (McClave et al., 2016).
6. Administration of an immune-modulating component (e.g., fish oil [FO], selenium) may be considered in patients beginning nutritional support in less than 24 hours in patients who underwent lengthy or complex cardiac surgery cases to decrease the inflammatory response (Stoppe et al., 2017).

Nutritional Support

Patients who should be considered to receive nutritional support include those who have identified deficits and those who are at risk, including patients with an actual or potential decrease in food intake and those with multiple organ dysfunction (Fairfield & Askari, 2017). Once it is determined that malnutrition is present or that the patient is at risk for its development, initiation of oral, enteral, or nutritional support is essential. Nurses should collaborate with a nutritionist and other members of the multidisciplinary team to determine which mode(s) of nutritional support is(are) indicated for the cardiac surgery patient. It is suggested that patients who have severe malnutrition preoperatively may benefit from a delay of surgery so that their nutrition status can be optimized (Fairfield & Askari, 2017).

Enteral Nutrition

The majority of patients who have undergone cardiac surgery are able to tolerate oral nutrition a few hours postoperatively. Those who are not able are at risk for malnutrition (Makikado, Lasierra, Pérez-Vela, & Gonzalez, 2014).

Enteral nutrition is the delivery of protein, calories, fluid, vitamins, minerals, electrolytes, and trace elements either orally or via a feeding tube. It is generally recommended over parenteral nutrition as it is safe and easy to administer and is associated with fewer complications and lower costs. The function of the mucosal barrier is maintained with EN (Fairfield & Askari, 2017). International data suggest that EN is favored over PN following cardiac surgery (Stoppe et al., 2017).

Enteral Nutrition and Hemodynamic Instability

When early EN is administered to hemodynamically unstable patients, it is primarily done to preserve the mucosal barrier (Yang, Wu, Yi, & Li, 2014). Enteral nutrition is felt to be contraindicated in hemodynamic failure due to associated decreases in splanchnic blood flow in relation to cardiac output. This is felt to put patients at risk for splanchnic ischemia (LaSierra et al., 2015). The ASPEN and European Society for Clinical Nutrition and Metabolism recommend withholding EN in patients with hemodynamic failure given this risk (McClave, Martindale, & Vanek, 2009).

Adequate blood supply and GI motility are required to safely begin early EN. When patients are hypotensive, blood shunts from the GI tract to protect the core (heart, brain, and lungs). Splanchnic perfusion may be further compromised if early EN is administered to patients with mesenteric ischemia and reduced peristalsis (Yang et al., 2014).

Some data support EN being administered to patients with hemodynamic instability and who are receiving vasopressors (Makikado et al., 2014). The data surrounding administration of early EN to patients with hemodynamic instability who are receiving vasopressor therapy, however, are conflicting. Both the benefits (e.g., restoration of splanchnic blood flow, decreased ICU length of stay, mortality, and infectious complications) and risk of complications (e.g., nonocclusive bowel necrosis) are reported in the literature (LaSierra et al., 2015; Yang et al., 2014).

Despite the aforementioned recommendations by ASPEN and the European Society for Clinical Nutrition and Metabolism, other data suggest that patients in the cardiac surgery ICU with hemodynamic failure may tolerate EN without serious adverse events (Makikado et al., 2014) as the gut is felt to be functional following cardiac surgery. In another study, postoperative cardiac surgery patients with hemodynamic failure (requiring two or more vasopressors, circulatory support, or both) and who required at least 24 hours of mechanical ventilation received EN. The most common complication reported was constipation. No serious adverse events were experienced. The researchers reported, however, it was difficult to deliver an adequate number of calories solely with EN. One patient developed a GI bleed with ischemic colon, which was attributed to the patient's history of vascular disease. They concluded that EN is feasible in patients with hemodynamic failure following cardiac surgery, including those who required extracorporeal membrane oxygenation (ECMO), intra-aortic balloon pump therapy, or mechanical assistance. The authors further reported challenges with attaining the required calories (LaSierra et al., 2015). This latter finding is consistent with earlier data reported by Berger and colleagues (2005).

Data reported by Khalid, Doshi, and DiGiovine (2010) suggest better outcomes when EN is initiated within the first 48 hours of admission to the ICU. The guidelines suggest that while EN may be used cautiously in patients who are stable on low-dose vasopressor therapy, it should be withheld on patients with a mean arterial pressure of less than 50 mmHg, in those who are having vasopressor therapy initiated for hypotension, and for those who are having vasopressor therapy titrated up to attain and maintain hemodynamic stability. Similarly, patients on vasopressor therapy who are manifesting symptoms suggesting EN intolerance (e.g., hypoactive bowel sounds, abdominal distention, decreased bowel movements or passing of gas, development of a metabolic acidosis) should be evaluated for ischemic bowel (McClave et al., 2016).

Earlier reports of decreased hospital and ICU lengths of stay, infectious complication rates, and mortality when EN nutrition is administered to patients with hemodynamic instability appear in the literature (Artinian, Krayem, & DiGiovine, 2006; Fernández-Ortega, Herrero Meseguer, & Martinez Garcia, 2011). These latter data, however, reflect findings of critically ill patients but not those who have undergone cardiac surgery.

Parenteral Nutrition

Parenteral nutrition is the administration of required nutrients via the intravenous route. It is indicated for patients who are not able to tolerate or receive EN.

A number of studies and meta-analyses have been published on the preoperative administration of PN. Data are conflicting, and the studies were not performed on patients undergoing cardiac surgery specifically. Some older studies and meta-analyses suggest that total PN may decrease postoperative complications (Bozzetti et al., 2000; Burden, Todd, Hill, & Lal, 2012; Heyland et al., 2001), while others report an increase in complication rate such as increased infection rate, ICU length of stay, and hospital costs (Heyland, 2012).

Earlier data suggest that use of PN with 10% intralipids in patients who underwent CPB did not cause negative hemodynamic sequela. Measured parameters included left ventricular stroke work, left ventricular filling pressure, cardiac output, systemic vascular resistance, mean arterial pressure, central venous pressure, and mean pulmonary artery pressure (Fisch & Abel, 1981).

Nutrients with Cardioprotective Properties

A number of studies have been conducted to investigate the role of antioxidants and various other nutrients with cardioprotective qualities (Sanchez et al., 2011). There are conflicting results of these studies. Given the inflammatory response associated with CPB with concomitant oxidative stress,

there is a potential for these sequelae to impact metabolism. Key nutrients such as the amino acids glutamine and arginine, omega-3 fatty acids, vitamins A, C, D, E, and micronutrients such as zinc and selenium were evaluated. While logical, data did not support their use in critically ill patients in the ICU (Bloos et al., 2016; Heyland et al., 2013; Stoppe et al., 2017; van Zanten et al., 2014; Ziegler et al., 2016). In the Ziegler study, it was suggested that the sample size may not have been adequate to fully determine differences in incidence of bloodstream infections or 6-month mortality of patients who did and did not receive glutamine supplementation (Fairfield & Aksari, 2017). Further, in one study glutamine supplementation was associated with the development of multiple organ dysfunction and death (Heyland et al., 2013).

In patients who underwent cardiac surgery, data from one earlier study suggested that administration of coenzyme Q10, magnesium, omega-3 fatty acids, and selenium resulted in decreased myocardial damage and decreased length of stay (Leong et al., 2010). More recent data do not support beneficial effects of the amino acid arginine or glycine (Visser et al., 2015).

Earlier studies have examined the effects of administration of the amino acid arginine or aspartate, or the neurotransmitter glutamate in patients who were undergoing cardiac surgery. Increased heart flow was reported in patients who received supplementation with arginine (Visser et al., 2011).

A number of meta-analyses have been performed to evaluate the effect of immunonutrition. This entails supplementing nutrition with arginine, glutamine, nonessential fatty acids, or branched chain fatty acids. The data are inconsistent. Results of some meta-analyses reflect a decrease in postoperative infections and hospital length of stay but no effect on mortality rates (Drover et al., 2011; Fairfield & Askari, 2017; Mazaki, Ishii, & Murai, 2015). The meta-analyses performed on this subject lacked strength; recommendations were unable to be made based on the results (Fairfield & Askari, 2017; Marik & Zaloga, 2008; Marimuthu, Varadhan, Ljungqvist, & Lobo, 2012).

Polyunsaturated Fatty Acids (PUFAs)

Data from studies evaluating administration of emulsions that contain fish oils to patients undergoing cardiac surgery suggest that the inflammatory response to surgery may be moderated (Berger et al., 2013). A more recent systematic review suggests that administration of FO emulsions in either EN or PN may significantly decrease postoperative infection rate, length of time on mechanical ventilation, and length of stay (Manzanares, Langlosi, Dhaliwal, Lemieux, & Heyland, 2015).

Conflicting results of clinical trials evaluating the effect of omega-3 PUFAs in patients undergoing cardiac surgery are reported. Omega-3 PUFAs are hypothesized to produce systemic anti-inflammatory effects and affect immune response (Langlios, Hardy, & Manzanares, 2017).

A recent systematic review of 14 randomized controlled trials revealed a decreased length of hospital stay and incidence of postoperative atrial fibrillation in patients who had undergone cardiac surgery. No significant differences in ICU length of stay or mortality rates were found. The anti-inflammatory effect of PUFAs was found to be most prevalent in patients who underwent CPB. The authors confirm that given the differences in doses of omega-3 PUFAs, types of surgery performed, and amount of time over which PUFAs were administered, a strong recommendation for PUFA administration could not be made for its use (Langlios et al., 2017).

Data from some earlier studies revealed no difference in ICU length of stay with administration of PUFAs (Berger et al., 2013; Bernabe-Garcia et al., 2013; Farquharson et al., 2011; Rodrigo et al., 2013; Yamamoto et al., 2014). Other data corroborated that hospital length of stay was significantly lower for patients who underwent cardiac surgery who received PUFAs (Berger et al., 2013; Castillo et al., 2011; Farquharson et al., 2011; Kolesnikov, Boeva, Yagoda, Danilova, & Danilov, 2014; Rodrigo et al., 2013; Sorice, Tritto, Sordelli, Gregorio, & Piazza, 2011; Yamamoto et al., 2014).

Data from several studies revealed a significant difference in incidence of postoperative atrial fibrillation in patients who underwent cardiac surgery and received PUFAs (Berger et al., 2013; Castillo et al., 2011; Farquharson et al., 2011; Kolesnikov et al., 2014; Leong et al., 2010; Lomivorotov et al., 2014; Mozaffarian et al., 2012; Rodrigo, Gutierrez, Fernandez, & Guzman, 2012; Rodrigo et al., 2013; Sandesara et al., 2012; Sorice et al., 2011; Wilbring, Ploetze, Bormann, Waldow, & Matschke, 2014; Yamamoto et al., 2014). Of note, patients who received PUFAs with parenteral nutrition had no significant decrease in incidence of postoperative atrial fibrillation; only patients who received omega-3 PUFAs via EN experienced this benefit (Langlios et al., 2017). Data also reflect no decrease in mechanical ventilation time with the administration of PUFAs to patients who underwent cardiac surgery (Berger et al., 2013; Leong et al., 2010).

▶ Nursing Interventions

Given the significant role that nutrition plays in the recovery of a patient who has undergone cardiac surgery, it is essential for nurses to collaborate with the multidisciplinary team to implement strategies to augment postoperative nutrition. **BOX 23.1** lists some suggested strategies. In addition, nurses should collaborate with the multidisciplinary team to initiate enteral feeds on any cardiac surgery patient who is unable to resume oral nutrition postoperatively. This is viewed as a proactive strategy that may serve to decrease the severity of an illness and ICU length of stay, and mitigate postoperative complications (McClave et al., 2016).

Nutritional support entails identifying patients at risk, providing patient and family education, and coordinating the administration of nutrition. Upon identifying patients at risk for malnutrition, it is essential for nurses to communicate their findings to the multidisciplinary team (Tyler & Guenter, 2017). Based on the assessment of nutritional risk, postoperative patients with hemodynamic instability, who have an increased length of stay in the ICU, or who are experiencing postoperative complications should receive EN or PN and physiotherapy (Stoppe et al., 2017).

BOX 23.1 Nursing Strategies to Augment Caloric Intake in Patients Undergoing Cardiac Surgery

Use of a tool to identify patients who lack proper nutrition preoperatively

Counsel patient about nutritional issues before surgery

Early postoperative mobilization

Encourage a high-calorie diet

Monitor daily caloric intake

Monitor for signs of gut ischemia

Consider additions to the patient's diet (e.g., lemon) to increase palatability

Prevent malnutrition

Prevent complications of malnutrition

Treat malnutrition in collaboration with the multidisciplinary team

Refer to the evidence guidelines of ASPEN.

Patients found to be at risk should be referred to a nutritionist

Note: ASPEN, American Society of Parenteral and Enteral Nutrition
Data from Hosain, Akter, Rasheed, Maruf, & Ahmed, 2009; LaSierra et al., 2015; Tyler & Guenter, 2017; van Venrooij et al., 2013

Nurses in the ICU should collaborate with the multidisciplinary team to ensure the patient receives adequate caloric, protein, macronutrient, and micronutrient intake. Logically, the nutrition plan of care should be derived from the nutrition assessment. Ongoing monitoring is key (Tyler & Guenter, 2017).

▶ Summary

Identifying patients at risk, collaborating with the multidisciplinary team to implement and manage a comprehensive plan of care, and conducting an ongoing evaluation of the nutritional status of patients undergoing cardiac surgery are essential elements of care that can optimize postoperative outcomes. More data from randomized controlled trials are needed to provide additional evidence for clinical practice guidelines in order to optimize the nutritional status of patients who undergo cardiac surgery. Identification of patients at risk for alterations in nutritional status is essential (Stoppe et al., 2017).

To mitigate some of the reported deleterious effects of cardiac surgery, nurses working in the outpatient and inpatient settings play a pivotal role in promoting optimal patient outcomes. As there are no established standards on how to decide which patients will gain the most from nutritional therapy (Stoppe et al., 2017), high levels of critical thinking and collaboration with the multidisciplinary team are critical.

🔍 CASE STUDY

A 70-year-old patient of Korean descent was admitted with a history of coronary artery disease, diabetes mellitus, hypertension, and tobacco use for 50 years. The patient reports leading a sedentary lifestyle. The most recent echocardiogram revealed a left ventricular ejection fraction of 30% compared to 3 years prior at 55%. He was admitted for a planned robotic assisted CABG ×1 and in situ left mammary artery to LAD as part of the first stage of a hybrid revascularization with planned PCI to circumflex.

His dietary pattern includes fish, rice, and fried vegetables prepared with typical Korean spices that contain high sodium levels.

Critical Thinking Questions

1. What risk factors does this patient have that predisposes him to postoperative nutritional deficits?
2. For which complications should the patient assess?
3. What is the nurse's role to help promote optimal nutrition in the patient postoperatively?

> ### Answers to Critical Thinking Questions
>
> 1. The patient has a lack of physical activity. He is also aging and has associated alterations in metabolism. He also has a history of diabetes. His diet lacks protein. He may also have cardiac cachexia associated with heart failure.
> 2. If the patient has nutritional deficits preoperatively, there is an increased risk of postoperative infection, increased length of ICU and hospital lengths of stay, readmission, pressure injury development, poor wound healing, decreased quality of life, and death.
> 3. Nurses should collaborate with a nutritionist and other members of the multidisciplinary team to determine which mode(s) of nutritional support is(are) indicated for the cardiac surgery patient. It is suggested that patients who have severe malnutrition preoperatively may benefit from a delay of surgery so that their nutrition status can be optimized.

Self-Assessment Questions

1. Which puts the cardiac surgery patient at risk for postoperative nutritional issues?
   A. Prolonged on-pump time
   B. Fasting for 24 hours preoperatively
   C. Exercising preoperatively
   D. Changes in metabolism from cardiac disease

2. Which patient is at greatest risk for alterations in nutrition? A patient with:
   A. weight loss of 15 pounds after dieting.
   B. obesity.
   C. preference for having a protein bar as a meal alternative.
   D. elevated transferrin levels.

3. Which patient should the nurse anticipate having a low prealbumin level? A patient with:
   A. serum creatinine 2.3 mg/dL.
   B. bilirubin 1 mg/dL.
   C. a resolved inflammatory process.
   D. low iron levels.

4. According to expert consensus, which patient can be considered to have malnutrition? A patient with:
   A. increased in edema.
   B. increased subcutaneous fat.
   C. caloric intake of 2,000/day.
   D. weight gain of 10 pounds in a month's time.

5. Which is a *contraindication* to receiving enteral nutrition? A patient:
   A. with left ventricular dysfunction.
   B. with taste sensitivity.
   C. receiving extracorporeal membrane oxygenation therapy.
   D. with splanchnic ischemia.

6. A postoperative cardiac surgery patient is receiving parenteral nutrition with fish oils and asks why the supplement was added. Which is the nurse's best response?
   A. "All of the data show that you will have a decreased length of stay with use of fish oils."
   B. "The fish oils will increase heart flow."
   C. "Fish oils decrease the risk of your developing multiple organ dysfunction syndrome."
   D. "Fish oils may decrease the inflammation associated with surgery."

7. Upon assessment of a preoperative cardiac surgery patient, the nurse notes the presence of decreased strength and stamina, edema, hair loss, and mouth sores. With whom should the nurse initially collaborate?
   A. The surgeon
   B. A nutritionist
   C. A physical therapist
   D. A dentist

8. Which should the nurse help assure the patient needs after cardiac surgery?
   A. Increased protein and increased calories
   B. Increased glycogen and decreased fat
   C. Increased carbohydrates and decreased antioxidants
   D. Decreased micronutrients and decreased calories

9. Which patient should be suspected of having undernutrition?

	Weight in January (in pounds)	Weight in July (in pounds)
A.	125	135
B.	130	145
C.	150	140
D.	140	125

10. A patient asks what it means when completing a nutritional risk scoring tool. The nurse's best response is, "The score will tell us _____."
    A. how much muscle loss to anticipate after surgery
    B. if you are at risk for malnutrition after surgery
    C. which postoperative complications you will develop
    D. your length of stay after surgery

Answers to Self-Assessment Questions

1. D. **changes in metabolism from cardiac disease**
   Rationale: A patient with alterations in metabolism from cardiac disease related to the presence of cardiac disease places the patient at risk. Prolonged on-pump time and fasting for 24 hours preoperatively are not risk factors. Lack of physical exercise puts the patient at risk.

2. B. **obesity**
   Rationale: A patient with a BMI of 25 kg/m^2 or greater is at risk for alterations in nutrition. Unintended weight loss is a factor, but the patient in option A had intended weight loss. Use of dietary supplements should be part of the nutritional assessment but is not necessarily a risk for alteration in nutrition. Serum transferrin levels can be used to evaluate a patient's protein status over the previous 2 to 4 weeks. It also reflects a patient's iron status. If a patient's iron level is within range, low serum transferrin levels can be used as an indicator of a patient's protein status.

3. A. **serum creatinine 2.3 mg/dL**
   Rationale: Production of prealbumin can be reduced with kidney disease. Liver disease can decrease prealbumin levels but the patient in option B has a bilirubin level within range. Inflammatory processes decrease production of prealbumin; the inflammatory process is resolved in the patient in option C. Serum transferrin levels are affected by iron levels.

4. A. **increase in edema**
   Rationale: Accumulation of fluid is a criterion for the diagnosis of malnutrition. Decreased subcutaneous fat, inadequate caloric intake, and weight loss are other criteria.

5. D. **with splanchnic ischemia**
   Rationale: Presence of gut ischemia is a contraindication for a patient to receive enteral nutrition based on the evidence. Data suggest that patients with left ventricular dysfunction can receive enteral nutrition. Taste changes are challenges to patients receiving adequate nutrition but are not a contraindication to enteral nutrition. Data suggest that patients on extracorporeal membrane oxygenation therapy can receive enteral nutrition.

6. D. "**Fish oils may decrease the inflammation associated with surgery.**"
   Rationale: Data suggest that the inflammatory response of surgery with cardiopulmonary bypass can be mitigated with fish oils. The data are not consistent that length of stay will decrease. Fish oils do not increase heart blood flow and do not decrease the risk of development of multiple organ dysfunction syndrome.

7. B. **a nutritionist**
    Rationale: This patient has symptoms consistent with malnutrition. Collaboration with a nutritionist is indicated. While surgery may be delayed in the face of malnutrition, collaboration with a nutritionist in indicated first. The decreased strength and stamina and mouth sores are likely related to malnutrition. Collaboration with a physical therapist or dentist is not indicated at this time.

8. A. **increased protein and increased calories**
    Rationale: Increased protein and calories are needed for the hypermetabolic state associated with cardiac surgery. The other macronutrients and micronutrients are not helpful in the face of a hypermetabolic state.

9. D. **140/125**
    Rationale: A weight loss of greater than 10% in 6 months is an indicator of presence of undernutrition. Weight gain is not necessarily an indicator of undernutrition. The patient in option C had a weight loss of less than 10%.

10. B. **if you are at risk for malnutrition after surgery**
    Rationale: The purpose of a nutritional risk assessment is to determine if a patient is at risk for developing alterations in nutrition postoperatively. It does not help predict muscle loss, determine which complications a patient is likely to experience postoperatively, or predict length of stay.

CLINICAL INQUIRY BOX

Question: What is the evidence about nutrition in patients undergoing cardiac surgery?

Reference: Hill, A., Nesterova, E., Lomivorotov, V., Efremov, S., Goetzenich, A., Benstoem, C., . . . Stoppe, C. (2018).

Objective: To describe the most recent evidence associated with nutrition in patients undergoing cardiac surgery.

Method: Systematic review

Results: Topics discussed included inflammation in cardiac surgery, importance of nutrition in cardiac surgery, and a systematic review of current nutritional practice.

Conclusion: There are low levels of evidence from small studies and heterogeneous patient populations, with different nutritional interventions used in the studies found. There is a need for adequate studies and for clinical guidelines.

References

American Society for Parenteral and Enteral Nutrition. (2015). *Improving patient outcomes: A.S.P.E.N.'s step-by-step guide to addressing malnutrition.* Silver Springs, MD: Author.

American Society for Parenteral and Enteral Nutrition. (2018). *Definitions.* Retrieved from https://www.nutritioncare.org/Guidelines_and_Clinical_Resources/Toolkits/Malnutrition_Toolkit/Definitions/

Artinian, V., Krayem, H., & DiGiovine, B. (2006). Effects of early enteral feeding on the outcome of critically ill mechanically ventilated medical patients. *Chest, 129,* 960–967.

Baracos, V., & Kazemi-Bajestani, S. M. R. (2013). Clinical outcomes related to muscle mass in humans with cancer and catabolic illnesses. *The International Journal of Biochemistry and Cell Biology, 45*(10), 2302–2308.

Berger, M. M., Delodder, F., Liaudet, L., Tozzi, P., Schlaepfer, J., Chioléro, R. L., . . . Tappy, L. (2013). Three short perioperative infusions of n-3 PUFAs reduce systemic inflammation induced by cardiopulmonary bypass surgery: A randomized controlled trial. *The American Journal of Clinical Nutrition, 97*(2), 246–254.

Berger, M. M., Revelly, J. P., Cayeux, M. C., & Chiolero, R. L. (2005). Enteral nutrition in critically ill patients with severe hemodynamic failure after cardiopulmonary bypass. *Clinical Nutrition, 24*(1), 124–132.

Bernabe-Garcia, M., Mansilla-Olivares, A., Maldonado-Hernandez, J., Blanco-Favela, L., Chavez-Sanchez, K., Chavez-Rueda, K., . . . Riera-Kinkel, C. (2013). Oral administration of n-3 long-chain fatty acids reduce inflammatory response and improve clinical outcomes in patients with cardiovascular surgery. *Experimental & Clinical Cardiology, 20,* 145–160.

Bloos, F., Trips, E., Nierhaus, A., Briegel, J., Heyland, D. K., Jashinski, U., . . . Reinhart, K. (2016). Effect of sodium selenite administration and procalcitonin-guided therapy on mortality in patients with severe sepsis or septic shock: A randomized clinical trial. *Journal of the American Medical Association, 176,* 1266–1276.

Bozzetti, F., Gavazzi, C., Miceli, R., Rossi, N., Mariani, L., Cozzaglio, L., . . . Piacenza, A. (2000). Perioperative total parenteral nutrition in malnourished, gastrointestinal cancer patients: A randomized, clinical trial. *Journal of Parenteral and Enteral Nutrition, 24*(1), 7–14.

Burden, S., Todd, C., Hill, J., & Lal, S. (2012). Pre-operative nutrition support in patients undergoing gastrointestinal surgery. *Cochrane Database of Systematic Reviews, 11,* CD008879.

Cangelosi, M. J., Rodday, A. M., Saunders, T., & Cohen, J. T. (2014). Evaluation of the economic burden of diseases associated with poor nutrition status. *Journal of Parenteral and Enteral Nutrition, 38*(2 Suppl), 35S–41S.

Castillo, R., Rodrigo, R., Perez, F., Cereceda, M., Asenjo, R., Zamorano, J., . . . Aguayo, R. (2011). Antioxidant therapy reduces oxidative and inflammatory tissue damage in patients subjected to cardiac surgery with extracorporeal circulation. *Basic & Clinical Pharmacology & Toxicology, 108*(4), 256–262.

Chermesh, I., Hajos, J., Mashiach, T., Bozhko, M., Shani, L., Nir, R. R., . . . Bolotin, G. (2014). Malnutrition in cardiac surgery: Food for thought. *European Journal of Preventive Cardiology, 21*(4), 475–483.

Costa, V. E. A., Ferolla, S. M., dos Reis, T. O., Rabello, R. R., Rocha, E. A. V., Couto, C. M. F., . . . Bento, A. (2015). Impact of body mass index on outcome in patients undergoing coronary artery bypass grafting and/or valve replacement surgery. *Brazilian Journal of Cardiovascular Surgery, 30*(3). doi:10.5935/1678-9741.20150027

Drover, J. W., Dhaliwal, R., Weitzel, L., Wischmeyer, P. E., Ochoa, J. B., & Heyland, D. K. (2011). Perioperative use of arginine-supplemented diets: A systematic review of the evidence. *Journal of the American College of Surgery, 212*(3), 385–399.

Fairfield, K. M., & Askari, R. (2017). *Overview of perioperative nutritional support.* Retrieved from http://www.uptodate.com/contents/overview-of-perioperative-nutritional-support

Farquharson, A. L., Metcalf, R. G., Sanders, P., Stuklis, R., Edwards, J. R., Gibson, R. A., . . . Young, G. D. (2011). Effect of dietary fish oil on atrial fibrillation after cardiac surgery. *American Journal of Cardiology, 108*(6), 851–856.

Fernández-Ortega, J. F., Herrero Meseguer, J. I., & Martinez Garcia, P. (2011). Guidelines for specialized nutritional and metabolic support in the critically ill patient: Update. Consensus SEMICYUC-SENPE: Indications timing, and routes of nutrient delivery. *Nutricion Hospitalaria, 26*(Suppl 2), S7–S11.

Fisch, D., & Abel, R. M. (1981). Hemodynamic effects of intravenous fat emulsions in patients with heart disease. *Journal of Parenteral and Enteral Nutrition, 5*(5), 402–405.

Gonçalves, L. de B., de Jesus, N. M. T., Gonçalves, M. de B., Dias, L. C. G., & Deiró, T. C. B. (2016). Preoperative

nutritional status and clinical complications in the postoperative period of cardiac surgeries. *Brazilian Journal of Cardiovascular Surgery, 31*(5), 371–380.

Gustafsson, U. O., Scott, M. J., Schwenk, W., Demartines, N., Roulin, D., Francis, N., . . . International Association for Surgical Metabolism and Nutrition (IASMEN). (2013). Guidelines for perioperative care in elective colonic surgery: Enhanced Recovery After Surgery (ERAS) Society recommendations. *World Journal of Surgery, 37*(2), 259–284.

Heyland, D. K. (2012). Early supplemental parenteral nutrition in critically ill adults increased infections, ICU length of stay, and cost. *Evidence-Based Medicine, 17*(3), 86–87.

Heyland, D. K., Dhaliwal, R., Wang, M., & Day, A. G. (2015). The prevalence of iatrogenic underfeeding in the nutritionally "at risk" critically ill patient: Results of an international, multicenter, prospective study. *Clinical Nutrition, 34,* 659–666.

Heyland, D. K., Montalvo, M., MacDonald, S., Keefe, L., Su, X. Y., & Drover, J. W. (2001). Total parenteral nutrition in the surgical patient: A meta-analysis. *Canadian Journal of Surgery, 44*(2), 102–111.

Heyland, D., Muscedere, J., Wischmeyer, P. E., Cook, D., Jones, G., Albert, M., . . . Day, A. G. (2013). A randomized trial of glutamine and antioxidants in critically ill adults. *The New England Journal of Medicine, 368,* 1489–1497.

Hosain, S. N., Akter, S. J., Rasheed, H., Maruf, F., & Ahmed, N. (2009). Effect of cardiopulmonary bypass on postoperative nutrition of cardiac surgery patients. *Bangladesh Medical Journal, 38*(2), 53–55.

Keith, M., Mokbel, R., San Emeterio, M., Song, J., & Errett, L. (2010). Evaluation of taste sensitivity in patients undergoing coronary artery bypass graft surgery. *Journal of the American Dietetic Association, 110*(7), 1072–1077.

Khalid, I., Doshi, P., & DiGiovine, B. (2010). Early enteral nutrition and outcomes of critically ill patients treated with vasopressors and mechanical ventilation. *American Journal of Critical Care, 19,* 261–268.

Kolesnikov, V. N., Boeva, O. I., Yagoda, A. S., Danilova, E. N., & Danilov, S. V. (2014). Prevention of new-onset atrial fibrillation after direct myocardial revascularization surgery: Randomized comparative study. *News of the North Caucasus, 10,* 120–127.

Langlios, P. L., Hardy, G., & Manzanares, W. (2017). Omega-3 polyunsaturated fatty acids in cardiac surgery patients: An updated systematic review and meta-analysis. *Clinical Nutrition, 36*(3), 737–746.

LaSierra, J. F. L., Pérez-Vela, J. L., Makikado, L. D. U., Sánchez, E. T., Gómez, L. C., Rodriguez, B. M., . . . González, J. C. M. (2015). Early enteral nutrition in patients with hemodynamic failure following cardiac surgery. *Journal of Parenteral and Enteral Nutrition, 39*(2), 154–162.

Leong, J.-Y., van der Merwe, J., Pepe, S., Bailey, M., Perkins, A., Lymbury, R., . . . Rosenfeldt, F. (2010). Perioperative metabolic therapy improves redox status and outcomes in cardiac surgery patients: A randomized trial. *Heart, Lung, & Circulation, 19*(10), 584–591.

Lomivorotov, V. V., Efremov, S. M., Boboshko, V. A., Nikolaev, D. A., Vedernikov, P. E., Deryagin, M. N., . . . Karaskov, A. M. (2013a). Prognostic value of nutritional screening tools for patients scheduled for cardiac surgery. *Interactive Cardiovascular and Thoracic Surgery*, 16(5), 612–618.

Lomivorotov, V. V., Efremov, S. M., Boboshko, V. A., Nikolaev, D. A., Vedernikov, P. E., Lomivorotov, V. N., . . . Karaskov, A. M. (2013b). Evaluation of nutritional screening tools for patients scheduled for cardiac surgery. *Nutrition*, 29(2), 436–442.

Lomivorotov, V.V., Efremov, S.M., Pokushalov, E.A., Romanov, A.B., Ponomarev, D.N., Chemiavsky, A. M., . . . Lomivorotov, V. N.214). Randomized trial of fish oil infusion to prevent atrial fibrillation after cardiac surgery: Data from an implantable continuous cardiac monitor. *Journal of Cardiothoracic and Vascular Anesthesia*, 28,(5), 1278-1284.

Lukas, G., Davies, A. R., Hilton, A. K., Pellegrino, V. A., Scheinkestel, C. O., & Ridley, E. (2010). Nutritional support in adult patients receiving extracorporeal membrane oxygenation. *Critical Care Resuscitation*, 12, 230–234.

Makikado, L. D. U., Lasierra, J. L. F., Pérez-Vela, J. L., & Gonzalez, J. C. M. (2014). Early enteral nutrition in postoperative cardiac surgery patients with severe hemodynamic failure and venoarterial (VA) extracorporeal membrane oxygenation (ECMO). *Diet and Nutrition in Critical Care*, 1–14. doi:10.1007/978-1-4614-8503-2_67-1

Manzanares, W., Langlosi, P. L., Dhaliwal, R., Lemieux, M., & Heyland, D. K. (2015). Intravenous fish oil lipid emulsions in critically ill patients: An updated systematic review and meta-analysis. *Critical Care*, 19. doi:10.1186/s13043-015-0888-7

Marik, P. E., & Zaloga, G. P. (2008). Immunonutrition in critically ill patients: A systematic review and analysis of the literature. *Intensive Care Medicine*, 34(11), 1980–1990.

Marimuthu, K., Varadhan, K. K., Ljungqvist, O., & Lobo, D. N. (2012). A meta-analysis of the effect of combinations of immune modulating nutrients on outcome in patients undergoing major open gastrointestinal surgery. *Annals of Surgery*, 255(6), 1060–1068.

Mazaki, T., Ishii, Y., & Murai, L. (2015). Immunoenhanced enteral and parenteral nutrition for gastrointestinal surgery: A multiple-treatments meta-analysis. *Annals of Surgery*, 261(4), 662–669.

McClave, S., Martindale, R. G., & Vanek, W. V. (2009). Guidelines for the provision and assessment of nutrition support therapy in the adult critically ill patient: Society of Critical Care Medicine (SCCM) and American Society for Parenteral and Enteral Nutrition (A.S.P.E.N.). *Journal of Parenteral and Enteral Nutrition*, 33, 277–316.

McClave, S. A., Taylor, B. E., Martindale, R. G., Warren, M. M., Johnson, D. R., Braunschweig, C., . . . Society of Critical Care Medicine, and the American Society for Parenteral and Enteral Nutrition. (2016). Guidelines for the provision and assessment of nutrition support in the adult critically ill patient: Society of Critical Care Medicine (SCCM) and American Society of Parenteral and Enteral Nutrition (A.S.P.E.N.) *Journal of Parenteral and Enteral Nutrition*, 40(2), 159–211.

Mozaffarian, D., Marchioli, R., Macchia, A., Silletta, M. G., Ferrazzi, P., Gardner, T. J., . . . Tognoni, G. (2012). Fish oil and postoperative atrial fibrillation: The omega-3 fatty acids for prevention of postoperative atrial fibrillation. (OPERA) randomized trial. *Journal of the American Medical Association*, 308, 2001–2011.

Ohkuma, R. E., Crawford, T. C., Brown, P. M., Grimm, J. C., Magruder, J. T., Kilic, A., . . . Whitman, G. J. R. (2017). A novel risk score to predict the need for nutrition support after cardiac surgery. *Annals of Thoracic Surgery*. doi:10.1016/j.athorasurg.2017.03.013

Pathirana, A. K., Lokunarangoda, N., Ranathunga, J., Santharaj, W. S., Ekanayake, R., & Jayawardena, R. (2014). Prevalence of hospital malnutrition among cardiac patients: Results from six nutrition screening tools. *SpringerPlus*, 3. Retrieved from http://www.springerplus.com/content/3/1/412

Puthucheary, Z. A., Rawal, J., McPhail, M., Connolly, B., Ratnayake, G., Chan, P., . . . Montgomery, H. E. (2013). Acute skeletal muscle wasting in critical illness. *Journal of the American Medical Association*, 310(15), 1591–1600.

Rahman, A., Agarwala, R., Martin, C., Nagpal, D., Teitelbaum, M., & Heyland, D. K. (2016). Nutrition therapy in critically ill patients following cardiac surgery: Defining and improving practice. *Journal of Parenteral and Enteral Nutrition*. doi:10.1177/0148607116661839

Rahman, A., Jafry, S., Jeejeebhoy, K., Nagpal, D., Pisani, B., & Agarwala, R. (2015). Malnutrition and cachexia in heart failure. *Journal of Parenteral and Enteral Nutrition*, 40(4), 475–486.

Rodrigo, R., Gutierrez, R., Fernandez, R., & Guzman, P. (2012). Ageing improves the antioxidant response against postoperative atrial fibrillation: A randomized controlled trial. *Interactive Cardiovascular Thoracic Surgery*, 15(2), 209–214.

Rodrigo, R., Korantzopoulos, P., Cereceda, M., Asenjo, R., Zamorano, J., Villalabeitia, E., . . . Gormaz, J. G. (2013). A randomized controlled trial to prevent post-operative atrial fibrillation by antioxidant reinforcement. *Journal of the American College of Cardiology*, 62(16), 1457–1465.

Sanchez, J. A., Sanchez, L. L., & Dudrick, S. J. (2011). Nutritional considerations in adult cardiothoracic surgical patients. *Surgical Clinics of North America*, 91(4), 857–875.

Sandesara, C. M., Chung, M. K., Van Wagoner, D. R., Barringer, T. A., Allen, K., Ismail, H. M., . . . Olshansky, B. (2012). A randomized, placebo-controlled trial of omega-3 fatty acids for inhibition of supraventricular arrhythmias after cardiac surgery: The FISH trial. *Journal of the American Heart Association*, 1, e000547.

Snider, J. T., Linthicum, M. T., Wu, Y., LaVallee, C., Lakdawalla, D. N., Hegazi, R., . . . Matarese, L. (2014). Economic burden of community-based disease-associated malnutrition in the United States. *Journal of Parenteral and Enteral Nutrition*, 38(2), S77–S85.

Sorice, M., Tritto, F. P., Sordelli, C., Gregorio, R., & Piazza, L. (2011). N-3 polyunsaturated fatty acides reduces postoperative atrial fibrillation incidence in patients undergoing "on-pump" coronary artery bypass graft surgery. *Monaldi Archives for Chest Disease, 76*(2), 93–98.

Stamou, S. C., Nussbaum, M., Stiegel, R. M., Reames, M. K., Skipper, E. R., Robicsek, F., . . . Lobdell, K. W. (2011). Effect of body mass index on outcomes after cardiac surgery: Is there an obesity paradox. *Annals of Thoracic Surgery, 91*(1), 42–47.

Stoppe, C., Goetzenich, A., Whitman, G., Ohkuma R., Brown, T., Hatzakorzian, R., . . . Heyland, D. K. (2017). Role of nutrition support in adult cardiac surgery: A consensus statement from an international multidisciplinary expert group on nutrition in cardiac surgery. *Critical Care, 21.* doi:10.1186/s13054-017-1690-5

Tepaske, R., Velthuis, H., Oudemans-van Straaten, H. M., Heisterkamp, S. H., van Deventer, S. J., Ince, C., . . . Keseciuglu, J. (2001). Effect of preoperative oral immune-enhancing nutritional support on patients at high risk of infection after cardiac surgery: A randomized placebo-controlled trial. *Lancet, 358*(9283), 696–701.

Thourani, V. H., Keeling, W. B., Kilgo, P. D., Puskas, J. D., Lattouf, O. M., & Guyton, R. A. (2011). The impact of body mass index on morbidity and short- and long-term mortality in cardiac vascular surgery. *The Journal of Thoracic and Cardiovascular Surgery, 142,* 1052–1061.

Tillquist, M., Kutsogiannis, D. J., Wischmeyer, P. E., Kummerien, C., Leung, R., Stollery, D., . . . Heyland, D. K. (2014). Bedside ultrasound is a practical and reliable measurement tool for assessing quadriceps muscle layer thickness. *Journal of Parenteral and Enteral Nutrition, 38*(7), 886–890.

Tyler, R. D., & Guenter, P. (2017). Identifying malnutrition: From acute care to discharge and beyond. *Nurse Practitioner, 42*(4), 18–24.

Vaduganathan, M., Lee, R., Beckham, A. J., Andrei, A. C., Lapin, B., Stone, N. J., . . . McCarthy, P. M. (2012). Relation of body mass index to late survival after valvular heart surgery. *American Journal of Cardiology, 110*(11), 1667–1678.

van Stijn, M. F., Korkic-Halilovic, I., Bakker, M. S., van der Ploeg, T., van Leeuwen, P. A., & Houdijk, A. P. (2013). Preoperative nutrition status and postoperative outcome in elderly general surgery patients: A systematic review. *Journal of Parenteral and Enteral Nutrition, 37*(1), 37–43.

van Venrooij, L. M., De Vos, R., Zijlstra, E., Borgmeijer-Hoelen, A. M., Leeuwen, P. A., & De Mol, B. A. (2011). The impact of low preoperative fat-free body mass on infections and length of stay after cardiac surgery: A prospective cohort study. *The Journal of Thoracic and Cardiovascular Surgery, 142,* 1263–1269.

van Venrooij, L. M., Verberne, H. J., De Vos, R., Borgmeijer-Hoelen, A. M., Van Leeuwen, P. A., & De Mol, B. A. (2012). Postoperative loss of skeletal muscle mass, complications and quality of life in patients undergoing cardiac surgery. *Nutrition, 28,* 40–45.

van Venrooij, L. M., Visser, M., de Vos, R., Leeuwen, P. A., Peters, R. J., & de Mol, B. A. (2013). Cardiac surgery-specific screening tool identifies preoperative undernutrition in cardiac surgery. *Annals of Thoracic Surgery, 95*(2), 642–647.

van Zanten, A. R. H., Sztark, F., Kaisers, U. X., Zielmann, S., Felbinger, T. W., Sablotzki, A. R., . . . Hofman, Z. (2014). High-protein enteral nutrition enriched with immune-modulating nutrients vs standard high-protein enteral nutrition and nosocomial infections in the ICU: A randomized clinical trial. *Journal of the American Medical Association, 312*(5), 514–524.

Visser, M., Davids, M., Verberne, H. J., Kok, W. E. M., Niessen, H. W. M., van Venrooij, L. M. W., . . . van Leeuwen, P. A. M. (2011). Rationale and design of a proof-of-concept trial investigating the effect of uninterrupted perioperative (par)enteral nutrition on amino acid profile, cardiomyocytes structure, and cardiac perfusion and metabolism of patients undergoing coronary artery bypass grafting. *Journal of Cardiothoracic Surgery, 6.* doi:10.1186/1749-8090-6-36

Visser, M., Niessen, H. W. M., Kok, W. E. M., Cochieri, R., Wisselink, W., van Leeuwen, P. A. M., . . . de Mol, B. A. J. (2015). Nutrition before and during surgery and the inflammatory response to the heart: A randomized controlled trial. *Journal of Nutrition and Metabolism.* doi:10.1155/2015/123158

Wilbring, M., Ploetze, K., Bormann, S., Waldow, T., & Motschke, K. (2014). Omega-3 polyunsaturated fatty acids reduce the incidence of postoperative atrial fibrillation in patients with history of prior myocardial infarction undergoing isolated coronary artery bypass grafting. *Thoracic & Cardiovascular Surgeon, 62,* 569–574.

Yamamoto, T., Kajikawa, Y., Otani, S., Yamada, Y., Takemota, S., Hirota, M., . . . Fijiwara, T. (2014). Protective effect of eicosapentaeroic acid on insulin resistance in hyperlipemic patients and on the postoperative course of cardiac surgery patients: The possible involvement of adiponectin. *Acta Medica Okayama, 68*(6), 349–361.

Yang, S., Wu, X., Yu, W., & Li, J. (2014). Early enteral nutrition in critical ill patients with hemodynamic instability: An evidence-based review and practical advice. *Nutrition in Clinical Practice, 29*(1), 90–96.

Ziegler, T. R., May, A. K., Hebber, G., Easley, K. A., Griffith, D. P., Dave, N., . . . Wischmeyer, P. E. (2016). Efficacy and safety of glutamine-supplemented parenteral nutrition in surgical ICU patients: An American multicenter randomized controlled trial. *Annals of Surgery, 263*(4), 646–655.

Web Resource

Guidelines for the Provision and Assessment of Nutrition Support in the Adult Critically Ill Patient: Society of Critical Care Medicine (SCCM) and American Society for Parenteral and Enteral Nutrition (A.S.P.E.N.): http://journals.sagepub.com/doi/pdf/10.1177/0148607115621863

CHAPTER 24

Depression, Anxiety, and Spirituality Among Patients Undergoing Cardiac Surgery

Muna Hassan Hammash, Amy Wimsatt

▶ Introduction

Coronary artery bypass graft (CABG) surgery is the gold standard treatment of coronary artery disease (CAD). The benefits of CABG surgery in relieving symptoms and decreasing mortality are extensively documented. Nevertheless, CABG is a traumatic event that causes considerable depression and anxiety for patients before and after surgery. It has also been documented that depression and anxiety are risk factors for cardiac morbidity, mortality, or both in patients who have undergone cardiac surgery. This chapter describes depression and anxiety associated with CABG procedures. Psychosocial considerations related to heart transplantation were discussed in Chapter 19.

▶ Depression

Depression in all its minor, moderate, and major forms is commonly reported by 15% to 61% of patients undergoing CABG surgery (Ravven, Bader, Azar, & Rudolph, 2013). It has been estimated that 35% to 45% of patients suffer from major depression and impaired quality of life (QoL) after CABG surgery (Ghoneim & O'Hara, 2016). Major depression after cardiac surgery is linked to increased risk of postoperative cardiac morbidity or mortality or both (Tully, Baumeister, Bennetts, Rice, & Baker, 2016). Findings from a number of studies showed that depressed patients after cardiac surgery with persistent (i.e., before as well as 6 months after a CABG) mild or moderate to severe depression had 1.5 to 2.5 relative risk of cardiac death compared to patients without depression within 6 to 12 months after surgery, even after controlling for other biomedical risk factors (Poole et al., 2017; Ravven et al., 2013).

Preoperative depression has been reported as the strongest predictor of postoperative depression, poor QoL, recurrent hospitalization, increased mortality, and prolonged pain up to 6 months after CABG surgery (Patron, Messerotti Benvenuti, & Palomba, 2014; Perrotti et al., 2016). Approximately half of patients with preoperative depression remain depressed for 1 year postoperatively. Depressed patients tend to have poor perception of perceived control over their illness, which leads to poor QoL and nonadherence to postoperative rehabilitation regimens (Kidd, Poole, Leigh, et al., 2016). Other reported risk factors of depression among patients undergoing cardiac surgery included female gender, unmarried status, unemployment, age, length of stay in the intensive care unit (ICU), and having not received preoperative CABG surgery education from a nurse (Hweidi, Gharabibeh, Al-Obeisat, & Al-Smadi, 2017).

▶ Anxiety

Patients undergoing CABG surgery experience considerable anxiety. Data suggest that 80% of patients were at their baseline level of anxiety immediately postoperatively, 10% were within baseline range at 6 to 8 weeks, and 94% were at range 12 months following CABG surgery (Kidd, Poole, Ronaldson, et al., 2016). Pathologic anxiety manifests as a feeling of impending doom, excessive worrying thoughts of being disabled, persistent palpitations, generalized muscular tension with inability to relax, breathlessness, hypervigilance, persistent headache, frequent urge to pass urine, butterflies in stomach, and persistent sleep disturbance. Frequently, such symptoms are either ignored or not asked/reported; however, they cause significant distress and may lead to adverse outcomes.

Waiting for surgery and fear of pain increases one's anxiety, feelings of vulnerability, and helplessness (Rosiek, Kornatowski, Rosiek-Kryszewska, Leksowski, & Leksowski, 2016). Patients who are anxious preoperatively tend to be anxious throughout the postoperative period and exhibit poorer outcomes postoperatively, including an increased risk of readmission, increased postoperative complications, and future cardiac events (Kidd, Poole, Ronaldson, et al., 2016). The cost and duration of the hospital stay of anxious cardiac patients is four times that of nonanxious patients. Therefore, anxiety should be routinely assessed before and after the surgery.

▶ Potential Mechanisms Linking Depression and Cardiac Events

Multiple behavioral and physiological factors may explain the link between depression and increased risk of morbidity and mortality after CABG surgery.

Behavioral Factors

Following cardiac surgery, patients are expected to engage in a rehabilitation program and adhere to multiple aspects of a treatment regimen, including diet, medication, exercise, smoking cessation, and alcohol intake restrictions. Patients who experience depression following CABG surgery report pain (48.9%) and physical surgical symptoms (90.3%) at 12 months postoperatively. Patients experienced major adverse cardiac events when depression was present postoperatively (Poole et al., 2017). Cardiac patients with depressive symptoms have a 2.5-fold increased risk of rehospitalization and death at 1-year follow-up in comparison to those without depressive symptoms. In addition, postoperative depression is associated with poor functional, physical, and emotional healing during recovery from CABG reflected by shorter walking distance, delayed wound healing, increased frequency of wound infection, and poor sense of perceived control over one's health.

Biologic Mechanisms

Multiple biologic mechanisms explain the relationship between depression and cardiac events, including elevated inflammatory activity, hypothalamo-pituitary-adrenal axis dysfunction, altered autonomic nervous system activity, decreased heart rate variability, and elevated platelet activation.

Inflammation

Systematic inflammatory response usually occurs with major operations. In CABG, this response is exaggerated by the use of cardiopulmonary bypass. The use of off-pump CABG in the early 1990s has helped to some extent in reducing this state of systemic inflammation. Yet, even without cardio-pulmonary bypass, a significant amount of proin-flammatory cytokines and cytotoxic enzymes are released into the circulation after the surgery (Jongman et al., 2014). Inflammatory cytokines are markedly increased after CABG surgery and have been linked with adverse clinical outcomes. Elevated C-reactive protein (CRP) has been posi-tively associated with a greater risk of postoperative mortality and extended hospital stay in patients undergoing CABG (Poole et al., 2014). Data sug-gest a relationship between depression and inflam-mation (Ciobanu & Baune, 2018; Inserro, 2018; Short, 2018). A meta-analysis by Howren, Lamkin, and Suls (2009) showed depressive symptoms to be positively associated with CRP, interleukin-1 (IL-1), and IL-6 in both community and clinical samples. Later data corroborate this relationship (Chocano-Bedoya et al., 2014). There is evidence to suggest that preoperative CRP levels predict depression experienced 6 months after CABG surgery (Yang et al., 2012) and interferon-gamma measured in the days following surgery predicts depression 12 months after surgery (Steptoe et al., 2015), after controlling for covariates.

Endothelial Dysfunction

Normal endothelium typically releases nitric oxide in response to serotonin to ensure adequate blood flow through the coronary arteries. Inflam-mation impairs endothelial nitric oxide release and results in vasoconstriction, myocardial isch-emia, and coronary thrombosis. Depression has been associated with impaired endothelial func-tion in healthy individuals and cardiac patients (Shi et al., 2015).

Altered Autonomic Nervous System Activity

Stress and depression are associated with increased sympathetic nervous system, reduced parasympa-thetic nervous system, or both (Hu, Lamers, de Geus, & Penninx, 2016; Won & Kim, 2016). These can lead to myocardial ischemia, arrhythmia, and sudden cardiac death.

Depression is associated with reduced heart rate variability (HRV), a measure that reflects increased sympathetic nervous system, reduced parasympathetic nervous system activity, or both in patients who underwent cardiac surgery (Patron et al., 2014). Depressed patients are in a constant state of perceived stress, which may potentiate reduced HRV. There is substantial evidence that decreased HRV causes arrhythmias and sudden cardiac death in patients with cardiac disease. The depression-reduced HRV association may further increase the risk of cardiac morbidity, mortality, or both in depressed patients after cardiac surgery (Nenna et al., 2017).

The Sympathetic-Adrenomedullary System

Increased norepinephrine secretion has been documented in patients with major depression. Norepinephrine increases the risk of thrombotic and ischemic cardiac events by increasing the occurrence of cardiac dysrhythmia, triggering platelets aggregation, and altering vasoactivity and vessel permeability (Nygren, Redfors, Thorén, & Ricksten, 2010; Tschuor et al., 2008).

Hypothalamic-Pituitary-Adrenal (HPA) Axis Abnormalities

Increased secretion of cortisol, alterations in the diurnal profile of cortisol, and elevated corticotropin-releasing hormone have been asso-ciated with major depression in patients with cor-onary heart diseases (Cowen, 2010). High cortisol levels have been shown to promote the devel-opment of atherosclerotic lesions and increase the risk of arterial hypertension and endothelial damage. Hypothalamic-Pituitary-Adrenal axis dysregulation has been associated with a greater risk of adverse cardiac events and mortality in depressed patients (Jokinen & Nordstrom, 2009). Poole and colleagues (2016) analyzed the cortisol slope in 171 patients awaiting first-time, elective CABG surgery. The authors indicated that cortisol slope measured 2 months after CABG surgery was predictive of depression status 12 months later. Elevated cortisol and pre-CABG dysregulated diurnal cortisol profiles predicted increased risk of death and adverse cardiac events in subsequent years (Ronaldson et al., 2015).

Identifying Depression in Patients Undergoing CABG Surgery

Depression is an important predictor of cardiac events and mortality in CABG patients and has a great influence on patients' adherence to the treatment regimen and rehabilitation programs. As preexisting depression is the most common predictor of postoperative psychological distress, patients should be screened for depression prior to surgery, routinely monitored, and appropriately treated. Identifying depressive symptoms postoperatively is also important but can be complicated by somatic symptoms of coronary heart disease and physical stressors of surgery. Therefore, the American Heart Association (AHA) has recommended routine assessment of depression and suicidal thoughts by self-administered questionnaires (Lichtman et al., 2008) such as the Patient Health Questionnaire (PHQ) to screen patients for depressive symptoms and suicidal thoughts. The brief version of this questionnaire (PHQ-2) includes 2 questions about major depressive symptoms (1) little interest or pleasure in daily activities; and (2) feeling down, depressed, or hopeless. It has been suggested that a positive response to either of the PHQ-2 questions should be followed up with administration of the PHQ-9. A score of 10 or higher on the PHQ-9 confirms the presence of moderate to major depression (Lichtman et al., 2008) and the patient should be referred to a psychiatrist or psychologist for a comprehensive assessment (Colquhoun et al., 2013).

Treatment

The high rates of depression after cardiac surgery highlight a requirement for appropriate support and intervention efforts. For better outcomes, clinicians should consider pharmacologic and psychotherapeutic interventions to treat depression in cardiac surgery patients, preferably before introducing any self-management or rehabilitation programs.

Pharmacological Treatment

Antidepressants are the first treatment choice for depression. Multiple randomized, placebo-controlled trials have demonstrated the efficacy of selective serotonin reuptake inhibitors (SSRIs), including sertraline (Zoloft®), citalopram (Celexa®), and fluoxetine (Prozac®) for depression treatment in coronary disease and CABG patients (Sepehripour, Eckersley, Jiskani, Casula, & Athanasiou, 2018) because of their lowest interactions with other drugs and safe profile among cardiac patients. Tricyclic antidepressants are effective in treating depression and anxiety, but their use has declined owing to their potential for cardiotoxicity (Tsai, 2017).

Statins

Statins are a group of lipid-lowering agents that act via competitive inhibition of the hydroxymethylglutaryl-CoA reductase enzyme that normally catalyzes the conversion of 3-hydroxy-3-methylglutaryl-coenzyme A to mevalonate, the rate-limiting enzyme in cholesterol biosynthesis. According to the American College of Cardiology Foundation and the AHA guidelines for CABG, the use of statins is recommended for all patients undergoing CABG (Hillis et al., 2012). Beyond their primary lipid-lowering role, statins had anti-inflammatory action that was demonstrated in clinical trials by a significant reduction in serum levels of CRPs, usually within 14 days of initiation of statin therapy, independent of serum low-density lipoprotein (LDL) level (Ridker, 2010). Data have confirmed the effectiveness of statin therapy in decreasing the systemic inflammatory response after CABG (Sodha & Sellke, 2015). Statins also promote endothelial function and have antithrombotic effects, which partly explain their role in reducing the incidence of in-stent restenosis. Furthermore, statins decrease atherosclerotic plaque neovascularization leading to plaque stabilization and a reduction in the risk of plaque rupture (Altun et al., 2014).

There is evidence of a link between inflammation and depression. Several studies showed elevated levels of proinflammatory cytokines and CRP in patients with depressed mood (Fernandes et al., 2016; Haapakoski, Mathieu, Ebmeier, Alenius, & Kivimaki, 2015). Statins have anti-inflammatory properties and thus have been effective in treating depression (Stafford & Berk, 2011). Two meta-analyses suggested that statins are associated with improvement in depressive mood and QoL (O'Neil et al., 2012; Parsaik et al., 2014). In a meta-analysis of 7 observational studies, use of statins was associated with a 32% risk reduction of developing depression (Parsaik et al., 2014). Stafford and Berk (2011) investigated the prevalence of depression 3 and 9 months after hospitalization in 193 patients with CAD, including 157 statin users (81.3%) who had recent myocardial infarction and underwent angioplasty or CABG surgery. The likelihood of depression was reduced by 69% and 79% in patients 3 and 9 months after discharge, respectively, following the initiation of statin therapy after controlling for potential confounders. Among different statins currently available, simvastatin (Zocor®) is known to possess the greatest ability to infiltrate the blood-brain barrier (BBB) (Wood, Eckert, Igbavboa, & Müller, 2010). In one study, the estimated potency of simvastatin in penetrating the BBB was six to seven times greater than atorvastatin, the most common statin used in the management of CAD patients (Sierra et al., 2011).

Psychotherapy

Several nonpharmacologic psychotherapeutic interventions have been proposed to relieve post–cardiac surgery anxiety and depression. These interventions include cognitive behavioral therapy (CBT), music therapy, and physical activity.

Cognitive Behavioral Therapy

Among various types of psychotherapy, CBT is the most heavily researched method for treating depressive symptoms (Ebert et al., 2015; Gould, Coulson, & Howard, 2012). The primary goal of CBT is to modify negative cognitive processes and maladaptive behaviors that are core elements of depression and other mental disorders. Cognitive behavioral therapy holds promise as an intervention to decrease depressive symptoms in patients with cardiovascular illness, including CABG patients. In addition to reducing depression, CBT has been found to be effective in treating HRV (Jang, Hwang, Padhye, & Meininger, 2017).

Music and Relaxation Therapy

Patients undergoing CABG experience moderate to severe anxiety before and after the surgery. Patients are often worried about the procedure, outcomes, pain, and risk of death. Anxiety increases the heart rate, cardiac output, and the need for oxygen (Khanade & Sasangohar, 2017). Therefore, lessening of anxiety is highly important for cardiac patients. Sedative-hypnotic drugs are commonly used in ICUs to improve patients' anxiety. However, anxiolytics are usually associated with many side effects. Hence, complementary and alternative methods such as music therapy have been investigated for improving patients' anxiety without causing serious side effects.

Music therapy is a complementary method that can help improve patients' anxiety and well-being by providing a calm atmosphere, improving the threshold of stress, distracting patients from negative thoughts, eliminating negative emotion, and making them feel relaxed (Comeaux & Comeaux, 2013). Several studies showed that music therapy could reduce the level of anxiety, heart rate, and systolic and diastolic blood pressures among patients undergoing CABG (Heidari et al., 2015; Phadke, Parkar, & Yardi, 2014). One of the varieties of music is nature sounds. Amiri, Sadeghi, and Negahban Bonabi (2017) investigated the effect of natural sounds on anxiety in CABG patients. These researchers reported that the mean anxiety level significantly decreased in the intervention group 30 minutes before surgery in the waiting room and 30 minutes following surgery.

▸ Educational Programs

The majority of patients develop depression at home after they have been discharged from the hospital. It may be difficult for immediate family members to fully understand mood changes after CABG surgery. Depressed patients experience fatigue, pain, insomnia, and anorexia during the postoperative period, and family members may falsely attribute the resultant symptoms of depression to surgical failure or complications.

Educational programs are paramount to improve patients' outcomes and adherence to their treatment regimen after hospital discharge. Audiotape educational programs were found to decrease the level of anxiety and depression and improve general health and quality of life in patients after CABG surgery. In a randomized clinical trial, including 70 patients undergoing CABG surgery, the data revealed that the audiotape educational program decreased the level of postoperative anxiety and depression (Hoseini, Soltani, Babaee Beygi, & Zarifsanaee, 2013).

The Bypassing the Blues randomized controlled trial investigated the impact of a telephone-delivered collaborative care intervention in post-CABG patients with depression. Patients in the intervention group received a tailored nurse-led telephone-delivered program for up to 8 months after surgery. The researchers reported significant improvements in health-related quality of life and mood in the intervention group compared to usual care control (Rollman & Belnap, 2011).

▸ Spirituality

Spirituality, an innate personally defined aspect from deep within an individual, is an important resource throughout one's transitions and during crisis (Campesino, Belyea, & Schwartz, 2009). Spirituality has been defined as a unifying force that gives meaning to one's life while being connected to self, others, and a higher power, which encourages deeper understanding and promotes the health of the individual (Bezerra, Gomes, Galvao, & Souza, 2018). Spirituality often

becomes more of a core issue when one is facing mortality (Diddle & Denham, 2010). The nature of one's spirituality varies and can produce either positive or negative emotions during stressful times (Reinert & Koenig, 2013). Spirituality may be perceived as a coping mechanism that provides mental and social support in an attempt to understand life circumstances. When individuals perceive support during life-threatening critical times, psychological distress can decrease and hope can thrive. So, spirituality can add a "protective influence" in patients undergoing open heart surgery (Ai, Hall, Pargament, & Tice, 2013).

Many aging Americans, due to growing diversity, have reported no expressed religious affiliation (Ai, Wink, & Shearer, 2011). However, most individuals have professed a belief in a higher power or transcendent source with spiritual energy (Ai et al., 2010), thus expressing spirituality and not religiosity.

Although CABG surgery can prolong life and reduce physical symptoms in those diagnosed with CAD, patients experience severe stress, contradictory feelings regarding life and self-image, and may have difficult recovery due to their fear of the unknown and psychologic distress regarding surgery and anesthesia (Rosiek et al., 2016). The negative prolonged emotions of depression and anxiety following surgery worsen patients' prognoses with maladjustment (Ai et al., 2010). Patients often have acute feelings and interpretations; and view the postoperative period as being given additional "time" (Ai, Hall, Pargament, & Tice, 2013). Positive emotions from spirituality and private prayer during this stressful encounter help to enhance one's coping process.

▸ Coping with Spirituality

Spirituality is viewed by the patient as a sense of protection prior to the surgery and during the recovery period (Ai et al., 2013). There is some agreement that religion and spirituality are connected concepts but still maintain their uniqueness through culture (Campesino et al., 2009). Positive religious coping can be empowering to those facing open heart surgery (Ai et al., 2013). Prayer use in open heart patients has been shown to assist with distress and reduce preoperative and postoperative complications (Ai et al., 2013, 2010). Faith gives individuals a sense of empowerment and personal control during times of crisis. Preoperative private prayer has been noted to assist in an individual's coping prior to open heart surgery by increasing perceived connectedness and enhancing growth (Ai et al., 2013). Faith-based prayer offers coping in the face of distress and adversity with an increase in outlook preoperatively when distress is peaked. Spirituality can provide patients with protective hope and determination during this critical time. Spirituality also can increase one's emotional strength and coping ability (Diddle & Denham, 2010). When individuals feel supported, quality of life and compliance to postoperative treatment will be enhanced (Ai et al., 2010).

▶ **Summary**

Multiple behavioral and physiological factors may explain the link between depression and increased risk of morbidity and mortality after CABG surgery. Nurses are in a position to identify depression preoperatively and postoperatively. While a number of interventions have been studied, most are costly and require a long-term approach postoperatively. There is a need to design interventions that are integrated into the primary care and cardiology visits. Interventions focused on spirituality are lacking in the literature. Emphasizing culture and religion in designing approaches to support patients and to reduce anxiety is critical to ensure an optimal recovery.

🔍 *CASE STUDY*

A 58-year-old patient was scheduled for a CABG. She has stated her fear about undergoing the surgery and her worry that she will not survive. The patient shares that she has been depressed over the past year since her husband left. She feels alone, especially since her son, who lives across the country, cannot be present for the surgery. Her history includes diabetes, overweight, and hypercholesterolemia.

Critical Thinking Questions

1. What is the strongest predictor of postoperative depression in this case?
2. Why is this patient at risk for poor postoperative outcomes?
3. What is the best treatment for this patient's postoperative depression?

Answers to Critical Thinking Questions

1. Preoperative depression has been reported as the strongest predictor of postoperative depression, poor QoL, recurrent hospitalization, increased mortality, and prolonged pain up to 6 months after the surgery. Approximately half of patients with preoperative depression remain depressed at 1 year postoperatively. Other reported risk factors of depression among patients undergoing cardiac surgery include younger age, female gender, living alone, lower education, and comorbidities.
2. Patients who are anxious preoperatively tend to be anxious throughout the postoperative period and exhibit poorer outcomes postoperatively, including increased risk of readmission, increased morbidity and mortality, and increased health care utilization.
3. For better outcomes, clinicians should consider pharmacologic and psychotherapeutic interventions to treat depression in cardiac surgery patients, preferably before introducing any self-management or rehabilitation programs. Antidepressants, specifically SSRIs, are the first treatment choice for this patient's depression.

Self-Assessment Questions

1. Which patient is at greatest risk of postoperative depression following cardiac surgery? A patient with:
   A. recurrent hospitalizations.
   B. poor quality of life.
   C. prolonged pain.
   D. preoperative depression.

2. Which is a sequela of postoperative depression following cardiac surgery?
   A. Decreased infection rate
   B. Walking longer distances
   C. Delayed wound healing
   D. Increased control over one's health

3. Which is a biologic mechanism that explains the relationship between depression and cardiac events?
   A. Decreased interleukin-6 levels
   B. Increased C-reactive protein
   C. Decrease in cytotoxic enzymes
   D. Decreased sympathetic nervous system stimulation

4. Secretion of which substance is associated with major depression?
   A. Norepinephrine
   B. Adrenocorticotropic hormone
   C. Dopamine
   D. Interleukin-2

5. Which should the nurse anticipate in a patient with major depression following cardiac surgery?
   A. Decreased platelet aggregation
   B. Increased vascular permeability
   C. Vasodilation
   D. Dysrhythmias

6. Which is a likely result of increased cortisol levels?
   A. Dysrhythmias
   B. Atherosclerotic lesions
   C. Hypotension
   D. Increased C-reactive protein levels

7. Which is considered the first treatment of choice for depression?
   A. Statin therapy
   B. Selective serotonin reuptake inhibitors
   C. Music therapy
   D. Tricyclic antidepressants

8. Which occurs concomitantly with anxiety?
   A. Persistent headache
   B. Decreased frequency of urination
   C. Decreased vigilance
   D. Occasional palpitations

9. Which statement should indicate to the nurse that additional patient teaching should be performed?
   A. "I need something to treat my depression so my surgical wound will heal better."
   B. "If I have less depression, I will feel more in control of my life."
   C. "I am glad I am having off-pump surgery, so I don't have to worry about depression."
   D. "My wife wants me to be treated for depression to decrease my chances of being brought back to the hospital after my cardiac surgery."

10. Which is the primary goal of cognitive behavioral therapy?
    A. Decrease C-reactive protein levels
    B. Modify maladaptive behaviors
    C. Promote relaxation
    D. Decrease interleukin-6 levels

Answers to Self-Assessment Questions

1. **D. preoperative depression**
   Rationale: Recurrent hospitalizations, poor quality of life, and prolonged pain are sequelae of postoperative depression. Preoperative depression is a risk factor for developing postoperative depression following cardiac surgery.

2. **C. delayed wound healing**
   Rationale: Postoperative depression can result in an increase in infection rate, ability to walk only short distances, and decreased control over one's health. It is associated with delayed wound healing.

3. **B. increased C-reactive protein**
   Rationale: Interleukin-6 and cytotoxic enzyme levels are increased in depression. Depression

is associated with an increase in sympathetic nervous system stimulation, which can promote myocardial ischemia. C-reactive protein levels are elevated with depression, which increases the risk of postoperative mortality and extended length of hospital stay.

4. A. **norepinephrine**
Rationale: Norepinephrine secretion is associated with major depression. Adrenocorticotropic hormone, dopamine, and IL-2 are not involved with autonomic nervous system alterations with depression.

5. D. **dysrhythmias**
Rationale: Dysrhythmias should be anticipated in postoperative cardiac surgery patients who are experiencing major depression. There is also an associated increase in platelet aggregation, which increases the risk of a thrombotic event, decreased vascular permeability, and vasoconstriction associated with major depression following cardiac surgery.

6. B. **atherosclerotic lesions**
Rationale: High cortisol levels have been shown to promote development of atherosclerotic lesions. Dysrhythmias and elevated C-reactive protein levels are not directly associated with elevated cortisol levels. Arterial hypertension is associated with elevated cortisol levels.

7. B. **selective serotonin reuptake inhibitors**
Rationale: Multiple trials have demonstrated the efficacy of SSRIs in treating depression. This group of drugs has the lowest number of reactions with other

drugs reported and the side effect profile demonstrates it is safe to administer to patients with cardiac disease. Statins are lipid-lowering agents. Music therapy is a complementary therapy that may be used to decrease anxiety. Use of tricyclic antidepressants has fallen out of favor due to their associated cardiotoxicities.

8. A. **persistent headache**
Rationale: Persistent headaches are reported to be associated with anxiety. Anxiety is also associated with increased frequency of urination, hypervigilance, and persistent palpitations.

9. C. **"I am glad I am having off-pump surgery, so I don't have to worry about depression."**
Rationale: Cytokines are released with off-pump procedures. The cytokines can contribute to the development of depression following cardiac surgery. The first statement is reasonable as decreased wound healing is associated with depression. The second statement is reasonable since depression is associated with decreased control over one's health. The last statement is reasonable as there is an increased risk of rehospitalization with the presence of depression.

10. B. **modify maladaptive behaviors**
Rationale: Cognitive behavioral therapy can modify negative cognitive processes. Cognitive behavioral therapy does not alter C-reactive protein or IL-6 levels. It does not promote relaxation. Relaxation may be promoted with music or relaxation therapy.

CLINICAL INQUIRY BOX

Question: What is the association between theoretical conceptualizations of depression and anxiety with major adverse cardiovascular and cerebrovascular events?

Reference: Tully, P. J., Winefield, H. R., Baker, R. A., Donollet, J., Pedersen, S. S., Wittert, G. A., . . . Turnbull, D. A. (2015). Depression, anxiety and major adverse cardiovascular and cerebrovascular events (MACCE) in patients following coronary artery bypass graft surgery: A five year longitudinal cohort study. *Biopsychosocial Medicine, 9.* doi:10/1186/s13030-015-0041-5

(continues)

CLINICAL INQUIRY BOX *(continued)*

Objective: To determine the association between theoretical conceptualizations of depression and anxiety with major adverse cardiovascular and cerebrovascular events.

Method: Patients (n=158) underwent a structured interview before CABG surgery to determine presence of depression and anxiety disorders. Patients also completed the Mood and Anxiety Symptom Questionnaire.

Time to MACCE (myocardial infarction, unstable angina, repeat revascularization, heart failure, sustained dysrhythmia, cerebrovascular event, left ventricular failure, and cardiac-related mortality) were determined.

Results: After covariate adjustment, there was an association between generalized anxiety disorder and MACCE. The distress was not associated with MACCE risk. No symptom dimensions were significantly associated with MACCE.

Conclusion: There was a relationship between the presence of preoperative generalized anxiety disorder and MACCE following CABG surgery.

References

Ai, A. L., Hall, D., Pargament, K., & Tice, T. N. (2013). Posttraumatic growth in patients who survived cardiac surgery: The predictive and mediating roles of faith-based factors. *Journal of Behavioral Medicine, 36,* 186–198.

Ai, A. L., Ladd, K. L., Peterson, C., Cook, C. A., Shearer, M., & Koenig, H. G. (2010). Long-term adjustment after surviving open heart surgery: The effect of using prayer for coping replicated in a prospective design. *The Gerontologist, 50,* 798–809.

Ai, A. L., Wink, P., & Shearer, M. (2011). Secular reverence predicts shorter hospital length of stay among middle-aged and older patients following open-heart surgery. *Journal of Behavioral Medicine, 34,* 532–541.

Altun, I., Oz, F., Arkaya, S. C., Altun, I., Bilge, A. K., Umman, B., . . . Turkoglu, U. M. (2014). Effect of statins on endothelial function in patients with acute coronary syndrome: A prospective study using adhesion molecules and flow-mediated dilatation. *Journal of Clinical Medicine Research,* 6(5), 354–361.

Amiri, M. J., Sadeghi, T., & Negahban, B. T. (2017). The effect of natural sounds on the anxiety of patients undergoing coronary artery bypass graft surgery. *Perioperative Medicine (London), 6.* doi:10.1186/s13741-017-0074-3

Bezerra, S., Gomes, E. T., Galvao, P., & Souza, K. V. (2018). Spiritual well-being and hope in the preoperative period of cardiac surgery. *Revista Brasileira de Enfermagem, 71,* 398–405.

Campesino, M., Belyea, M., & Schwartz, G. (2009). Spirituality and cultural identification among Latino and non-Latino college students. *Hispanic Health Care International, 7.* doi:10.1891/1540-4153.7.2.72

Chocano-Bedoya, P. O., Mirzaei, F., O'Reilly, E. J., Lucas, M., Okereke, O. I., Hu, F. B., . . . Ascherio, A. (2014). C-reactive protein, interleukin-6, soluble tumor necrosis factor α receptor 2 and incident clinical depression *Journal of Affective Disorders, 163,* 25–32.

Ciobanu, L. G., & Baune, B. T. (2018). Gene expression of inflammation markers in depression. In B. T. Baune (Ed.), *Inflammation and immunity in depression* (pp. 199–222). Cambridge, MA: Academic Press.

Colquhoun, D. M., Bunker, S. J., Clarke, D. M., Glozier, N., Hare, D. L., Hickie, I. B., . . . Branagan, M. G. (2013). Screening, referral and treatment for depression in patients with coronary heart disease. *Medical Journal of Australia, 198,* 483–484.

Comeaux, T., & Comeaux T. (2013). The effect of complementary music therapy on the patient's postoperative state anxiety, pain control, and environmental noise satisfaction. *MEDSURG Nursing, 22*(5), 313–318.

Cowen, P. J. (2010). Not fade away: The HPA axis and depression. *Psychological Medicine, 40,* 1–4.

Diddle, G., & Denham, S. A. (2010). Spirituality and its relationships with the health and illness of appalachian people. *Journal of Transcultural Nursing, 21,* 175–182.

Ding, C., Hu, M., Yong-Jian, W., & Tomlinson, B. (2015). Achievement of specified lipid and high-sensitivity C-reactive protein levels with two statins in Chinese patients with hypercholesterolaemia. *Lipids in Health and Disease, 14.* doi:10.1186/s12944-015-0116-0

Ebert, D. D., Zarski, A. C., Christensen, H., Stikkelbroek, Y., Cuijpers, P., Berking, M., . . . Riper, H. (2015). Internet and computer-based cognitive behavioral therapy for anxiety and depression in youth: A meta-analysis of randomized controlled outcome trials. *PloS One, 10,* e0119895.

Fernandes, B. S., Steiner, J., Bernstein, H. G., Dodd, S., Pasco, J. A., Dean, O. M., . . . Berk M. (2016). C-reactive protein is increased in schizophrenia but is not altered by antipsychotics: Meta-analysis and implications. *Molecular Psychiatry, 21,* 554–564.

Ghoneim, M. M., & O'Hara, M. W. (2016). Depression and postoperative complications: An overview. *BMC Surgery, 16.* doi:10.1186/s12893-016-0120-y

Gould, R. L., Coulson, M. C., & Howard, R. J. (2012). Cognitive behavioral therapy for depression in older people: A meta-analysis and meta-regression of randomized controlled trials. *Journal of the American Geriatric Society, 60,* 1817–1830.

Haapakoski, R., Mathieu, J., Ebmeier, K. P., Alenius, H., & Kivimaki, M. (2015). Cumulative meta-analysis of inter-leukins 6 and 1β, tumour necrosis factor α and c-reactive protein in patients with major depressive disorder. *Brain, Behavior, and Immunity, 49,* 206–215.

Heidari, S., Babaii, A., Abbasinia, M., Shamali, M., Abbasi, M., & Rezaei, M. (2015). The effect of music on anxiety and cardiovascular indices in patients undergoing coronary artery bypass graft: A randomized controlled trial. *Nursing and Midwifery Studies, 4*(4), e31157. doi:10.17795/nmsjournal31157

Hillis, L. D., Smith, P. K., Anderson, J. L., Bittl, J. A., Bridges, C. R., Byrne, J. G., . . . Winniford, M. D. (2012). 2011 ACCF/AHA guideline for coronary artery bypass graft surgery: Executive summary: A report of the American College of Cardiology Foundation/American Heart Association Task Force on practice guidelines. *Anesthesia and Analgesia, 114,* 11–45.

Hoseini, S., Soltani, F., Babaee Beygi, M., & Zarifsanaee N. (2013). The effect of educational audiotape programme on anxiety and depression in patients undergoing coronary artery bypass graft. *Journal of Clinical Nursing, 22,* 1613–1619.

Howren, M. B., Lamkin, D. M., & Suls, J. (2009). Associations of depression with C-reactive protein, IL-1, and IL-6: A meta-analysis. *Psychosomatic Medicine, 71,* 171–186.

Hu, M. X., Lamers, F., de Geus, E. J., & Penninx, B. W. (2016). Differential autonomic nervous system reactivity in depression and anxiety during stress on type of stressor. *Psychosomatic Medicine, 78*(5), 562–572.

Hweidi, I. M., Gharabibeh, B. A., Al-Obeisat, S. M., & Al-Smadi, A. M. (2017). Prevalence of depression and its associated factors in patients post-coronary artery bypass graft surgery. *Journal of Research in Nursing, 23*(1). doi:10.1177/1744987117728314

Inserro, A. (2018). *Depression: Not an inflammatory disease, but inflammation plays a huge role.* Retrieved from https://www.ajmc.com/conferences/psychcongress2018/depression-not-an-inflammatory-disease-but-inflammation-plays-a-huge-role

Jang, A., Hwang, S.-K., Padhye, N. S., & Meininger, J. C. (2017). Effects of cognitive behavior therapy on heart rate variability in young females with constipation-predominant irritable bowel syndrome: A parallel-group trial. *Journal of Neurogastroenterology and Motility, 23*(3), 435–445.

Jokinen, J., & Nordstrom, P. (2009). HPA axis hyperactivity and cardiovascular mortality in mood disorder inpatients. *Journal of Affective Disorders, 116,* 88–92.

Jongman, R. M., Zijlstra, J. G., Kok, W. F., van Harten, A. E., Mariani, M. A., Moser, J., . . . van Meurs, M. (2014). Off-pump CABG surgery reduces systemic inflammation compared with on-pump surgery but does not change

systemic endothelial responses: A prospective randomized study. *Shock, 42,* 121–128.

Khanade, K., & Sasangohar, F. (2017). Efficacy of using heart rate measurements as an indicator to monitor anxiety disorders: A scoping literature review. *Proceedings of the Human Factors and Ergonomics Society.* Retrieved from https://journals.sagepub.com/doi/pdf/10.1177/1541931213601927

Kidd, T., Poole, L., Leigh, E., Ronaldson, A., Jahangiri, M., & Steptoe A. (2016). Health-related personal control predicts depression symptoms and quality of life but not health behaviour following coronary artery bypass graft surgery. *Journal of Behavioral Medicine, 39,* 120–127.

Kidd, T., Poole, L., Ronaldson, A., Leigh, E., Jahangiri, M., & Steptoe, A. (2016). Attachment anxiety predicts depression and anxiety symptoms following coronary artery bypass graft surgery. *British Journal of Health Psychology, 21*(4). doi:10.1111/bjhp.12191

Lichtman, J. H., Bigger Jr., J. T., Blumenthal, J. A., Frasure-Smith, N., Kaufmann, P. G., Lesperance, F., . . . Froelicher, E. S. (2008). Depression and coronary heart disease: Recommendations for screening, referral, and treatment: A science advisory from the American Heart Association Prevention Committee of the Council on Cardiovascular Nursing, Council on Clinical Cardiology, Council on Epidemiology and Prevention, and Interdisciplinary Council on Quality of Care and Outcomes Research: Endorsed by the American Psychiatric Association. *Circulation, 118,* 1768–1775.

Nenna, A., Lusini, M., Spadaccio, C., Nappi, F., Greco, S. M., Barbato, R., . . . Chello, M. (2017). Heart rate variability: A new tool to predict complications in adult cardiac surgery. *Journal of Geriatric Cardiology, 14*(11), 662–668.

Nygren, A., Redfors, B., Thorén, A., & Ricksten, S.-E. (2010). Norepinephrine causes a pressure-dependent plasma volume decrease in clinical vasodilatory shock. *Acta Anaesthesiologica Scandinavica.* doi:10.1111/j.1399-6576.2010.02244x.

O'Neil, A., Sanna, L., Redlich, C., Sanderson, K., Jacka, F., Williams, L. J., . . . Berk. M. (2012). The impact of statins on psychological wellbeing: A systematic review and meta-analysis. *BMC Medicine, 10.* doi:10.1186/1741-7015-10-154

Parsaik, A. K., Singh, B., Murad, M. H., Singh, K., Mascarenhas, S. S., Williams, M. D., . . . Rummans, T. A. (2014). Statins use and risk of depression: A systematic review and meta-analysis. *Journal of Affective Disorders, 160,* 62–67.

Patron, E., Messerotti Benvenuti, S., Favretto, G., Gasparotto, R., & Palomba, D. (2014). Depression and reduced heart rate variability after cardiac surgery: The mediating role of emotion regulation. *Autonomic Neuroscience, 180,* 53–58.

Patron, E., Messerotti Benvenuti, S., & Palomba, D. (2014). Preoperative and perioperative predictors of reactive and persistent depression after cardiac surgery: A three-month follow-up study. *Psychosomatics, 55*(3), 261–271.

Perrotti, A., Mariet, A. S., Durst, C., Monaco, F., Vandel, P., Monnet E., . . . Chocron, S. (2016). Relationship between depression and health-related quality of life in patients undergoing coronary artery bypass grafting: A MOTIV-CABG. *Quality of Life Research, 25*(6), 1433–1440.

Phadke, S. D., Parkar, H., & Yardi, S. (2014). Effect of music intervention on immediate post operative coronary artery bypass graft surgery (CABG) patients. *Indian Journal of Physiotherapy & Occupational Therapy, 8*(4), 106–111.

Poole, L., Kidd, T., Leigh, E., Ronaldson, A., Jahangiri, M., & Steptoe, A. (2014). Depression, C-reactive protein and length of post-operative hospital stay in coronary artery bypass graft surgery patients. *Brain, Behavior, and Immunity, 37*, 115–121.

Poole, L., Kidd, T., Ronaldson, A., Leigh, E., Jahangiri, M., & Steptoe, A. (2016). Depression 12-months after coronary artery bypass graft is predicted by cortisol slope over the day. *Psychoneuroendocrinology, 71*, 155–158.

Poole, L., Ronaldson, A., Kidd, T., Leigh, E., Jahangiri, M., & Steptoe, A. (2017). Pre-surgical depression and anxiety and recovery following coronary artery bypass surgery. *Journal of Behavioral Medicine, 40*(2), 249–258.

Ravven, S., Bader, C., Azar, A., & Rudolph, J. L. (2013). Depressive symptoms after CABG surgery: A meta-analysis. *Harvard Review of Psychiatry, 21*(2), 59–69.

Reinert, K. G., & Koenig, H. G. (2013). Re-examining definitions of spirituality in nursing research. *Journal of Advanced Nursing, 69*, 2622–2634.

Ridker, P. M. (2010). Statin therapy for elevated hsCRP: What are the public health implications? *American Journal of Managed Care.* Retrieved from https://www.ajmc.com/journals/issue/2010/2010-08-vol16-n08/ajmc_10aug_ridker_561to562

Rollman, B. L., & Belnap, B. H. (2011). The bypassing the blues trial: Collaborative care for post-CABG depression and implications for future research. *Cleveland Clinic Journal of Medicine, 78*(Suppl 1), S4–S12.

Ronaldson, A., Kidd, T., Poole, L., Leigh, E., Jahangiri, M., & Steptoe, A. (2015). Diurnal cortisol rhythm is associated with adverse cardiac events and mortality in coronary artery bypass patients. *Journal of Clinical Endocrinology and Metabolism, 100*, 3676–3682.

Rosiek, A., Kornatowski, T., Rosiek-Kryszewska, A., Leksowski, L., & Leksowski, K. (2016). Evaluation of stress intensity and anxiety level in preoperative period of cardiac patients. *BioMed Research International, 2016.* doi:10.1155/2016/1248396

Sepehripour, A. H., Eckersley, M., Jiskani, A., Casula, R., & Athanasiou, T. (2018). Selective serotonin reuptake inhibitor use and outcomes following cardiac surgery—a systematic review. *Journal of Thoracic Disease, 10*(2), 1112–1120.

Shi, H., Feng, G., Wang, Z., Zhou, C., Zhong, G., Hu, Y., . . . Wang, G. (2015). Relationships between depressive symptoms and endothelial function among outpatients of a general hospital in China. *Medical Science Monitor, 21*, 1812–1819.

Short, E. B. (2018). The inflamed mind: A radical new approach to depression. *Nature, 557*, 633–634.

Sierra, S., Ramos, M. C., Molina, P., Esteo, C., Vazquez, J. A., & Burgos, J. S. (2011). Statins as neuroprotectants: A comparative in vitro study of lipophilicity, blood-brain-barrier penetration, lowering of brain cholesterol, and decrease of neuron cell death. *Journal of Alzheimer's Disease, 23*, 307–318.

Sodha, N. R., & Sellke, F. W. (2015). The effect of statins on perioperative inflammation in cardiac and thoracic surgery. *The Journal of Thoracic and Cardiovascular Surgery, 149*(6), 1495–1501.

Stafford, L., & Berk, M. (2011). The use of statins after a cardiac intervention is associated with reduced risk of subsequent depression: Proof of concept for the inflammatory and oxidative hypotheses of depression? *Journal of Clinical Psychiatry, 72*, 1229–1235.

Steptoe, A., Poole, L., Ronaldson, A., Kidd, T., Leigh, E., & Jahangiri, M. (2015). Depression 1 year after CABG is predicted by acute inflammatory responses. *Journal of the American College of Cardiology, 65*, 1710–1711.

Tsai, V. (2017). *Tricyclic antidepressant toxicity medication.* Retrieved from https://emedicine.medscape.com/article/819204-medication

Tschuor, C., Asmis, L. M., Lenzlinger, P. M., Tanner, M., Härter, L., Keel, M., . . . Stover, J. F. (2008). In vitro norepinephrine significantly activates isolated platelets from healthy volunteers and critically ill patients following severe traumatic brain injury. *Zurich Open Repository and Archive.* Retrieved from https://www.zora.uzh.ch/id/eprint/10617/2/Tschuor_Crit_CareV.pdf

Tully, P. J., Baumeister, H., Bennetts, J. S., Rice, G. D., & Baker, R. A. (2016). Depression screening after cardiac surgery: A six month longitudinal follow up for cardiac events, hospital readmissions, quality of life and mental health. *International Journal of Cardiology, 206*, 44–50.

Won, E., & Kim, Y. K. (2016). Stress, the autonomic nervous system, and the immune-kynurenine pathway in the etiology of depression. *Current Neuropharmacology, 14*(7), 665–673.

Wood, W. G., Eckert, G. P., Igbavboa, U., & Müller, W. E. (2010). Statins and neuroprotection: A prescription to move the field forward. *Annals of the New York Academy of Sciences, 1199*, 69–76.

Yang, L., Wang, J., Zhang, L., Hou, J., Yuan, X., Hu, S., . . . Zheng Z. (2012). Preoperative high-sensitivity C-reactive protein predicts depression in patients undergoing coronary artery bypass surgery: A single-center prospective observational study. *The Journal of Thoracic and Cardiovascular Surgery, 144*, 500–505.

Web Resource

Patient Health Questionnaire: http://www.phqscreeners.com/sites/g/files/g10016261/f/201412/PHQ-9_English.pdf

CHAPTER 25

Rehabilitation and Care of the Cardiac Surgery Patient

Kathy Lee Bishop

▶ Introduction

Coronary heart disease (CHD) is the single most common cause of death in the world (Anderson et al., 2016). In the United States, approximately 790,000 adults suffer from a myocardial infarction (MI) each year with as many as 210,000 being recurrent events (Fang, Ayala, Luncheon, Ritchey, & Loustalot, 2017). Exercise-based cardiac rehabilitation (CR) has been shown to reduce cardiovascular mortality and improve health-related quality of life (HRQOL) compared to no participation in CR (Anderson et al., 2016). The clinical benefit of CR has been correlated to increases in overall fitness and related physiologic effects on coronary endothelial function, blood pressure, insulin resistance, fibrinolytic state, and inflammatory markers (Ades et al., 2017). Close to 12 million individuals could benefit from enrollment in CR if all the eligible cardiac diagnostic groups were combined (Alexander & Smith, 2016; Benjamin et al., 2017; Kohan & Annex, 2015; Thomas et al., 2018) (**TABLE 25.1**). Despite evidence to support CHD patients being referred for CR, the referral rate remains low. Physician encouragement about the benefit and value of CR is most likely the

single most important connection for a patient's enrollment (Lavie, Bennett, & Arena, 2017). This provider conversation has been shown to increase a patient's willingness to participate.

Overall use of cardiac rehabilitation ranges from 19% to 34% nationally with state to state geographic variations (Ades et al., 2017; Fang et al., 2017). Following coronary artery bypass surgery, patients are more likely to participate than after an MI as are nonminorities, men, and those with higher socioeconomic status. The lowest participation rates are in the southern states with the midwestern states having the highest (Ades et al., 2017). An unpublished report from a large southern health care system reviewed discharge data over a 13-month period (3/2016–3/2017). Over 1,750 patients were eligible for referral following either a percutaneous coronary intervention (PCI) or MI, but only 51% of the men and 49% of the women were referred (Bishop, 2017). Having the connection from electronic referral to actual enrollment for CR is an ongoing opportunity that is a focus of a current national initiative.

Over time, traditional exercise-based CR programs have evolved to focus on the importance of secondary prevention and disease management.

TABLE 25.1 Primary Diagnoses and Potential Patients Who Would Benefit from Cardiac Rehabilitation in the United States

Diagnosis	Potential CR Patient Candidates
Stable angina	9,000,000
Myocardial infarction (MI), non–ST segment elevation MI (NSTEMI), ST segment elevation MI (STEMI)	790,000
Angioplasty with or without percutaneous coronary intervention (PCI)	954,000
Heart valve repair/replacement	102,000
Coronary artery bypass graft (CABG)	400,000
Heart failure (Class II–IV) – stable >6 weeks (no elective or emergency hospital admissions)	960,000
Heart transplant or heart/lung transplant	3,200

Data from Alexander & Smith, 2016; Benjamin et al., 2017; Kohan & Annex, 2015; Thomas et al., 2018.

Medication adherence, lifestyle management, and comorbidity management of diabetes, depression, stress, hypertension, and smoking cessation are key components of an efficacious CR program (Ades et al., 2017). The *Million Hearts Initiative* was launched in 2012 and renewed in 2017 to focus on preventing 1 million cardiovascular events over 5 years. Using the acronym ABCS to focus on **A**spirin use as appropriate, **B**lood pressure control, **C**holesterol management, and **S**moking cessation makes CR an ideal partner to help provide education and be supportive of these aspects of cardiovascular care (Ades et al., 2017). Referral, enrollment, and adherence in CR are the anchors for a strong connection to improve outcomes for individuals with cardiovascular disease.

▶ Definition

In 1995, the Cardiac Rehabilitation Clinical Practice Guidelines were published by the U.S. Department of Health and Human Services (Wenger et al., 1995). The definition of CR was established as "comprehensive, long-term programs involving medical evaluation, prescribed exercise, cardiac risk factor modification, education, and counseling" (Wisconsin Society for Cardiovascular and Pulmonary Health & Rehabilitation, 2018). These programs are designed to limit the physiologic and psychologic effects of cardiac illness, reduce the risk for sudden death or reinfarction, control cardiac symptoms, stabilize or reverse the atherosclerotic process, and enhance the psychosocial and vocational status of selected patients (Wenger et al., 1995). There are seven primary diagnoses approved by the Centers for Medicare and Medicaid Services (CMS) to benefit from CR. These include stable angina, MI, angioplasty with or without stenting (PCI), heart valve repair or replacement, coronary artery bypass graft (CABG), chronic stable heart failure (HF) with reduced ejection fraction (HFrEF), and heart and or heart/lung transplant (CMS, n.d.; Medicare.gov, n.d.) (see Table 25.1). Cardiac rehabilitation is considered a class I recommendation for CABG, ST elevation MI, non–ST elevation MI, valvular heart disease, and chronic stable angina (Thomas et al., 2018). Patients with HF who are able to participate in exercise training have been shown to improve endothelial and diastolic function, increase exercise capacity, reduce inflammatory cytokines, improve HRQOL, and reduce mortality (Forman, Sanderson, Josephson, Raikhelkar, & Bittner, 2015; Park, Schopfer, Zhang, Shen, & Whooley, 2017). Eligible cardiovascular patients may be seen along a continuum of inpatient through outpatient care for CR.

▶ Cardiac Rehabilitation Phases

Phase I

Phase I CR pertains to when the patient is still in the hospital (American Association of Cardiovascular and Pulmonary Rehabilitation, 2013) (**TABLE 25.2**). The delivery model of Phase I has changed over past decades due to shorter hospitals stays on one hand and survival of more complicated patients on the other end of the spectrum. For the uncomplicated patient, Phase I may be focused primarily on education and setting up follow-up provider appointments, including a connection to outpatient CR. If time permits, bedside teaching or group teaching will focus on newly prescribed or updated medications, an introduction to a nutrition plan, symptoms and when to call the provider, and getting started or resuming physical activity. The hospital stay may be as short as 6 hours to several days and extending to weeks depending on complications and the need for further workup to prevent additional heart damage

TABLE 25.2 Phases of Cardiac Rehabilitation			
Secondary Prevention			
Cardiac Event	**Phase 1**	**Phase 2**	**Phases 3/4**
Treatment in hospital	**Inpatient CRP**	**Outpatient CRP**	**Maintenance phase (s)**
Immediate Focus on: ■ Triage ■ Testing ■ Medication ■ Intervention	**Usually 6 Hours–Days?** Focus on: ■ Basic Information (medications, symptoms, incision site, sleep, shower, ADLs, resuming work, initiate low-level walking or movement program, contact phone number) ■ Supportive counseling ■ Guidelines for mobilization ■ D/C planning ■ F/up provider appt ■ Referral to outpatient CRP	**Usually 4–12 Weeks** Focus on: ■ Assessment review and follow-up ■ Patient-centered goals ■ Update medications ■ Physical activity and exercise training ■ Nutrition and psychological counseling ■ Education on behavior modification strategies and lifestyle management	**Lifetime** Focus on: ■ Sustained heathy activities, lifestyle, and behaviors ■ Reduction in risk of future coronary and/or cerebrovascular events ■ Strategies for delaying progression of underlying ASCVD and clinical deterioration ■ Strategies for reduction in morbidity and mortality ■ Strategies for sustaining and progressing exercise

Notes: ADL, activity of daily living; appt, appointment; ASCVD, atherosclerotic cardiovascular disease; CRP, cardiac rehabilitation program; D/C, discharge; F/up, follow-up.
Data from Guidelines for Cardiac Rehabilitation and Secondary Prevention Programs. (2013). *American Association of Cardiovascular and Pulmonary Rehabilitation.* (5th Ed). Champaign, IL: Human Kinetics.

as well as the management of other comorbidities such as diabetes, HF, and renal disease (American Heart Association, n.d.). Discharge from the hospital may be delayed if further treatment intervention (e.g., staged stent placement, bypass surgery, valve repair, or valve replacement) is needed. Heart failure, whether new onset or chronic, will take more specific education and follow-up coordination before hospital discharge. The foci will include medication, salt and fluid intake, nutrition, activity guidelines, symptom awareness, and weight gain.

In the case of the complicated cardiovascular patient (e.g., with cardiogenic shock, acute HF, uncontrollable dysrhythmias, or multisystem organ failure), the initial medical focus is on patient survival (medications such as inotropes; mechanical support interventions such as intra-aortic balloon pump [IABP], ventricular assist devices [VADs]; surgical intervention; or any combination of these). Once the critically ill cardiovascular patient is deemed hemodynamically stable, early mobilization in the intensive care unit (ICU) provides interventions for reducing long-term functional and cognitive impairment.

Intensive Care Unit–Acquired Weakness

Intensive care unit–acquired weakness (ICUAW) is a common complication for critically ill patients who have prolonged mechanical ventilation, sepsis, multiorgan system failure, systemic inflammatory response syndrome, or hyperglycemia (Hermans & Van den Berghe, 2015). Generalized weakness is documented with no other possible causes other than ill-defined inflammation. Muscle mass loss can occur as early as 7 days after initiation of mechanical ventilation. Residual impairments may persist following discharge from the ICU: Cognitive, psychological, reduced physical function and decreased quality of life (Hermans & Van den Berghe, 2015).

Early Mobilization

Early hospital care of the cardiac patient has changed drastically over the past 80 years. In the 1930s, Sir Thomas Lewis stated, "On the

treatment of myocardial infarction: the patient is to be guarded by day and night nursing and helped in every way to avoid voluntary movement and effort" (Magder, 1985, p. 442). Even in the early 1960s, bed rest was still being used for immediate treatment of acute myocardial infarction (Duke, 1971). Prolonged bed rest is associated with increased risk for prolonged ventilation, ventilator-associated events, increased risk for pressure injury development, higher risks for falls, increased workload on the cardiovascular system, higher occurrences of delirium, and adverse impact on quality of life following hospital discharge (Parry & Puthucheary, 2015). An uncomplicated cardiac surgical patient could be fast-tracked and out of bed to chair and even walking as early as postoperative day 1.

Early progressive mobility in the ICU is considered a standard of care with the reduction in the risk for venous thromboembolism and pulmonary emboli, improvements in airway clearance, decreased length of stay, and reduced need for rehabilitation postdischarge (Parry & Puthucheary, 2015). Determining the timing for out-of-bed early mobilization is based on many factors, especially if the patient has a complicated cardiovascular course. The considerations include hemodynamic status, use of vasoactive medications, cognitive status (Confusion Assessment Method-ICU score), sedation level, and level of ventilatory support (Cassina, Putzu, Santambrogio, Villa, & Licker, 2016; Santos, Ricci, Suster, Paisani, & Chiavegato, 2016). An example of how to determine if early mobilization should be restricted is if there have been increases in mechanical ventilation requirements within the previous 12 hours: fraction of inspired oxygen (FiO_2) greater than 0.60, oxygen saturation less than 90%, mean arterial pressure less than 65 mmHg on vasoactive medication (Green, Marzano, Letidschke, Mitchell, & Bissett, 2016).

Mechanical Circulatory Support

Patients may be placed on mechanical circulatory support (MCS) devices to allow for several possibilities for "unloading" of the heart: a temporary bridge to recovery, a bridge to transplant, or for destination therapy if heart transplantation is not an option (Shekar, Gregory, & Fraser, 2016). These devices typically are implanted to support recovery of the left ventricle. Whether the devices are placed temporarily (external) or implanted, early mobilization allows for improved organ perfusion, increased tolerance to exercise, improved cardiac index, and the potential for remodeling of the left ventricle (Tozzi & Hullin, 2016). Improved post–heart transplant outcomes have been demonstrated in patients who engage in early progressive mobilization with MCS devices. Placement of the access catheters for the MCS will impact the ability to mobilize the patient. If the cannulas are placed in the femoral vessels, out-of-bed activities will be restricted due to hemodynamic status and risk of decannulation.

Phase II

Phase II CR (see Table 25.2) is considered immediately after hospital discharge and up to 1 year after the cardiac event. Typically, 36 visits are allowed for this outpatient service, but there is some variation in insurance carriers and timing dependent on when patients achieve their program goals. Barriers for referral and enrollment into Phase II CR are well documented (Lavie et al., 2017; Oosenbrug et al., 2016) (**TABLE 25.3**). Barriers to Phase II CR are broken down into essentially two categories: provider and patient. If there is an automatic electronic ordering process, there is a higher referral and attendance rate. Educating the hospital and ambulatory providers on the benefits of Phase II CR should be a regular occurrence to ensure patient referrals and thus better long-term outcomes for patients.

The enrollment process of a candidate for CR should include an initial evaluation to review recent hospital discharge documentation, laboratory results, pertinent diagnostic tests (e.g., catheterization, echocardiogram, 12-lead electrocardiogram, nuclear studies), current medication list, assessing comorbidities and cardiovascular risk factors,

TABLE 25.3 Barriers to Referral and Adherence for Cardiac Rehabilitation

Provider Barriers	Patient Barriers
Unfamiliar with CRP benefits Unfamiliar with EMR referral tool External CRPs to health care system do not accept EMR referral Patient considered high risk Patient too well	"Doctor doesn't think I need it" "My doctor never mentioned it" Fear Lower socioeconomic status Unmarried status (women) Lower education level (≤12 years) Ease of accessing program (transportation, location) Financial (co-pay, co-insurance, deductibles) Minorities Multiple comorbidities (previous stroke, DM, HF, cancer)
Lower Rates of Adherence/Attendance	**Higher Rates of Referral and Attendance**
Lower levels of physical function Less physically active Lower socioeconomic status Multiple comorbidities (e.g., smoking, diabetes)	Automatic referral/electronic order Direct recommendation by provider Reduced time to enrollment Offering gender-specific classes Alternative delivery models Wider variety of exercise Younger

Notes: CRP, cardiac rehabilitation program(s); DM, diabetes mellitus; EMR, electronic medical record; HF, heart failure.
Data from Lavie, Bennett, & Arena, 2017; Oosenbrug et al., 2016.

establishing baseline hemodynamic/biometric status (vital signs, heart rhythm, body mass index, waist circumference or waist/hip measurement, body fat measurement), quality of life, screening for depression, prior/current level of activity, current nutrition intake (Rate Your Plate®), goal setting, and establishing an individualized treatment plan (ITP) (**TABLES 25.4** and **25.5**). All certified CR programs need an ITP established at program initiation; this plan must be reviewed every 30 days until the program is completed to support medical necessity and patient progression (American Association of Cardiovascular and Pulmonary Rehabilitation, 2013).

TABLE 25.4 Essential Evaluation and Components of Cardiac Rehabilitation and Secondary Prevention Programs

Component	

Patient Assessment	**Evaluation:**
	■ Detailed health history questionnaire
	■ Current medications
	■ Current over-the-counter medications
	■ Recent test results:
	  • Catheterization; 12-lead electrocardiogram (ECG); lab work, including fasting lipid panel
	  • Recent hospital discharge document and/or most recent physician or provider office note
	■ Physical activity assessment
	  • Entry stress test; Duke Activity Scale Index (DASI)
	  • Risk stratification (determines number of visits: low risk 6–18; moderate risk 12–24; high risk 18–36)

Nutrition Counseling	**Rate Your Plate®**
Weight Management	■ Waist circumference and/or waist-to-hip measurement ■ Weekly weight and daily weight for heart failure
Blood Pressure Management	■ Resting and exercise blood pressure (BP) ■ Present intervention regiment
Lipid Management	■ Baseline fasting labs and post–cardiac rehabilitation (CR) fasting labs
Diabetes Management	■ Baseline HbA$_{1c}$ ■ Daily blood glucose (BG) measurements in CR
Tobacco Cessation	
Psychosocial Management	**Quality of Life:** ■ Ferrans and Powers Quality of Life Index ■ Medical Outcomes Trust Short Form 36 or 12 (SF-36/SF-12) ■ Patient Health Questionnaire-9 (PHQ-9)

Nutrition Counseling	Rate Your Plate®
Physical Activity Counseling	■ Steps/day ■ Walk a pet (type of pet) ■ Fitbit® or other tracking devices ■ Community resources
Exercise Training/ Medical Supervised Program	**American College of Sports Medicine:** ■ Frequent, intensity, time, type of exercise, volume, and progress (FITT-VP)
Medication Counseling	
Individualized Treatment Plan	■ Initial, 30 days, 60 days, 90 days reassessment of goals: Exercise, nutrition, psychosocial, education

Data from American Association of Cardiovascular and Pulmonary Rehabilitation. (2013). *Guidelines for Cardiac Rehabilitation and Secondary Prevention Programs* (5th ed.). Champaign, IL: Human Kinetics.

TABLE 25.5 Individualized Treatment Plan (ITP) Phase II Cardiac Rehabilitation Example			
Program Name:	Initial	Start Date:	
Patient Name:	MRN	Age	DOB
Referring Physician:	Primary Cardiac Diagnosis:		
	Secondary Diagnoses:		
Hospital Admission/Discharge	Risk Stratification (circle): Low/Moderate/High		

Core Categories			
Exercise	**Nutrition**	**Education**	**Psychosocial**
Initial level of fitness: *Stress test results* Date of test: Peak METs: THRR: TMR: BP Initial Peak Recovery	Lipids Initial Date: Total Cholesterol HDL Non-HDL LDL Triglyceride Diabetes Y/N	Barriers Identified (circle) Speech Hearing Vision Language Literacy Cognitive Tobacco Use: Y/N #cigarettes/day Smokeless Tobacco: Y/N Date Quit: Quit Date Set: Family Support Y/N	Tool: PHQ-9 Score: Other Tools: Sleep Assessment: Epworth Score PSQI Score Other

(continues)

TABLE 25.5 Individualized Treatment Plan (ITP) Phase II Cardiac Rehabilitation Example *(continued)*			
Core Categories			
Exercise	**Nutrition**	**Education**	**Psychosocial**
HR Initial Peak Recovery Rhythm Initial During Recovery *6 MWT results* Distance walked Time walked BP Initial Peak Recovery HR Initial Peak Recovery	Date: HbA$_{1C}$ Diabetes Therapy (circle) Oral Medication Insulin Diet Plan Weight Management Wt (lbs): Ht: BMI: Waist Circumference: Hip Circumference:		
Exercise Prescription Mode 1: Duration Intensity Mode 2: Duration Intensity Mode 3: Duration Intensity	Referred to Diabetes Education Y/N Dietitian Consult Y/N Weight Management Class Y/N	Intervention Refer to Smoking Cessation Class Y/N Education (√ **all that apply**) Self-pulse Safety Symptoms Low Na$^+$ Diet BP Education Angina RPE scale Equip orient Diabetes Hypertension Basic nutrition Benefit of exercise Strength training Warmup Cool Down Physical activity Education class Other:	Intervention (√ **all that apply**) Psych Consult MD Referral Medication Stress Mgmt. Skills Support Group Other: Repeat PHQ-9 MD informed
Goals ST: LT: Pt. Goals HEP Discussed/Date Comments Stage of Readiness:	Goals ST: LT: Pt. Goals HEP Discussed/Date Comments Stage of Readiness:	Goals ST: LT: Pt. Goals HEP Discussed/Date Comments Stage of Readiness:	Goals ST: LT: Pt. Goals HEP Discussed/Date Comments Stage of Readiness:

Core Categories			
Exercise	**Nutrition**	**Education**	**Psychosocial**

Plan of Care: Monitored exercise session 2 to 3 times/week until completion of 36 sessions as long as patient continues to improve. Will progress workloads based on hemodynamic response to exercises. Patient to attend education risk factor class and individual consult with registered dietitian.

Continue CR: Yes/No	D/C CR and rationale:
Staff Signature/Date:	MD Signature/Date:

Notes: BMI, body mass index; BP, blood pressure; CR, cardiac rehabilitation; DOB, date of birth; HbA$_{1c}$, hemoglobin A$_1$C; HDL, high density lipoprotein; HEP, home exercise program; HR, heart rate; Ht, height; ITP, individualize treatment plan; lbs., pounds; LDL, low density lipoprotein; LT, long term; MD, medical doctor; MET, metabolic equivalent; Mgmt., management; MRN, medical record number; MWT, minute walk test; Na$^+$, sodium; PHQ, patient health questionnaire; PSQI, Pittsburgh Sleep Quality Index; RPE, rating of perceived exertion; ST, short term; THRR, total heart rate range; TMR, total metabolic equivalent range; Wt, weight. Data from American Association of Cardiovascular and Pulmonary Rehabilitation. (2013). *Guidelines for Cardiac Rehabilitation and Secondary Prevention Programs* (5th ed.). Champaign, IL: Human Kinetics.

Program Components

The three areas focused on in Phase II are the three *E*s: education, emotional support, and exercise (**FIGURE 25.1**). Education and emotional support can be performed in a group setting or individually (American Association of Cardiovascular and Pulmonary Rehabilitation, 2013) (see Tables 25.4 and 25.5). To best fit patients' needs, educational options should be available to have the education delivery model in person, online, through mobile applications, or any combination of these. Education must be fluid and comprehension reassessed regularly because strategies for risk factor modification

and lifestyle changes are continuously evolving. Primary areas for education are risk factor identification and reduction (e.g., tobacco, stress, diabetes, nutrition level, weight, sedentary lifestyle, blood pressure, and cholesterol), strategies for maintaining and sustaining a healthier lifestyle, and benefits of lifestyle changes and regular exercise.

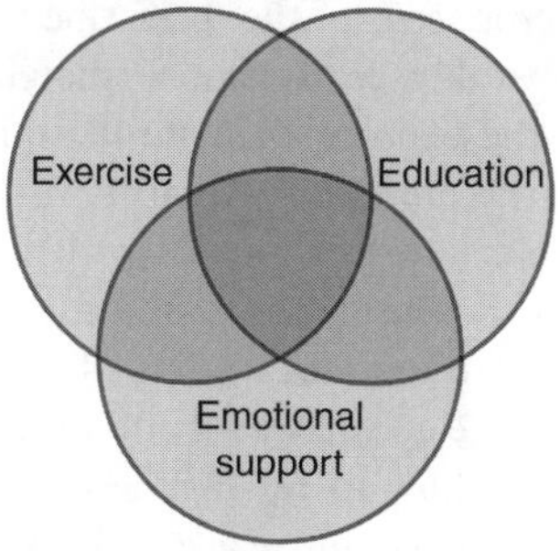

Emotional support should also take on different formats depending on the individual's needs. For example, team-run support groups are viable options, but there should be consideration for gender-specific groups if staffing, space, and time allow. Another option is to seek other community resources to meet the emotional needs of the individual. Patients may need to be referred back to their primary care provider if their emotional needs are beyond the scope of the CR team. A screening tool given at the time of entry to the program to assess depression is recommended because of the relationship of heart disease and depression (Steward & Rollman, 2014). A simple tool such as the Patient Health Questionnaire (PHQ-9) by Pfizer® can be administered in fewer than 2 minutes. The PHQ-9 allows for a screening score and a determining point whether the patient needs additional psychosocial help beyond the program's resources.

FIGURE 25.1 Focus of Cardiac Rehabilitation Programs: The 3 *E*s.

Sleep is an important factor in the recovery and day-to-day health of the patient. A screening tool to assess sleep habits is valuable in designing the plan of care. A simple tool such as the Epworth Sleep Scale, which assesses daytime sleepiness, or the Pittsburgh Sleep Quality Index (PSQI), which is a tool for self-reported sleep quality, are easy ways for the patient and team to identify barriers to sleep. Reduced physical functioning, sleep-related symptoms, and sleep disturbances are common in HF and contribute to poor HRQOL. Similar findings related to sleep are seen in patients with diabetes mellitus (DM), including poor sleep quality, fragmented sleep, and reduced sleep time (Fritschi & Redeker, 2015).

Obstructive sleep apnea (OSA) has been shown to have an increased incidence of 30% to 50% in patients with cardiovascular disease. Upwards of 80% of patients with OSA have stenosis in at least two coronary vessels (Javadi, Jililolghadr, Yazdi, & Majd, 2014). C-reactive protein levels and fibrinogen can be elevated in OSA leading to the early stages of thrombosis in the coronary arteries. The influence of quality of sleep continues to evolve as a component of risk factor management in the CR patient.

Team

Qualified health care personnel are key to the success of a CR program. Physician coverage is twofold: a medical director to oversee the program and an assigned physician for day-to-day coverage. Core competencies are required for any CR program that qualifies for certification through the American Association of Cardiovascular and Pulmonary Rehabilitation (2013). The team members (e.g., nurses, registered dietitians, exercise physiologists, physical therapists, occupational therapists, pharmacists) working in direct collaboration with the medical director should demonstrate advanced cardiovascular knowledge in secondary prevention of cardiac disease and emergency procedures and demonstrate annual competency in patient assessment, nutrition counseling, management of blood pressure, weight, diabetes, lipids, psychosocial management, tobacco cessation, exercise

training evaluation, and physical activity counseling (American Association of Cardiovascular and Pulmonary Rehabilitation, 2013). Development of medical and educational strategies to identify steps for behavior change related to "readiness for change" and barriers for change are paramount for patients to achieve realization of lifestyle changes.

Monitored Exercise Sessions

Supervised exercise sessions are designed based on cardiac diagnosis (see Table 25.1) for program admission, risk stratification, fall risk, prior level of function (PLOF), comorbidities (e.g., diabetes mellitus, heart failure, peripheral vascular disease, stroke, cancer, orthopedic disorders, Parkinson's, morbid obesity), mechanical or surgically implanted or wearable devices (e.g., external wearable cardioverter defibrillators, ventricular assist devices, peripherally inserted central venous catheters, dialysis ports, prosthetic limbs), home inotropes, or results of an entry stress test (American Association of Cardiovascular and Pulmonary Rehabilitation, 2013). A combination of aerobic exercise, strength training, and flexibility are fundamental mainstays of the exercise program design. Heart rate range, target metabolic equivalent range (MET), and a rating of perceived exertion (RPE) are helpful in designing the individualized program (American Association of Cardiovascular and Pulmonary Rehabilitation, 2013; American College of Sports Medicine, 2014) (**TABLE 25.6**; also see Table 25.5).

Progression and pace of progression of the exercise program are dependent on patient hemodynamic responses to the prescribed program. Daily and weekly reassessment should be performed by the team to evaluate these responses, including any symptoms (e.g., cardiovascular, musculoskeletal, and neurologic) the patient may have experienced. Because risk stratification, fall risk, and PLOF are important aspects of the prescription for safety (e.g., getting on and off equipment, understanding how to set up the equipment for workload, patient cognitive level), determining the type of equipment for the patient to use is critical. Another consideration in design of the exercise

TABLE 25.6	Aerobic Exercise Evidence-Based Recommendations
FITT-VP	**Evidence-Based Recommendations**
Frequency	5+ days/week of moderate exercise or 3+ days/week vigorous or combination 35 days/week
Intensity	Moderate +/or vigorous intensity for most adults Light to moderate beneficial for deconditioned individuals
Time	30–60 min/day—purposeful moderate exercise or 20–60 min/day of vigorous exercise or combination for most adults under 20 min/day—previously sedentary individuals
Type	Regular, purposeful exercise involving large muscle groups; continuous; rhythmic
Volume	Target volume of 500–1,000 MET/min/week Increasing pedometer step counts 2,000+/day to reach 7,000+/day Below this level may still be beneficial if unable or unwilling to do the above levels
Pattern	Continuous session/day; or multiple sessions of 10+ minutes to accumulate desired duration and volume/day Bouts of 10+ minutes/day may still yield favorable adaptations in deconditioned individuals
Progression	Gradual progression of volume by adjusting duration, frequency, +/or intensity until desired goal attained Approach may enhance adherence and reduce risks of musculoskeletal injury and adverse cardiac events

Data from American College of Sports Medicine. (2014). *ACSM's Guidelines for Exercise Testing and Prescription* (9th ed.). Philadelphia, PA: Wolters Kluwer Health/Lippincott Williams & Wilkins.

prescription is if the patient is a novice user of exercise equipment or has never participated in an exercise program versus an experienced, regular exerciser to a highly trained athlete. The challenge in the design of the program is to meet the needs of each individual to accomplish the best aerobic conditioning outcome to help reduce secondary cardiovascular events.

Patients in Phase II wear a telemetry monitor. This allows the staff to observe the heart rate and rhythm response to progressive exercise. The staff also monitors blood pressure response to exercise and RPE. Blood glucose response to exercise as well as oxygen saturation are additional measurements assessed when appropriate. Patients are asked early in their CR program to start checking their own pulse. If this is a difficult task, they are encouraged to use self-monitoring devices for accuracy

(e.g., Fitbit™, Polar™ oxygen saturation monitor, or mobile device applications such as AliveCor®).

The amount and type of equipment available in a given program will also impact the makeup of the exercise prescription (**FIGURE 25.2**). Patients should be asked at the entry appointment what type of equipment they will have available to them in the home setting or their normal gym facility and at the time of discharge of the Phase II program. This information should also play a role in the development of the exercise prescription by the CR team. Each individualized exercise prescription should be based on a model that focuses on frequency, intensity, time, type, volume, and progress (FITT-VP) (American College of Sports Medicine, 2014) (see Table 25.6). Patients will have an individualized exercise prescription that will start and progress at their own level or pace.

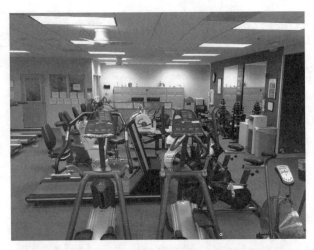

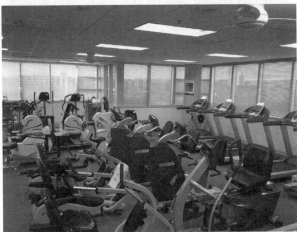

FIGURE 25.2 Typical Equipment and Exercise Area Setup for Phases II–IV Outpatient Cardiac Rehabilitation Programs.

Comorbidities, medication changes, hemodynamic responses to medications, new onset of symptoms, rhythm or heart rate abnormalities are just a few challenges patients face to progress within their own exercise program.

One of the benefits of group supervised exercise sessions and group education classes is the building of camaraderie among patients. This allows for a built-in level of support from day 1 of Phase II. Celebrating patient accomplishments such as exercise milestones or program completion allows each patient to see a success point and how completing the program in this supportive environment is an achievement. This augments program adherence. Group education classes allow patients time to get to know one another in a structured setting. Building a supportive, positive environment is important for the team that works in Phase II, which adds to the patients' desire to want to complete their sessions and be healthier.

Assigning a case manager to each patient to track the patient's progress and give individual feedback also leads to success with adherence and lifestyle changes. Beyond the value of the individual case manager is having as many staff members as possible learn to address each patient by name. This also helps to build the emotional bond and support for that patient by the CR team.

An exit assessment from Phase II allows the patient to see documented changes in risk factors, progress with exercise, and gain a better understanding of weight, diabetes, stress, and tobacco management. The other benefit of this exit assessment is establishing a transitional plan to allow the patient to continue to make healthier lifestyle choices. If patients are not staying within a CR program to progress to Phases III/IV (see Table 25.2), a home exercise plan of care as well as documentation of their achievements is given to them to take and continue either at their own gym or home. Patients should also offer opinions of their treatment course to enable ongoing program improvements.

Community resources (e.g., support groups, available gym facilities in the area, smoking cessation programs) should be shared with patients so that they receive support and direction following conclusion of the monitored Phase II program. A caveat about CR is that to be eligible for Phase II, patients with HF must be stable following hospital discharge for 6 weeks (CMS, n.d.).

Phases III/IV

Phases III/IV of CR are considered transitional (see Table 25.2). Most insurance companies do not pay for these phases of CR. There are some insurances that will pay for "health maintenance." Patients are encouraged to contact their insurance company to see if this is offered. The foci of Phases III/IV are on making patients more independent with their exercise prescription and to continue to support them as they continue to make lifestyle changes to reduce their risk for another cardiac event. Once patients complete the prescribed Phase II monitored sessions and transition to Phases III/IV, some CR programs offer continued supervision, but without telemetry monitoring. Blood pressure, pulse checks, quick looks via a defibrillator for rhythm assessment, and progressing the patients' exercise prescription to allow patients to continue to make gains are key to sustaining the established link to a healthier lifestyle. Patients are encouraged to continue to attend education classes and utilize staff to help with questions or problems that may arise during this evolution to independence.

▶ Rehabilitation Challenges of the Cardiac Surgery Patient

Immediate In-Hospital Postoperative Rehabilitation

The immediate in-hospital postoperative rehabilitation challenges for the post–cardiac surgery patient will be dependent on the surgical approach, preexisting cardiovascular diagnoses, and whether there was full revascularization in the case of CABG. The traditional CABG approach is via a medial sternotomy and may or may not use a cardiopulmonary bypass machine during the procedure (American Association of Cardiovascular and Pulmonary Rehabilitation, 2013). Some of the challenges of this approach include incisional care, pain, airway clearance, orthostatic hypotension, cognitive impairment and delirium, dysrhythmias, and resuming activities of daily living (ADL) as well as early mobility (Cassina et al., 2016). Patients may initially have soreness and limitation of range of motion (ROM) near the joint where the vein or artery was harvested for the bypass. Valve repair or replacement surgery has a similar approach to traditional CABG, but patients may also require prophylactic anticoagulation for mechanical valves and prophylactic antibiotics following discharge (American Association of Cardiovascular and Pulmonary Rehabilitation, 2013). This patient cohort tends to be more symptomatic and deconditioned prior to surgery, which may prolong length of stay and may require inpatient and home health rehabilitation postoperatively prior to starting outpatient CR. Patients undergoing transcatheter aortic valve implantation (TAVI) tend to also be older, frailer, and have comorbidities that originally precluded them from surgical aortic valve replacement. This population is also symptomatic and may be functionally limited prior to surgery. Once symptoms occur, they have as high as a 60% mortality rate after 2 years of the onset of symptoms (Genta et al., 2017).

The baseline distance walked on a 6-minute walk test for TAVI recipients has been shown to predict long-term mortality. Cardiac rehabilitation has been shown to be safe, feasible, and improve physical performance significantly following the less invasive TAVI in this high-risk population (Voller et al., 2015).

The minimally invasive coronary artery bypass (MIDCAB) and PCI patients also have a potential risk for thrombosis and reocclusion (American Association of Cardiovascular and Pulmonary Rehabilitation, 2013). The patient may still report chest wall pain, impaired airway clearance, difficulty with ADLs, cognitive impairment, delirium, and dysrhythmias. Education is key to understanding antiplatelet and anticoagulation management, as well as learning about recognizing signs and symptoms of vascular reocclusion versus musculoskeletal soreness at rest and with movement (American Association of Cardiovascular and Pulmonary Rehabilitation, 2013). This cohort of patients may not be as deconditioned as a patient undergoing a traditional CABG or valve surgery.

Patients undergoing a midsternal approach for cardiac surgery are instructed in sternal precautions. Sternal precautions include universal guidelines to limit stress on the sternum during the initial days and weeks following surgery. There is no consensus on the exact list of sternal precautions, but they generally include no lifting, pulling, or pushing more than 10 pounds, limit above 90 degrees of unilateral shoulder flexion/abduction, limit above 90 degrees of bilateral shoulder flexion/abduction, and no driving for at least 4 weeks after discharge (Katijjahbe et al., 2018). Patients feel better when their chest incision is supported. Using a pillow, a blanket, or even crossing their hands across the incision helps brace during a cough or sneeze, or when moving. Having patients "breathe" through the movement seems more comfortable than holding their breath. Instructing in pursed lip breathing (PLB) with activity is an easy way to incorporate this into ADLs. When patients are getting out of bed, out of a chair, off a commode or toilet, they should utilize their stronger leg muscles. Moving to the front of the chair (commode/toilet) and closer to the edge of the bed will help reduce some of the stress on the sternal incision. Once the patient is able to be out of bed and ambulating, this will help with airway clearance and the patient will no longer focus as much on the incisional areas.

Evaluating for orthostatic blood pressure with position change (supine, sit, or stand) as well as monitoring patient symptoms is valuable to help with their early mobilization progression and reduction of fall risk. If patients are symptomatic, having a physical therapy consult for safety, balance, and gait progression is key to preparing them for discharge. Evaluating patients for readiness for bathing, showering, and standing at the sink activities (e.g., brushing teeth, combing hair, washing face, or shaving) should also be completed before discharge to home. An occupational therapist may need to be consulted if there are challenges with any of these ADLs, which may limit a level of independence prior to discharge. Patient and caregiver education on energy conservation, a walking program, wound care, medications, and comfort positions for sleep are important aspects for addressing quality of life before hospital discharge.

Cognitive Impairment

One of the most common post–cardiac surgery impairments is postoperative cognitive dysfunction (POCD), which has a major impact on quality of life as well as social and financial well-being. Approximately 50% of post-CABG patients experience cognitive decline at time of hospital discharge and up to 4 weeks following discharge. This cognitive decline has been shown to persist in upwards of 25% of individuals at 5 years (Bhamidipati et al., 2017). A core battery of tests that assess motor skill, verbal memory, attention, concentration, as well as evaluating effects of anxiety and depression have been recommended to be tested at 3 months following surgery (Indja et al., 2017). Some tools that have been used to assess this population are the California Verbal Learning Test (CVLT), which is a measure of delayed verbal and immediate memory; the Purdue Pegboard, which tests manual dexterity; and the Trail Making Test A and B, which is a test of abstraction and mental flexibility (Tully, Baune, & Baker, 2013). One of the challenging questions knowing the high incidence of POCD is, Should cognitive function also be tested prior to surgery if time allows to identify preexisting deficits and highlight the need to allocate specific resources postoperatively?

Preoperative risk factors for cognitive decline are age, type II diabetes mellitus, underlying vascular disease, temporal lobe gray matter volume, posttraumatic stress disorder, preoperative cognitive function, and preexisting psychiatric disorders such as depression (Bhamidipati et al., 2017). Perioperative risk factors include inflammation, microemboli, anesthetic regimen, intraoperative oxygen saturation, surgical and cross-clamping technique, body temperature, and rewarming. Off-pump procedures have not revealed a significant difference in cognitive outcomes at 3- and 6-month follow-ups (Bhamidipati et al., 2017). Postoperative cognitive dysfunction was discussed in more detail in Chapter 16.

Discharge from Hospital

When the patient is discharged from the hospital, care should be used with transferring to and from a low car seat. A general suggestion is to have patients turn themselves perpendicular to the car seat and then slowly lower into or out of the seat. Patients should be reminded to PLB or at least not hold their breath during the transfer to and from the seat. Once sitting on the car seat, they should bring one leg and then the other leg into the car. This should be reversed when exiting the vehicle. Patients should be instructed not to pull up on the car door and not to have a family member or caregiver pull on their arms to help them get out of the car. Patients may require a home health assessment and follow-up if they are not independent with ADLs and have functional impairments determined at the time of discharge.

Symptom Management

Patients should be educated on signs and symptoms they may experience once discharged as well as a battery of other valuable tips for home. These include when to initiate a low-level walking program on level surfaces, when to take a bath versus a shower, how to identify incision infection or poor healing, and how to manage medications. Persistent postoperative pain following sternotomy has been reported to range from 23% to 56% up to 1 year following surgery (Veal, Bereznicki, Thompson, Peterson, & Orlikowski, 2016). How to manage symptoms such as chest wall soreness versus persistent chest pain or recurrent chest pain are key to help with anxiety and stress at the time of discharge. A discharge instruction sheet is typically given with contact numbers, follow-up appointments, and an emergency number to call after hours. The patient's primary caregiver receives specific instructions to help ease the transition from hospital to home. The patient and caregiver should understand the difference between cardiovascular pain and musculoskeletal pain from the actual surgical incision. Some typical patient complaints are "My chest hurts when I take a deep breath or when I cough" and "I cannot find a comfortable position for sleep."

Resuming Driving and Regular Physical Activities

Resuming driving is dependent on the presence of any cognitive impairment, delirium, rate of healing, safety concerns, or functional limitations in the postoperative phase. Driving has been documented as early as 21 days following the traditional sternotomy surgery, although being cautious and waiting until the follow-up visit with the surgeon is recommended (Afflerbach, 2018). Evaluating sternal healing, persistent chest wall pain, ROM restrictions in the cervical and thoracic spine, and for the presence of any persistent cognitive impairments is key to safety and resuming this valued activity. Patients undergoing robotically assisted totally endoscopic CABG (TECAB) have been reported to return to activity level closer to 6 weeks compared to 12 weeks via a sternotomy. Resuming driving has been reported as early as 16 days after TECAB surgery. The ability to drive a car requires psychomotor, cognitive, and sensory skills. Safety for the patient and others on the road should be the first concerns when patients seem frustrated to regain this functional activity prior to medical clearance.

Complications and Comorbidities After Discharge

Complications and comorbidities (e.g., poor wound healing, poorly controlled diabetes, obesity) may extend beyond the time of the sternal precautions—sometimes as long as 6 to 12 months following surgery. One example may be a patient's desire to return to playing golf. Golf is not considered an intense activity and is especially suitable for older individuals to improve their health and stay active (Murray et al., 2017). The challenge after a sternotomy is that a full golf swing adds a tremendous amount of torque on the thoracic and lumbar spine (Lindsay & Vandervoort, 2014). Putting or chipping may be easier to return to within the first 6 months rather than using a "full swing with a driver." If the patient has had any type of persistent chest wall soreness or poor healing 3 to 6 months following the surgery, the surgical team should reevaluate the surgical area and consider referral to a musculoskeletal expert such as a physical therapist. The conservative recommendation is always to "listen to your body" once the surgeon has cleared the patient to resume regular physical activity.

For higher level physical activity such as tennis, swimming (crawl/butterfly), a full golf swing, or vigorous yard work, easing into resuming these activities is strongly recommended. Living in an area with extreme temperatures and humidity should also be calculated into resuming higher level physical activities. Hydration, sun exposure, and heat exhaustion are aspects of a home exercise program that should be discussed either by the CR team or attending physician. There are instances when high-intensity exercise has been used postoperatively because the patients' occupations required a higher fitness level to resume their job. Checking with the surgeon prior to resuming high-intensity exercise, driving, or work is recommended. Patients should be evaluated individually to see how their program should be established and progress. Poor wound healing and persistent chest wall soreness should be considered at each stage of the activity progression.

▶ Summary

Cardiac rehabilitation is recommended for all patients following cardiac surgery to promote secondary prevention and full return to prior functional level and higher exercise capacity. Most hospitals have an automatic referral process at the time of discharge. The CR team will individualize the program; take into consideration sternal precautions, persistent chest wall soreness, and restrictions of the cervical and thoracic spine; and identify any safety issues that may persist. The ultimate goal is to have patients return to their same level of function prior to surgery or, better yet, a higher level of function and quality of life.

🔍 CASE STUDY

An 80-year-old male was admitted to the hospital with increasing shortness of breath (SOB) and fatigue over the past 6 months. His recent 12-lead ECG showed a left bundle branch block, which led to a stress test. The stress test was abnormal so the patient underwent a left heart catheterization. The catheterization revealed a 99% proximal left anterior descending to first diagonal occlusion as well as 95% of the circumflex. His echocardiogram was 35% to 40% compared to 3 years prior at 55%. He was admitted for symptom management resulting in planned robotic assisted CABG ×1 and in situ left mammary artery to LAD as part of the first stage of a hybrid revascularization with planned PCI to circumflex.

His past medical history included chronic AF, h/o CVA ×3, type II DM, HTN, bilateral peripheral neuropathy, BPH with urinary retention, HF—NYHA class II, PAD, h/o skin CA, and a prior seizure related to Keppra.

Prior level of function: The patient lives alone in a townhouse with 1 flight of stairs to his bedroom. Independent ambulatory without assistive device, and he drives.

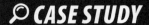

CASE STUDY

Postoperative medications: apixaban, atorvastatin, clopidogrel, docusate, furosemide, glimepiride, insulin-lispro, levetiracetam, metformin, metoprolol, pantoprazole, potassium chloride, and tamsulosin.

5 days after admission data are: weight 104.4 kg; HR 93 bpm; RR 18 bpm; SpO$_2$ 98% on 2 L/min nasal cannula; BP 136/58 (76) mmHg; temp 36.6° C.

6 days after admission data are: weight 94.3 kg; HR 84 bpm; RR 18 bpm; SpO$_2$ 98% on RA; BP 117/72 (84) mmHg; temp. 36.3° C; groin site: CDI. Chest x-ray (CXR) in comparison to previous day: Right-sided central venous catheter (CVC) terminating in cavoatrial junction; cardiomegaly, tortuous unfolded aorta; no consolidation, pleural effusion, or pneumothorax (PTX); impression stable cardiomegaly with stable right-sided CVC.

Lab data are: glucose 142 mg/dL; BUN 23 mg/dL, creatinine 1.01 mg/dL, U:C 23; WBC 9.4; Hgb 10.6 gm, hematocrit 32.8%; platelet 241.

Critical Thinking Questions

1. What would at least three indications be to request a bedside consult by physical therapy for this patient?
2. What concerns should the nurse have when preparing to complete discharge education with the patient and his daughter about his medications?
3. The physical therapist wants to assess the patient's ambulation to determine safety and planning for discharge follow-up care. What criteria should be discussed with the nurse and team prior to progressing to hallway ambulation in the ICU?

Answers to Critical Thinking Questions

1. The patient has had a prior stroke, HF, type II DM, and bilateral PN. Even though he stated he was independent prior to hospital discharge, he may be a safety risk after being at bed rest for nearly 5 days prior to surgery and cognitive impairments related to the surgery. The patient is also anemic and may demonstrate an excessive HR response to position change and limited activity, which would be challenging to his cardiovascular system postoperatively. He has had a significant fluid shift as demonstrated by his weight change; this may impact how he responds hemodynamically to position changes and ambulation. After open heart surgery, teaching and observing the patient to safely do bed mobility, transfers, and gait with sternal precautions will help with chest wall discomfort and risk for prolong wound healing.
2. The primary concern is that the patient lives alone and he is on 13 medications. This also places him at a greater fall risk. Evaluating understanding of dosing and timing of medication will be the key to safety. Making sure the patient has a home health evaluation and follow-up outpatient cardiac rehabilitation referral will help with medication management. Also, the medical team placed him back on a medication that had led to a seizure within the past 3 years. This should be discussed with the surgical team and pharmacist. Observing the patient preparing his own insulin dose and delivering will also help to confirm his comprehension and motor skills following surgery.
3. The therapist should discuss with the nurse the most current vital signs to determine hemodynamic stability as well as cognitive impairment concerns. The therapist and nurse should review the lab data for signs of blood glucose management and timing of therapy, levels of anemia, and heart failure. Also determining whether the CVC is still in place or has recently been discontinued is important for postdischarge management. If the CVC has recently been discontinued, it should be determined if the patient has had a CXR to confirm no pneumothorax or possible pericardial effusion.

Self-Assessment Questions

1. Which is a benefit of cardiac rehabilitation?
    A. Increased insulin resistance
    B. Increased release of inflammatory mediators
    C. Decreased effect on coronary arteries
    D. Increased overall fitness
2. For which condition is cardiac rehabilitation a Class I recommendation?
    A. STEMI
    B. Nonischemic cardiomyopathy
    C. Unstable heart failure
    D. Unstable angina
3. Which patient statement indicates understanding of the goals of Phase I cardiac rehabilitation?
    A. "I will learn about risk reduction for future cardiac events."
    B. "I look forward to the supportive counseling I will receive."
    C. "I will have a decreased risk of death by attending rehab."
    D. "My medication list will be updated in these sessions."
4. Which patient statement indicates understanding of the goals of Phase II cardiac rehabilitation?
    A. "I am glad my hospital discharge planning will be coordinated by someone."
    B. "My follow-up provider appointments will be coordinated for me."
    C. "It is a real benefit to have patient-centered goals coordinated with me."
    D. "The progressive exercise program will really help me get well."
5. Which patient statement indicates understanding of the goals of Phases III/IV cardiac rehabilitation?
    A. "There will be guidelines for me to follow for moving out of bed."
    B. "I am looking forward to beginning exercise training."
    C. "The behavior modification strategies they will share with me will be helpful."
    D. "I will learn strategies to decrease my risk of future cerebrovascular events."

6. Which patient is at risk for intensive care unit acquired weakness? A patient:
    A. with SIRS.
    B. with serum calcium level of 8 mg/dL.
    C. who was extubated in 6 hours postoperatively.
    D. with blood glucose 70 mg/dL.
7. A patient with which set of values should be considered ready for early extubation?

	FiO_2	SpO_2	Mean arterial pressure (MAP)
A.	0.65	91%	60
B.	0.50	94%	67
C.	0.45	88%	70
D.	0.70	95%	63

8. Which patient is at greatest risk for sleep disturbances following cardiac surgery? A patient with increased:
    A. low-density lipoproteins.
    B. fibrinogen.
    C. HbA_{1c}.
    D. C-reactive protein.
9. Which patient should the nurse anticipate needing inpatient rehabilitation prior to starting cardiac rehabilitation? A patient who underwent:
    A. mitral valve replacement.
    B. on-pump CABG.
    C. percutaneous coronary intervention.
    D. minimally invasive coronary artery bypass (MIDCAB).
10. Which patient is at greatest risk for postoperative cognitive dysfunction? A patient with:
    A. fever.
    B. HbA_{1c} 5.3.
    C. depression.
    D. three-vessel disease.

Answers to Self-Assessment Questions

1. D. **increased overall fitness**
    Rationale: One of the benefits of cardiac rehabilitation is to improve overall fitness. There will be an anticipated decrease in insulin resistance and release of

inflammatory mediators and a decreased effect on coronary endothelium.

2. A. **STEMI**
    Rationale: According to the Centers for Medicare and Medicaid Services, STEMI is a Class I recommendation for cardiac rehabilitation. The other three options are not acceptable indicators for cardiac rehabilitation by CMS.

3. B. **"I look forward to the supportive counseling I will receive."**
    Rationale: Supportive counseling is one of the goals of Phase I of cardiac rehabilitation. Risk reduction for future coronary events and morbidity and mortality reduction are goals of Phases III/IV. Medication update is a goal of Phase II.

4. C. **"It is a real benefit to have patient-centered goals coordinated with me."**
    Rationale: Development of patient-centered goals is a focus of Phase II of cardiac rehabilitation. Discharge planning and making of follow-up provider appointments are the foci of Phase I. Sustaining and progressing exercises is a focus of Phases III/IV.

5. D. **"I will learn strategies to decrease my risk of future cerebrovascular events."**
    Rationale: Risk reduction for cerebrovascular events is a focus of Phases III/IV cardiac rehabilitation. Guidelines for mobilization is a focus of Phase I. Exercise training and behavior modification strategies are the foci of Phase II.

6. A. **with SIRS**
    Rationale: Patients with systematic inflammatory response syndrome are at noted risk for development of ICU-acquired weakness. Hypocalcemia is not a risk factor for this condition. Prolonged mechanical ventilation and hyperglycemia are known risk factors.

7. B. **0.50/94%/67**
    Rationale: Early extubation should be considered on patients with a MAP of at least 65 mmHg, SpO_2 at least 90%, and on FiO_2 of less than 0.60.

8. C. **HbA_{1c}**
    Rationale: Diabetes is a risk factor for sleep disturbances following cardiac surgery. Elevated low-density lipoproteins is not a risk factor for sleep disturbances. Fibrinogen and C-reactive protein levels are elevated in patients with obstructive sleep apnea, but elevation in these levels on their own is not a risk factor for sleep disturbances.

9. A. **mitral valve replacement**
    Rationale: Patients who undergo valve repair or replacement tend to be more symptomatic and deconditioned prior to surgery than those patients undergoing other procedures. As such, inpatient rehabilitation may be required for patients undergoing valve repair or replacement prior to enrolling in cardiac rehabilitation.

10. C. **depression**
    Rationale: Data suggest that patients with depression are at risk for POCD. Patients with three-vessel disease are not at risk. Fever and diabetes are known risk factors for POCD.

CLINICAL INQUIRY BOX

Question: What are the barriers for women to participate in cardiac rehabilitation?

Reference: Supervia, M., Medina-Inojosa, J. R., Yeung, C., Lopez-Jimenez, F., Squires, R. W., Pérez-Terzic, C. M., . . . Thomas, R. J. (2017). Cardiac rehabilitation for women: A systematic review of barriers and solutions. *Mayo Clinic Proceedings*. doi: 10.1016/j.mayocp.2017.01.002

Objective: To identify evidence-based barriers and solutions for women's participation in cardiac rehabilitation.

(continues)

CLINICAL INQUIRY BOX *(continued)*

Method: Systematic review

Results: Twenty-four studies evaluated barriers for women's participation in cardiac rehabilitation. Patient-related barriers included lower education level, multiple comorbid conditions, non-English native language, lack of social support, and high burden of family responsibilities. Some data suggest that incentive-based strategies and home-based programs may improve attendance at cardiac rehabilitation and augment completion rates of these programs.

Conclusion: Use of an automatic referral for cardiac rehabilitation helped to overcome barriers for referral for women. Automatic referral should be implemented into clinical practice.CLINICAL INQUIRY BOX

References

Ades, P. A., Keteyian, S. J., Wright, J. S., Hamm, L. F., Lui, K., Newlin K., . . . Thomas, R. J. (2017). Increasing cardiac rehabilitation participation from 20% to 70%: A road map from the Million Hearts cardiac rehabilitation collaborative. *Mayo Clinic Proceedings, 92*(2), 234–242.

Afflerbach, A. (2018). Fitness to drive after sternotomy. *Deutsches Ärzteblatt International, 115*(11). doi:10.3238/arztebl.2018.011b. Retrieved from https://www.aerzteblatt.de/int/archive/article/196922/Fitness-to-Drive-After-Sternotomy

Alexander, J. H., & Smith, P. K. (2016). Coronary-artery bypass grafting. *New England Journal of Medicine, 374,* 1954–1964.

American Association of Cardiovascular and Pulmonary Rehabilitation. (2013). *Guidelines for cardiac rehabilitation and secondary prevention programs* (5th ed.). Champaign, IL: Human Kinetics.

American College of Sports Medicine. (2014). *ACSM's guidelines for exercise testing and prescription* (9th ed.). Philadelphia, PA: Lippincott Williams & Wilkins.

American Heart Association. (n.d.). *Cardiac rehabilitation.* Retrieved from http://www.heart.org/idc/groups/heart-public/@wcm/@mwa/documents/downloadable/ucm_497590.pdf

Anderson, L., Thompson, D. R., Oldridge, N., Zwisler, A. D., Rees K., & Taylor, R. S. (2016). Exercise-based cardiac rehabilitation for coronary heart disease. *Cochrane Database of Systematic Reviews, 5*(1), CD001800.

Benjamin, E. J., Blaha, M. J., Chiuve, S. E., Cushman, M., Das, S. R., Deo, R., . . . Muntner, P. (2017). Heart disease and stroke statistics—2017 update: A report from the American Heart Association. *Circulation, 135*(10), e146–e603.

Bhamidipati, D., Goldhammer, J. E., Spering, M. R., Torjman, M. C., McCarey, M. M., & Whellan, D. J. (2017). Cognitive outcomes after coronary artery bypass grafting. *Journal of Cardiothoracic and Vascular Anesthesia 31,* 707–718.

Bishop, K. L. (2017). Cardiac rehabilitation in women: Emory data. Quarterly Sex-Specific Cardiovascular Health and Medicine Conference. Presented at Emory University Hospital, Atlanta, GA, August 22.

Cassina, T., Putzu, A., Santambrogio, L., Villa, M., & Licker, M. J. (2016). Hemodynamic challenge to early mobilization after cardiac surgery: A pilot study. *Annals of Cardiac Anaesthesia, 19*(3), 425–432.

Center for Medicare and Medicaid Services. (n.d.). *Welcome to the Medicare coverage database.* Retrieved from https://www.cms.gov/medicare-coverage-database/details/nca-decision-memo.aspx?NCAId=270

Duke, M. (1971). Bed rest in acute myocardial infarction A study of physician practices. *American Heart Journal, 82*(4), 486–491.

Fang, J., Ayala, C., Luncheon, C., Ritchey, M., & Loustalot, F. (2017). Use of outpatient cardiac rehabilitation among heart attack survivors—20 states and the District of Columbia, 2013 and four states, 2015. *Morbidity and Mortality Weekly Report, 66*(33), 869–873.

Forman, D. E., Sanderson, B. K., Josephson, R. A., Raikhelkar, J., & Bittner, V. (2015). Heart failure as a newly approved diagnosis for cardiac rehabilitation. Challenges and opportunities. *Journal of the American College of Cardiology, 65,* 2652–2659.

Fritschi, C., & Redeker, N. A. (2015). Contributions of comorbid diabetes to sleep characteristics, daytime symptoms, and physical function among patients with stable heart failure. *Journal of Cardiovascular Nursing, 30*(5), 411–419.

Genta, F. T., Tidu, M., Bouslenko, Z., Bertolin, F., Salvetti, I., Comazzi, F., . . . Giannuzzi, P. (2017). Cardiac rehabilitation after transcatheter aortic valve implantation compared to patients after valve replacement. *Journal of Cardiovascular Medicine, 18,* 14–120.

Green, M., Marzano, V., Leditschke, I. A., Mitchell, I., & Bissett, B. (2016). Mobilization of intensive care patients: A multidisciplinary practical guide for clinicians. *Journal of Multidisciplinary Healthcare, 9,* 247–256.

Hermans, G., & Van den Berghe, G. (2015). Clinical review: Intensive care unit acquired weakness. *Critical Care, 19*(1), 274. doi:10.1186/s13054-015-0993-7

Indja, B., Seco, M., Seamark, R., Kaplan, J., Grieve, S. M., & Vallely, M. P. (2017). Neurocognitive and psychiatric issues post cardiac surgery. *Heart, Lung and Circulation 26,* 779–785.

Javadi, H. R., Jalilolghadr, S., Yazdi, Z., & Majd, Z. R. (2014). Correlation between obstructive sleep apnea syndrome and cardiac disease severity. *Cardiovascular Psychiatry and Neurology, 2014*. Article ID 631380.

Katijjahbe, M. A., Granger, C. L., Denehy, L., Royse, A., Royse, C., Bates, R., . . . El-Ansary, D. (2018). Standard restrictive sternal precautions and modified sternal precautions had similar effects in people after cardiac surgery via median sternotomy ("SMART" Trial): A randomized trial. *Journal of Physiology, 64*(2), 97–106.

Kohan, L., & Annex, B. H. (2015). Clinical outcomes of patients with stable angina. *Journal of the American College of Cardiology*. Retrieved from http://www.acc.org/latest-in-cardiology/articles/2015/05/28/09/03/clinical-outcomes-of-patients-with-stable-angina

Lavie, C. J., Bennett, A., & Arena, R. (2017). Enhancing cardiac rehabilitation in women. *Journal of Women's Health, 26*(8), 817–819.

Lindsay, D. M., & Vandervoort, A. A. (2014). Golf-related low back pain: A review of causative factors and prevention strategies. *Asian Journal of Sports Medicine, 5*(4), e24289.

Magder, S. (1985). Assessment of myocardial stress from early ambulatory activities following myocardial infarction. *Chest, 87*, 442–447.

Medicare.gov. (n.d.). *Your Medicare coverage*. Retrieved from https://www.medicare.gov/coverage/cardiac-rehab-programs.html

Murray, A. D., Daines, L., Archibald, D., Hawkes, R. A., Schiphorst, C., Kelly, P., . . . Mutrie, N. (2017). The relationships between golf and health: A scoping review. *British Journal of Sports Medicine, 51*(1), 12–19.

Oosenbrug, E., Marinho, R. P., Zhang, J., Marzolini, S., Colella, T. J., Pakosh, M., . . . Grace, S. L. (2016). Sex differences in cardiac rehabilitation adherence: A meta-analysis. *Canadian Journal of Cardiology, 32*(11), 1316–1324.

Park, L. G., Schopfer, D. W., Zhang, N., Shen, H., & Whooley, M. A. (2017). Participation in cardiac rehabilitation among patients with heart failure. *Journal of Cardiac Failure, 23*(5), 427–431.

Parry, S. M., & Puthucheary, Z. A. (2015). The impact of extended bed rest on the musculoskeletal system in the critical care environment. *Extreme Physiology & Medicine, 4*. doi:10.1186/s13728-015-0036-7

Santos, P. M. R., Ricci, N. A., Suster, É. A. B., Paisani, D. M., & Chiavegato, L. D. (2016). Effects of early mobilization in patients after cardiac surgery: A systematic review. *Physiotherapy, 103*(91), 1–12.

Shekar, K., Gregory, S. D., & Fraser, J. F. (2016). Mechanical circulatory support in the new era: An overview. *Critical Care, 20*. doi:10.1186/s13054-016-1235-3.

Steward, J. C., & Rollman, B. L. (2014). Optimizing approaches to addressing depression in cardiac patients: A comment on O'Neil et al. *Annals of Behavioral Medicine, 48*(2), 142–144.

Thomas, R. J., Balady, G., Banka, G., Beckie, T. M., Chiu, J., Gokak, S., . . . Wang, T. Y. (2018). ACC/AHA clinical performance and quality measures for cardiac rehabilitation. A report of the American College of Cardiology/American Heart Association Task Force on Performance Measures. *Journal of the American College of Cardiology*. Retrieved from http://www.acc.org/latest-in-cardiology/ten-points-to-remember/2018/03/28/16/17/2018-acc-aha-clinical-performance-and-quality-measures-for-cr

Tozzi, P., & Hullin, R. (2016). Mechanical circulatory support for destination therapy. *Swiss Medical Weekly, 146*. doi:10.1044/smw.2016.14267

Tully, P. J., Baune, B. T., & Baker, R. A. (2013). Cognitive impairment before and six months after cardiac surgery mortality risk at median 11 year follow-up: A cohort study. *International Journal of Cardiology 168*, 2796–2802.

Veal, F. C, Bereznicki, L. R. E., Thompson, A. J., Peterson, G. M., & Orlikowski, C. E. (2016). Pain and functionality following sternotomy: A prospective 12-month observational study. *Pain Medicine, 17*, 1155–1162.

Völler, H., Salzwedel, A., Nitardy, A., Buhlert, H., Treszl, A., & Wegscheider K. (2015). Effect of cardiac rehabilitation on functional and emotional status in patients after transcatheter aortic-valve implantation. *European Journal of Preventive Cardiology, 22*(5), 568–574.

Wenger, N. K., Froelicher, E. S., Smith, L. K., Ades, P. A., Berra K., Blumenthal, J. A., . . . DeBusk, R. F. (1995). Cardiac rehabilitation as secondary prevention. Agency for Health Care Policy and Research and the National Heart, Lung, and Blood Institute. *Clinical Practice Guideline. Quick Reference Guide for Clinicians, 17*, 1–23.

Wisconsin Society for Cardiovascular and Pulmonary Health & Rehabilitation. (2018). *What is cardiac rehabilitation*. Retrieved from https://wiscphr.wisc.edu/Content.aspx?cmspageid=698

Web Resources

2018 ACC/AHA Clinical Performance and Quality Measure for Cardiac Rehabilitation. 2018 ACC/AHA Clinical Performance and Quality Measure for Cardiac Rehabilitation

American Association of Cardiovascular and Pulmonary Rehabilitation. https://www.aacvpr.org/About-AACVPR

Million Hearts. https://millionhearts.hhs.gov/tools-protocols/tools/cardiac-rehabilitation.html

Glossary

A

ABCDEF bundle The ABCDEF bundle elements individually and collectively can help reduce delirium. The A Element refers to assessing, preventing, and managing pain. The B Element focuses on setting a time(s) each day to stop sedative medications, orient the patient to time and day, and conduct an SBT in an effort to liberate the patient from the ventilator. The C Element focuses on constructing a safe and effective medication regimen for the management of pain and agitation in critically ill adults, consistent with ICU pain, agitation, and delirium (PAD) guideline recommendations. The D Element refers to assessing, preventing, and managing delirium. The E Element focuses on understanding the physical deficits that ICU survivors face, and identifying strategies for successful implementation of early mobilization programs. The F Element focuses on examining the concept of family presence in the ICU and identifying strategies to create family engagement and empowerment.

Afterload The resistance against which the left ventricle must pump to move blood forward. The pressure of the arterial systemic circulation produces afterload. Smooth muscle tone in the arterioles can increase the resistance to blood flow and increase afterload. Medications can alter the amount of resistance that arteriolar smooth muscle generates.

Alcohol septal ablation (ASA) A procedure performed in the catheterization lab to remove hypertrophied heart muscle. It entails injection of 100% alcohol into one of the branches of the coronary artery that leads to the enlarged septum and the hypertrophied myocardium; it is left in place for a few minutes. This results in immediate cell death to that area. The end result is improved blood flow as the hypertrophied myocardium is no longer obstructing blood flow.

Allograft The transfer of an organ from one person to another. The donor is not a twin but is of the same species.

Allograft coronary artery disease (ACAD) Development of coronary artery disease in heart transplant patients. It can be described based on the degree of stenosis of the affected vessel(s). This disease is often associated with graft failure.

Alveolar-arterial oxygen gradient (A-a gradient) A method of measuring intrapulmonary shunt. The calculation is the difference between the concentration of alveolar oxygen entering the alveoli and the concentration of oxygen diffused into the arterial blood.

Ankle-brachial index An assessment used to evaluate arterial blood flow to the lower extremities. Results of this calculation are used to rate the degree of peripheral artery disease and to determine if the saphenous vein is suitable for use during cardiac surgery.

Annuloplasty Surgical repair of an ineffectual heart valve.

Aortic regurgitation Incomplete closure of the aortic valve leaflets, resulting in a backflow of blood. There is a reflux of blood from the aorta into the left ventricle (LV) during diastole because the valve leaflets fail to close completely and remain tightly closed during diastole. Acute aortic regurgitation imposes a large volume load on the LV, which a normal heart cannot accommodate. The sudden increase in end-diastolic volume (preload) will result in increased left ventricular end-diastolic pressure and decreased cardiac output. Aortic regurgitation is identified by the presence of an early diastolic murmur that can be heard at the second and third intercostal spaces at the right sternal border and the second and fourth intercostal spaces at the left sternal border. The murmur of aortic regurgitation usually decreases in intensity and disappears before S1.

Aortic stenosis Narrowing or constriction of the aortic valve that creates a pressure gradient. The aortic valve does not open completely, which creates a left ventricular outflow tract obstruction and increases both the workload and afterload of the left ventricle. The calcification of aortic stenosis is regarded as a proliferative and inflammatory process, similar to atherosclerosis.

Aortopathy Any disease or malfunction of the aorta. There are five main aortopathic conditions that have clinical focus: Marfan syndrome, Loeys–Dietz syndrome, Ehlers–Danlos syndrome (Types I/II, IV, and VI), idiopathic thoracic aneurysm/dissection, and coarctation of the aorta.

Arterial pulse contour continuous cardiac output monitoring A method that estimates cardiac output by use of pulse contour analysis; it is an indirect method based on analysis of the arterial pressure pulsation waveform. The key underlying concept is that the contour of the arterial pressure waveform is proportional to stroke volume. The arterial pressure waveform is used to calculate cardiac output, stroke volume variance, intrathoracic volumes, and extravascular lung water. These data may predict response to fluid therapy.

Assisted aortic end-diastolic pressure The pressure in the aorta at the end of diastole when counterpulsation has assisted the cardiac cycle. It is usually lower than the unassisted end-diastolic pressure.

Assisted systole The systolic aortic pressure when counterpulsation has assisted the cardiac cycle. It is usually lower than the unassisted systole due to the action of balloon deflation.

Atrial septal defect (ASD) An opening between the right and left atria. Oxygenated blood leaves the left atrium and returns to the right atrium through this opening rather than continuing forward to deliver oxygen to cells, organs, muscles, and tissues throughout the body.

B

Balloon valvotomy/valvuloplasty Use of a balloon to stretch open a narrowed heart valve or to break adhesions in a scarred valve.

Beating heart surgery *See* **off-pump coronary artery bypass.**

Bicaval technique A method used during heart transplantation in which the anastomoses are made in the superior and inferior vena cavae.

Biologic valves Valves that are constructed from bovine, porcine, and human cardiac tissue.

Biventricular assist device (BiVAD) A type of mechanical support for the heart. It is used when both the right and left ventricles are failing. Blood is drained from each ventricle through cannulae to centrifugal pumps, which provide circulatory support in severely decompensated heart failure patients until a heart transplant can be performed. A BiVAD is typically used when a left ventricular assist device does not provide sufficient circulatory support.

Bridge to recovery Use of a mechanical circulatory device (ventricular assist device [VAD]) to support circulation in patients with heart failure. If myocyte damage is not permanent, myocardial cells may regain their ability to function. The VAD supports the patient until heart function improves and is adequate without mechanical support.

Bridge to transplantation Use of a mechanical circulatory device (ventricular assist device) to support circulation in patients with severe heart failure until a donor heart becomes available and a transplant can be performed.

C

Cardiac allograft vasculopathy A type of stenosis caused by plaque in the coronary arteries. The lesions contain inflammatory cells (including T cells). Coronary artery vasculopathy is a major cause of long-term morbidity and mortality in heart transplant patients who survive past the first year. Innate and adaptive immune responses result in development of vascular lesions.

Cardiac catheterization An invasive diagnostic test whereby a catheter is inserted and advanced into the heart chambers or coronary arteries. It reveals information about the blood pressure of the heart and the heart's ability to pump, blood flow in the heart chambers, presence and degree of narrowing of the coronary arteries, and valve function.

Cardiac rehabilitation A comprehensive, long-term program involving medical evaluation, prescribed exercise, cardiac risk factor modification, education, and counseling. These programs are designed to limit the physiologic and psychological effects of cardiac illness, reduce the risk for sudden death or re-infarction, control cardiac symptoms, stabilize or reverse the atherosclerotic process, and enhance the psychosocial and vocational status of selected patients.

Cardiac tamponade Cardiac tamponade results from an accumulation of pericardial fluid under pressure, leading to impaired cardiac filling and hemodynamic instability.

Cardiac output (CO) A measure of the amount of blood that is ejected by the heart each minute. It is affected by the individual's preload, afterload, and contractility.

Cardiogenetics The specialized focus on genetics related to the cardiovascular system within humans.

Cardiomyopathies A heterogeneous group of diseases of the myocardium associated with mechanical or electrical dysfunction, or both, that usually (but not invariably) exhibit inappropriate ventricular hypertrophy or dilatation and are due to a variety of causes that are frequently genetic. There are two categories of cardiomyopathies: primary and secondary. (*See* **primary cardiomyopathy** and **secondary cardiomyopathy**.)

Cardioplegia A method of intentionally arresting the heart's motion with infusion of a solution to facilitate performance of cardiac surgery. The solution contains potassium (to decrease myocardial oxygen consumption and the rate of anaerobic metabolism while the heart is ischemic), magnesium (to decrease myocardial oxygen consumption), calcium (to decrease the chance of reperfusion injury), procaine (vasodilator and antiarrhythmic; may decrease dysrhythmias following aortic cross-clamping), bicarbonate (to counter the metabolic acidosis that occurs secondary to anaerobic metabolism while the heart is in arrest), hypothermia (decreases myocardial oxygen consumption and increases the heart's tolerance to ischemia), mannitol (to decrease edema related to hypothermia and ischemia, and may minimize reperfusion injury), dextrose (to counter edema due to hypothermia and ischemia, and for continued energy production), amino acids (for energy production, may minimize reperfusion injury, and has a role as a scavenger for oxygen free radicals), and oxygenated blood (to optimize the heart's metabolic environment and minimize reperfusion injury). The patient's circulation is diverted to a heart–lung machine that takes over the function of these two organs. The heart is isolated from the body with cross-clamping of the aorta. A cold cardioplegic solution is then instilled to decrease myocardial oxygen consumption and increase the heart's tolerance to ischemia, thereby preventing heart damage during the procedure.

Cardiopulmonary bypass (CPB) The temporary rerouting of blood from the right atrium to the aorta via an oxygenator (bypass machine), thereby bypassing the heart and lungs during the surgical procedure.

Carotid bruit A sound associated with turbulent blood flow that may indicate arterial stenosis.

Central venous oxygen saturation (ScvO$_2$) A method used to determine how much oxygen the tissues are extracting. It entails analysis of a blood sample from a central venous catheter.

Commissurotomy A procedure that opens commissures (the contact area for the valve leaflets), which have developed scarring and do not open to allow blood to flow.

Contractility The rate and ability of the myocardial muscle to shorten itself, or the amount of strength evidenced by the myocardium when it ejects blood. It is influenced by heart rate, neural factors, and certain metabolic states.

Coronary artery bypass grafting (CABG) *See* **surgical revascularization**.

Coronary artery vasculopathy see cardiac allograft vaculopathy.

Cox Maze III procedure A modification of a procedure that interrupts the reentrant pathways required for atrial fibrillation using surgical incisions. The Cox Maze III procedure remains the standard surgical therapy for atrial fibrillation. It entails a number of incisions being made on the right and left atria. "Maze" refers to the pattern of incisions made in the atrium. The incisions cause scarring, which does not conduct electricity, stops irregular electrical activity, and eradicates atrial fibrillation. The scarring also prevents future irregular electrical signals from developing.

Cox Maze IV procedure A procedure that uses radio-frequency ablation to eradicate atrial fibrillation.

D

Deep sternal wound infection Infection of the sternum and underlying structures.

Deep sternal wound injury *See mediastinitis*.

Delirium An acute confusional state characterized by an alteration of consciousness with reduced ability to focus, sustain, or shift attention. There are three subtypes of delirium that can occur anytime during the postoperative period: hypoactive, hyperactive, and mixed.

Destination therapy Use of a ventricular assist device in patients with severe heart failure who are not candidates for or have declined a heart transplant.

Diastolic augmentation The increase in pressure in the aorta above the balloon catheter that results with balloon inflation during diastole. This phenomenon increases perfusion in the coronary arteries and myocardial oxygen supply.

Dicrotic notch When referring to an intra-aortic balloon pump or intra-arterial pressure monitoring, an area on the downstroke of the arterial waveform that results from the slight pressure increase created by closure of the aortic valve.

Dilated cardiomyopathy (DCM) One of the main causative factors for congestive heart failure. Dilated cardiomyopathy is characterized by dilatation and systolic dysfunction of one or both ventricles, with specific detriment to left ventricular function.

Drug-eluting stent (DES) A metal tube or "scaffold" inserted into a coronary artery following dilation of the vessel with a balloon (balloon angioplasty). The tube is coated with a drug to prevent reblockage (restenosis) of the vessel.

Dynamic response test *See* **square wave test.**

E

Ejection fraction (EF) The percentage of blood volume of the left ventricle that is ejected with each contraction. A normal ejection fraction is approximately 65% to 70%.

Electrical bioimpedance A noninvasive method to determine cardiac output. Using this technology, cardiac output is identified by changes in impedance that take place as blood is ejected from the left ventricle into the aorta and is calculated from changes in thoracic impedance. Change in thoracic blood volume during the cardiac cycle can be used to calculate cardiac output.

Ethanol septal ablation A procedure for relieving outflow obstruction symptoms that is accomplished by infusing ethanol into the first septal branch of the left anterior descending coronary artery via an angioplasty catheter. This technique reduces outflow tract obstruction, increases exercise capacity, and improves symptoms.

Ex-Maze procedure A cutting-edge technique for the Maze procedure. It is performed endoscopically on the outside of a beating heart. The ablation device uses unipolar radiofrequency energy with vacuum-maintained contact and suction-controlled saline perfusion to ensure uniform energy transmission and transmural lesion development. Because the procedure is performed on a beating heart, atrial function can be monitored during treatment. Patients can convert to normal sinus rhythm during the procedure or within 6 weeks. The Ex-Maze procedure is less invasive and does not require cardiopulmonary bypass. It is safer, associated with less postoperative pain, and has fewer complications.

Extracorporeal membrane oxygenation (ECMO) Use of a machine that can provide oxygen to the blood while it is circulating outside of the body. Blood is removed from the body via a catheter, pumped through a machine to be oxygenated by an artificial lung, and returned to the body through another catheter. The heart and lungs are bypassed, providing both hemodynamic and respiratory support. Blood oxygenation is a distinct advantage with this technique.

F

Fast flush *See* **square wave test.**

G

Graft closure Failure of the harvested vein (graft) to maintain patency, usually due to platelet aggregation. Antithrombotic therapy is initiated to prevent this complication of coronary artery bypass surgery.

H

Heterotopic method A heart transplantation technique utilizing end-to-end anastomoses of the donor to the superior vena cava, pulmonary artery, and aorta. The donor heart is placed "piggyback" to the recipient heart. This method may be used in patients with severe pulmonary hypertension or if there is a mismatch between the donor and recipient heart size. It is rarely used.

Hypertrophic cardiomyopathy (HCM) A condition in which the myocardium becomes abnormally thick or hypertrophied. The thickened myocardium makes it more difficult for the heart to pump blood. It is a common genetic cardiovascular disease characterized by abnormal myocytes leading to hypertrophy without dilatation and preserved systolic function. Hypertrophy is most severe in the ventricular septum. It is asymmetrical and usually occurs at the level of the left ventricular outflow tract, leading to subaortic stenosis or asymmetrical HCM. In addition, abnormal systolic anterior motion of the mitral valve contributes to the outflow obstruction.

Hypothermia A decrease in internal (core) body temperature below normal values. Often, a temperature less than 95°F (35°C) is considered hypothermia.

I

Infective endocarditis A condition that occurs when bacteria attach to and destroy the surface of a valve leaflet or chordae. If a valve is damaged, immune cells, platelets, and fibrin migrate to the site to initiate healing of the valve. If bacteria become trapped under layers of these cells, "clumps" of tissue (called vegetations) can develop on the valves and within the heart muscle (endocarditis). Vegetations may break off and become emboli.

Intensive care unit acquired weakness A common complication for critically ill patients who have prolonged mechanical ventilation, sepsis, multi-organ system failure, systemic inflammatory response syndrome, or hyperglycemia.

Internal thoracic artery (ITA) An artery in the chest located adjacent to the left anterior descending coronary artery. There is one ITA on either side of the sternum. This artery is resistant to cholesterol buildup (atherosclerosis), which makes it a good choice for use as a graft in coronary artery bypass surgical procedures.

Intra-aortic balloon pump (IABP) A mechanical device that is used to improve cardiac function on a temporary basis. It increases blood flow, oxygen delivery to the heart, and cardiac output, and decreases the amount of work the heart must do to eject blood through a process called counterpulsation.

Intrapulmonary shunt (IPS) The percentage of cardiac output that does not participate in gas exchange. This portion of blood passes through the lungs but is not exposed to ventilated alveoli, so gas exchange does not take place and the blood leaves the lungs desaturated.

L

Left-to-right shunting Diversion of blood from the left heart to the right heart, rather than forward into the systemic circulation. Oxygenated blood from the arterial circulation mixes with deoxygenated blood from the venous system. Chronic left-to-right shunting may cause right ventricular failure, tricuspid regurgitation, atrial arrhythmias, paradoxical embolization, and cerebral abscesses.

Left ventricular assist device (LVAD) A type of mechanical support for the left ventricle. Blood is drained from the apex of the left ventricle to a pump via an inflow cannula. It is returned to the body via an outflow cannula, which is attached to the aorta. The pump is housed in the pre-peritoneal space of the abdomen, near the stomach. A percutaneous driveline that is tunneled across the pre-peritoneal space to the left side of the body carries an electrical cable and air vent to the electrical controller outside the patient's body.

Lower and Shumway method A method used during heart transplantation in which the donor heart is anastomosed to the left atrium, right atrium, pulmonary artery, and aorta.

M

Malnutrition An acute, subacute, or chronic state of nutrition in which a combination of varying degrees of overnutrition or undernutrition (with or without inflammatory activity) have led to a change in body composition and diminished function.

Maze procedure *See* **Cox Maze III procedure**.

Mean arterial pressure (MAP) The driving force for peripheral blood flow and the preferred pressure to be evaluated in unstable patients. It is measured electronically by first integrating the area under the arterial pressure waveform and then dividing by the duration of the cardiac cycle.

Mechanical cardiac assist device A device used to support cardiac function over the short or long term. Mechanical circulatory support has three primary functions: bridge to transplantation, bridge to recovery, and destination therapy. Short-term, temporary devices are often used as a bridge to recovery in the setting of acute cardiogenic shock or cardiopulmonary arrest. Under these circumstances, circulatory assistance provides immediate hemodynamic support, restoring blood flow to vital organs while decompressing the heart, avoiding pulmonary edema, and minimizing cardiac workload to maximize the patient's chances of recovery.

Mediastinitis Inflammation of the mediastinum. A postoperative sternal wound infection. It is characterized by fever, tachycardia, chest pain, sternal instability, redness, and purulent drainage from the mediastinum. The chest pain is typically out of proportion to what should be experienced so many days out from surgery in the post-ICU setting. Patients may also experience some edema and crepitus of the chest wall. Laboratory and diagnostic findings will show leukocytosis, mediastinal widening or air may also be noted on radiological tests.

Minimally invasive cardiac surgery (MICS) An approach to coronary artery bypass grafting surgery that entails use of a laparoscopic procedure to perform cardiac surgery. Minimally invasive cardiac surgery has also been defined as cardiac surgery without the use of cardiopulmonary bypass or sternotomy; rather, smaller incisions are made. This term also refers to various procedures used to bypass blocked coronary arteries.

Minimally invasive direct coronary artery bypass (MIDCAB) An approach to traditional coronary artery bypass grafting (CABG). Differences between the two approaches are threefold. First, the incision size is much smaller for MIDCAB; several 3- to 5-inch incisions are made between the ribs as compared to a 10- to 12-inch median sternotomy incision in conventional CABG procedures. Second, because MIDCAB is a beating heart procedure, no cardioplegia is instilled to stop the heart. Third, because MIDCAB is a beating heart surgery and no cardioplegia is instilled, cardiopulmonary bypass is not required for MIDCAB procedures. These procedures are performed on patients with one or two blockages to the right coronary artery, left anterior descending coronary artery, or its branches on the front of the heart.

Minimally invasive direct view Techniques that were developed to repair or replace the mitral valve and repair or replace the aortic valve. The main benefit of minimally invasive direct view valve surgery is the avoidance of a median sternotomy. An 8-cm incision is made and cartilage is removed to allow for direct visualization of the valves.

Minute ventilation The volume of gas exchange (inhaled and exhaled) in 1 minute. It is measured by multiplying respiratory rate and tidal volume.

Mitral regurgitation Incomplete closure of the mitral valve leaflets, resulting in a backflow of blood into the left atrium during ventricular systole.

Mitral stenosis Narrowing or constriction of the mitral valve that creates a pressure gradient. The narrowing creates resistance to the forward flow of blood into the left ventricle during diastole.

Myocardial revascularization Restoration of blood supply to the myocardium. It may be accomplished by either percutaneous intervention or surgery.

Myectomy A procedure that involves excision of a section of subaortic septal muscle approximately 3 to 7 cm long and 3 to 12 g in weight, with or without mitral valve replacement. Left ventricular myectomy is recommended for patients with drug-refractory symptomatic outflow obstruction (peak gradient > 50 mmHg under resting conditions and/or gradient > 50 mmHg measured). Surgery may also be considered in symptomatic patients with documented outflow obstruction under physiologic exercise but with absent or very mild resting obstruction. One additional subset of patients may benefit from left ventricular myectomy: young, asymptomatic patients with documented severe outflow tract obstruction (gradient 75–100 mmHg).

Myxoma A benign cardiac tumor. It causes obstruction of blood flow, which leads to the clinical presentation of heart failure; signs of central nervous system embolization; and constitutional symptoms such as fever, weight loss, fatigue, weakness, arthralgia, myalgia, or any combination of these. Tumor resection is the only effective treatment.

N

Negative inspiratory pressure Also referred to as negative inspiratory force. The amount of negative pressure that the patient generates during a forced inspiration when working against an obstruction to flow. It is a reflection of a patient's ability to take a deep breath and generate a cough that is strong enough to clear secretions.

Nitric oxide (NO) A product that is released by endothelial cells. It produces vasodilation and increased vascular permeability.

O

Obesity Obesity is defined based on body mass index (BMI). Obesity is defined as a BMI greater than 30 kg/m^2. Obese class I corresponds with a BMI of 30 to 34.99 kg/m^2, class II is a BMI of 35 to 39.99 kg/m^2, and class III is a BMI greater than 40 kg/m^2.

Obesity hypoventilation syndrome (OHS) A condition in which a person with obesity has a CO_2 level greater than 45 mmHg while awake.

Off-pump coronary artery bypass (OPCAB) Also known as a beating heart procedure. This type of minimally invasive cardiac surgery entails a median sternotomy or thoracotomy incision; no bypass machine is required. The surgeon sews the grafts onto the beating heart using specialized instruments to stabilize the myocardial tissue. Off-pump coronary artery bypass may be performed on patients needing four or five vessels repaired, when compared with minimally invasive direct coronary artery bypass, where only one or two vessels can be repaired. With OPCAB, an artery or vein from the lower extremities is used to make the bypass.

Orthotopic heart transplant A heart transplant approach that entails replacing the recipient heart with the donor heart.

Overdamped waveform A situation in which a pressure waveform is sluggish and has an exaggerated or falsely widened and blunt tracing. It will cause the patient's systolic pressure to be recorded as falsely low and the diastolic pressure to be recorded as falsely high.

Oxygen consumption The amount of oxygen used by the body's tissues.

Oxygen delivery The amount of oxygen that is carried to the body's tissues each minute.

P

PaO$_2$/FiO$_2$ ratio An index of oxygenation. A PaO$_2$/FiO$_2$ ratio of less than 200 is associated with a significant intrapulmonary shunt.

Paroxysmal nocturnal dyspnea (PND) A feeling of shortness of breath that awakens the patient. It is usually relieved when the patient assumes an upright position.

Percutaneous balloon mitral valvotomy (PBMV) *See* **commissurotomy**. This technique has very successfully reduced left atrial gradient, increased mitral valve area, and improved symptoms of mitral stenosis.

Percutaneous transluminal coronary angioplasty (PTCA) A technique that uses an arterial catheter and various mechanical means to increase the diameter of diseased coronary arteries, thereby improving blood flow.

Pericardiectomy Surgical removal of part of the membrane that surrounds the heart (pericardium). It is usually performed to treat inflammation and prevent collection of fluid in the pericardial sac (between the pericardium and heart), which can cause hemodynamic compromise from poor cardiac filling and emptying.

Pharmacogenetics The study of how genetic differences in a single gene influence variability in drug response (e.g., efficacy, toxicity). Components of both pharmacogenomics and pharmacogenetics include drug targets and transporters, drug-metabolizing enzymes, pharmacodynamics, and pharmacokinetics.

Pharmacogenomics The study of how genes affect the person's response to drugs.

Phlebostatic axis An anatomic landmark located at the fourth intercostal space, midpoint of the anterior–posterior diameter. Leveling at the phlebostatic axis is

performed to eradicate the effects of hydrostatic forces on the hemodynamic pressures.

Phrenic nerve injury A complication following cardiac surgery with cardiopulmonary bypass. The extent of injury can range from neuropathy to paralysis of the diaphragm. It is often reported to be attributed to the use of hypothermia, application of ice slush around the heart, and harvesting of the internal thoracic artery that occur during surgery.

Pleural effusion Collection of fluid in the pleural space.

Post intensive care syndrome (PICS) Impairment in cognition, mental health, and physical function. A grouping of post-critical care complications that includes persistent cognitive dysfunction, acquired weakness, and intrusive memories akin to post-traumatic stress disorder.

Postoperative cognitive dysfunction A subtle disorder of thought processes, which may influence isolated domains of cognition such as verbal memory, visual memory, language comprehension, executive function, and the speed of processing information.

Postpericardiotomy syndrome An immune phenomenon that occurs after an incision of the pericardium. It is often characterized by a new pericardial effusion and fever.

Preload The pressure found in the left ventricle at the end of diastole. It is sometimes referred to as left ventricular end-diastolic pressure. Right-sided preload is the pressure found in the right atrium at the end of diastole.

Primary cardiomyopathy The heart is predominantly the main organ affected. Primary cardiomyopathies are then subdivided into those that are genetic, mixed (predominantly nongenetic or less commonly genetic), or acquired. The most commonly known cardiomyopathies include dilated cardiomyopathy, hypertrophic cardiomyopathy (HCM), left ventricular non-compaction cardiomyopathy (LVNCC), arrhythmogenic right ventricular cardiomyopathy (ARVC), and restrictive cardiomyopathy. Hypertrophic cardiomyopathy, LVNCC, and ARVC are classified as genetic cardiomyopathies.

Prosthetic heart valve endocardis A potential risk for any patient who has had cardiac surgery. In early infection, microorganisms can come in contact with the valve prosthesis by contamination intraoperatively or via hematogenous spread during the initial days and weeks after surgery. The mechanisms of endocarditis involve the disposition of fibrin and platelets at the site of endothelial damage or at the location of the sutures, at the valve sewing ring, or both of these. The organisms can adhere to these structures and initiate infection.

Prosthetic valves (mechanical valves) Valves that are manufactured from manmade materials such as metal alloys, pyrolytic carbon, and Dacron. Mechanical prosthetic valves are more durable and last longer than biologic valves.

Pulmonary hypertension High blood pressure in the arteries that supply the lungs and right side of the heart. It develops when these vessels become constricted or obstructed, which slows blood flow. The result is an increase in pressure in the pulmonary arteries, making it more difficult for the right ventricle to eject blood to the pulmonary arteries. An elevated mean arterial pressure at least 25 mmHg at rest.

Pulmonary stenosis Narrowing or constriction of the pulmonic valve that creates a pressure gradient.

Pulse oximetry A noninvasive method of monitoring the percentage of hemoglobin that is saturated with oxygen.

Pulse pressure variation (PPV) An alternative, less invasive method of evaluating cardiac output. It may be used as a means for determining the patient's ability to respond to fluid. Pulse pressure variation is the difference between the maximum and minimum values of the arterial pulse pressure during one mechanical breath divided by the mean of the two values. In the evaluation of the Frank-Starling curve, an increase in preload causes a decrease in PPV; decreasing preload causes an increase in PPV and contractility.

Pulsus alternans An exaggeration of the normal variation in the pulse during the inspiratory phase of respiration, in which the pulse becomes weaker as the person inhales and stronger as the person exhales. It is an indicator of the presence of severe ventricular systolic failure and decreased myocardial contractility.

R

Right-to-left shunting The flow of blood from the right to left side of the heart, usually through an opening between the two atria or ventricles. Great vessels in the chest may be affected as well. Right-to-left shunting can be attributed to a patent foramen ovale, especially with conditions that increase right atrial pressure (e.g., tricuspid stenosis). An example is a patient with an atrial septal defect. The affected patient may have periods of cyanosis.

Right ventricular assist device (RVAD) A type of mechanical support for the right ventricle. Blood is drained through a pump from the right ventricle to the pulmonary artery.

Robot-assisted coronary artery bypass A cutting-edge surgical technique. Unaccommodating places is what robot-assisted surgery is about; the human surgeon is not optimized for tiny spaces. In RACAB, the surgical robot consists of a collection of wristed tools called manipulators, which receive digital instructions from an interfaced computer. The surgeon, who is seated at a computer console with a three-dimensional display, acts as the "driver" of the computer. The surgeon initiates the digital instructions by controlling the hand grips. By using the hand grips, the surgeon's hand movements at the console are then duplicated in the robot, with software filtering out physiologic hand tremors.

S

Saphenous vein A vein in the patient's leg that runs near the leg's surface. It is used as a graft for coronary artery bypass procedures. There are actually two saphenous veins in the leg—the great (large) and small veins. When harvested for bypass procedures, long incisions are usually made. Almost directly upon harvest, the surface of the saphenous vein becomes vulnerable to platelet aggregation because of the loss of the vascular endothelium. For this reason, patients require antithrombotic therapy to prevent graft closure.

Serum transferrin A lab test that reflects a patient's iron status. If a patient's iron level is within range, low serum transferrin levels can be used as an indicator of a patient's protein status.

Square wave test Also referred to as a fast flush or dynamic response test; a test that is performed to ensure that the waveforms that appear on the monitoring screen accurately reflect pressures. It is accomplished by pulling and releasing the "pigtail" or squeezing the button of the flush device so that the flow through the tubing increases (from 3 mL/hr obtained with a pressure bag inflated to 300 mmHg). The sudden rise in pressure in the system generates a square wave on the monitor oscilloscope.

Stabilizer A device used in minimally invasive cardiac surgery that provides a direct view of the operating field, dampens the movement of the epicardium, and permits the surgeon to maintain a nontraumatic grip on the beating heart. The device helps the surgeon isolate the diseased vessel and stabilizes the localized region of epicardium for anastomosis.

Stroke volume The amount of blood ejected by the left ventricle with each contraction. Stroke volume is affected by the amount of blood in the ventricle and by the force of contraction of the ventricle. It can also be affected if the aortic valve restricts flow out of the left ventricle.

Stroke volume variation (SVV) An alternative, less invasive method of evaluating cardiac output. It may be used as a means for determining the patient's ability to respond to fluid. Stroke volume variation occurs due to changes in intrathoracic pressure during spontaneous breathing. It produces data on changes in preload that occur with mechanical ventilation. Stroke volume variation is the difference between the maximum and minimum stroke volume during one mechanical breath relative to the mean stroke volume.

Sudden cardiac death The sudden cessation of cardiac activity with hemodynamic collapse, typically due to sustained ventricular tachycardia or ventricular fibrillation.

Surgical revascularization Also known as coronary artery bypass grafting (CABG). Use of arterial or venous vessels to create a new pathway for blood to reach the coronary arteries, thereby "bypassing" a stenosis.

Sympathomimetics Agents that activate adrenergic receptors by direct receptor binding, promotion of norepinephrine (NE) release, blockade of NE reuptake, and inhibition of NE inactivation.

Systolic pressure variation (SPV) An alternative, less invasive method of evaluating cardiac output. It may be used as a means for determining the patient's ability to respond to fluid. SPV is the difference between the maximum and minimum systolic blood pressure during one mechanical breath.

T

Tidal volume The amount of air inhaled during a normal breath (versus a forced inhalation).

Total artificial heart (TAH) A treatment alternative for patients with biventricular failure who are hospitalized candidates for heart transplant. A TAH replaces the function of both ventricles and the four heart valves. It is implanted in the patient's chest and attached to the atria. Tubes from the ventricles continue from the patient's chest to a power-generating console. The TAH can deliver cardiac output at a rate as high as 9.5 L/min.

It reportedly augments renal and hepatic blood flow and improves survival of heart transplant patients with preoperative biventricular failure.

Totally endoscopic coronary artery bypass (TECAB) A method of performing off-pump coronary artery bypass grafting. It entails using endoscopy, as opposed to the minimally invasive direct coronary artery bypass approach, which uses small thoracotomy incisions.

Transfusion-associated circulatory overload (TACO) Pulmonary edema after transfusion of blood products. It is a form of circulatory volume overload that can occur with transfusion of any blood component (e.g., packed red blood cells, platelets, fresh frozen plasma, cryoprecipitate).

Transfusion-related acute lung injury (TRALI) Noncardiogenic pulmonary edema following transfusion of blood or blood products.

Transmyocardial laser revascularization (TMR) A procedure whereby transmyocardial channels are created from the epicardium into the ventricle via a laser. The channels then allow blood from the ventricle to reach the myocardium directly.

Transplantation The surgical removal of a diseased heart and replacement with a healthy donor heart.

Transplant vasculopathy Accelerated coronary artery disease in the transplanted heart.

Tricuspid regurgitation Incomplete closure of the tricuspid valve leaflets, resulting in a backflow of blood.

Tricuspid stenosis Narrowing or constriction of the tricuspid valve, which creates a pressure gradient.

Tricuspid valve The heart valve that is located between the right atrium and ventricle, near the atrioventricular node, right coronary artery, and coronary sinus. Its function is to maintain forward flow of blood. The tricuspid valve has an annular ring and three leaflets connected via chordae tendineae to papillary muscles that are integrated with the right ventricle.

U

Unassisted aortic end-diastolic pressure The pressure in the aorta at the end of diastole when counterpulsation via the balloon pump has not assisted that cardiac cycle.

Unassisted systole The systolic aortic pressure when counterpulsation has not assisted the cycle.

Underdamped waveform A situation in which a pressure waveform has an overresponse, revealed visually as an exaggerated, narrow, and artificially peaked tracing. In this case, the waveform overestimates the patient's systolic pressure and underestimates the diastolic pressure.

Undernutrition Presence of 10% or more weight loss in the six months prior to cardiac surgery and a low free-fat mass index.

V

Valvuloplasty A procedure that entails insertion of a balloon to stretch or enlarge the valve opening.

Venous oxygen saturation (SvO₂) A method used to determine how much oxygen the tissues are extracting. Venous oxygen saturation reveals the association between oxygen delivery (the amount of oxygen that is carried to the tissues each minute) and oxygen consumption (the amount of oxygen used by the tissues).

Ventricular assist device (VAD) A device used for longer term mechanical circulatory support. This implanted mechanical pump is used in patients with end-stage heart disease. Ventricular assist devices assist a weakened heart by pumping blood throughout the body.

Ventricular septal defect (VSD) An opening in the wall (septum) between the right and left ventricles. The result of this opening is the return of oxygenated blood in the left ventricle to the right ventricle, rather than the blood continuing forward into the systemic circulation to deliver oxygen to the cells, organs, muscles, and tissues. A VSD also results in an increase in ventricular workload because greater volumes of blood are being circulated; this effect ultimately leads to heart failure.

Vital capacity The amount of air that can be exhaled forcibly following a full inspiration.

Z

Zero balance A process of establishing atmospheric pressure as zero to obtain accurate hemodynamic values.

Index

Note: Page numbers followed *b*, *f* and *t* indicates box, figure and table respectively.